PULMONARY REHABILITATION

The Obstructive and Paralytic Conditions

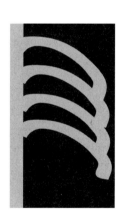

PULMONARY REHABILITATION

The Obstructive and Paralytic Conditions

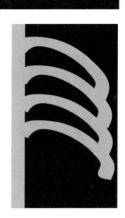

Edited by
John R. Bach, MD
Professor and Vice Chairman
Department of Physical Medicine
  and Rehabilitation
University of Medicine
  and Dentistry of New Jersey
New Jersey Medical School
Newark, New Jersey

HANLEY & BELFUS, INC. / Philadelphia

MOSBY/ St Louis • Baltimore • Boston • Carlsbad • Chicago • London
Madrid • Naples • New York • Philadelphia • Sydney • Tokyo • Toronto

Publisher: HANLEY & BELFUS, INC.
                                      210 South 13th Street
                                      Philadelphia, Pa 19107
                                      (215) 546-7293
                                      FAX (215) 790-9330

North American and worldwide sales and distribution:

                                      MOSBY
                                      II830 Westline Industial Drive
                                      St Louis, MO 63146

In Canada: Times Mirror Professional Publishing, Ltd.
                                      130 Flaska Drive
                                      Markham, Ontario L6G 1B8
                                      Canada

Library of Congress Cataloging-in-Publication Data

Pulmonary rehabilitation : the obstructive and paralytic conditions /
  [edited by] John R. Bach.
      p.   cm.
  Includes bibliographical references and index.
  ISBN 1-56053-109-6 (hard : alk. paper)
  1. Respiratory therapy. 2. Lungs--Diseases--Patients-
-Rehabilitation. I. Bach, John R., 1950-
  [DNLM: 1. Lung Diseases, Obstructive--rehabilitation. WF 600
P9864 1995]
RC735.I5P85 1995
616.2'0043--dc20
DNLM/DLC
for Library of Congress   95-50018
                                                                     CIP

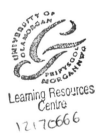

PULMONARY REHABILITATION: THE OBSTRUCTIVE
AND PARLYTIC CONDITIONS   ISBN 1-56053-109-6

Last digit is printed number: 9 8 7 6 5 4 3 2 1

Dedication

This book is dedicated to Augusta Alba, M.D., for her mentorship in the field of physical medicine respiratory muscle aids. It is dedicated to Mr. Ira Holland and Mr. James Starita, who, even more than the many others who doggedly refused to undergo tracheostomy for long-term ventilatory support, succeeded in convincing me that they were right to do so. Last, but not least, it is dedicated to my son Gaveric for his inspiration and assistance (seen below) in the preparation of this book.

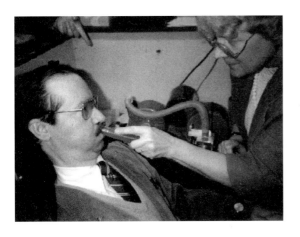

Dr. Augusta Alba (right) applying mechanical insufflation-exsufflation to Mr. Ira Holland.

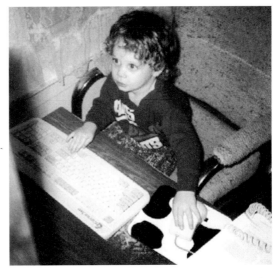

Gaveric Alexandre Bach at 27 months of age in the process of deleting my word processor, presumably for the purpose of installing an updated version.

Contents

THE PARALYTIC/RESTRICTIVE CONDITIONS

Contributors

Thomas K. Aldrich, MD
Professor and Acting Director, Pulmonary Medicine Division, Albert Einstein College of Medicine and Montefiore Medical Center, Bronx, New York

John R. Bach, MD
Professor and Vice Chairman, Department of Physical Medicine & Rehabilitation, University of Medicine and Dentistry of New Jersey—New Jersey Medical School, Newark, New Jersey

Vicki Barnett, PhD
Assistant Professor, Department of Physical Medicine & Rehabilitation, University of Medicine and Dentistry of New Jersey—New Jersey Medical School, Newark, New Jersey

Michael J. Belman, MD
Associate Professor, Division of Pulmonary Medicine, Cedars Sinai Medical Center, Los Angeles, California

Bartolome R. Celli, MD
Professor, Department of Medicine, Tufts University, Boston, Massachusetts

Kenneth R. Chapman, MD, MSc, FRCPC, FACP
Associate Professor of Medicine, Division of Respiratory Medicine, University of Toronto, Toronto, Ontario, Canada

Michael T. Dealy, PhD
Associate Professor of Psychology, New York University School of Medicine, Fordham University, Pace University, New York, New York

Joel A. DeLisa, MD, MS
Professor and Chairman, Department of Physical Medicine and Rehabilitation, University of Medicine and Dentistry of New Jersey—New Jersey Medical School, Newark, New Jersey

Karen J. Dikeman, MA, SLP
Department of Speech Pathology, Silvercrest Extended Care Facility, Jamaica, New York

Alfred P. Fishman, MD
Professor, Department of Rehabilitation Medicine, University of Pennsylvania Medical Center, Philadelphia, Pennsylvania

Susan L. Garritan, MA, PT, CCS
Supervisor, Department of Physical Therapy–Cardiopulmonary, New York University Medical Center, New York, New York

Christian Gilardeau, MD
Consulting Physician for the Association Francaise contre les Myopathies, Evry, France

Karen Glenn, RRT
Outcomes Study Coordinator, National Jewish Center for Immunology and Respiratory Medicine, Denver, Colorado

Roger Goldstein, MB, ChB, FRCP(UK), FRCP(C), FCCP
Associate Professor and Director, Divisional Programme in Respiratory Rehabilitation, Division of Respiratory Medicine, Department of Medicine, University of Toronto, Toronto, Ontario, Canada

Seth Gottlieb, MD
Pulmonary Fellow, Boston University School of Medicine, Boston, Massachusetts

Ditza Gross, MD
Department of Anesthesia, Hadassah University Hospital, Jerusalem, Israel

Susan L. Guzzardo, PT, MA
Senior Physical Therapist, Department of Pediatrics, Rusk Institute, New York University Medical Center, New York, New York

Robert E. Hillberg, MD
Assistant Professor, Department of Medicine, Tufts University; Clinical Instructor, Department of Medicine, Harvard University Medical School, Boston, Massachusetts

Margaret E. Hodson, MD
Director, Department of Cystic Fibrosis, Royal Brompton Hospital, London, England

Robert M. Kaplan, PhD
Professor, Department of Family and Preventive Medicine, University of California at San Diego, LaJolla, California

Marta S. Kazandjian, MA, SLP
Department of Speech Pathology, Silvercrest Extended Care Facility, Jamaica, New York

Theresa Keegan, MA, CRC
Director, Career Guidance and Placement Services, Kessler Institute for Rehabilitation, West Orange, New Jersey

Gerhardus Hermannus Koëter, MD, PhD
Professor, Department of Pulmonary Diseases, University of Groningen, Groningen, The Netherlands

Michael I. Lewis, MD
Associate Profesor, Pulmonary/Critical Care Division, Department of Medicine, University of California at Los Angeles School of Medicine, Los Angeles, California

Brendan P. Madden, MD, MSC, FRCPI
Consultant, Thoracic and Transplant Physician, Senior Lecturer in Transplant Medicine, Department of Cardiological Science, St. Georges Hospital Medical School, London, England

Barry Jay Make, MD
Professor, Division of Pulmonary Sciences and Critical Care Medicine, University of Colorado School of Medicine, Denver, Colorado

William D. Marino, MD
Associate Professor, Department of Medicine, New York Medical College, Our Lady of Mercy Medical Center, Bronx, New York

W. Clinton McSherry, PhD
Chief, Counseling Psychology Section, Perry Point Veterans Affairs Medical Center, Perry Point, Maryland

Jean Navarro, MD
Service de Gastroenterologie et de Nutrition Pediatrique, Hopital Robert Debre, Paris, France

Horacio D. Pineda, MD
Clinical Assistant Professor, Department of Rehabilitation Medicine, New York University Medical Center, New York, New York

Dirkje Sjoukje Postma, MD, PhD
Professor, Department of Pulmonary Diseases, University Hospital Groningen, Groningen, The Netherlands

Cynthia S. Rand, PhD
Associate Professor, Department of Medicine, Johns Hopkins University, Baltimore, Maryland

Andrew L. Ries, MD, MPH
Professor, Division of Pulmonary and Critical Care Medicine, Department of Medicine, University of California at San Diego, San Diego, California

Bruce Kalman Rubin, MSurg, MD, FRCP(C), FCCP
Associate Professor, Department of Pediatrics, St. Louis University, St. Louis, Missouri

Marca Leonise Sipski, MD
Associate Professor, Department of Physical Medicine and Rehabilitation, University of Medicine and Dentistry of New Jersey—New Jersey Medical School, Newark, New Jersey

Joseph P. Valenza, MD, MCE
Clinical Instructor, Department of Physical Medicine & Rehabilitation, University of Medicine and Dentistry of New Jersey—New Jersey Medical School, Newark, New Jersey

Thomas W. van der Mark, PhD
Associate Professor, Department of Lung Function, University Hospital Groningen, Groningen, The Netherlands

Cees P. van der Schans, PT, PhD
Department of Rehabilitation, University Hospital Groningen, Groningen, The Netherlands

Venance Varille, MD
Service de Gastroenterologie et de Nutrition Pediatrique, Hopital Robert Debre, Paris, France

Thiébaut Noël Willig, MD
Association Francaise contre les Myopathies, Evry, France

Preface

In this era of cost containment, physical medicine, rehabilitation, and general medicine interventions are expected to be both efficacious and cost-effective. Both survival and quality of life are considered in equations designed to justify the cost-benefit for any prospective intervention. Interestingly, studies involving the rehabilitation of patients with chronic obstructive pulmonary disease have consistently demonstrated increasing exercise tolerance, while decreasing dyspnea and hospitalization rates. The latter may be at least in part responsible for the fact that some studies have suggested that rehabilitation may prolong survival independently of any effects of concurrent supplemental oxygen administration. Likewise, the functional benefits and sense of well-being derived from taking part in a well-designed pulmonary rehabilitation program suggest an improved quality of life for these patients. The fact that effective programs can be inexpensive, indeed less expensive than the hospitalizations and emergency room visits that would otherwise result, attests to their cost-effectiveness.

Although Dr. Fishman's definition of pulmonary rehabilitation in Chapter 1, and all other widely accepted definitions, apply equally well to individuals with chronic obstructive pulmonary disease as for ventilator users with paralytic-restrictive pulmonary syndromes, the latter are infrequently considered in pulmonary rehabilitation publications. This is unfortunate because these patients require attention to both pulmonary and habilation status, and physical medicine interventions can be very beneficial for them. They can greatly prolong survival and facilitate airway secretion elimination without the need to resort to tracheostomy; they can facilitate discharge to the community; significantly reduce hospitalization rates and the cost of home mechanical ventilation; and can improve quality of life. Further, the great majority of severely physically impaired individuals who require continuous ventilator use report life satisfaction comparable to that of the general population. Many of these patients also remain extremely active and gainfully employed even though living the majority of their lives as ventilator users.

This book is unique in presenting and evaluating the results of physical medicine and rehabilitation for both patients with obstructive and paralytic/restrictive pulmonary syndromes.

John R. Bach, MD

The Chest Physician and Physiatrist:
Perspectives on the Scientific Basis of Pulmonary Rehabilitation and Related Research

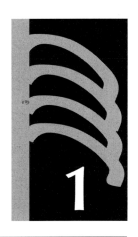

Alfred P. Fishman, MD

REHABILITATION RESEARCH

Background

For individuals with disabilities, rehabilitation medicine is both a medical speciality and a provider of primary care. It is committed to improving the functioning and the quality of life of the population that it serves. Because of the diversity of impairments (the physiologic deficits), disabilities (the performance deficits of the whole person), and handicaps (the societal disadvantages) in this population, rehabilitation medicine draws not only on the services of physicians, but also of other specialists in the allied health sciences and the biologic, social, and behavioral sciences. Each, operating from a somewhat different vantage, brings to rehabilitation medicine a different perspective and views the consumer (patient/client) somewhat differently. The feedback loop is completed by tempering input from the consumer. All concerned parties have in common the commitment to

work together to improve the quality of life and the functional capability of the consumer.

The domain of rehabilitation medicine is exceedingly wide. Indeed, its concepts and practice have ramifications throughout each of the subspecialties of medicine. Because of its relative novelty and wide expanse, however, it is not yet deeply vested in science and relies heavily on experience and empiric practice.

Rehabilitation medicine and chest medicine have overlapping interests in pulmonary rehabilitation. Convergence of the two specialties, however, has been from strikingly different directions. The approach of the chest physician is rooted in chest medicine, a subspecialty of internal medicine that is deeply steeped in science, especially physiology and pathology. The domain of the specialty is sharply circumscribed, and its practitioners are fairly homogeneous in their training and in their clinical practice. As a rule, care of the patient is dominated by the traditional *medical model*, that is, highly concentrated on the physician-patient relation-

1

ship using clinical observations and physiologic testing as indices of success in management.

In contrast, rehabilitation medicine is more empiric in orientation and outlook and less anchored in science, although traditionally committed to human research from the perspective of evaluation of functional outcomes and quality of life. Moreover, born and raised on the team concept, the rehabilitation physician is more long-term and expansive in outlook, weighing into the balance the societal, social, and familial influences that shape outcome.

The specialists that result from these different backgrounds and training see life, their goals, and their obligations quite differently: (1) The chest physician is tuned to being a medical specialist, occasionally calling for help on others in allied fields (e.g., a nurse or respiratory therapist); in contrast, the rehabilitation physician operates as the leader of a team. (2) The outlook of the chest physician is to treat the individual as a patient, curing or ameliorating a disease, whereas the rehabilitation physician takes the longer view, concerned with optimizing functional outcome and quality of life, even after the individual has become a client instead of a patient. (3) To accomplish the broader goals, the rehabilitation physician takes fuller advantage not only of other health professionals, but also of a variety of societal agencies and bodies.

Over the years, chest and rehabilitation physicians have applied themselves intensively to chronic bronchitis and emphysema—chronic obstructive pulmonary diseases (COPD). This focus warrants the heavy commitment of both specialties because of the prevalence of these disorders. In recent years, the attention of both specialties has differed somewhat: The horizons of chest medicine have widened to include larger representation from other disorders, such as interstitial lung diseases, global alveolar hypoventilation, sleep apneas, neuromuscular disorders, and pulmonary hypertensive diseases. In turn, rehabilitation physicians have had to take responsibility for populations of their own. For example, quadriplegic individuals are largely the purview of the rehabilitation physician, who has to prevent as well as treat respiratory complications, to which this population is particularly vulnerable (e.g., pneumonia, atelectasis, and respiratory failure). Rehabilitation physicians are also more likely to face up to individuals with neuropathies, myopathies, postpoliomyelitis syndromes, and muscular dystrophies. In addition, the rehabilitation physician is both the specialist and the generalist for a wide range of developmental and acquired disorders of infancy and childhood that persist into adulthood. The latter disorders call for special talents in *habilitation* rather than in rehabilitation.

A recent development has been increased emphasis on the part of both specialties on the need to practice preventive medicine. Both specialties are strong advocates of smoking cessation, not only for its relationship to COPD and carcinoma of the lung, but also for its role in aggravating any underlying pulmonary disorder. Proper nutrition and physical conditioning are also recognized to be essential preventive measures, not only in managing critically ill patients, but also in preparing individuals for surgical interventions and for long-term health care.

Success in achieving goals is easier to demonstrate for the chest physician than for the rehabilitation physician. The chest physician, committed to reversing or arresting pathogenetic mechanisms, is often rewarded with self-evident abatement of symptoms and signs, reinforced by physiologic testing to demonstrate improvement. In contrast, the traditional rehabilitation physician's end points of improving function and quality of life rely on less easily quantifiable indices.

The Workshop

Increasing awareness on the part of two major components of the National Institutes of Health (NIH)—the Division of Lung Diseases of the National Heart, Lung, and Blood Institute (NHLBI) and the recently formed National Center for Medical Rehabilitation Research (NCMRR)—led to the convening of a workshop in April 1993 to consider areas of congruity and prospects for research. The meeting was attended by chest physicians with proven records of interest in pulmonary rehabilitation and by a diverse group of health professionals who have special interests and talents in rehabilitation medicine and generally share in the *team effort* that characterizes rehabilitation medicine. The diversity of the group contributed greatly to the broad perspective of the deliberations.

Definition of Pulmonary Rehabilitation

As a start, the participants were asked to consider the appropriateness of the definition espoused by the American College of Chest Physicians and the American Thoracic Society. This definition, widely quoted in textbooks, refers to pulmonary rehabilitation as "an art of medical practice. . . ." The participants, based on their different vantages, expressed reservations about the adequacy of this definition. Although many definitions were tendered, the consensus was that a definition that regarded pulmonary rehabilitation as "an art . . ." no longer sufficed. After considerable debate and balloting during the course of the meeting, the post-meeting writing group settled on the following definition:

> Pulmonary rehabilitation is a multidimensional continuum of services directed to persons with pulmonary disease and their families, usually by an interdisciplinary team of specialists, with the goal of achieving and maintaining the individual's maximum level of independence and functioning in the community.

Conceptually, this comprehensive definition underscores the wide sweep of pulmonary rehabilitation—from prevention to functional outcome and quality of life, the involvement of families in the rehabilitation process, the team concept, and the goals of independent living and functioning. This definition also underscores the need for reappraisal of current practice. For example, what is meant by *the team* that is engaged in pulmonary rehabilitation? Do a physician and a nurse constitute a proper team? May the composition of the team vary during the course of the patient's/client's lifetime? Can a physician, nurse, and physical therapist suffice? How should the composition of the team vary according to the course and outcome of the interventions? Is return to gainful employment a realistic outcome for some who undergo pulmonary rehabilitation but not for others? If so, which group of patients with pulmonary disease can profitably undergo vocational rehabilitation? Few successful attempts at vocational rehabilitation have been reported for individuals with COPD. Does this failure reflect, at least in part, inadequacies in the selection of patients for vocational rehabilitation? Moreover, what relevance does the experience with COPD have for individuals with other types of respiratory disorders, such as the alveolar hypoventilation and sleep apnea syndromes?

Functional Assessment

Not only the physical disabilities, but also their emotional and social consequences have to be taken into account in functional assessment. The emotional and social consequences affect importantly the ability of the patient to perform many of the activities of daily living, including personal care, household tasks, childbearing, and vocational tasks. Adjustments to the demands of the activities of daily life are not only complex, but also apt to vary with time. Evaluation of the effectiveness of pulmonary rehabilitation requires a method of evaluation that goes beyond somatic and physiologic issues (i.e., a method that would account for, quantify, and monitor variables that are important determinants of a patient's quality of life).

Functional assessment provides a systematic and comprehensive inventory of the activities and attitudes that shape the patient's daily living. If, in the analysis of function, impairments do not account entirely for the disability or handicap (and they commonly do not), other intervening factors must be considered. The ultimate goal of functional assessment and analysis is to identify unmet medical, psychosocial, and environmental needs and to intervene appropriately to achieve optimal function and health-related quality of life. The functional approach not only is useful for monitoring the individual's functional status, but also enables the rehabilitation team to set and achieve goals for improvement in the health-related quality of the individual's life.

Unfortunately the task of gathering comprehensive data for functional assessment is formidable. In addition to quantifying physical, emotional, and social functioning, the social role of the individual and the subjective sense of the individual's well-being has to be addressed. Moreover, clinical data have to be collected effectively and economically and promptly analyzed and the results fed back to the individual and to the health care providers.

Because of practical obstacles to this comprehensive approach, attention has turned to task-specific indices; for example, can the patient feed himself or herself? Physiologic measurements have also been related to specific functions, for example, the oxygen cost of dressing in patients with COPD. From the perspective of practicality, however, dyspnea has emerged as a critical manifestation of pulmonary disease that can be used in assessing the health-related quality of life.

Quantification of dyspnea as part of functional assessment is no easy matter. A variety of measures have been directed at quantification (e.g., the Borg Dyspnea Rating Scale, the Chronic Respiratory Questionnaire, and the Baseline and Transition Dyspnea Indices). Despite its elusiveness, quantification of dyspnea affords several attractive prospects: insights into the pathogenesis and pathophysiology of dyspnea, a basis for assessing functional limitation, definition of realistic (achievable) goals in the process of pulmonary rehabilitation, specification of appropriate therapeutic interventions, and evaluation of outcomes. One approach to pulmonary rehabilitation that centers on the relief of dyspnea is illustrated for an individual with obstructive airways disease in Table 1–1.

Outcomes Research in Pulmonary Rehabilitation

The study of outcomes in pulmonary rehabilitation is important for two related reasons: (1) the need to ascertain the effectiveness of pulmonary rehabilitation in general and of specific interventions in particular and (2) the responsibility of the medical and scientific community to provide data that helps society to allocate optimally its scarce health care resources. In general, participants in the workshop, drawing on personal experiences, agreed that pulmonary rehabilitation epitomizes medical *caring* and is beneficial for certain patients with pulmonary disease. Proof of this supposition, however, can be challenged: Much of the research in support of this view suffers from methodologic problems, such as small sample size, the lack of ade-

TABLE 1–1
Domains Relevant to Pulmonary Rehabilitation in Patients with Dyspnea*

Domain	Example
Pathophysiology	Obstructive airways disease
Impairment	Breathless, cough, sputum; malnutrition; depression
Functional limitation	Limited exercise tolerance; requires O_2 for the activities of daily life and sleep; weakness
Disability	Cannot do constructive work; deterioration of sex life and intimate relationships; loss of recreation
Societal limitation	Cannot find employment; difficulty with health, life, or disability insurance; architectural barriers

*Illustrated for patient with COPD.
Modified from Research Plan for the National Center for Medical Rehabilitation Research, National Institutes of Health, National Institute of Child Health and Human Development, NIH Publication No. 93-3509, 1993.

quate control populations, incompletely validated outcome measures, or the absence of prospective data collection. Moreover, long-term benefits from pulmonary rehabilitation have yet to be proved. Because of the lack of consensus about long-term benefits, many medical care payers do not feel compelled to provide for pulmonary rehabilitation.

The range of therapeutic interventions used in pulmonary rehabilitation is exceedingly broad. It includes diverse exercise regimens, techniques for the retraining of breathing patterns, education and assorted strategies for behavior modification, smoking cessation, and psychosocial support. The more rigorous studies of effectiveness suggest that the more effective programs are comprehensive in nature and emphasize exercise programs, relief of symptoms, and modification of behavior. Which of these components, however, is responsible for achieving desirable outcomes and the relative contributions of each remain unproven.

Evaluation of success in pulmonary rehabilitation has been based on a variety of indices: improvement in the health-related quality of life, decrease in debilitating respiratory symptoms, increase in exercise tolerance, increase in the level of physical activity, weaning from a ventilator to independent ventilation, improvement in physiologic measurements, improvement in health-related behavior (e.g., smoking cessation; greater mobility; ability to function independently at home using supplemental oxygen; improved physical, mental, emotional, and social functioning), a perception of well-being, and improved cost-benefit relationships.

In general, these end points have been measured qualitatively. The 1990 Report of the Task Force on Medical Rehabilitation Research identified certain needs for quantification of rehabilitation in general that apply to pulmonary rehabilitation. Among these is the need to "develop meaningful, quantitative measures of impairments, disabilities, and handicaps . . . ." It also called for "standards and guidelines for the design and application of evaluative tools." Although many studies have dealt with some of the end points enumerated and have concluded that pulmonary rehabilitation does benefit the patient in one way or another, the great majority of the studies have not been pursued with scientific rigor.

As noted previously, most studies in pulmonary rehabilitation have centered around individuals with COPD. Although COPD does merit considerable attention because of its prevalence and social and economic impacts, it is uncertain whether the criteria for successful pulmonary rehabilitation that are applied to these patients can be applied to patients with other types of respiratory disease. For example, in certain diseases of the lungs or thorax, the major criteria for success might be a decrease in the work of breathing, improvement in pulmonary function, a change for the better in the pattern of breathing, alleviation of dyspnea, and normalization of the arterial blood gases. In others, a reasonable criteria for success might be an increase in the efficiency of energy utilization, improved nutrition, and brightening of the patient's outlook.

Another challenge to those engaged in the practice of pulmonary rehabilitation is the cost-effectiveness of the team that is needed for pulmonary rehabilitation. Is the traditional full team of physicians and allied health professionals necessary, or could a smaller team suffice? Another important question is the distinction between exercise, education, or psychological intervention as the most important factor in promoting functional improvement in a program of pulmonary rehabilitation. By what criteria can benefit from interdisciplinary care be proved? Should cost analysis be an integral part of the study design? From whose perspective is the study or analysis being conducted: the patient/client, the payer, or society?

Studies of clinical effectiveness and economic impact are under way in virtually all aspects of rehabilitation medicine. With respect to pulmonary rehabilitation, certain general measures of outcome can be readily identified: mortality, disability, morbidity, indices of quality of life, and physiologic indices. In addition, certain indices have particular applicability to COPD: the frequency of exacerbations of disease, hospitalizations, and medical use of emergency care services; respiratory symptoms; physical, neurophychological, and social functioning; the perception of well-being; caregiver burden; and the need for assistive devices.

INTERVENTIONS IN PULMONARY REHABILITATION

Relieving, Arresting, or Reversing Pathogenetic Mechanisms

Conventional physiologic interventions in pulmonary rehabilitation include administration of oxygen, physical exercise conditioning, breathing exercises; respiratory muscle training is a more recent modality. Among these, only the administration of oxygen has been shown to prolong life.

Physical exercise training improves exercise capacity, the ability to walk, and the sense of well-being, even in hypercapnic patients. Different types of exercise have proven to be effective (e.g., high intensity and low frequency on the one hand and low intensity and high frequency on the other; also, exercise involving legs, arms, cycling, walking, and stair climbing). Virtually all of these observations concerning exercise, however, have been gained from patients with COPD. The extent to which they apply to other types of patients (e.g., with neuromuscular or chest wall abnormalities) is unclear.

A variety of other physiologically oriented strategies have been advocated to improve outcome from pulmonary rehabilitation. Respiratory muscle strength and endurance improve in response to inspiratory muscle resistive training or threshold load training. Dyspnea is only marginally relieved, however, and the capacity for the activities of daily living is only slightly improved. The value of other breathing exercises has not been assessed in controlled studies. Unique types of breathing training (glossopharyngeal breathing, cough training) seem to have their place in special situations, but both value and limits remain to be defined.

Patients with low ventilatory reserve often require mechanical ventilatory support for prolonged periods. Familiarity with the methods and features of devices used for ventilatory assistance is essential for their proper use. For example, some allow better quality of life than others by permitting greater mobility, safety, or comfort. Provision of mechanical ventilatory support without intubating the trachea is a major concern of proper management. Sometimes, attention focuses on ventilatory support that can alternate with spontaneous breathing. To accomplish the goal of avoiding intubation, one can use body ventilators, positive pressure devices delivering air via facial interfaces, and other methods. Although long-term mechanical ventilatory support can reduce morbidity, decrease duration of hospitalization, and prolong life in neuromuscular and chest wall diseases, its value in COPD is less certain. The process of weaning from mechanical ventilators is anchored in physiologic principles and clinical observations. The process is not always successful, however, and the reasons for failure are not always understood. Other mechanical aids in common use but of unproven value are continuous positive airway pressure (CPAP) and devices used to facilitate airway secretion elimination.

Other supportive measures include nutritional repletion and treatment with anabolic agents (i.e., steroids, growth hormone, or growth factors). Although improvements in strength and body weight have been reported following these interventions, the functional and long-term benefits are uncertain. Indeed, risks of excessive nutritional repletion are now well-known, and the prospect that long-term use of anabolic steroids may exact an unwarranted price is not far-fetched.

Although each of the physiologic interventions identified is based on insight into the pathophysiology of the disease process, assessment of the effectiveness of these may not be readily accomplished by conventional physiologic testing. For example, although mechanical ventilation in severe pulmonary disease may fail to restore autonomous breathing capacity, it can sustain life and contribute to a continued productive life. Indeed, physiologic parameters often fail as indices of outcome. Instead, more meaningful indices may be the performance of the activities of daily living and other social and occupational aspects of functional capacity.

Modifying Psychosocial Influences

Psychosocial factors (*psychosocial assets*) important in the recovery and rehabilitation process include emotional and personality characteristics. In general, the better endowed the individual with psychosocial assets, the better the adaptation to stress, the more positive the responses to psychological interventions such as group therapy, and the more likely is adherence to medical and behavioral regimens. With respect to pulmonary rehabilitation, the better endowed individuals experience less dyspnea, require less medication, adapt more readily to physical medicine interventions, and survive longer than do patients with fewer psychosocial assets.

Psychosocial interventions afford the prospect of enhancing the patient's health-related quality of life and psychosocial functioning, increasing adherence to behavioral and medical treatment regimens, and enhancing physical recovery and survival. Types of psychosocial interventions include education of patients and family members as to the nature of the disease and the use of preventive and self-management strategies; counseling and therapy, whether group or individually oriented; stress management and relaxation techniques; specific cognitive and behavioral modification techniques; and provision of support to patients and their families. The role of these interventions in a pulmonary rehabilitation program requires dissection and evaluation.

Improving coping skills has the potential for improving outcome in individuals undergoing pulmonary rehabilitation. Coping skills may be cognitive (e.g., enhancing self-confidence and positive attitudes) or behavioral. Interventions that focus on enhancing coping skills are directed at increasing the patient's ability to meet the demands imposed by the disease by enhancing feelings of mastery and control, leading to improvement in physiologic and psychological functioning. Behavioral and cognitive techniques used in conjunction with an exercise program and measures to combat depression have been successfully applied in pulmonary patients with COPD.

Psychological and Cognitive Dysfunction

Although dyspnea often cannot be fully relieved, interventions directed at changing the affective component (i.e., the patient's response to the symptom) may change the patient's perception of the intensity of the symptom without changes in the physiologic cause. A decrease in the intensity of dyspnea and the distress associated with the symptom may be one of the most significant goals for patients in pulmonary rehabilitation.

Certain emotional states (fear, anxiety, anger) can increase dyspnea. The increase in breathlessness is accompanied by an increase in energy expenditure, ventilation, oxygen consumption, and skeletal muscle tension. In turn, the increase in dyspnea promotes greater anxiety, which contributes to its pathophysiologic underpinnings. Clearly, psychosocial interventions at the emotional level would have as their goal the interruption of this destructive cycle.

One hypothesis concerning the origin of dyspnea is a purported relationship between the perceived and the actual effort expended in breathing. Although psychosensory scales based on this relationship can be used to quantify dyspnea during specific activities, dyspnea arising during the activities of daily living must be quantified differently (i.e., using the patient's/client's historical information and psychological assessment techniques).

Patients with COPD seem to be able to differentiate the sensory component of dyspnea (i.e., the intensity of the symptom) from its affective component (the distress and anxiety associated with the symptom). The patient's self-efficacy (defined as the belief in one's capability to perform a specified task) is related to dyspnea. Increasing patients' self-efficacy and confidence through systematic desensitization, or *guided mastery* techniques, holds promise for decreasing both the intensity of dyspnea and the distress associated with it.

RECOMMENDATIONS FOR RESEARCH IN PULMONARY REHABILITATION

The recommendations of the NIH Task Force can be sorted into four groups: interventions based on pathogenetic mechanisms, interventions based on psychosocial considerations, functional assessments, and evaluation of outcomes.

Interventions Based on Pathogenetic Mechanisms

Exploration of physiologically based interventions in pulmonary rehabilitation have only recently begun and have largely been confined to COPD. In addition, limitations in the performance of specific physical tasks, such as walking, stair climbing, or showering, should be analyzed with respect to particular physiologic parameters. The instruments used for these assessments need to be evaluated with respect to validity, reliability, and responsiveness (capability of an instrument to measure changes over time).

Distinctions should be drawn between the results of tests that show what *can* be achieved physically and how much of this accomplishment is actually maintained for long periods. Instruments for assessing long-term effects of pulmonary rehabilitation on the quality of life need to be developed or applied. Until now, the benefits of pulmonary rehabilitation do not appear to be long lasting. Although this conclusion may prove to be valid, it may also reflect inadequacy of current instruments for assessment.

Attention has already been called to the need for standardized instruments for measuring health-related quality of life in adults. The situation is even more critical for children. In applying and developing such instruments, distinctions have to be maintained between habilitation of the growing child and rehabilitation in the adult.

Dyspnea

The mechanisms responsible for dyspnea and a strategy for its quantification are of para-

mount importance to pulmonary rehabilitation. Some questions regarding its mechanisms are as follows: How do interactions between lung and chest wall mechanics, respiratory muscle function, and gas exchange operate to produce dyspnea? What is the role of lung hyperinflation? How are the physiologic and psychological manifestations of dyspnea related? Does psychological distress magnify perceived dyspnea, as quantified by physiologic scales?

With respect to quantification of dyspnea, what is the relationship between physiologic dyspnea scores and questionnaire dyspnea ratings? How can the language of dyspnea be classified and related to physiologic variables or to other scoring measures?

Physical Exercise Training (Conditioning or Reconditioning)

Even in COPD, *fundamental knowledge* is still lacking. Although both high-intensity and low-intensity training have been reported to improve exercise performance in COPD, questions remain. For example, by what objective criteria has physical exercise training proved to be of benefit? In which populations of patients with COPD? What are optimal regimens for initial conditioning and for its maintenance? What types of exercise (e.g., arm, leg) or combinations of exercise are optimal for different categories of patients/clients? What are the effects of exercise training on dyspnea; capacity for activities of daily living; and overall psychological, functional, and societal status?

The same sorts of queries apply to respiratory muscle training. In addition, other questions can be identified: Are combinations of respiratory muscle training regimens (e.g., strength, endurance, and increase in tidal volume) more effective than conventional regimens? Does combining respiratory muscle training with physical exercise training confer more benefit? Is it possible to increase diaphragmatic excursion by training? Does respiratory muscle training delay the onset of ventilatory failure? Is it possible by training to increase the effectiveness of the cough mechanism? How effective are breathing exercises?

Mechanical Ventilation

Certain key questions can be raised about the choice of method used for mechanical ventilation. How should patients be selected for newly discovered and rediscovered techniques? What pattern of mechanical ventilation is most comfortable, and why? What are the optimal ways of delivering mechanical ventilation to different types of patients? What psychological factors determine a person's acceptance of any given mode of mechanical ventilation?

Long-term mechanical ventilation poses a different set of questions: What are the clinical, physiologic, and psychological criteria for initiating long-term ventilatory support? What is the optimum schedule for each type of patient? What are the most important outcomes? What factors most interfere with long-term ventilatory support, and how can they be ameliorated? Similar questions can be posed with regard to other forms of mechanical support (e.g., CPAP and mechanical insufflation-exsufflation).

Nutritional Repletion and Anabolic Agents

Nutritional repletion rebuilds muscles, improves function of vital organ systems, and restores immune competence. Key questions about nutritional repletion are: What is the minimum prescription needed for repletion? What is needed to maintain the gains of repletion? What are the optimal routes of enteral administration? What should be the relative contributions of components for restoring nitrogen versus potassium? What factors prevent patients from complying with nutritional repletion or maintenance? With respect to the use of anabolic substances, what are the optimal initial and maintenance prescriptions? What are the long-term side effects?

Interventions Based on Psychosocial Considerations

Psychosocial interventions need to be integrated with physiologic interventions in pulmonary rehabilitation programs. It is unclear, however, which psychosocial interventions produce the best outcomes. One goal of research along this line would be to determine if there is a minimal psychosocial intervention or set of interventions that can be incorporated into pulmonary rehabilitation programs for all patients (i.e., a *core* set of interventions). Also, which psychosocial interventions are most effective and most cost-effective, either alone or along with physiologic interventions? Are interventions that improve the health-related quality of life for patients, clients, and caregivers also cost-effec-

tive (e.g., as a result of decreases in emergency services and hospitalizations)?

Identification of Proper Patients/Clients

One corollary of defining the optimal psychosocial and physiologic interventions is the identification of those patients for whom particular interventions would be most effective. To this end, screening measures for psychosocial factors have to be developed. Among these could be mood and emotional state, ability to process information, and cognitive function. Screening should also include measures to evaluate the patient's/client's emotional and cognitive state with respect to the ability to benefit from pulmonary rehabilitation.

Although motivation is generally held to be an important predictor of outcomes, the understanding of the construct of motivation and its effects is lacking. Who is a *motivated* patient or client? Are patients who are traditionally labeled as *unmotivated* simply motivated toward different values or outcomes? Can standard criteria be developed to determine who is motivated and who is not, or who is differently motivated?

Psychosocial Support and Education

Adherence to behavioral and medical regimens is a prerequisite for individuals to benefit fully from rehabilitation programs. What interventions are most effective in increasing the individual's adherence to behavioral or medical regimens? What are the major barriers to the adherence of the patient/client to specific components of rehabilitation (e.g., exercise, medications)?

Although psychosocial support can improve outcomes for individuals with pulmonary disease, the optimal way to use psychosocial support in pulmonary rehabilitation is unclear. Can the patient/client be trained to take better advantage of available supports? What methods are most suited to provide support for spouses and other caregivers? What is the impact of the pulmonary disease on family functioning? Are interventions involving group support for family members beneficial to both the family and the patient?

The education of patients and their families is a necessary part of any rehabilitation program. Understanding of the illness for which the patient is being treated can help to relieve anxiety and improve the quality of life. No studies, however, have systematically tested the effects of providing different types of information (e.g., different materials, modes of delivery) to patients with chronic pulmonary disease.

Affective Component of Dyspnea

Several aspects of the affective component warrant investigation: What kinds of interventions decrease the affective component of dyspnea? Does decreasing the affective component improve outcome? Where does attention to the affective component fit into the overall program of pulmonary rehabilitation? What are the optimal *dosage* and combination of components of pulmonary rehabilitation (e.g., exercise, education) needed to decrease dyspnea and make significant differences in psychological outcomes?

Depression

Although depression is prevalent in individuals with chronic pulmonary disease, little is known about the natural history of depression in such patients and its impact on rehabilitation outcomes. Among the uncertainties are the following: What factors are predictors of depression in individuals with respiratory disease? Does it help to treat their depression, and what are the optimal strategies for treatment (i.e., pharmacologic, nonpharmacologic, or combination of the two)? Should depression be treated before or within the rehabilitation program? Are current measures capable of distinguishing between somatic symptoms and depression, or will new measures be needed?

Smoking Cessation

Stopping smoking is essential for a successful outcome of pulmonary rehabilitation no matter how outcome is measured. What is the optimal use of nicotine replacement therapy? Should community-based COPD prevention programs be initiated to increase public awareness of the risks of COPD, increase smoking cessation among patients with early signs of pulmonary impairment, and, in time, decrease morbidity and mortality? The Lung Health Study is an efficacy study. Should this model be translated to a community setting?

Timing of Psychosocial Interventions

Little is known about the proper timing of psychosocial interventions. How early in the course of pulmonary rehabilitation should psychosocial interventions be started? For example, when should psychosocial support be provided in the intensive care unit? What is the optimal length of psychosocial intervention and follow-up?

Training and Support of Health Care Providers

The training of physicians and other health professionals involved in the management of individuals with chronic pulmonary disease should provide for exposure to the concepts and practice of pulmonary rehabilitation. The optimal size and composition of the *pulmonary rehabilitation team* needs definition. Provision should be made for support of the members of the team, taking due account of burnout and stress on these personnel.

Vocational Rehabilitation

This aspect of pulmonary rehabilitation has received scant attention. Both state and federal agencies can be helpful in this regard. The patient's/client's outlook would brighten considerably by the prospect of a productive nonsedentary existence. Inventory has to be taken of the role of vocational rehabilitation in patients/clients with chronic pulmonary disease and strategies developed for optimal interplay between health care deliverers and governmental agencies concerned with vocational rehabilitation.

Functional Assessment

Instruments for assessing the health-related quality of life are currently being evaluated. Their application for the evaluation of the efficacy and effectiveness of pulmonary rehabilitation is still in its infancy. Nonetheless, these instruments should be applied, and accounts must be taken of the fact that health-related quality of life is multidimensional and that its assessment should include measures of the activities of daily life (e.g., emotional, physical, social, mental, occupational). If existing instruments should prove inadequate, they should be refined or new instruments developed.

With respect to the types of measuring instruments to be applied or developed, the relative effectiveness of disease-specific instruments should be compared with that of generic instruments. Generic instruments for evaluation of general health status have the advantage of being reducible to a single or small number of scores and applicable to a variety of conditions. Their disadvantage is that they may not deal adequately with specific aspects of health status, such as dyspnea. Disease-specific or symptom-specific measures have the advantage of being closely related to the clinical manifestations of a particular disorder so that they are more responsive than general instruments to changes effected by an intervention. Disease-specific instruments, however, suffer the disadvantage of not providing a single measure that can be applied to different diseases and treatments. Whether a combination of generic and disease-specific scales will provide the best approach remains to be explored.

Dyspnea as a Special Focus

The case for focusing on dyspnea in assessing the health-related quality of life has already been presented. One immediate application of available instruments would be to discriminate quantitatively between the affective and the other components of dyspnea. Because of its high frequency, dyspnea in patients with COPD merits special attention.

Functional Versus Quality of Life Assessment

Functional assessment, the individual's ability to perform certain tests (e.g., pulmonary function, exercise tolerance, timed walk tests, functional status questionnaires), and the assessment of health-related quality of life can be used. Improvement in the quality of life can be achieved without improvement in pulmonary function. The mechanisms responsible for improvement in health-related quality of life brought about by pulmonary rehabilitation need to be clarified. For example, does improvement reflect desensitization to dyspnea, or improved emotional state, or improved ventilatory muscle strength, or improved endurance?

Evaluation of Outcomes

Evaluation of success in pulmonary rehabilitation has been based on diverse indices, such as improvement in health-related quality of life; decrease in debilitating respiratory symptoms;

increase in the level of physical activity; weaning from a ventilator; improvement in physiologic measurements; improvement in health-related behavior (e.g., smoking cessation); improved physical, mental, emotional, and social functioning; and improved cost-benefit relationships. In general, these end points have been measured qualitatively.

The need for quantitative measures is self-evident. Because of the sheer weight of the numbers of patients with chronic obstructive airway diseases, the evaluation of the effectiveness of pulmonary rehabilitation in these patients continues to be a top priority. It might appear that one immediate approach might be a clinical trial. The time for this type of study is not yet ripe. Conventional clinical trials, such as those used in the evaluation of drugs, rarely provide for assessment of outcomes. In addition, several essential elements for a meaningful clinical trial are not yet at hand. Quantitative measures, such as for performance, health-related quality of life, physiologic state, and behavior, are still in short supply, and criteria are lacking for identifying those individuals who would be the best candidates for a pulmonary rehabilitation program. In addition, certain categories of pulmonary disorders, such as COPD, would benefit greatly from subgrouping based on physiologic criteria. Until such uncertainties are eliminated, a clinical trial would run the grave risk of producing type II errors (i.e., no difference in outcome would be uncovered between treatment groups even though, in reality, differences would exist). In light of these considerations, preliminary steps should be taken to develop measures necessary for a meaningful clinical trial of the effectiveness of pulmonary rehabilitation.

Long-Term Benefits of Pulmonary Rehabilitation in COPD

That pulmonary rehabilitation provides long-term benefits has been difficult to prove. The long-term benefits of pulmonary rehabilitation in patients/clients with COPD should be evaluated.

Effectiveness of Different Components of a Pulmonary Rehabilitation Program in COPD

The respective contributions to the successful outcome of the components of an effective pulmonary rehabilitation program need to be sorted out. Among those that need to be examined individually are exercise, breathing retraining, and psychosocial interventions.

Cost-Effectiveness of Pulmonary Rehabilitation in COPD

Evaluation of the cost-effectiveness of pulmonary rehabilitation for persons with COPD should be incorporated into studies of efficacy. The analytic perspective (e.g., the patient's, the payer's, or society's), the kinds of costs (e.g., indirect, direct), opportunities lost or gained, and the time frame (short-term versus long-term) should be addressed separately. Whenever possible, these analyses should use measures of health-related outcomes that apply to other illnesses.

Pulmonary Rehabilitation in Diseases Other than COPD

Not only should the essential components of an effective pulmonary rehabilitation program be defined for COPD and methods established for assessing the outcomes of the interventions, but also a similar approach should be applied to other pulmonary conditions (e.g., cystic fibrosis, neuromuscular disease, interstitial and other restrictive lung diseases, pulmonary vascular disease, lung transplantation, and the ventilator-dependent patient).

CONCLUSION

These recommendations have drawn heavily on the workshop convened by the Division of Lung Diseases of the NHLBI and the NCMRR. In doing so, it defined two particular goals as being of high priority. First is the development of suitable instruments for measurement. In this process, the question arises of how different health domains are interrelated. For example, what is the relationship between dyspnea and depression? Similarly the development of suitable instruments may help to distinguish between the affective and pathophysiologic aspects of dyspnea. Research directed at such questions promises not only to orient and anchor the rehabilitation process, but also to improve the specificity of interventions.

The second goal is to apply these instruments for assessing the health-related quality of life in clinical trials. These instruments will greatly en-large the scope of clinical trials with respect to outcomes; that is, they will enable account to be taken of such elements as behavior, functional capacities, exercise tolerance, self-feeding, and ability to work.

For the chest physician, the meeting was a reminder that pulmonary rehabilitation meant much more than chronic pulmonary care. The role of other health professionals in providing health care was clearly outlined as the subject passed from being a patient, to becoming a client, and back and forth between the two states. Psychosocial influences surfaced as major elements in the rehabilitation program. Cost-benefits were raised as part of the evaluation of outcomes. Vocational rehabilitation received short shrift largely because of previous disappointing experience in returning patients with severe COPD to employable status. The possibility was left open, however, that earlier intervention in certain patients/clients with COPD might be more effective and that vocational rehabilitation in non-COPD patients/clients might make reemployability a reasonable goal of pulmonary rehabilitation.

The meeting illustrated that pulmonary rehabilitation could well serve as a model for medical rehabilitation in general. With respect to pulmonary rehabilitation in particular, it was also clear that this first encounter among diverse professionals with a common cause was only a beginning. The joint sponsorship of the meeting by two distinct units of the NIH—the Division of Lung Diseases of the NHLBI and the NCMRR—has the potential for building bridges and for promoting productive interactions. With respect to research, the Division of Lung Diseases is deeply steeped in the sciences of physiology, biochemistry, and pathology. In contrast, the NCMRR is deeply vested in other sciences—psychology, social sciences, and evaluative sciences. Also, the orientation of the NCMRR leans heavily toward functional assessment, measurements of the quality of life, and outcomes research. The two components of the NIH seem to have a great deal to learn from each other by joining forces in pulmonary rehabilitation.

Currently, comprehensive pulmonary rehabilitation programs are not widely practiced. Certain questions remain to be answered if such programs are to be part of the emerging national agenda for health care. For example, which elements of a pulmonary rehabilitation program can withstand scientific scrutiny for effectiveness? Can essential components of the program be handled, cost-effectively, at a primary care level? For example, is it possible for nonprofessional health care workers or for professionals who cross the traditional lines, working under the direction of a primary care physician, to accomplish outcomes equal to those effected by a more traditional interdisciplinary team of highly trained specialists? Can programs directed at smoking cessation that are run by primary care physicians be linked with pulmonary rehabilitation programs? If so, does the linkage improve outcomes more than each does separately?

Finally the workshop underscored the need to cross-train physicians in both chest medicine and physiatry. To promote research in pulmonary rehabilitation, special provision has to be made in the NIH peer-review mechanisms to recognize the diversity of research interests that emerge in the practice of rehabilitation medicine.

Acknowledgments

This Introduction has drawn heavily on the workshop sponsored by the Lung Division of the National Heart, Lung, and Blood Institute and the Center for Medical Rehabilitation Research. A full account, which includes the names of the participants, can be obtained from the Division of Lung Diseases, NHLBI, Bethesda, MD 20892.

Particular recognition should be paid to the editorial group that prepared the final report; including Theodore M. Cole, M.D.; Marcus J. Fuhrer, Ph.D.; David B. Gray, Ph.D.; Suzanne S. Hurd, Ph.D.; Louis A. Quatrano, Ph.D.; J. Sri Ram, Ph.D.; Dudley F. Rochester, M.D.; and the following reviewers of the edited version: Michael J. Belman, M.D.; Bartolome R. Celli, M.D.; Suzanne M. Czajkowski, Ph.D.; T. Andrew Dodds, M.D., M.P.H.; Carl V. Granger, M.D.; Barry J. Make, M.D., F.A.C.P., F.C.C.P.; Andre L. Ries, M.D.; Hilary Siebens, M.D.; and Cynthia C. Zadai, P.T., M.S.

Overview of Rehabilitation, General Evaluation Principles, and the Rehabilitation Team

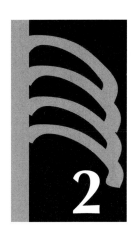

2

Joel DeLisa, MD
John R. Bach, MD

Rehabilitation has been defined as the development of the individual to the fullest physical, psychological, social, vocational, avocational, and educational potential consistent with his or her physiologic or anatomic impairment and environmental limitations. Rehabilitation programs include prevention; early recognition; and inpatient, outpatient, and extended care. Anticipated patient outcomes of a comprehensive, integrated rehabilitation program include increased independence, fewer hospitalizations or shortened length of stays, and improved quality of life.[10] The difference between disease, impairment, disability, and handicap should be understood.

DISEASE, IMPAIRMENT, DISABILITY, AND HANDICAP

Disease is a pathologic condition of the body with a unique set of symptoms and signs. Most disease results in impairment. Although impairment often leads to functional deficit, functional deficit is not a necessary result.

As defined by the World Health Organization (WHO), impairment is any loss or abnormality of psychological, physical, or anatomic structure or function.[12] When an impairment prohibits one from accomplishing a task required for personal independence or physical well-being, disability is created.

According to WHO, disability is any restriction or lack resulting from an impairment of ability to perform an activity in the manner or within the range considered normal for a human being.[12] For example, impairment of respiratory muscle function, airway obstruction, or anatomic destruction of the lungs can disable the cough mechanism. To assess the status of the general abilities needed by all people, rehabilitation specialists apply various classifications of activities of daily living (ADL) to the impaired person. These activities are the endeavors that individuals accomplish on a daily basis to maintain personal independence. The abilities to breathe, eat, bathe, groom, toilet, move about, and communicate all have an impact on the capacity of the individual to live independently. When one cannot accomplish some or all of these activities, independence is compromised or lost.

When an impairment or a disability disadvantages a person's social functioning, it results in a handicap. According to WHO, a handicap is a disadvantage for a given individual resulting from an impairment or a disability that limits or prevents the fulfillment of a role that is normal (depending on age, sex, social, and cultural factors) for that individual.[12] A patient may be handicapped in social terms without being disabled. A child receiving full ventilatory support via an indwelling tracheostomy tube may be banned from certain schools or even from returning home because third-party payer regulations may prohibit *wound care* and tracheal suctioning by other than the patient's family members or health care professionals. The same patient receiving full ventilatory support by noninvasive means might be permitted to return to the community.[1,5]

For patients with pulmonary impairment, disability can be due to muscle dysfunction, musculotendinous contractures, primary skeletal or cardiopulmonary pathology, poor endurance, other associated disease pathology, or some combination of impairments. The patient can be further handicapped by architectural barriers, public policies, inadequate finances, family support, or education. Therefore, for rehabilitation to be successful, the rehabilitation professional must identify and differentiate the disease process, impairments, disabilities, and handicaps so that remedial strategies can be determined. Each impairment should be listed and its possible functional consequences addressed so that the handicapped person is returned to the fullest possible physical, mental, social, and economic independence.

REHABILITATION EVALUATION

The rehabilitation evaluation is a comprehensive *total person* evaluation that must include the person's family, financial resources, vocational and social activities, avocational interests, and plans for the future.

History

The history is obtained by interviewing the patient and family. It may also be helpful to contact the patient's other physicians and personal care attendants or nurses when involved. The chief complaint; history of present and past illnesses; functional, social, and psychological histories; review of systems; and family history should be documented.

The patient's chief complaint is usually an impairment in the form of a symptom, a disability, or a handicap. Chief complaints that include mention of disability or handicap are most apt to be associated with chronic disease of the musculoskeletal, neurologic, or cardiopulmonary systems.

History of Present Illness

The present illness review should include inquiry into the ability to perform the following basic functions and the factors that limit them: (1) breathing, (2) ambulation and functional mobility, (3) dressing, (4) eating and communication, (5) personal hygiene, and (6) transfers. Dependency in the performance of ADL is quantified by observing the patient and questioning the family or caregivers about the nature of the assistance provided. Endurance and symptom-limiting factors are taken into account.

Patients may accomplish tasks independently, with the use of equipment, or with personal assistance. When equipment is needed, it is important to describe its use. An example of a patient who is independent performing a task with the use of equipment is that of a patient with a neuropathy such as Charcot-Marie-Tooth disease that significantly impairs only the common peroneal nerve, who ambulates safely only when wearing an ankle-foot orthosis but can get the orthosis, put it on, and take it off without assistance. Another example is that of a postpoliomyelitis patient with limited upper extremity function who requires ventilatory support when reclining. The patient may not be able to independently don the strap retention systems usually used with nasal or lipseal ventilation but can independently don and use ventilatory support via a strapless oral-nasal interface.

Personal assistance may be standby assistance in which the assistant "stands by" to ensure that the patient performs the task safely. He or she may provide verbal cues. With partial physical assistance, the patient may only be able to do part of a task by himself. For example, the assistant may buckle the patient's belt after the patient has put on his or her pants, or the assistant may position a sliding transfer board so that the patient can transfer into bed. Total physical assistance is required when the assistant has to perform the entire task. Many people with severe physical disabilities, however, can efficiently direct the assistant in the performance of all ADL.

Cardiopulmonary History

Many pulmonary and neuromuscular patients have cardiac impairment both secondary to respiratory impairment and as a primary concomitant condition (e.g., arteriosclerotic heart disease for patients with chronic obstructive pulmonary disease [COPD], cardiomyopathy for patients with myopathies). Cardiac impairment must be differentiated from pulmonary impairment because rehabilitation strategies are different. The reasons for, timing, and extent of all previous cardiopulmonary hospitalizations should be sought. Particular attention should be given to any previous episodes of pneumonia, endotracheal intubation, bronchoscopies, or ventilator use. Symptoms of respiratory impairment should be sought and their association with pulmonary dysfunction, hypoxia, and hypercapnia determined. Primary cardiac causes may need to be ruled out by physical examination, electrocardiogram, Holter monitoring, evaluation of cardiac stroke volumes, clinical exercise testing, and other studies when indicated. The extent of breathing impairment needs to be considered when the patient is erect, supine, prone, and sidelying and when using a thoracolumbar orthosis if applicable.

Besides questions directed to explore for the presence of symptoms related to hypoxia and hypercapnia, other questions concerning pulmonary function include:

1. Which activities cause shortness of breath?
2. Do you have difficulty coughing up secretions and, if so, when?
3. What assistive devices or techniques do you use to help you cough or breathe, and under what circumstances do you use them?

Ambulation and Functional Mobility

Functional mobility includes not only walking, but also wheelchair travel and even crawling. To assess the extent of disability in these areas, ambulation and functional mobility in different environments, endurance, and factors limiting these activities such as inefficiency and instability are analyzed. Representative questions are:

1. Do you use equipment such as canes, crutches, a walker, or braces?
2. Do you use a standard or motorized wheelchair? If the latter, how is it operated?
3. Is your mobility limited inside or outside the home? Why?
4. Can and do you go out visiting friends, restaurants, theaters, and stores?
5. Do you feel unsteady or fall? On what terrain? With what frequency?
6. Do you go upstairs and downstairs with or without assistance?

7. Do you drive a car? If yes, do you use hand controls or other automobile modifications?
8. Can you use public transportation without assistance?

Communication and Eating

Effective communication is necessary for any rehabilitation intervention. Severe hearing, speech, and language deficiencies are obvious. Representative questions are:

1. Do you have difficulty hearing?
2. Do you use a hearing aid?
3. Do you have difficulty reading?
4. Do you need glasses to read?
5. Do others find it hard to understand what you say?
6. Do you have difficulty finding words?
7. Can you write?
8. Can you type?
9. Do you use any communication aids?
10. Do you get short of breath speaking?

The presence of motor difficulties that result in impaired verbal communication also suggests the possible presence of swallowing difficulties and aspiration. Loss of the ability to feed oneself may result in malnutrition, aspiration pneumonia, or depression and is devastating to self-image. Dysphagia and significant aspiration also imply that bulbar muscle function is inadequate for the use of noninvasive ventilatory assist methods rather than tracheal intubation. Eating skills include the use of fork, spoon, and knife; the handling of cups and glasses; and possibly the use of assistive devices, such as a balanced forearm orthosis, overhead sling, or robotics. Representative questions include:

1. Can you eat without help?
2. Can you cut meat?
3. Do you have difficulty holding glasses and cups?
4. Do you have trouble opening containers or pouring liquids?
5. Do you have problems chewing?
6. Do you have difficulty swallowing solids or liquids?
7. Are any of these activities limited by shortness of breath?

Dressing History

We dress for protection, warmth, self-esteem, and pleasure. The ability to doff and don clothes must be assessed. A disabled individual may have abandoned the use of shoes, socks, pants, clothes with buttons, and close-fitting undergarments. Representative questions are:

1. Can you put on, without assistance, your shirt, pants, dress, undergarments, socks, and shoes?
2. Are you able to fasten buttons and tie shoes?
3. Do you use clothing modifications?
4. Are these activities limited by shortness of breath?

Personal Hygiene History

Personal hygiene activities include toothbrushing, hair combing, shaving, the use of tub and shower, perineal care, and successful bowel and bladder management. To the cognitively intact person, incontinence of stool or urine can be the most psychologically devastating deficit of personal independence. Socially acceptable elimination does not necessarily require that the systems be physiologically intact. Patients with catheters can develop a successful system by emptying collecting bags and satisfactorily hiding the collecting system under clothes.

Difficulty with one's body image can negatively affect self-esteem and social and vocational options. Cleanliness and grooming skills, therefore, have far-reaching psychosocial implications. In addition, deficits in cleaning can result in skin maceration and ulceration, skin and systemic infections, and the spread of disease. Representative questions include:

1. Can you shave and comb your hair unaided?
2. Can you take a tub bath or shower without assistance?
3. Can you brush your teeth without help?
4. Can you apply your make-up independently?
5. Can you use a toilet without assistance?
6. Are bladder and bowel accidents a problem?
7. Do you need help with clothing when toileting?
9. Do these activities cause shortness of breath?

Transfer History

Transfers are movements that involve changes of position and place. They include going from a bed to a wheelchair or regular chair; going from a wheelchair to a toilet, bathtub, shower, or car; and going from a wheelchair, regular chair, or toilet seat to a standing position. Low seats without arm supports can present a much greater problem for transfers and

for coming to a standing position than straight-backed chairs with arm supports. All transfer activities and any associated shortness of breath are explained.

General Principles in Determining Disability in Basic Functions

In exploring for disability in the basic functions, several principles should be kept in mind:

1. When the patient reports he or she is not independent, determine the extent of assistance required: equipment only, standby, partial physical, or total physical.
2. Determine who is supplying the assistance.
3. Separately interview the people who are providing the assistance. The assistant may indicate that the degree of assistance is actually greater than reported by the patient.
4. When it is expected or anticipated that the patient may be dependent, questions of the "Can you . . . " or "Do you . . . " type should be rephrased to "Who helps you . . . ." Questions asked in this manner may yield more information.
5. When the disability is of acute onset, such as during or immediately following an acute exacerbation of pulmonary disease, the inquiry is made into the premorbid level of independence. This information is particularly important in the older patient. Earlier disease or trauma may have left some residual dependency. Therapeutics brought to bear on the new problems are not likely to increase premorbid independence levels.
6. If dependency is present and the disease is progressive, determine the time course of the loss of independence. Therapeutics are more likely to remove disability in more recently lost functions.

When the inquiry into basic self-care functions is complete, a specific disability problem list is formed. Each functional problem is listed separately even though the problems are secondary to a specific disease.[11]

Past Medical History

Past illnesses, trauma, or medical conditions can affect the present level of function. These must be understood to permit the establishment of the baseline functional level. An effective directed inquiry requires an understanding of the full range of rehabilitation interventions. Failure to resolve previous impairments entirely may circumscribe present rehabilitation goals. Examples may help clarify this principle. (1) When 11 years old, a patient with Duchenne muscular dystrophy refused to undergo spinal instrumentation to prevent or reverse early scoliosis. Now at age 17, he has severe back deformity. He presents with an upper respiratory tract infection and severe weakness of respiratory musculature. Because of scoliosis, the use of abdominal thrusts for assisted coughing is ineffective to achieve adequate cough flows to eliminate airway secretions. Unless mechanical insufflation-exsufflation can be used effectively, the risk of pulmonary complications and need for resort to tracheal intubation or an indwelling tracheostomy increase greatly. Tracheostomy, in turn, impairs swallowing and communication. Scoliosis also reduces the number of noninvasive respiratory muscle aid options available to the patient. (2) Similar patients with a past medical history of seizures,[2] or a fractured nose and subclinical nasal obstruction, may be unable to achieve adequate insufflation volumes reliably when using intermittent positive-pressure ventilation (IPPV) via a nasal interface. This, too, would increase the likelihood of need to resort to an indwelling tracheostomy. (3) A 37-year-old muscular dystrophy patient who was unable to walk and who had severe ventilatory insufficiency and ventilator dependency with nasal IPPV when reclining was hit by a truck while driving his motorized wheelchair. The resulting tibial fracture was surgically set, but he could not be weaned from IPPV via an endotracheal tube while supine following the general anesthesia and subsequently died from pulmonary complications. The physician failed to elicit the need for supine or nocturnal ventilatory support in the history of associated illnesses.

Review of Systems

Concomitant disorders can adversely affect rehabilitation outcome. This is particularly true for infectious and certain metabolic, neurologic, musculoskeletal, cardiovascular, gastrointestinal, and genitourinary disorders and disorders of the special senses. Good nutritional status is extremely important both for achieving general rehabilitation goals[14] and in maintaining autonomous ventilatory function. The ability to swallow and to control saliva and adequate airway patency are important to permit the use of physical medicine interventions for respiratory muscle dysfunction. Symptoms suggestive of pulmonary and cardiovascular diseases should be sought and, when present, treated to optimize cardiopulmonary reserve and endurance. The elderly or diabetic patient should be asked about claudication and any tendency to develop foot ulcers, which can impede ambulation.

Gastrointestinal disease or the malabsorption that occurs with advancing age can result in vitamin and nutritional deficiencies. Further, the incidence of constipation is high, and incontinence is not uncommon in patients with pulmonary disorders. A history of incontinence, laxative use, and bowel management routines should be sought.

Most spinal cord–injured individuals have neurogenic bladders. Others who may not be incontinent but who have lost extremity function may have ADL curtailed by assistance needs for micturition. For all of these patients, fluid intake, voiding schedules, and bladder emptying techniques should be reviewed. The ADL of continent but severely physically disabled individuals can be facilitated by the use of a condom catheter drainage system. Other symptoms and signs to consider include frequency, urgency, dysuria, flank pain, incontinence, retention, incomplete emptying, pyuria, hematuria, and passage of calculi. Sexual functioning is explored elsewhere in this text.

Psychological function needs to be assessed as well as intellectual function and premorbid life-style. Because the organic pathology may be irreversible, stress may be considerable. For example, a patient who loses the use of his or her legs has to adjust not only to this loss, but also, perhaps, to the secondary stress of the loss of a job. The physical requirements of the job may be incompatible with the activity limitations of wheelchair use. A review of the patient's previous responses to stress facilitates understanding and modification of his or her current responses to illness or trauma. The patient and family may have to relinquish established goals and old ways of doing things. The patient may also have to learn new behaviors and ways to protect his or her health, such as avoiding alcohol consumption, that are not consistent with his or her personality. An understanding of what is likely to motivate the patient and reinforce new learning is necessary.

SOCIAL PROFILE

The social and vocational history provides information about the patient's interaction with the environment. Coping mechanisms, social milieu, education, and vocational and avocational background are explored.

Chronic illness places enormous stress on the family unit. If the family unit is already facing other difficulties with interpersonal relations, health, or finances, the potential for decompensation is even greater. Family support, however, is probably the most important factor in patient social reintegration and life satisfaction.[3,4] The patient's marriage history and status is determined and the possible support of others explored. It is important to understand specific roles, for example, who does the housework and who manages the finances. For all potential caregivers, willingness, ability to participate, and availability are determined.

The patient's home and source of transportation must be evaluated. Is the home owned or rented, urban or rural, and how far from critical services? The home and each room in it should also be evaluated for patient accessibility. Plans should be drawn up to eliminate architectural barriers between rooms and to appliances. The number of steps into the home and between rooms should be determined as well as the potential for entry ramps when indicated. Representative questions to begin a search for problems in social functioning include:

1. Where do you live? (urban, suburban, rural)
2. Do you rent or own?
3. Are the bedroom, bathroom, and kitchen on the same floor?
4. Are there entrance stairs or stairs within the home?
5. Who else is at home? Their ages? Do any of them go to work or school? Are they in good health? Are the children having difficulty in school?
6. Do your relatives live in the area? Do you maintain contact with them?
7. Are you (how long have you been) married? Is this your first marriage?
8. What activities and functions did you do at home for the family that you can no longer do? (Examples are discipline, financial management, chores, sexual functions, avocational activities.) How are these functions now handled?
9. Where were you born?
10. Where else have you lived?
11. What did (or do) your parents and siblings do for a living?
12. When did you leave your parents' home?

Educational accomplishments and further needs must be determined and special skills, degrees, licenses, and certifications noted. Discussion of vocational history and future plans indicates specific skills testing and help in planning appropriate training. The vocational or homemaker history provides an idea of the patient's ambition, reliability, and self-discipline. A chronologic employment history including job descriptions and titles should be obtained, reasons for job changes, and whether architectural barriers exist in the patient's current place of work. Not only do many COPD patients return to work following their rehabilitation, but many severely disabled ventilator users are married and gainfully employed.[3,4,9] Specific expectations relating to kitchen, shopping, home maintenance, and child-rearing activities should be determined, and the rehabilitation team should have an understanding of the patient's financial resources. Representative questions to determine if the disease and the lost function in ADL are compatible with employment are:

1. Describe specifically what you did or do on the job. Start with when you first arrive in the morning.
2. Was (is) your income sufficient to support your family, or do you have other sources? Do you have debts?
3. What kind of work do you plan to do in the future?

For the homemaker who is not employed outside the home, or for anyone living alone, inquire:

1. Did you do the cooking? Shopping? Light housekeeping? Heavy cleaning?
2. Who does these things now?
3. Is this arrangement satisfactory for you and your family?

Avocational activities are also an important aspect of a patient's function. Many patients derive more of their enjoyment of life from avocational rather than vocational activities. To seek problems in this area, the patient should be asked what he or she does with leisure time alone and with his or her family.

PHYSICAL EXAMINATION

The physical examination serves three functions. First, it is a search for deviations from normal structure and function that along with the patient's history and laboratory data yield the disease diagnoses. Second, the physician searches for signs that signify secondary problems that are not necessarily direct consequences of the disease. Such secondary problems may occur as a result of a lack of preventive measures. Third, the residual strengths in the systems or parts of systems unaffected by the disease are assessed. The patient and physician build on these strengths to remove disability and *train around* the impairment induced by the chronic disease. The physical examination, especially the neuromusculoskeletal examination, is concentrated on function and how it relates to outcome.

In evaluating vital signs, supine, sitting, and standing blood pressures should be obtained when possible to rule out orthostasis in any patient with unexplained falls, lightheadedness, or dizziness. Tachycardia can be the initial manifestation of sepsis in a patient with high-level tetraplegia, can suggest pulmonary embolism, or can be a manifestation of severe cardiomyopathy, especially in the myopathy patient. Chronic hypertension can be associated with sleep-disordered breathing or with the use of negative pressure body ventilators to treat chronic alveolar hypoventilation. Effectively treating the primary process can normalize arterial tensions.[8]

Nutritional status can be estimated from the patient's weight, serum albumin, total protein levels, hematocrit, and body habitus. Malnutrition and obesity are common in both COPD and paralytic/restrictive pulmonary patients.

Decubitus ulcers are the most serious and possibly the most frequently encountered skin lesions in patients with chronic ventilatory failure. They usually result from pressure and are more likely to occur when there is impaired sensation, altered consciousness, peripheral vascular disease, or corticosteroid use.

The head is inspected for evidence of craniofacial abnormalities, which might interfere with the use of interfaces for assisted ventilation. Vision and hearing are assessed and refraction deficits and hearing deficits corrected when possible. A routine examination of the nose and documentation of nasal patency generally suffice.

The mucosa of the upper airway is inspected for hygiene and infection. Good dentition or dentures is important for eating. Patients with poor or changing dentition are not candidates for the use of strapless oronasal interfaces for IPPV.[6] The temporomandibular joint is commonly involved in patients with trauma, arthritis, or neuromuscular disease severe enough to affect respiratory function. It should be examined for tenderness, crepitation, swelling, and range of motion (ROM). An inadequately open bite can hamper eating and the use of mouthpiece IPPV.

ROM of the neck is evaluated once neck stability has been ascertained. In patients with neuromusculoskeletal disorders, active ROM may be critical for the optimal use of mouthpiece IPPV as well as for performing ADL. There may also be scars from previous tracheostomy sites.

Many individuals given a diagnosis of COPD have primarily cardiac disease or, not infrequently, a restrictive pulmonary condition. A cardiac evaluation should be performed as described earlier. Right ventricular strain patterns on the electrocardiogram and ventricular dilation often signal cor pulmonale. This is unfortunately all too common in inadequately treated patients with obstructive and, especially, restrictive conditions. Identification of arrhythmias is particularly important for patients with Emery-Dreifuss muscular dystrophy and those with other severe cardiomyopathies. An evaluation of ventricular ejection fraction can help to prognosticate survival by ventilator use for patients with cardiomyopathies.[16]

The respiratory system is considered in other sections of this book.

The genitalia and rectum should be examined. Cystocele, rectocele, and prostatic hypertrophy can interfere with bladder and bowel function. Hydrocele and other causes of scrotal swelling can impede condom catheter utilization, thereby complicating bladder management; lead to skin maceration; and possibly restrict ADL. An intact bulbocavernosus reflex indicates that the S-2 to S-4 level of the sacral conus of the spinal cord is intact. The afferent component is elicited by pressure on the clitoris or glans or a tug on the urinary drainage catheter when present. The efferent response is contraction of the external sphincter.

Every pulmonary patient should undergo a full neurologic examination. The mental status and cognitive examination include evaluation of recent memory, perception, affect, and judgment. Good recent memory function is critical because rehabilitation requires learning new ways of functioning and often the use of new equipment. The severely disabled self-directed patient needs to understand the care plan and management needs sufficiently to be able to direct and train others in his or her care. When recent memory is diminished, much repetition is needed.

Perception includes the process by which the patient organizes sensory input into information about the environment. Subtle disturbances commonly involve the interpretation of visual inputs of form, space, and distance. Such visual inputs require correct interpretation for the patient to be able to make a correct motor response to them. For example, a patient in a wheelchair about to make a transfer onto a bed needs to interpret correctly that both feet are on the floor, that he or she is close enough to the bed, and that nothing is in the way. Similarly a patient about to put on a shirt needs first to interpret correctly the inside and outside parts of the shirt and to determine that both sleeves are right side out. Disturbances in perception can be sought by asking the patient to copy figures or reproduce them from memory. Asking a patient to put on a shirt that is presented rolled up with one sleeve inside out is also a useful test. When perception disturbances exist, the examiner recognizes that the teaching of basic self-care skills by demonstration will not be as successful as verbal instruction.

A reactive depression is common following sudden onset of new disability or following a relatively sudden additional functional loss in long-standing disease. It is a healthy response, indicating that the patient is able to recognize his or her losses and therefore is more likely to apply himself or herself to the rehabilitation program. A reactive depression requires remedial action if it interferes with cooperation.

Judgment difficulties most often occur in the presence of brain injury. Such patients have difficulties monitoring their behavior.

Individuals with chronic hypoxia or hypercapnia should undergo more complete neuropsychological examination. Patients with obstructive pulmonary syndromes may have neurologic, cognitive, and psychological aberrations resulting from hypoxia and the use of steroids and other treatments. Patients with restrictive pulmonary syndromes often have generalized neurologic deficits. Most myopathy patients have subtle cognitive deficits.

The cranial nerves, language functions, articulation, visual and auditory reception, and verbal and written expression are evaluated. Anosmia is often the only obvious sensory finding in patients with amyotrophic lateral sclerosis (ALS). For ALS patients and other patients with severe neuromuscular disease, residual oculomotor and eyelid movements may provide the only means possible to operate a computer, voice synthesizer, and printer for communication and environmental control. Poor balance or ataxia, vertigo, and bulbar muscle weakness can also hamper rehabilitation efforts.

The sensory examination should include at least superficial touch and pain, deep pain, position sense, and two-point discrimination. Extremity sensation is critical for walking, performing most ADL, and avoiding decubitus ulcers.

Muscle stretch reflexes and superficial reflexes are helpful in localizing lesions, and pathologic reflexes indicate central nervous system involvement. The appearance of involuntary movements or convulsions can also hamper the rehabilitation process and render the use of noninvasive respiratory muscle aids unsafe.

The functional unit of the musculoskeletal system is the joint and its associated structure: synovial membrane, capsule, ligaments, and skeletal muscles that cross it. Articular ROM, skeletal deformities, muscle and joint pain, stiffness, swelling, and muscle atrophy or hypertrophy can have a direct bearing on function and should be thoroughly evaluated. A screening examination is useful for all patients. For conditions that may result in major disability, individual joint examinations are necessary. Such examinations include inspection, palpation, passive and active ROM, stability, and muscle strength evaluations.

Inspection is done for scoliosis, abnormal kyphosis, and lordosis; joint deformity, amputation, and asymmetry of body parts; soft tissue swelling, masses, scars, and other defects; and muscle fasciculations, atrophy, hypertrophy, and ruptures. Localized abnormalities should be palpated to ascertain the structural origin of tenderness and deformity.

Joint stability is determined by evaluating the bony congruity, cartilaginous and capsular integrity, ligaments and muscle strength, and joint function. It is important to determine whether a pathologic condition of the bone, capsule, or ligament is causing abnormal movement, subluxations, or dislocations. The joint should be moved under stress in the direction in which it is not supposed to move by virtue of its contour, ligaments, and capsule, with the patient at rest. Tears in ligaments or laxity of the capsule results in abnormal mobility.

Joint motion can be measured using the anatomic position as the baseline (zero angle starting point). The midway point between the normal rotation range is usually chosen as the zero starting point for rotation measurements. There is a wide range of normal joint motion depending on age, sex, body habitus, conditioning, and genetics. When ROM is less than normal, it must be determined whether the ROM is restricted by joint surface incongruities; joint fluid excess or loose bodies; or capsule, ligament, or muscle contractures.

Examination of active ROM should be performed before strength tests in the event that pain is a problem. Muscle tension and joint compressions induced by an active movement are less than in a strength test. If pain is minimal in the active ROM, the examiner can more easily proceed with a manual muscle test. When active ROM is less than passive ROM, the examiner must decide between true weakness, hysterical weakness, joint instability, pain, or malingering.

Musculotendinous contractures in themselves can hamper walking and the performance of both upper extremity[15] and lower extremity ADL. They can cause premature loss of ambulation for neuromuscular disease patients[7]; once a patient is wheelchair dependent, such contractures can hamper transfers, personal hygiene, sitting balance, comfort, and other functions.

Manual muscle testing is crucial in any disability evaluation. The many factors that can affect effort, such as age, sex, pain, fatigue, motivation, fear, misunderstanding, and concomitant lower or upper motor neuron disease, should be kept in mind.

Lower motor neuron diseases result in flaccid or paretic muscles. Upper motor neuron diseases often result in spastic muscles, which make precise voluntary muscle strength determination difficult. Spasticity or contractures can both resist the action of the muscle being tested.

Grading systems are based on the ability of the muscle to move a joint against the force of gravity.

Grade 5—normal strength: The muscle can move the joint through a full ROM against gravity and against *full* resistance applied by the examiner.

Grade 4—good strength: The muscle can move the joint through a full ROM against gravity with only *moderate* resistance applied by the examiner.

Grade 3—fair strength: The muscle can move the joint through a full ROM against gravity only (with no resistance).

Grade 2—poor strength: The muscle can move the joint through a full ROM if the part is positioned so that the force of gravity is not acting to resist the motion.

Grade 1—trace strength: Muscle contraction can be seen or palpated but is insufficient to produce motion.

Grade 0—zero strength: No visible or palpable contraction.

Grade 3 or greater strength is needed for most ADL, and only muscles with greater than grade 3 strength can be strengthened by resistive exercise. Muscles with less than grade 3 strength may require the external support of orthoses to accomplish functional activities, and the joints served by these muscles are prone to develop contractures.

Muscle strength can be further differentiated into a 1 to 5 +/− system for greater precision.[13] Use of a dynamometer further improves the precision with which muscle strength can be quantitated.[18]

FUNCTIONAL NEUROMUSCULAR EXAMINATION

The functional examination is the actual translation of the objective neurologic and musculoskeletal examinations into performance. Adequate cardiopulmonary function is also needed for the endurance to perform many activities. The functional examination can improve even when cardiopulmonary, neurologic, and musculoskeletal parameters do not.

Sitting balance is a prerequisite for most transfer skills. It is tested by placing the patient in the sitting positions with the feet on the floor, back supported, and hands on the lap. If the patient can hold this position, he or she should be nudged in various directions and his or her ability to recover observed. Sitting balance can permit patients who are unable to walk to use motorized scooters rather than wheelchairs.

Abilities to be examined include turning from supine to prone and back, rising to a sitting position, transfers, and functional mobility. Standing balance is a prerequisite for safe ambulation. It should be assessed with support and, if balance is present, with side-to-side nudging.

Eating skills can be assessed by demonstration of hand-to-mouth abilities using various objects or by means of actual observation at meal time. Use of orthotic or robotic aids should be tried and evaluated when appropriate.

Dressing skills are easily assessed in the examining room. If the examiner remains in the examining room while the patient undresses and does not leave before the patient dresses, much information on patient skill and patient/family interaction can be obtained.

Personal hygiene skills evaluation involves the observation of the motions necessary for face, perineal, and back care. Direct observation of specific tasks may be necessary.

Walking is observed if the patient has standing balance. It is inspected with and without street shoes, from the front and back as well as from the side with the patient appropriately disrobed. Abnormalities and discomfort are described in relation to the phases of the gait. Observe for:

1. Cadence (rate, symmetry, fluidity, and consistency).
2. Trunk posture and movements in the anterior, posterior, and lateral planes.
3. Arm swing (protective positioning or posturing).
4. Hip hiking or dropping (Trendelenburg) or lateral thrust.
5. Genu valgum, varum, or recurvatum.
6. Excessive inversion or eversion of the ankle and foot.
7. Stride width and knee and ankle clearance.
8. Stride length for each leg.
9. Synchronization of knee and ankle dorsiflexion during swing phase and rule out excessive abduction or circumduction.
10. Stance phase heel strike, foot flat, and push off.
11. Knee and ankle stability and coordination.

The appropriateness of fit, construction, and use of any orthotic devices are evaluated. If walking is not possible, wheelchair ambulation is evaluated. The patient's ability to produce straight line travel and to negotiate turns is observed whether using a standard or a motorized wheelchair.

REHABILITATION TEAM

Because rehabilitation is a holistic and comprehensive approach to medical care, the combined expertise of an interdisciplinary team is necessary. There are many ways of organizing a team, and many differences exist with respect to integration, collaboration, hierarchical organization, and individual responsibilities.

The rehabilitation team is usually led by the rehabilitation physician specialist. This person needs specific skills in the evaluation of neuromuscular, musculoskeletal, cognitive, and cardiopulmonary systems. The physician should also be trained in cardiopulmonary and exercise fitness, ventilator management, and treatment of functional deficits. The physician is responsible for both the medical treatment and the rehabilitation programs. He or she must know how to organize, motivate, and direct the team; oversee the goals; and be willing to defer appropriately to the opinions of team members. The patient is the most important member and co-manager of the team. A successful team maintains coordination, cooperation, and open communication. Each member also needs to have knowledge regarding the general principles of each other member's approach.

The following members are usually present on each pulmonary rehabilitation team. They are listed, and their expertise is summarized.[10]

Physical Therapist

The physical therapist:

1. Provides exercises to maintain or increase ROM.
2. Performs manual muscle testing and offers exercises to increase strength, endurance, and coordination.
3. Evaluates sitting and standing balance, functional mobility, transfers, and stair climbing and provides training in these areas with or without mechanical aids as appropriate.
4. Uses therapeutic temperature, fluid, electricity, massage, and traction modalities to decrease pain and increase ROM.
5. Does home evaluations to suggest equipment to optimize ADL and provides plans to decrease barriers.
6. Assesses the patient's wheelchair needs and assists in the individualized prescription.

Occupational Therapist

The occupational therapist:

1. Evaluates and trains the patient in energy conservation, including the use of home management techniques and assistive devices to minimize fatigue.
2. Evaluates and trains the patient in self-care activities using assistive equipment and orthoses when necessary.
3. Trains patients and caregivers in the use and maintenance of adaptive equipment.
4. Fabricates and fits custom interfaces and strap retention systems for the noninvasive delivery of IPPV.
5. Explores vocational and avocational interests in conjunction with the vocational counselor.
6. Aids in maintaining and improving joint ROM, muscle strength, endurance, and coordination.
7. Evaluates and trains in the use of environmental control systems and robotics for upper extremity ADL.

8. Trains the patient to compensate for specific deficits.
9. Evaluates the home and suggests modifications to eliminate barriers to optimal function.
10. Assesses driving skills and retrains with the appropriate car modifications when necessary.

Prosthetist-Orthotist

The prosthetist-orthotist designs, fabricates, and fits extremity braces and prostheses as appropriate. Orthotics laboratories can also assist in the fabrication of custom interfaces for providing ventilatory support by noninvasive IPPV.[14]

Prosthodontist

The prosthodontist designs, fabricates, and fits orthodontic bite plates and constructs custom acrylic nasal and oronasal interfaces for ventilatory support by noninvasive IPPV.[13]

Rehabilitation Nurse

The rehabilitation nurse:

1. Is often the principal provider of and trainer in the use of prescribed medications, personal hygiene, skin care, pulmonary toilet, and adaptive equipment for ADL.
2. Minimizes immobility and dependence and integrates the multidisciplinary team's interventions into daily activities.
3. Educates the patient and family regarding the patient's impairments and the team's strategies for decreasing disability.
4. Maintains the patient's environment conducive to achieving the rehabilitation goals.

Speech Pathologist

The speech pathologist:

1. Evaluates verbal production and communication and provides vocal reeducation or augmentative communication.
2. Evaluates for dysphagia, performs methylene blue swallowing tests, and assists in barium swallow video fluoroscopic swallowing evaluations.
3. Provides appropriate family education and assists in cognitive retraining.

Psychologist

The psychologist performs the appropriate diagnostic testing to evaluate cognitive and affective functioning. This includes the evaluation of judgment, perception, memory, and coping mechanisms. The psychologist helps the patient and family develop effective coping skills.

Social Worker

The social worker:

1. Discusses financial options and informs the patient and family about community resources.
2. Evaluates disposition options and advises about possible lifestyle changes to accommodate residual disabilities.
3. Facilitates communication and cooperation between the patient, family, and rehabilitation team.

Vocational Counselor

The vocational counselor:

1. Evaluates vocational interests, experience, aptitudes, skills, and potential future opportunities.
2. Prepares a program for sharpening marketable skills.
3. Facilitates communication between the patient and employment and training agencies and counsels potential employers.

Respiratory Therapist

The respiratory therapist:

1. Institutes any prescribed respiratory treatments.
2. Presents or prepares noninvasive IPPV interfaces and instructs the patient in their use and preparation.
3. Trains the patient, family, and medical staff, as appropriate, in the use of ventilators, exsufflators, and other respiratory muscle assistive devices.
4. Trains in oximetry biofeedback and monitors the success of ventilator applications and assisted coughing on blood gases.
5. Performs pulmonary function and clinical exercise testing for assessing patient status and for documenting the results of the rehabilitation program.

Other Team Members

Other key team members include the nutritionist, recreation therapist, dentist, and audiologist.

PROBLEM LIST

Once the initial evaluation is complete, the physician summarizes the findings, constructs a problem list, and formulates a plan. An example of problem list construction following an appropriate workup follows.

A 26-year-old single woman has high-level tetraplegia owing to a fractured cervical spine as the result of a driving accident. The patient was hospitalized for a short period on an acute neurosurgical service and then transferred for acute rehabilitation. Her problem list included:

1. C-2 fracture dislocation.
2. C-2 complete sensorimotor tetraplegia.
3. Ventilator dependence with no ventilator free time.
4. Tracheostomy dependent.
5. Impaired cough/airway clearance mechanisms.
6. Impaired verbal communication.
7. Cervical spine instability.
8. Dependent for all functional mobility and transfers.
9. Eating, dressing, and personal hygiene skills dependent.
10. Neurogenic bowel dysfunction.
11. Neurogenic bladder dysfunction.
12. Potential for pressure ulcers.
13. Potential for thrombophlebitis.
14. Reactive depression.
15. Home architecture incompatible with paralysis.
16. Financially dependent.
17. Estranged from parents.
18. Unemployed, no prior work history.
19. Homemaking skills deficient.
20. Transportation dependent.

Problems 1 through 5 and 10 through 13 are of the character of *classic* medical problems. Problems 7 through 9, and 20, although also a direct result of the trauma, relate to the patient's physical disabilities. Problem 14 relates to the patient's psychological condition, and problems 15, 16, 17, and 19 to the social sphere. Problem 18 identifies the vocational disability. Problems 5 and 6 are in large part iatrogenic.

One might argue that most of the problems are secondary to the first, C-2 fracture dislocation, and hence this one alone should be sufficient. Such an approach would be valid if there were a therapeutic technique that could reverse the spinal cord damage and restore full nervous system function. Unfortunately, such a technique does not exist. There does exist, however, a set of physical medicine and rehabilitation therapeutic interventions for all of the individual problems. The interventions can be used to minimize the severity of, and in the case of problems 3 through 7 resolve, the problems without any physiologic recovery, hence the importance of their identification. Problems 3 through 6, 8, and 14 through 19 among others can apply equally to individuals with advanced COPD.

Diagnosis of the disease alone is often insufficient for planning a comprehensive treatment program. Diagnosing and managing the disability—that is, the specific losses in physical, social, vocational, and psychological functions—requires investigations and interventions not ordinarily considered in the treatment of acute short-term disease.

References

1. Bach JR: Update and perspectives on noninvasive respiratory muscle aids: Part 1—the inspiratory muscle aids. Chest 105:1230–1240, 1994.
2. Bach JR, Alba AS: Noninvasive options for ventilatory support of the traumatic high level quadriplegic. Chest 98:613–619, 1990.
3. Bach JR, Campagnolo D: Psychosocial adjustment of post-poliomyelitis ventilator assisted individuals. Arch Phys Med Rehabil 73:934–939, 1992.
4. Bach JR, Campagnolo DI, Hoeman S: Life satisfaction of individuals with Duchenne muscular dystrophy using long-term mechanical ventilatory support. Am J Phys Med Rehabil 70:129–135, 1991.
5. Bach JR, Intintola P, Alba AS, Holland I: The ventilator-assisted individual: Cost analysis of institutionalization versus rehabilitation and in-home management. Chest 101:26–30, 1992.
6. Bach JR, McDermott I: Strapless oral-nasal interfaces for positive pressure ventilation. Arch Phys Med Rehabil 71:908–911, 1990.
7. Bach JR, McKeon J: Orthopedic surgery and rehabilitation for the prolongation of brace-free ambulation of patients with Duchenne muscular dystrophy. Am J Phys Med Rehabil 70:323–331, 1991.
8. Bach JR, Penek J: Obstructive sleep apnea complicating negative pressure ventilatory support in patients with chronic paralytic/restrictive ventilatory dysfunction. Chest 99:1386–1393, 1991.
9. Bach JR, Wang TG: Pulmonary function and sleep disordered breathing in traumatic tetraplegics: A longitudinal study. Arch Phys Med Rehabil 75:279–284, 1994.
10. DeLisa JA, Martin GM, Currie DM: Rehabilitation

medicine: Past, present, and future. In DeLisa JA (ed): Rehabilitation Medicine: Principles and Practice, ed 2. Philadelphia, JB Lippincott, 1993, pp. 3–25.

11. Erickson RP, McPhee MC: Clinical evaluation. In DeLisa JA (ed): Rehabilitation Medicine: Principles and Practice, ed 2. Philadelphia, JB Lippincott, 1993, pp. 51–95.

12. International Classification of Impairments, Disabilities, and Handicaps: A Manual of Classification Relating to the Consequences of Disease. Geneva, World Health Organization, 1980.

13. Kendall FP, McCreary EK: Muscles Testing and Function, ed 3. Baltimore, Williams & Wilkins, 1983.

14. McDermott I, Bach JR, Parker C, Sortor S: Custom-fabricated interfaces for intermittent positive pressure ventilation. Int J Prosthod 2:224–233, 1989.

15. Newmark SR, Sublett D, Black J, Geller R: Nutritional assessment in a rehabilitation unit. Arch Phys Med Rehabil 62:279–282, 1981.

16. Willig TN, Bach JR, Rouffet MJ, et al: Correlation of flexion-contractures with upper extremity function for spinal muscular atrophy and congenital myopathy patients. Am J Phys Med Rehabil, 74:33–38, 1995.

17. Stewart CA, Gilgoff I, Baydur A, et al: Gated radionuclide ventriculography in the evaluation of cardiac function in Duchenne's muscular dystrophy. Chest 94: 1245–1248, 1988.

18. Stuberg EA, Metcalf AK: Reliability of quantitative muscle testing in healthy children and in children with Duchenne muscular dystrophy using a hand-held dynamometer. Phys Ther 68:977–982, 1988.

Chronic Obstructive Pulmonary Disease: Causes and Clinicopathologic Considerations

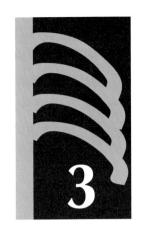

3

Robert E. Hillberg, MD

EPIDEMIOLOGY

In the United States, more than 7.5 million individuals have chronic bronchitis, 2.3 million have pulmonary emphysema, and 7.9 million have bronchial asthma. More than 70,000 deaths annually result from chronic obstructive pulmonary disease (COPD), which is the fifth leading cause of death and represents 3% of all deaths.[27,43] The direct costs attributed to COPD are estimated by the National Heart, Lung, and Blood Institute to be in excess of $5 billion annually. When indirect costs as a result of loss of productivity from morbidity and mortality are calculated, another $35 billion in annual losses are estimated.

Death rates owing to COPD have been increasing in elderly men. There is currently an annual incidence of about 600 deaths per 100,000 population for men over 75 years old. Below 75 years of age, however, death rates in men have leveled off, and in the younger cohort of 45- to 54-year-olds, deaths have been decreasing.[27] For women, however, the situation is entirely different. In all age groups of women from 45 through 85 years of age, the death rates from COPD continue to rise.[26]

EMPHYSEMA

Pulmonary emphysema has been characterized in pathologic terms as a permanent abnormal enlargement of any part of the acinus accompanied by destruction of respiratory tissue. The acinus is the bronchoalveolar unit distal to the first appearance of alveoli in the respiratory bronchiole. When emphysematous lungs are examined pathologically, the alveoli are irregularly distended and form large cystic areas. Elastic recoil is reduced, and the lungs empty air poorly. Cigarette smoking is the most common causative factor in the development of pulmonary emphysema.

Current thoughts of pathogenesis of pulmonary emphysema implicate neutrophil-derived elastase as the agent of alveolar destruction. This enzyme is present in polymorphonuclear leukocytes, which occur in large numbers at the bases of normal human lungs. The neutrophil-derived elastase punches small holes in biologic membranes such as basement membranes allowing the neutrophil to approach sites from which neutrophil chemotaxic factor is emanating. This enzyme is extremely proteolytic and can fragment important structural proteins of the pulmonary parenchyma, such as elastin, reticulin, and fibrin. It has an important biologic role in the defense mechanisms of the lung by allowing neutrophils rapid access to areas of pulmonary inflammation and probably by aiding in the resolution of the inflammatory process. It has been shown that when elastase is instilled into the tracheas of rats, rabbits, and dogs, a pathologic process similar to panacinar pulmonary emphysema quickly develops.

Most humans do not develop the pathologic changes of pulmonary emphysema because of the presence of alpha$_1$-antiprotease. This molecule is produced in the liver and is a 291-amino-acid chain. Its active group appears to be a methionine group. The enzyme is stored in the pulmonary interstitium, and its primary biologic function appears to be stereotactic inactivation of neutrophil-derived elastase. Individuals with a genetically determined deficit of alpha$_1$-antitrypsin develop pulmonary emphysema in their third or fourth decades.[14] If these individuals also smoke cigarettes, a particularly aggressive and virulent form of pulmonary emphysema occurs early in life.[24]

Most patients with COPD have no demonstrable intrinsic defect in alpha$_1$-antitryspin. Smoking, however, results in an acquired deficit. Cigarette smoke contains dozens of toxins, including many oxidants such as ozone, superoxide, hydroxyl ions, and peroxidase. These oxidants can react with the methionine on the alpha$_1$-antitrypsin molecule and change the shape of the molecule so that it can no longer inactivate neutrophil-derived elastase. Consequently, free elastase can destroy structural protein, and

over several decades, the pathology of pulmonary emphysema develops.[13]

Normally the terminal bronchioles, which are less than 2 mm in diameter and have no cartilage in their walls, are held open throughout the respiratory cycle as a result of the elastic recoil of surrounding alveoli, which are tethered on the bronchiolar wall.[32] If alveolar septa are destroyed by elastase, the respiratory bronchioles collapse during exhalation, and airway obstruction develops. Thus, a pathologic process that is primarily alveolar in nature results in a clinical syndrome manifested by airway obstruction.

Cigarette smoking usually results in changes in the distribution of resting alveolar ventilation after several years. As a result of small airway disease, ventilation tends to shift to the upper parts of the lung. This can be detected by observation of an increased closing volume of the lung. Over the next several decades, in 15% to 20% of smokers, centrilobular emphysema develops, usually more severely in the upper lobes. In inherited alpha$_1$-antitrypsin deficiency, the resulting emphysema is panacinar and is more severe in the lower lobes.

The chest radiograph of the pulmonary emphysema patient shows pulmonary hyperinflation, flattening of the diaphragm, and often anterior displacement of the sternum (Fig. 3–1).

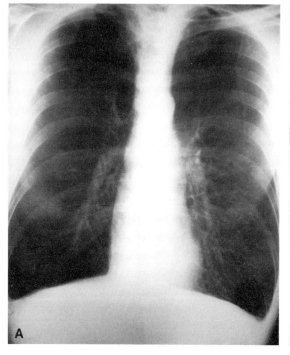 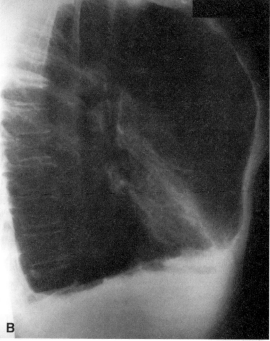

FIGURE 3–1 Pulmonary emphysema. *A,* Marked thoracic distortion resulting from pulmonary hyperinflation. *B,* Flattened diaphragm and anterior displacement of the sternum.

ASTHMA

Five percent of the population has asthma. Asthma is an illness characterized by reversible bronchospasm that usually develops early in life. Wheezing, dyspnea, coughing, and sputum production are present in most cases. A disproportionately large number of cases occur in poor inner-city districts, suggesting that contact with household antigens (i.e., danders, insect proteins, mites, or household air pollution such as secondary cigarette smoke) plays an important role in causation. Most asthmatic children have increased serum IgE levels, and 75% have positive skin tests on allergy testing.[8] Genetic factors appear to influence IgE production. The controlling gene is thought to be present on the long arm of chromosome 11.[11]

Once an individual has asthma, airway hyperactivity usually persists for life with intermittent flare-ups being common. New cases can occur at any age, however, even in the elderly. Asthma can be mild and episodic with normal respiratory function between attacks, or it can be chronic and severe. Individual attacks can occur abruptly or can develop gradually and insidiously. The course of any one case is highly variable and unpredictable.

Attacks are often precipitated by exposure to fumes, odors, dust, or smoke. Most asthmatics report increased wheezing after a viral upper respiratory infection. A subset of asthmatics note that symptoms worsen after vigorous exercise. Others report increased wheezing after exposure to cold air. Some individuals are hypersensitive to any of a large number of organic and inorganic fumes and dust.

Biopsy specimens of bronchial mucosa in asthmatics show hypertrophy and hyperplasia of goblet cells and bronchial glands. Capillary dilatation is prominent. The mucosa is usually swollen and infiltrated with polymorphonuclear lymphocytes, eosinophils, mast cells, and plasma cells. Biochemical assays show increased concentrations of a variety of inflammatory mediators.

Granules from eosinophils release basic protein and eosinophilic cationic protein that are toxic to respiratory epithelial cells and cause sloughing.[5] CD4+ lymphocytes release cytokinins, interleukins, and granulocyte-macrophage colony-stimulating factor. These not only amplify the inflammatory response, but also actively recruit other inflammatory cells, especially eosinophils. Interleukin-4 stimulates B lymphocytes to produce IgE.[34] Other mediator substances, such as platelet-activating factor and leukotrienes, have strong bronchoconstrictor effects and result in hyperresponsiveness of bronchial smooth muscle.[2]

An increased amount of collagen is usually deposited beneath the basement membrane giving the impression that the basement membrane itself is hypertrophied. The smooth muscle of the airways is hypertrophied. Goblet cell hyperplasia and hypertrophy of mucosal glands lead to excessive mucus production. In some fatal cases of asthma, extensive mucus plugging of the bronchi is seen on necropsy. The relationship between airway inflammation and bronchospasm is currently under intensive study. It is hoped that as specific inflammatory mediators are identified, useful antagonists can be developed.

Although inflammatory cells clearly mediate airway inflammation, the basic defect in asthma appears intrinsic to the lungs themselves. Corris and Dark[12] have reported that when two patients with severe asthma received lung transplants from nonatopic hosts, no clinical asthma developed in the transplanted lungs even after 3 years, by which point the transplanted lungs presumably had been well infiltrated by the atopic host's inflammatory cells. Two other nonasthmatic patients received lung transplants from donors with a history of atopic asthma, and these patients promptly developed asthma despite receiving large doses of immunosuppressive drugs.

In a study of 2499 asthmatic patients, asthma was reported to be the cause of death for 4% of them.[54] Other studies report an increasing death rate from asthma, and currently about 5000 asthma-associated deaths per year occur in the United States. Mortality from asthma has been associated with failure to seek medical care despite increasing symptoms, poverty, inadequate treatment, and noncompliance.[36] Undertreatment rather than overtreatment is a factor in most fatal cases.

Bronchial asthma may persist for decades. This makes patient education essential to minimize morbidity. Patients should be carefully taught to recognize inspissated mucus, bronchospasm, and the presence of lower respiratory infection. Patients need to change their behavior to minimize exposure to potential attack-provoking situations. It is desirable to instruct the patient in the proper use of oral and aerosolized bronchodilators, antibiotics, mucolytics, and steroids. In general, all of these medications should be used in full therapeutic doses to control exacerbations but should be tapered between flare-ups. Many patients can use a peak flowmeter to detect worsening airway obstruction and increase their medication doses early enough to minimize exacerbations. Such *adjusted therapy* necessitates an active partnership between the patient and physician. The use of a peak flowmeter in different environments or job situations or after exposure to specific allergens is often helpful in identifying specific asthma-causing agents.

Pneumothorax, bleb formation, pneumome-

diastinum, and interstitial emphysema occur sporadically (Figs. 3–2 and 3–3) and are probably caused by sudden increases in alveolar pressure distal to obstructed bronchioles during vigorous coughing. Tussive rib fractures can also occur, especially in patients who have been taking steroids long-term (Fig. 3–4).

Some patients with severe intractable asthma have become colonized with and develop hy-

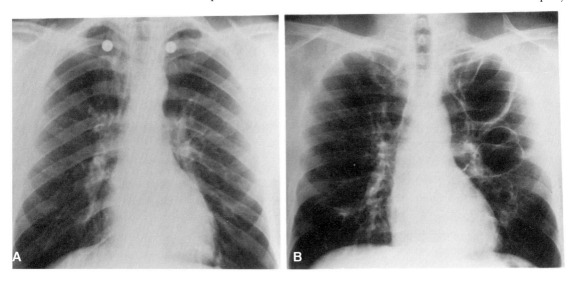

FIGURE 3–2 Complications of asthma. *A,* Subcutaneous emphysema in the right supraclavicular area indicates the presence of pneumomediastinum in an asthmatic patient. *B,* Development of pneumatoceles after an episode of pneumonia.

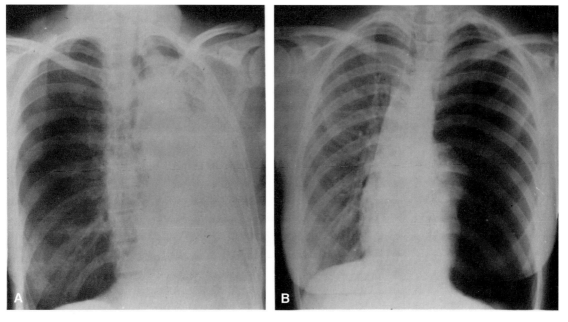

FIGURE 3–3 Complications of COPD. *A,* A complete collapse of the left lung with compensatory hyperinflation of the right lung caused by a mucus plug in the left main bronchus. *B,* Left tension pneumothorax in an asthmatic.

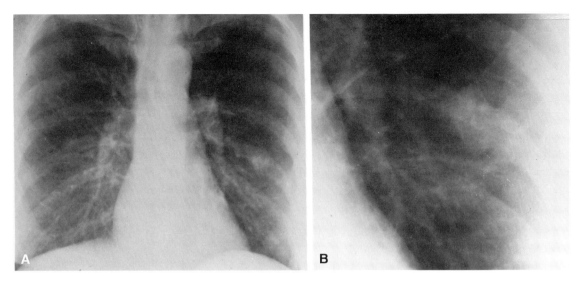

FIGURE 3–4 Complications of asthma. *A,* Chest radiograph of an asthmatic patient 2 months after developing left chest wall pain shows exuberant callus indicating a previous tussive rib fracture. *B,* Close-up detail.

persensitivity to *Aspergillus* species. These patients have elevated IgE levels and serum precipitins for *Aspergillus* as well as positive skin tests to aspergillin. Such patients develop patchy interstitial infiltrates and worsening asthma. The immune response to *Aspergillus* can result in destructive inflammation of the bronchial walls with the development of a form of bronchiectasis that is saccular in shape and involves the proximal segmental bronchi (Fig. 3–5).

Asthmatics are often physically deconditioned because of inactivity owing to fear of triggering an acute episode, fear of dyspnea, and possibly weakness associated with intermittent use of glucocorticoids. Besides using the educational interventions noted, some centers are exploring the use of exercise reconditioning and other aspects of comprehensive pulmonary programs for these patients.

CHRONIC BRONCHITIS

Chronic bronchitis is defined clinically as a productive cough occurring daily for at least 3 months in 2 successive years. Increased mucus production is the hallmark of this illness. Mucus hypersecretion appears to be a nonspecific response to irritating airborne substances, and cigarette smoking is the most important epidemiologic association. Cases have been reported in individuals living in homes heated by wood-burning stoves. Industrial exposure to high concentrations of smoke and dust as well as air pollution can both cause and aggravate chronic bronchitis. Why cigarette smoking causes chronic bronchitis in some individuals and pulmonary emphysema in others remains unclear. Most adult cigarette smokers who develop COPD, however, have elements of both chronic bronchitis and emphysema.

Hypersecretion of hypertrophied submucosal mucus glands produces most of the abnormal mucus in cases of chronic bronchitis. Pathologically, this glandular hypertrophy can be quantitated by determining the ratio of the mean width of the glands to the width of the bronchial wall, that is, the Reid index. A high gland-to-wall ratio, greater than 0.5, occurs in virtually all cases of chronic bronchitis and often occurs even before clinical symptoms develop.[49]

Some individuals with a chronic productive cough for many years never develop airway obstruction. These individuals with simple bronchitis also have abnormal hypertrophy of mucus glands. Additionally, even when bronchospasm is not a clinical feature, some smooth muscle hyperplasia can usually be found. In other cases, definite airway obstruction occurs. A bronchogram shows poor peripheral filling of terminal bronchi and distinct irregularities of the bronchial wall. These abnormalities are present even in individuals with mild clinical disease. Normally, goblet cells compose about 1% of bronchial epithelial cells. Their number is greatly increased in COPD.

Sputum can be separated in a centrifuge into gel and sol layers. It is thought that the cilia of

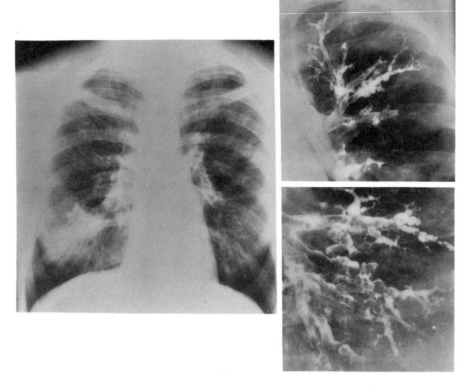

FIGURE 3–5 Allergic bronchopulmonary aspergillosis. Patient with perennial asthma developed worsening symptoms and transient pulmonary infiltrates. Bronchogram shows saccular bronchiectasis, primarily involving the proximal segmental bronchi. Skin test was positive for aspergillin.

the columnar respiratory epithelial cells beat in the sol layer, and the gel layer, with trapped particulate matter, floats like a blanket above. Additionally, in chronic bronchitis, Clara cells are lost, which are believed to be important in the production of airway surfactant. Loss of surfactant leads to the development of atelectasis. Peribronchiolar fibrosis has been identified in postmortem specimens of patients with chronic bronchitis and may stabilize small airways and prevent their collapse. Another pathologic finding in chronic bronchitis is the loss or diminution of cartilage in some of the small airways. This contributes to airway instability and predisposes to collapse during expiration. The cause of this is unclear, but it is thought to be a reaction to chronic inflammation.[41]

Disability associated with COPD is related to the extent of disease in the small bronchioles. Because they are small, these structures are easily blocked by mucus. Mucostasis often results in lower airway colonization by pathogenic organisms that incite an inflammatory response and a further increase in mucus production. Airway obstruction progresses relentlessly, and usually by the time the individual consults a physician, moderate-to-severe airway obstruction is present.

Episodes of acute decompensation with increased cough, sputum production, and dyspnea frequently occur during viral upper respiratory infections. Despite the presence of large quantities of purulent sputum, fever and leukocytosis are usually absent. The most common bacteria associated with exacerbation of chronic bronchitis are *Streptococcus pneumoniae, Haemophilus influenzae,* and *Moraxella catarrhalis.* This flora often changes to nosocomial pathogens during hospitalization for acute exacerbation and exposure to broad-spectrum antibiotics.

With progressive bronchial inflammation and scarring, ventilation-perfusion mismatching occurs and results in hypoxemia. Hypoxic vasoconstriction develops in the areas of the pulmonary arterial bed exposed to the poorly ventilated acini. Pulmonary artery pressure increases, causing right ventricular strain, hypertrophy, and dilatation. As the right ventricle dilates, the intraventricular septum often bulges into the left ventricle, decreasing left ventricular output. Once cor pulmonale develops, there is a greatly increased risk of mortality.

BRONCHIECTASIS

Before the development of antibiotics, bronchiectasis was a fairly common illness. Bronchiectasis is not a specific disease process but describes a final common pathway of a variety of destructive bronchial processes. Bronchiectasis most frequently results from lower respiratory infections that have not been properly or adequately treated.[9] As a result of intense inflammatory activity, the structural integrity of the bronchial walls is locally disrupted with resultant cylindric, saclike, or varicosity-like dilatation. Generally the segmental bronchi are involved with damage to the muscular, fibrous, and cartilaginous components of the wall. Distal to the bronchiectatic areas, the bronchi are filled with mucus and inflammatory cells. During coughing, high intrathoracic pressures collapse bronchiectatic segments, and expectoration is severely impaired. Areas of bacterial colonization and localized areas of invasive infection develop. Distal respiratory bronchioles and alveoli become atelectatic and eventually fibrotic, resulting in areas of right-to-left shunting of blood and hypoxemia. Additionally, there is a remarkable increase in the blood supply to these fibrotic and ectatic areas. Hemoptysis frequently occurs in association with acute infections, or it may occur spontaneously. The hemoptysis is usually self-limiting, but occasionally fatalities occur.

After bacterial colonization, bronchitis develops, and copious purulent sputum production becomes prominent. A cup of sputum from such a ptient often settles into three layers. The top layer is clear and frothy. The second layer is usually watery. The bottom layer is usually opaque and thick and when examined microscopically consists of a variety of inflammatory cells, epithelial cells, and sometimes submucosal cellular elements.

The lower lobes are most commonly involved, especially the left lower lobe, probably because of its anatomic disadvantage with regards to secretion removal. In aspiration syndromes, the right lower lobe is most commonly involved.[55] Upper lobe bronchiectasis often follows tuberculosis or severe upper lobe pneumonia. Often, upper lobe bronchiectasis is not associated with increased sputum production and is called *dry bronchiectasis*. Although sputum production is generally not a problem in upper lobe

bronchiectasis, episodes of hemoptysis are fairly frequent. The right middle lobe, because of the abrupt origin of the segmental bronchus and its ring of lymph nodes, is frequently the source of repetitive infections with resultant scarring, atelectasis, and localized bronchiectasis. This is the so-called right middle lobe syndrome.

Almost all cases of bronchiectasis are acquired, and most follow recognizable viral, mycoplasmal, bacterial, or mycobacterial infections. Some cases, however, have no recognizable antecedent infection. Some of these can be attributed to inhalation of toxic fumes, gases, or dust. Sulfur oxides,[39] anhydrous ammonia fumes, cork, and other inhalations have resulted in documented cases. Some cases appear to be the result of autoimmune inflammatory phenomena. Bronchiectasis has been reported in cases of Hashimoto's thyroiditis,[53] primary biliary cirrhosis, ulcerative colitis,[38,53] rheumatoid arthritis,[59] and sarcoidosis.[21] Kartagener's syndrome,[52] an autosomal recessive disorder with primary ciliary dyskinesia,[56] is associated with bronchiectasis, situs inversus, and sinusitis. In Young's syndrome,[25] men have obstructive azoospermia, chronic sinus and pulmonary infections, and a high incidence of bronchiectasis. The basic defect is not yet known. Patients with panhypoglobulinemia[57] often repeatedly have lower repsiratory infections and develop bronchiectasis. In the yellow nail syndrome,[28] lymphatic hypoplasia resuls in lymphedema, pale yellow dystrophic nails, and frequent pleural effusions, often associated with bronchiectasis and sinusitis. In Swyer-James syndrome,[37] a unilateral, small, hyperlucent lung is apparent on chest radiograph. This is believed to be a sequela of chldhood injury to the bronchi, such as from bronchopneumonia or bronchiolitis, and bronchography often shows areas of bronchiectasis. Bronchiectasis is also often associated with asthma, chronic bronchitis, and emphysema. Some patients with severe bronchial asthma develop a form of proximal saccular bronchiectasis associated with colonization of *Aspergillus* and resultant hypersensitivity (See Fig. 3–4).[29] Finally, bronchiectasis is sometimes first noted after a heroine overdose[3] or after expectoration of a large mucus plug.

Advanced cases of bronchiectasis can usually be identified by the radiographic appearance of characteristic ringlike saccular fluid-filled areas distal to the segmental bronchi, which tend to cluster centrally. Cases not apparent on chest radiograph can be identified by bronchography or computed tomography scanning. Bronchography has been an important test to determine the nature, extent, and anatomic distribution of the illness, but it is associated with considerable morbidity with many patients developing respiratory distress after the procedure. Computed tomography is becoming an increasingly popular alternative to identify areas of bronchiectasis. The thickened, crowded, and dilated bronchi are readily apparent using this technology.[23]

Pulmonary function testing generally shows a combined restrictive and obstructive ventilatory defect. On physical examination, coarse crackles, rhonchi, and occasionally wheezes are present.[42]

Treatment consists of prompt antibiotic treatment for episodes of infection and chest physical therapy when secretions are in excess of 30 mL per day. Bronchodilators are used if reversible bronchospasm is present. If the disease is localized, surgical removal is sometimes possible. Episodes of hemoptysis are usually first treated with antibiotics. Although sometimes alarming, generally, bleeding subsides without surgical intervention. Occasionally the bleeding site can be tamponaded with a balloon-tipped catheter inserted via a bronchoscope.[22] Bronchial artery embolization has been used successfully in patients with massive hemoptysis and a contraindication to surgery. Spinal cord infarction, however, is a potential complication of this procedure. Untreated, patients with bronchiectasis repeatedly develop lower respiratory infections, have episodes of hemoptysis, and develop pulmonary hypertension and cor pulmonale, which result in a significantly shortened life expectancy.[6]

BRONCHIOLITIS OBLITERANS

Bronchiolitis obliterans is another condition that results in severe airway obstruction. It has been estimated to be present in at least 4% of patients clinically labeled with COPD. It can often be distinguished from cigarette-induced airway obstruction by a history of rapidly progressive dyspnea on exertion, usually over a period of only several months. Cough is usually present, but sputum production is not a prominent feature. Bronchiolitis obliterans should be suspected when severe airway obstruction occurs in a nonsmoker or a light smoker and if other conditions, such as asthma, alpha$_1$-antitrypsin deficiency, and chronic bronchitis, are ruled out. A lung biopsy is often necessary for a definite diagnosis. On physical examination, tachypnea and prolonged expiratory phase along with evidence of pulmonary hyperinflation and acces-

sory muscle use are present. Wheezes are sometimes present. Pulmonary function testing usually shows a severe obstructive defect and a normal or decreased diffusion capacity. The chest radiograph shows pulmonary hyperinflation with occasional interstitial infiltrates. Generally, patients do not improve on bronchodilators.

Several known causes exist for bronchiolitis obliterans. Individuals who have been exposed to nitrogen dioxide, sulfur dioxide,[39] cocaine,[45] or other toxic agents have developed this syndrome. Additionally, infections with agents such as mycoplasma, *Nocardia*, legionella, and certain viruses have been reported to antedate the development of this syndrome.[4] Bronchiolitis obliterans can occur in rheumatoid arthritis, scleroderma, and systemic lupus erythematosus[35] and is a major cause of mortality after lung[7] and bone marrow[51] transplants.

Pathologically, medium-sized and small-sized bronchi are completely occluded with polypoid masses of granulation tissue. Distal to completely occluded bronchi, alveoli become ectatic and fibrotic. The earliest lesions contain an abundance of neutrophils and lymphocytes. Bronchoalveolar lavage fluid white blood cell counts usually include more than 25% neutrophils, in contrast to normal lavage fluid, which contains about 90% macrophages and fewer than 1% neutrophils.[18] For comparison, in chronic bronchitis, neutrophils may compose 10% to 15% of recovered cells, and in cases of fibrosing alveolitis and other interstitial lung diseases, mostly lymphocytes are present. Current evidence indicates that after an initial insult to the bronchial mucosa, neutrophils migrate to the area and damage the airway structures with their proteolytic and oxidative activities. There is resultant fibroblast proliferation, collagen deposition, and granulation tissue formation.

Treatment is with large doses of prednisone for several months or until significant clinical improvement develops.[1,18] Prednisone is then tapered and maintained for a prolonged period. In patients who respond to steroids, the percentage of neutrophils decreases in bronchoalveolar lavage fluid so this technique can be used to monitor patients. Unfortunately, most patients are not diagnosed early enough or fail to respond to treatment and succumb to progressive respiratory insufficiency.

CYSTIC FIBROSIS

Cystic fibrosis is the most common chronic respiratory condition in young adults. About

30,000 Americans have this inherited disorder, which develops in individuals homozygous for the defective gene. Chloride concentration is markedly elevated in the sweat of afflicted individuals. A sweat chloride level over 60 mEq/L, together with the presence of chronic pulmonary disease or pancreatic insufficiency, leads to establishment of the diagnosis.[15] The presence of *Psudomonas aeruginosa* in sputum is characteristic and in fact has been proposed as a diagnostic criterion. In most cases, sinusitis is present, and males are usually azoospermic. There may be a history of meconium ileus as a baby, and gallstones and liver function abnormalities are common.

The basic defect is a resistance to chloride permeability in epithelial cells that prevents the reabsorption of chloride along the sweat duct tubules.[10,47] The relationship of this cellular abnormality to chronic lung disease, however, is unclear. There appears to be no pulmonary damage in utero and autopsies of babies dying of meconium ileus indicate normal lungs.

Shortly after birth, infection with bacterial pathogens becomes established and it soon becomes impossible to eradicate these pathogens in many cases. *Staphylococcus aureus* usually becomes established first and may be instrumental in causing the bronchiectasis that eventually develops. *P. aeruginosa* colinization usually follows quickly. Initial *Pseudomonas* infection is with nonmucoid organisms, but this often switches to a variety that produces alginate, an expolysaccharide that forms a gel enmeshing the bacteria and protecting them from host defenses.[46] A related species, *Pseudomonas cepacia*, is becoming increasingly common.[31,58]

Lung disease begins in the bronchioles with evidence of intense inflammation. Gradually the larger and more central airways become affected. Mucus-secreting glands hypertrophy, and thick secretions plug the airways. The structural integrity of the bronchi is disrupted, and cystic and cylindric bronchiectasis develops. The chest radiograph shows pulmonary hyperinflation with evidence of peribronchial thickening and cystic changes. Patchy fibrotic areas develop, usually initially in the upper lobes. It is theorized that the chloride permeability defect may result in abnormal hydration of mucus or abnormal periciliary fluid and that this results in impaired mucociliary clearance. Many cystic fibrosis patients develop clubbing; hemoptysis is common in patients over 10 years of age. Occasionally, bronchial bleeding is fatal. The likelihood of pneumothoraces increases over time, and these are usually poorly tolerated. Eventu-

ally, hypoxemia, pulmonary hypertension, and cor pulmonale develop. Median survival is now over 20 years.[15]

Treatment programs emphasize the need to use postural drainage and chest percussion to aid in clearing secretions.[17,40] Although not of proven efficacy, aerosols are sometimes used before chest physical therapy. Deep breathing exercises, directed coughing, and regular exercise are usually prescribed.[16] Yearly immunization with influenza vaccine and the usual childhood vaccinations are indicated. It is unclear whether long-term antibiotic therapy is effective in decreasing the frequency of exacerbations. Most physicians prescribe antibiotics based on the results of cultures and sensitivities. About half of the patients have reactive airway disease, and aerosolized bronchodilators are prescribed.[33] Episodic treatment with steroids is sometimes useful, and some patients benefit from long-term steroid use in addition to compulsive attention to secretion clearance, infections, and bronchospasm.[20] Because DNA from disintegrating inflammatory cells contributes greatly to the increased viscosity of sputum, aerosolized human recombinant DNAase (rhDNAase) can be used to loosen sputum. DNAase has been shown to improve lung function and quality of life.[48] Studies are underway to determine if there are benefits from the use of salt transport regulators, such as the potassium-sparing diuretic amiloride.

The gene for cystic fibrosis has been isolated on the long arm of chromosome 7 and has been characterized. This gene codes for a protein called cystic fibrosis transmembrane conductance regulator. Many mutations of this gene have been described.[50] Gene therapy is currently under clinical investigation using attenuated adenovirus that has been inculcated with normal cystic fibrosis genes. The virus is delivered by aerosol to the tracheobronchial mucosa. The adenovirus infects epithelial cells allowing the normal gene to produce cystic fibrosis transmembrane conductance regulator and, thus, restore normal chloride ion transport. Because the life span of respiratory epithelial cells is between 40 and 60 days, periodic treatment is probably necessary when this method becomes available for general clinical use.

Lung transplantation has become available for patients with end-stage cystic fibrosis and is considered elsewhere in this text. Because of the presence of chronic infection, usually with multiply-resistant organisms, bilateral lung transplantation may be necessary to avoid spillover infection from a remaining cystic fibrosis lung.

RESPIRATORY PATHOMECHANICS

As a result of airway obstruction, expiratory airflow is impeded, and pulmonary hyperexpansion develops. This can be dramatic and may result in the flattening of the diaphragm into a relatively useless respiratory muscle. Normally the diaphragm accounts for 70% of resting ventilation. Its primary action is to abut its muscular central tendon against the resistance offered by the abdominal viscera with the result that its costal fibers pull upward and elevate the ribs. The central tendon descends, increasing abdominal pressure, which is transmitted laterally and results in an outward displacement of the lower rib cage. When the diaphragm is flat, its costal fibers are arranged horizontally instead of vertically. With contraction, the lower ribs move inward (Hoover's sign[30]).

The metabolic cost of pulmonary hyperinflation is high. The respiratory muscles of patients with advanced pulmonary emphysema may consume as much as 30 mL of oxygen per minute as opposed to the normal consumption of 2.5 mL. Normally, 1% to 2% of total body O_2 consumption is for breathing, but a patient with advanced chronic lung disease can use as much as 15%. Likewise, resting minute ventilation is normally 5% of maximum breathing capacity as opposed to as much as 40% for many COPD patients.

ACCESSORY MUSCLES OF RESPIRATION

Hyperinflated patients use accessory muscles of respiration. These are primarily the small strap muscles of the neck—the anterior, medial, and posterior scalenes, which arise from the third, fourth, and fifth cervical vertebrae and insert onto the first and second ribs. These muscles were formerly thought to be active only with increased breathing effort, but studies using intramuscular electrodes have shown that the scalenes are also active during normal quiet breathing. Their function is to elevate the first and second ribs. As pulmonary hyperinflation progresses, the sternocleidomastoid is recruited. This muscle is normally innervated by the 11th cranial nerve along with motor nerves from C-1 through C-3. When assisting breathing, it elevates the medial aspects of the clavicle and the manubrium. The pectoralis major, especially the cephalad portion, and the pectoralis minor are also useful for elevating the sternum. Posteriorly the trapezius and posterior serratus muscles have the effect of elevating the

ribs during inspiration. These trunk muscles all have an origin on or near the rib cage and insertion at or near the shoulder. They can function as accessory muscles of respiration only if the shoulders are kept immobile. This explains the commonly observed picture of respiratory patients leaning forward on their elbows to brace their shoulders. Leaning forward also appears to result in a more favorable shape of the diaphragm[19] and a better position for the contraction of accessory muscles in general. As the disease progresses, patients tend to perform less strenuous upper extremity activities and adopt a progressively restricted lifestyle.

Abdominal muscles are normally used for such functions as coughing, sneezing, and laughing and as expiratory muscles during strenuous activities. Ninane and Colleagues[44] used concentric needle electrodes to obtain electromyograms of the transversus abdominis and found that most patients with severe COPD had consistent expiratory transversus abdominis activity related to the development of intrinsic positive end-expiratory pressure (PEEP). Thus, for most patients with severe COPD, expiration is a mechanically active process.

The abdominal muscles also have important inspiratory functions. As a result of increased abdominal muscle tone in the upright position, the abdominal viscera are forced cephalad and act as a fulcrum for the central tendon of the diaphragm. The cephalad displacement of the diaphragm allows it to assume an optimal length for tension generation. Without this central fulcrum, the diaphragm would be virtually useless as a respiratory muscle for COPD patients. When the abdominal muscles are impaired, such as after abdominal surgery or with spinal cord injury, the risk of morbidity is increased especially for patients with underlying COPD.

As a result of prolonged elbow leaning, ulnar neuropathy can develop from pressure damage to the ulnar nerve as it traverses the elbow. This presents as numbness or weakness of the fourth and fifth digits and is often bilateral. Patients may also develop elbow cellulitis, cysts, and occasionally osteomyelitis. The use of elbow pads can decrease the risk of these conditions.

PULMONARY REHABILITATION AND INTERSTITIAL LUNG DISEASE

A large number of diverse conditions can result in inflammation, infiltration, and fibrosis of the pulmonary interstitium and lead to the development of stiff, fibrotic lungs. The interstitial lung diseases are characterized physiologically by a reduction in vital capacity with a proportional decrease in expiratory flow rates. There is a maldistribution of compliance with stiff fibrotic areas adjacent to normally compliant areas. The fibrotic or infiltrated areas are underventilated, and the resultant ventilation-perfusion mismatching causes hypoxemia. Even in patients with normal resting arterial blood oxygenation, exercise-induced hypoxemia is common. Generally, hypercapnia is not a prominent feature until the terminal phases of these illnesses.

Restrictive interstitial lung diseases include idiopathic fibrosing alveolitis, most of the pneumoconioses such as silicosis and asbestosis, pulmonary lung disease secondary to autoimmune disorders, fibrosis as a sequela of the diffuse alveolar injury of adult respiratory distress syndrome, hypersensitivity alveolitis, and other inflammatory and infiltrative conditions.[21]

Progressive dyspnea and exercise intolerance are prominent, and usually sputum production and wheezing are absent. Pulmonary hyperinflation does not develop; instead the lungs are generally small. Usually, coarse crackles are present on auscultation over the involved areas of the lung. If the disease process is unchecked, pulmonary hypertension and cor pulmonale develop and shorten survival.

Although not as intensively studied as COPD, the techniques of pulmonary rehabilitation, in the author's experience, are frequently successful in allowing these patients to adapt more successfully to ventilatory limitations. These patients tend to adopt a rapid, shallow breathing pattern and have many misconceptions about their illness, prognosis, treatments, and the role of exercise. Many patients report less dyspnea when employing pursed-lip breathing, relaxation, energy conservation, and pacing techniques.

Although these diseases are interstitial and result in a restrictive ventilatory impairment, the use of aerosolized bronchodilators, anticholinergics, and corticosteroids occasionally results in symptomatic improvement. These can be tried individually and continued if there is subjective or objective evidence of improvement. Oxygen requirements at rest, during exercise, and during sleep should be determined and supplemental oxygen prescribed to correct hypoxemia. Upper and lower extremity exercise may decrease the risk of steroid-induced myopathy in patients taking large doses of corticosteroids, and patients can be taught to recognize signs and symptoms of lower respiratory

infection to head off an acute exacerbation. In general, the multidisciplinary rehabilitation program offered to COPD patients should also be applied to these patients. More outcomes research, however, is necessary in this area.

References

1. Allen MD, Burke CM, McGregor CGA, et al: Steroid-responsive bronchiolitis after human heart-lung transplantation. J Thorac Cardiovasc Surg 92:449–451, 1986.
2. Arm JP, Spur BW, Lee TH: The effects of inhaled leukotriene E_4 on the airway responsiveness to histamine in subjects with asthma and normal subjects. J Allergy Clin Immunol 82:654–660, 1988.
3. Banner AS, Muthuswamy P, Shah R, et al: Bronchiectasis following heroin-induced pulmonary edema. Chest 69:552–555, 1976.
4. Barnett TB, Knowles MR: Diffuse bacterial bronchiolitis with bronchiolar pneumonia in adults. South Med J 80:10–15, 1987.
5. Bousquet J, Chanez P, Lacoste JY, et al: Eosinophilic inflammation in asthma. N Engl J Med 323:1033–1039, 1990.
6. Bradshaw HH, Putney FJ, Clerf LH: The fate of patients with untreated bronchiectasis. JAMA 116:2561–2563, 1941.
7. Burke CM, Theodore J, Dawkins KD, et al.: Post-transplant obliterative bronchiolitis and other late lung sequelae in human heart-lung transplantation. Chest 86:824–826, 1984.
8. Burrows B, Martinez FD, Halonen M, et al: Association of asthma with serum IgE levels and skin-test reactivity to allergies. N Engl J Med 320:271–277, 1989.
9. Cherniack NS, Dowling HF, Carton RW, et al: The role of acute lower respiratory infection in causing pulmonary insufficiency in bronchiectasis. Ann Intern Med 66:489–497, 1967.
10. Collins FS: Cystic fibrosis: molecular biology and therapeutic implications. Science 256:774–779, 1992.
11. Cookson WOCM, Sharp PA, Faux JA, et al: Linkage between immunoglobin E responses underlying asthma and rhinitis and chromosome 11q. Lancet 1:1292–1295, 1989.
12. Corris PA, Dark JH: Aetiology of asthma: Lessons from lung transplantation. Lancet 341:1369–1371, 1993.
13. Crystal RG: 1-Antitrypsin deficiency, emphysema, and liver disease: Genetic basis and strategies for therapy. J Clin Invest 85:1343–1352, 1990.
14. Crystal RG, Brantly ML, Hubbard RC, et al: The alpha$_1$-antitrypsin gene and its mutations: Clinical consequences and strategies for therapy. Chest 95:196–208, 1989.
15. Davis PB, di Sant'Agnese PA: Diagnosis and treatment of cystic fibrosis: An update. Chest 85:802–809, 1984.
16. DeBoeck C, Zinman R: Cough versus chest physiotherapy: A comparison of the acute effect on pulmonary function in patients with cystic fibrosis. Am Rev Respir Dis 129:182–184, 1984.
17. Desmond KJ, Schwenk WF, Thomas E, et al: Immediate and long-term effects of chest physiotherapy in patients with cystic fibrosis. J Pediatr 103:538–542, 1983.
18. Dorinsky PM, Davis WB, Lucas JG, et al: Adult bronchiolitis: Evaluation by bronchoalveolar lavage and response to prednisone therapy. Chest 88:58–63, 1985.
19. Erwin WS, Zolov D, Bickerman HA: The effect of posture on respiratory function in patients with ob-

structive pulmonary emphysema. Am Rev Respir Dis 94:865–872, 1966.

20. Fiel, SB: Clinical management of pulmonary disease in cystic fibrosis. Lancet 341:1070–1074, 1993.

21. Freundlich IM, Libshitz HI, Glassman LM, et al: Sarcoidosis. Clin Radiol 21:376–383, 1970.

22. Gottleib LS, Hillberg RE: Endobronchial tamponade therapy for intractable hemoptysis. Chest 67:482–483, 1975.

23. Grenier P, Maurice F, Musset D, et al: Bronchiectasis: Assessment by thin-section CT. Radiology 161:95–99, 1986.

24. Guidelines for the approach to the patients with severe hereditary alpha$_1$-antitrypsin deficiency. Am Rev Respir Dis 140:1494–1497, 1989.

25. Handelsman DJ, Conway AJ, Boylan LM, et al: Young's syndrome: Obstructive azoospermia and chronic sinopulmonary infections. N Engl J Med 310:3–9, 1984.

26. Higgins MW, Keller JB: Trends in COPD morbidity and mortality in the United States. Am Rev Respir Dis 140 (suppl):S9–S18, 1984.

27. Higgins MW, Thom T: Incidence, prevalence, and mortality: Intra- and intercountry differences. In Hensley MJ, Saunders NA (eds): Clinical Epidemiology of Chronic Obstructive Pulmonary Disease. New York, Marcel Dekker, 1989, pp. 23–39.

28. Hiller E, Rosenow EC, Olsen AM: Pulmonary manifestations of the yellow nail syndrome. Chest 61:452–458, 1972.

29. Hoehne JH, Reed CE, Dickie HA: Allergic bronchopulmonary aspergillosis is not rare. Chest 63:177–181, 1973.

30. Hoover CF: The diagnostic significance of inspiratory movements of the costal margin. Am J Med Sci 159:633–646, 1920.

31. Isles A, Machesky I, Corye M, et al: *Pseudomonas cepacia* infection in cystic fibrosis: An emerging problem. J Pediatr 104:206–208, 1984.

32. Jeffery PK: Morphology of the airway wall in asthma and in chronic obstructive pulmonary disease. Am Rev Respir Dis 143:1152–1158, 1991.

33. Kattan M, Mansell A, Levison H, et al: Response to aerosol salbutamol, SCH 1,000 and placebo in cystic firbrosis. Thorax 35:531–535, 1980.

34. Kay AB: "Helper" (CD4$^+$) T cells and eosinophils in allergy and asthma. Am Rev Respir Dis 145:S22–S26, 1992.

35. Kinney WW, Angelillo VA: Bronchiolitis in systemic lupus erythematosus. Chest 82:646–649, 1982.

36. Lang DM, Polansky M: Patterns of asthma mortality in Philadelphia from 1969 to 1991. N Engl J Med 331:1542–1546, 1994.

37. MacLeod WM: Abnormal transradiancy of one lung. Thorax 9:147–153, 1954.

38. Moles KW, Varghese G, Hayes JR: Pulmonary involvement in ulcerative colitis. Br J Dis Chest 82:79–83, 1988.

39. Morgenroth K: Morphological alterations to the bronchial mucosa in high-dose long-term exposure to sulfur dioxide. Respiration 39:39–48, 1980.

40. Murray JF: The ketchup bottle method. N Engl J Med 300:1155–1157, 1979.

41. Nagai A, West WW, Thurlbeck WM: The National Institutes of Health intermittent positive-pressure breathing trial: Pathology studies. II. Correlation between morphologic findings, clinical findings and evidence of expiratory airflow obstruction. Am Rev Respir Dis 132:946–953, 1985.

42. Nath AR, Capel LH: Lung crackles in bronchiectasis. Thorax 35:694–699, 1980.

43. National Center for Health Statistics: Current estimates from the National Health Interview Survey, United States. Vital and Health Statistics, Series 10, No. 164. Washington, D.C., DHHS (PHS) 897–1592, 1986.

44. Ninane V, Yernault JC, De Troyer A: Intrinsic PEEP in patients with chronic obstructive pulmonary disease. Am Rev Respir Dis 148:1037–1042, 1993.

45. Patel RC, Dutta D, Schonfeld SA: Free-base cocaine use associated with bronchiolitis obliterans and organizing pneumonia. Ann Intern Med 107:186–187, 1987.

46. Pedersen SS: Lungg infection with alginate-producing mucoid *Pseudomonas aeruginosa* in cystic fibrosis. APMIS 28(suppl):1–79, 1992.

47. Quinton PM: Missing Cl conductance in cystic fibrosis. Am J Physiol 251:C649–C652, 1986.

48. Ramset BW, Astley SJ, Aitken ML, et al: Efficacy and safety of short-term administration of aerosolized recombinant human deoxyribonuclease in patients with cystic fibrosis. Am Rev Respir Dis 148:145–151, 1993.

49. Reid LM: Correlation of certain bronchographic abnormalities seen in chronic bronchitis with the pathological changes. Thorax 10:199–204, 1955.

50. Rommens JM, Iannuzzi MC, Kerem B, et al: Identification of the cystic fibrosis gene: Chromosome walking and jumping. Science 245:1059–1065, 1989.

51. Rosenberg ME, Vercellotti GM, Snover DC, et al: Bronchiolitis obliterans after bone marrow transplantation. Am J Hematol 18:325–328, 1985.

52. Rott HD: Kartagener's syndrome and the syndrome of immotile cilia. Hum Genet 46:249–261, 1979.

53. Shneerson JM: Lung bullae, bronchiectasis, and Hashimoto's disease associated with ulcerative colitis treated by colectomy. Thorax 36:313–314, 1981.

54. Silverstein MD, Reed CE, O'Connell EJ, et al: Long-term survival of a cohort of community residents with asthma. N Engl J Med 331:1537–1541, 1994.

55. Sladen A, Zanca P, Hadnott WH: Aspiration pneumonitis, the sequelae. Chest 59:448–450, 1971.

56. Sturgess JM, Chao J, Wong J, et al: Cilia with defective radial spokes: A cause of human respiratory disease. N Engl J Med 300:53–56, 1979.

57. Suhs RH, Dowling HF, Jackson GG: Hypogammaglobulinaemia with chronic bronchitis or bronchiectasis. Arch Intern Med 116:29–39, 1965.

58. Thomassen ML, Demko CA, Klinger L, et al: *Pseudomonas cepacia* colonization among cystic fibrosis patients: A new opportunist. Am Rev Respir Dis 131:791–796, 1985.

59. Walker WC, Wright V: Pulmonary lesions and rheumatoid arthritis. Medicine 47:501–520, 1968.

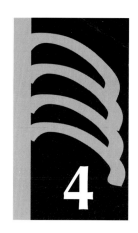

Smoking Cessation for the Pulmonary Patient

4

Cynthia S. Rand, PhD
W. Clinton McSherry, PhD

Smoking is the primary cause of preventable chronic lung disease. Smoking cessation is the single most important recommendation a physician can make to a patient with pulmonary disease who smokes. All too often, however, physicians have little knowledge about the process of smoking cessation and few counseling skills to assist patients in initiating this demanding behavioral change. Behavioral and pharmacologic research over the past 20 years has added significantly to understanding of smoking as an addictive disorder and underscored the role of the physician in assisting patients to quit smoking. Today's practitioner has available an effective armamentarium of behavioral and pharmacologic strategies that have been demonstrated to be effective aids to smoking cessation, ranging from simple directive physician advice to intensive interventions such as nicotine replacement therapy combined with a structured behavioral group program. This chapter reviews the current state-of-the-art research on smoking cessation in the medical care setting. In addition, smoking cessation research from the Lung Health Study (LHS) is reviewed, the largest study to date to evaluate the long-term efficacy of a structured smoking cessation program in initiating and sustaining smoking cessation in men and women at high risk for developing lung disease.

ASSOCIATION BETWEEN SMOKING AND LUNG DISEASE

Cigarette smoking is the leading preventable cause of pulmonary disease and is associated with increased morbidity and mortality risk for asthma, chronic obstructive pulmonary disease (COPD), and lung cancer. Estimates[11] have indicated that children whose mothers smoked were 10 times more likely to develop asthma than were children of nonsmoking mothers. Some researchers[27] have suggested that as many as 85% of current COPD cases (or 23,375,000 in the United States) are attributable to smoking. The Surgeon General's office reported that 85% of lung cancer cases are due to cigarette smoking.[64] Estimates[8] have placed the excess annual mortality rates due to cigarette smoking in the United States at 430,000 (Fig. 4–1), a number that is greater than the sum of total annual deaths due to alcohol, homicide, suicide, automobile accidents, acquired immunodeficiency syndrome, and all other illegal drugs combined.[13] Given this information, it is no wonder that the Surgeon General has stated that smoking cessation is "the single most important step that smokers can take to enhance the length and quality of their lives."[63]

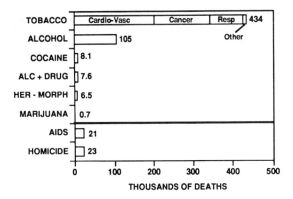

FIGURE 4–1. Estimated annual mortality in the United States, drug and related problems (about 1990). Alc + Drug = alcohol in combination with another drug; Her − Morph = heroin or morphine. (From Crowley TJ: Any man's death: Presidential Address. Washington, D.C., NIDA Research Monograph 140, NIH Pub. No. 94-3748, 1993, pp 5–10, with permission.)

SMOKING CESSATION METHODS

Smoking cessation for patient populations can be subdivided into the following categories: (1) methods that are suitable for primary care settings and (2) methods that are suitable for patients with chronic disease. Regardless of the specific setting or cessation method employed, however, physicians should recognize that there are numerous determinants of smoking and should therefore not expect to "cure" all or even most of their nicotine-addicted patients. Despite the odds, increased, improved, and persistent efforts on the part of physicians could potentially result in millions of Americans quitting, which would save millions of lives and billions of dollars in excess health care costs.

Although some research[61] has suggested that physicians in general have low confidence in their ability to counsel patients to quit smoking, other research has consistently found that a strong message to quit delivered by a physician doubles quit rates from approximately 5% to 10%,[26,46] and in some trials to as high as 15%.[10] Because 70% of smokers visit their physicians at least one time per year,[43] and many smokers visit their physicians as often as four times per year, increased rates of physician counseling would likely result in many more smokers attempting to quit. For example, the National Cancer Institute (NCI) is currently engaged in a program to train 100,000 U.S. physicians in smoking cessation techniques.[24] If each of these physicians' efforts results in a 10% cessation rate, that will produce an additional 3 million ex-smokers each year in the United States.[36]

Primary Care Settings

Primary care settings represent an ideal venue for both prevention and cessation inter-

ventions, yet research[1,22,68] has consistently revealed only a moderate rate (45% to 50%) of physician smoking cessation counseling in these settings. Patient demographic characteristics such as gender, age, education, and race have been found to be related to physician counseling rates,[22] yet the groups that are typically found to receive less counseling are precisely the groups that have experienced lower declines in prevalence rates over the last 20 years. Overall, physicians tend to counsel men, older smokers, more educated smokers, and whites at higher rates than women, younger smokers, less educated smokers, and nonwhites; demographic studies,[19,51,52] however, have indicated that smoking prevalence rates are declining at significantly lower rates among the latter groups. Reminders to counsel smoking patients have been found to increase physicians' rates of counseling,[10] and the authors have found that specific reminders may serve to eradicate some of these inequities of current counseling patterns. Clearly, physician education concerning smoking cessation counseling needs to include messages that will increase physician counseling to these specific groups if adequate and equitable public health is to be achieved.

One reason that primary care visits are an ideal opportunity for cessation counseling is provided by Prochaska and DiClemente's[53] process-oriented model of behavior change, known as stage theory. According to stage theory, smokers progress through a sequence of six stages of readiness to quit smoking. In order of increasing readiness, the first five stages are called: precontemplation, contemplation, preparation, action, and maintenance. The sixth and final stage does not represent increased readiness but is appropriately called relapse. Because smokers do appear to exhibit varying levels of readiness to quit, repeat encounters with a physician who provides individualized and highly credible advice to quit can help motivate smokers to move to the next stage of readiness until they finally quit successfully and permanently. Over these repeat visits, the physician counseling can be matched to the patient's stage of readiness, with the goals of counseling focused on motivating and assisting the patient to progress to the next stage of readiness.

Another approach to outpatient cessation counseling is physician-initiated, nurse-assisted counseling.[28,29] By this method, the physician is cued by a chart note on all smokers' medical charts to provide a brief (less than 30 seconds) stop-smoking message, which includes comments concerning the increased risks associated with smoking, the health benefits of quitting, advice to stop as soon as possible, and a request to meet with the counseling nurse. This approach offers the advantages of minimizing physicians' time involvement, while maximizing the likelihood that smokers will receive appropriate levels of cessation counseling. Hollis and coworkers[29] used a randomized, controlled trial with 12-month follow-up comparing three nurse-assisted treatment groups to an advice-only control group and found that all three treatments resulted in superior cessation rates as compared with the control group. Furthermore, an earlier report[28] indicated that the intervention was well received by patients and was both practical and sustainable. Other nurse-managed interventions have been designed and evaluated for cardiac patients[60] and are discussed in a later section.

In a meta-analytic comparison of the effectiveness of various smoking cessation methods,[66] it was found that although physician advice alone resulted in a 7% increase in quit rates, physician interventions that consisted of more than just advice resulted in an 18% increase in quit rates. Schwartz[57] reported that median quit rates increased from 6% for simple counseling to 22.5% for counseling plus some additional component. Clearly, interventions that consist of additional components appear to result in substantially increased quit rates as compared to physician advice alone. *Additional components* should not be interpreted as adding large amounts of time to the physician's workload because many additional components require little or no time involvement by physicians. Examples of additional components that have been shown to increase quit rates are warnings during physical examination, regularly scheduled follow-up visits, demonstration and explanation of expired breath carbon monoxide levels, a written contract to quit, and,

the most effective addition, nicotine replacement therapy.

Nicotine Replacement Therapy

As perhaps the most common form of additional component for smoking cessation provided by physicians, nicotine replacement therapy represents one of the most practical and powerful interventions for achieving smoking abstinence. Nicotine polacrilex gum became commercially available in the 1980s and has been widely used in medical clinics as a pharmacologic agent to assist smokers to achieve abstinence. Clinical results have generally been somewhat disappointing, owing in large part to inadequate physician and patient understanding of the correct use of the gum. Although nicotine gum has been shown in numerous clinical studies to be an effective aid to smoking cessation,[57] inappropriate gum use in a clinical setting (insufficient dose, rapid chewing, premature discontinuation) often results in unpleasant side effects and smoking relapse. With proper usage and adequate dosage, however, nicotine gum remains a highly cost-effective form of nicotine replacement therapy and may offer the only alternative for certain individuals, such as those with dermatologic, cardiovascular, or other contraindications for transdermal nicotine patches.

Currently the most popular clinical aid to smoking cessation is the use of transdermal nicotine replacement therapy. Transdermal nicotine, or nicotine patches, are typically worn for either 16 or 24 hours per day (depending on which brand is used), and higher doses (21 mg) provide plasma nicotine levels approximately one half those obtained by cigarette smoking. In earlier reports on the efficacy of nicotine patches,[62] both 21-mg and 14-mg patches resulted in significantly higher abstinence rates than placebo at both 6-week and 12-week follow-ups (21 mg: 61% and 39% versus 27% and 16% for placebo; 14 mg: 48% and 27% versus 27% and 16% for placebo), whereas at 24-week follow-up, only the 21-mg patch was associated with significantly higher abstinence (26% versus 12% for placebo; Fig. 4–2).

Since nicotine patches were introduced, both pharmaceutical manufacturers and the Food and Drug Administration have instructed physicians that patches should not be prescribed in the absence of a behavioral counseling program. A meta-analysis of 17 randomized, placebo-controlled nicotine patch studies,[20] however, indicated that patches alone are effec-

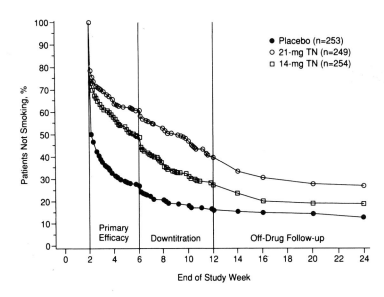

FIGURE 4–2. Time to smoking for the pooled database. The first 2 study weeks were not considered in the analyses for efficacy. TN = Transdermal nicotine. (From Transdermal Nicotine Study Group: Transdermal nicotine for smoking cessation: Six-month results from two multicenter controlled clinical trials. JAMA 266: 3133–3138, 1991, with permission.)

tive for a significant portion of smokers, and this research thus warrants that this issue be reevaluated. If future research confirms that patches without behavioral counseling are effective for a sizable portion of the smoking population, and especially if this subgroup can be identified *a priori* either by a measure of nicotine dependence or some other characteristic, that finding would suggest that physicians in primary care settings should administer smoking cessation treatments in a stepped-care approach. For example, if patients are amenable to quitting and wish to use the patch, the first step would be for the physician to prescribe the patch and schedule a follow-up visit to confirm smoking status. If patients are unable to quit using the patch alone (after some reasonable time period), they could then be referred to a behavioral counseling program, and a new prescription could be provided. In this manner, many more smokers who are uncomfortable attending counseling sessions would be likely to agree to make a quit attempt, and, at least initially, the least intensive (and less costly) intervention necessary for cessation and continued abstinence could be used.

Smoking Cessation for Patients with Chronic Disease

Although smoking cessation for healthy smokers is secondary prevention, cessation for patients identified with serious chronic illness is tertiary prevention. Perhaps because smoking is primarily associated with markedly increased risk for cardiovascular and pulmonary diseases, most research on smoking cessation in patients with chronic disease exists in these two disease categories.

Cardiovascular Disease

A 35-year-old male heavy (>25 cigarettes per day) smoker has a 7% chance of dying of coronary heart disease (CHD) by age 65 and an 11.5% chance by age 85, compared to 0.4% and 2.5% for never-smokers.[37] In other words, male heavy smokers are 17.5 times more likely to die of CHD by age 65 than nonsmokers and are 4.6 times more likely to die of CHD by age 85 than nonsmokers. Former smokers, however, were estimated to have a 1.7% chance of dying of CHD by age 65 and a 5.5% chance of dying by age 85; these incidences correspond to increased mortality risks of only 4.25 and 2.2.[37] Thus, quitting smoking by age 35 can reduce relative risk of premature CHD mortality by 75% at age 65 and nearly 50% at age 85. Similarly, once a smoker has developed cardiovascular disease, cessation remains a powerful avenue for subsequent risk reduction. In fact, at least one study reported that individuals who stop smoking after acute myocardial infarction (MI) have half the mortality of those who continue to smoke.[39]

Given that smoking cessation for patients with cardiovascular disease is an important risk-reduction goal, the question remains as to how best to effect cessation. More than 20 years ago, it was observed that an intervention as simple as stern advice from one's physician combined with written information and follow-up visits following a MI resulted in more than doubling of the cessation rate observed in a control group that was provided only conventional advice.[7] This relatively simple, easy, and inexpensive intervention remains one of the potentially most effective tools for increasing smoking cessation and abstinence rates in patients with known smoking-related disease.

Several reports have attempted to identify characteristics of smoking MI patients that predict successful smoking cessation. Duration of hospital stay greater than 19 days (but not duration of stay in coronary care unit) and peak creatine phosphokinase (CPK) elevation greater than 500 U/L were found to predict cessation in a sample of 80 Italian MI survivors.[15] In an attempt to validate the stages of change model in cardiac patients, Kristeller and associates[33] compared patients enrolled in the Coronary Artery Smoking Intervention Study (CASIS) to a nonmedical sample and concluded that cardiac patients used the various stages of change (e.g., contemplation, action) in a manner similar to the nonmedical sample. These results may help explain the consistent finding that patients with more severe disease tend to quit at higher rates than those with less severe disease,[3,45] suggesting that greater disease severity may motivate individuals to higher levels of readiness to quit.

The intervention used in the CASIS trial[45] included a single 30-minute inpatient counseling session provided by master's level health educators, one individual outpatient visit, and three to four follow-up counseling telephone calls in the 3 to 4 months following hospitalization. Only about 50% of these post–coronary arteriography patients attended the follow-up visit, thereby weakening the overall effect of the intervention. Consequently, although both 6-month and 12-month cessation rates, whether self-reported or biochemically validated, for the intervention group showed improvement of between 20% and 35% over the *advice only* control group, none of the improvements were statistically significant.

In a 6-month, randomized, nurse-managed smoking cessation program[60] that focused on the benefits of quitting, the dangers of smoking, and relapse prevention, intervention patients met once with a nurse while in the hospital and received written materials and audiotapes. Following discharge, patients were provided additional counseling by telephone once a week for 2 to 3 weeks then monthly for the next 4 months. At 12 months post-MI, cessation rates were significantly higher (71%) in the intervention group compared to the usual care group (45%). This study demonstrated that nurse-managed cessation programs can have significant effects on a population of smokers for whom cessation is critically important.

Although relatively little smoking cessation research has been conducted with coronary artery bypass graft (CABG) surgery patients, one 5-year, randomized, controlled clinical trial[54] found no difference in 1-year and 5.5-year follow-up smoking rates between a three-session, in-hospital, nurse-delivered smoking cessation intervention group and a control group. Self-reported nonsmoking was validated by saliva cotinine assay, which revealed identical abstinence rates in both groups (51% at 1 year; 44% at 5.5 years). Because these abstinence rates are remarkably similar to post-MI abstinence rates, these findings suggest two possible interpretations: (1) that CABG patients are similar to post-MI patients in terms of self-quitting and (2) that a three-session, in-hospital, nurse-delivered intervention is not intense enough to effect significant increases in cessation rates in this population of patients. Compared to the Taylor et al[60] study that used a post-discharge design with eight total nurse contacts, which resulted in a 58% increase in 1-year abstinence rates over control group rates, the failure of the Rigotti et al[54] study to find differences in abstinence rates indicates that there may exist some minimum threshold of intervention intensity for this group of smokers.

Smoking cessation following diagnosis of cardiovascular disease can significantly improve one's prognosis. Research has revealed that certain personal characteristics, such as degree of disease[3] and length of hospital stay,[15] affect one's likelihood of quitting after an acute MI. Findings from several studies with various types of cardiac patients[15,32,54,60] indicate that individualized inpatient counseling followed by post-discharge follow-up that focuses on relapse prevention may produce the greatest probability for continued abstinence.

Although a diagnosis of cardiovascular disease or an acute hospitalization for a MI or CABG surgery appears to have a motivating effect, often a diagnosis of pulmonary disease does not result in a significant increase in cessation rates.[23] Perhaps the comparatively slow, insidious onset of pulmonary diseases such as COPD belies the seriousness of the disease, thereby removing the motivational "benefit" of a single, identifiable event such as a MI.

Pulmonary Disease

COPD affects approximately 11% of the adult population of the United States, and smoking is the primary cause of morbidity and mortality due to COPD.[17] Smoking cessation for patients with chronic pulmonary disease has been shown to be of significant benefit in both short-term (6 months)[18] and long-term (6 years or greater)[6,34,55] studies. Smoking cessation results in significant reversibility of airways injury,[59] including increased activity of alveolar macrophages,[58] increases in maximum midexpiratory flow (MMF),[18] increased carbon dioxide diffusing capacity,[56] and reduced rates of decline in FEV_1.[6,35] Increases in MMF were maintained for at least 6 months.[18] Over a 6- to 7-year period in the Multiple Risk Factor Intervention Trial (MRFIT), in the smoking cessation intervention group there was a slower rate of decline in FEV_1 (11 mL per year slower, one-tailed $t < 0.05$) and a higher final FEV_1 (90 mL higher, one-tailed $t < 0.05$) for previously heavy smokers who were not using beta-blockers for high blood pressure as compared to the control group not offered smoking cessation help.[6] Two population studies in Poland and the United States found that symptoms of COPD, such as chronic cough, phlegm, wheeze, and dyspnea, were reduced by 50% by smoking cessation.[34] In a 20-year longitudinal study of 1445 male smokers, those who quit smoking were found to experience 7% less total mortality, 13% less cardiac mortality, and 11% less incidence of lung cancer as compared to continuing smokers.[55] Halpern and coworkers[25] reported that smoking cessation results in significantly reduced relative risk of lung cancer, not only for those who quit early in their smoking career, but also for smokers who quit in their mid-60s. This study revealed that although smoking cessation earlier in life (before age 50) results in significantly greater reductions in health risk and is therefore clearly preferable to quitting later in life, significant reductions in relative and absolute risk are possible for older (over 50) individuals as well, who often believe that smoking cessation will not result in reduced risk (Fig. 4–3). This study is important because it was the first to demonstrate that age at quitting has significant impact on relative risk of lung cancer mortality, whereas other studies have focused primarily on number of years since quitting.

Earlier studies indicated that several descriptive and treatment variables were predictive of smoking cessation among pulmonary patients. Pederson and colleagues[48] found that patients who had a primary diagnosis of COPD, were not middle-aged, and women (in decreasing order of predictive power) were more likely to quit successfully. In a study of patients with COPD, Daughton and colleagues[14] reported that the only predictor of long-term cessation (5 to 55 months posthospitalization) was pack-years of smoking history.

In two prospective studies of 308 pulmonary

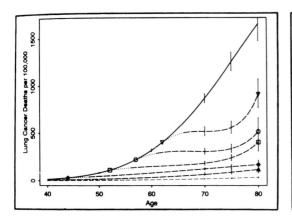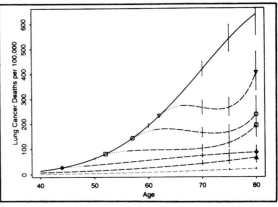

FIGURE 4–3. Model estimates of lung cancer death rates by age for male (*left*) and female (*right*) current, former, and never smokers. Estimates were based on male smokers who started at age 17.5 and smoked 26 cigarettes/day and female smokers who started at age 18.5 and smoked 22 cigarettes/day. Estimates are plotted for current smokers (*solid line*), never smokers (*dotted line*), and former smokers (*dashed lines*). The five age-at-quitting cohorts are distinguished by the following symbols on the graphs at the age of quitting and also at age 80: Δ 30–39, ◇ 40–49, □ 50–54, ○ 55–59, ▽ 60–64. (From Halpern MT, Gillespie BW, Warner KE: Patterns of absolute risk of lung cancer mortality in former smokers. J Natl Cancer Inst 85:457–464, 1993, with permission.)

patients,[47,48] predictors of successful quitting included patients' self-efficacy for quitting, older age, wanting to quit, higher socioeconomic status, and being married. Results of the Pederson et al[48] study are noteworthy because it was a multivariate investigation of predictors of compliance following physician advice to quit smoking. In that study, four separate logistic regression models were developed, and patients' prediction of cessation was the strongest predictor of actual 6-month cessation in three out of four models. In a follow-up investigation,[49] 6-month cessation was found to be the strongest predictor of long-term (4 to 7 years) cessation. The only other baseline predictor of long-term (4 to 7 years) cessation was smoking for reasons "other than addiction."

In a controlled, randomized trial designed to assess whether early intervention for 1445 men at high risk for cardiorespiratory disease would affect cessation rates, Rose and Colwell[55] provided four 15-minute counseling sessions over a 6-month period, combined with two self-help booklets. Although smoking status was measured only by self-report at 1 and 3 years posttreatment, 1-year complete tobacco abstinence rates were 38% and 8% for the intervention (n = 714) and control (n = 731) groups. At 3 years, abstinence rates were 23% and 10%.

In a study that examined the impact of physician advice to quit smoking on chronic bronchitis patients,[21] men who visited a physician about their bronchitis were more than twice as likely to quit or reduce their smoking than men who did not visit their physician. Furthermore, men who visited their physician *and received advice* to quit were 2.28 times more likely to quit or reduce their smoking than men who did not receive advice. Finally, when men and women in this study were analyzed together, those who received advice were 1.75 times more likely to quit than those who did not receive advice (63.6% versus 36.4%).

In a review of physician advice to quit smoking for four patient groups (general practice, pregnant, pulmonary, and cardiac patients), Pederson and coworkers[48] concluded that advanced disease and the more imminent the threat posed by continued smoking, the more likely it was that patients would quit smoking. At least one prospective study of more than 2500 primary practice patients,[16] however, revealed that patients with more smoking-related diagnoses were less likely to quit smoking. In the Duncan et al[16] 1-year physicians' counseling study comparing successful quitters (n = 245) with continuing smokers (n = 2247), 90% of quitters had one or more smoking-related symptoms (M = 3.2) and 47% of quitters had at least one smoking-related diagnosis. In a multiple logistic regression using baseline predictors, more diagnoses and smoking within 15 minutes of awakening were both associated with a significantly *decreased* probability of quitting 1 year later. Perhaps the combination of stronger addiction (indicated by smoking within 15 minutes of awakening) and more smoking-related diagnoses resulted in smokers resigning themselves to continue the habit, as if there were no point in quitting because they perceived themselves as already irrevocably damaged or diseased.

Analyses of nearly 1200 women and 1500 men smokers enrolled in the Framingham Heart Study[23] revealed that although recent hospitalization or diagnosis of CHD was predictive of smoking cessation, neither FEV_1 nor change in FEV_1 was predictive of cessation. These findings led Freund and associates[23] to conclude "that the development of acute symptoms, such as chest pain or medical conditions requiring hospitalization, is more important in facilitating smoking cessation than is insidious or chronic disability, such as obstructive pulmonary disease. The data also suggest that the perceived benefit of quitting smoking on one's symptoms or illness may affect smoking behavior" (p. 963).

THE LUNG HEALTH STUDY

In 1983, the National Heart, Lung and Blood Institute initiated LHS, a randomized clinical trial that was designed to test the hypothesis that smoking cessation intervention and the use of an inhaled bronchodilator (ipratropium bromide) would slow the decline in lung function in smokers with mild-to-moderate COPD.[12] The LHS is the largest study ever completed of smoking cessation in individuals with early lung impairment. Close to 4000 men and women participated in the treatment group at the 10 LHS clinical centers.

Lung Health Study Eligibility and Design

Eligible participants were men and women between the ages of 35 and 60 years who were regular cigarette smokers and who were found to have mild-to-moderate airflow obstruction, with a FEV_1/FVC ratio less than 0.7 or 70%, and a FEV_1 between 55% and 90% of predicted normal. All participants entering the study had to express interest in quitting smoking. The primary end point of the study was the rate of decline in FEV_1. Secondary end points were smoking cessation rates, morbidity, and mortality.

After providing informed consent, participants were randomly assigned to one of three treatment groups: usual care (UC), special intervention (SI) with active drug, or SI with placebo. A total of 5887 people were enrolled: 1964 into UC and 3923 into SI groups. The UC group returned annually for spirometric evaluation only. All SI participants were offered a 12-week smoking cessation program and were asked to return for visits with a health educator every 4 months in addition to the annual spirometric evaluation. Cotinine and expired carbon monoxide samples were collected at annual visits to provide biochemical verification of smoking status. Baseline characteristics of SI participants are shown in Table 4–1.[42]

Lung Health Study Physician's Smoking Cessation Message

Based on the known effectiveness of physician advice in motivating smoking cessation, an important first step was an individual meeting with a study physician for the participants in the SI groups. All study physicians were trained to deliver a standardized, authoritative smoking cessation message at this meeting and to discuss the study's goals. The content of the message emphasized the participant's impaired pulmonary function, the seriousness of COPD, the participant's personal risk, and the potential benefits, both scientific and personal, to be derived from immediate and complete smoking cessation. Pulmonary function results were used to underscore the risk of rapidly declining lung function. Study physicians focused on the participant's current pulmonary impairment and the likelihood of its continued decline with continued smoking, leading to premature disability and death. Participants were strongly encouraged to take full advantage of the smoking cessation program. Nicotine gum was prescribed at this time, for use only during the cessation program, and participants were immediately referred to a smoking cessation interventionist to set a quit date and discuss further participation. The smoking cessation interventionist discussed strategies for preparing to quit smoking (e.g., nicotine tapering, cigarette diaries, brand-switching) and set a firm quit date. Participants

were officially enrolled into the LHS smoking cessation program within 1 month of randomization into the study.[42]

Lung Health Study Smoking Cessation Group Program

Previous research has suggested that individuals with COPD have greater difficulty than most smokers in quitting smoking.[16] Smokers with COPD may include a disproportionately large number of "hard-core" smokers—that is, smokers who fail to quit even when faced with an increasing number of smoking-related symptoms. Such smokers are likely to need intensive behavioral and pharmacologic support to quit smoking successfully. For these reasons, the LHS SI smoking cessation program was designed to maximize sustained cessation rates by using a combination of the strongest available interventions from the outset of the study. In addition, a social learning, behavioral approach was designed and used to teach smokers the skills necessary to avoid relapse. Nicotine gum (nicotine polacrilex) was provided while the subjects acquired these new behavioral skills. Nicotine gum was provided free of charge throughout the program, and tapering was not initiated until at least 3 months after cessation.

This 12-week, 13-session program began with an orientation meeting designed to help participants prepare to quit, followed within 7 days by a quit week, which included four group meetings on consecutive days, with the first meeting designated as the quit day. Initial group sessions focused on learning the correct use of nicotine gum and cognitive-behavioral strategies for handling withdrawal and cravings. Because all participants in the program knew that they had pulmonary function impairment and a high risk of worsening lung impairment if they continued to smoke, the group shared a strong motivation to succeed in quitting. This common bond, coupled with reliance on the group for encouragement during the first weeks of quitting, made the group a powerful source of support. Later group sessions worked on relapse prevention skills, stress management, social support, and weight management. Nicotine gum was dispensed at the group meetings, and gum use technique and side effects were monitored by the interventionists. At the conclusion of the group program, participants were offered ongoing maintenance activities, such as relapse prevention support groups, weight loss, and ex-

TABLE 4–1
Baseline Characteristics of Special Intervention Participants in the Lung Health Study

Means and Standard Deviations of Selected Characteristics

	Male (n = 2448; 62.4%)		Female (n = 1475; 37.6%)		All SI (n = 3923)	
	Mean	SD	Mean	SD	Mean	SD
Ppt's age at entry	48.5	7.0	48.5	6.5	48.5	6.8
Beginning smoking age	17.0	4.1	18.2	4.5	17.5	4.3
Avg No. of cigs/day	32.8	13.3	29.0	11.9	31.4	12.9

Distributions of Selected Characteristics

	Male		Female		All SI	
	n	%	n	%	n	%
Used other tobacco products?						
Yes	307	12.5	15	1.0	322	8.2
No	2141	87.5	1460	99.0	3601	91.8
Ever used nicotine gum?						
Yes	834	34.1	626	42.4	1460	37.2
No	1614	65.9	849	57.6	2463	62.8
No. of quit smoking attempts						
None	297	12.1	203	13.8	500	12.8
1–3 times	1257	51.4	851	57.7	2108	53.7
4 or more times	894	36.5	421	28.5	1315	33.5
Longest time off cigs						
Less than 1 wk	396	18.4	305	24.0	701	20.5
1 wk to 6 mon	1161	53.9	676	53.1	1837	53.7
More than 6 mon	594	27.7	291	22.9	885	25.8
No. of other cigarette smokers in the house						
No other	1506	61.5	855	58.0	2361	60.2
1 other	777	31.7	482	32.7	1259	32.1
2 or more others	165	6.8	138	9.3	303	7.7
Educational level						
High school or less	952	38.9	718	48.7	1670	42.6
More than high school	1496	61.1	757	51.3	2253	57.4
Marital status						
Never married	118	4.8	67	4.5	185	4.7
Married	1912	78.1	911	61.8	2823	71.9
Widowed	30	1.2	86	5.8	116	3.0
Separated/divorced	388	15.9	411	27.9	799	20.4

(From O'Hara P, Grill J, Ridgon MA, et al: Design and results of the initial intervention program for the Lung Health Study. Prev. Med. 22:304–315, 1993, with permission.)

ercise programs. Restart smoking cessation programs were available throughout the 5-year study for participants who relapsed.[42]

Based on the work of Mermelstein and others,[9,38] the LHS smoking cessation intervention program placed great value on the importance of social support from family and friends. Participants were encouraged to bring a spouse or other support person with them to the program. Family members, friends, and even coworkers were invited to quit smoking along with the participant. Nonsmoking support persons were in-

structed on how best to encourage and sustain the participant's efforts at smoking cessation. The value of this component of the intervention was supported by the finding that participants who lived in nonsmoking households and those who attended the initial intervention meeting with a support person were also more likely to remain nonsmokers throughout the first year. The relationship between sustained smoking cessation and the presence of a social support network has been reported in a number of treatment programs.[44]

Lung Health Study Smoking Cessation and Pulmonary Function Results

Smoking status was determined by self-report at 4- and 8-month follow-up visits and validated by cotinine or expired carbon monoxide measurements at annual visits. At the first 4-month follow-up, 46.4% of the SI participants self-reported not having smoked since their quit day. By 1 year, 40.1% of the SI participants reported that they were nonsmoking, compared with 10.7% of the UC participants. Using biochemical validation, these 12-month abstinence rates dropped to 33.9% for the SI group and 8.7% for the UC group.[42] Throughout the trial, similar classification errors (3% to 6%) were observed, indicating a small but significant socially desirable bias in self-reporting smoking cessation.[40]

Participants' long-term smoking status was classified as either continuing (smoking at each annual visit), intermittent (nonsmoking at some annual visits), or sustained nonsmoking (nonsmoking at each annual visit). Figure 4–4 shows the biochemically validated smoking cessation rates throughout the study. Because the sustained nonsmoker category reflects only those individuals who quit during the initial cessation period and maintained abstinence at all subsequent visits, this category naturally declined over the course of 5 years. By the end of the study, approximately 22% of SI participants remained nonsmoking, without a relapse, compared with about 5% of the UC participants.

Cross-sectional rates of nonsmoking reflect the number of participants not smoking at a given annual visit, regardless of their smoking status at a previous visit. Cross-sectional rates of validated nonsmoking for SI participants were about 35% at the first annual visit and increased only slightly over the study, whereas cross-sectional rates for UC participants doubled from 10% to 20% by the fifth annual follow-up.[2]

Figure 4–5 shows the rate of decline in mean postbronchodilator FEV_1 for sustained quitters and continuing smokers (SI—placebo participants only). On average, FEV_1 increased slightly after smoking cessation, with a mean increase of 57 mL at the first annual visit. Rate of decline was dramatically slowed by sustained nonsmoking, whereas continuing smoking resulted in a decline of 63 mL per year from the first to the fifth follow-up. The total average decline over the 5 years in FEV_1 was 301 mL in the continuing SI smokers, compared with a loss of 72 mL in the sustained nonsmokers. Thus, LHS demonstrated that an intensive smoking cessation intervention offered to smokers with early pulmonary impairment could result in high rates of smoking cessation and significantly slow, or even reverse, the lung damage caused by smoking.

Similar to studies of the general population,[31] this study of individuals with mild-to-moderate COPD found that older, educated married men were most likely to quit smoking in the SI group. Consistent with the research of Duncan and coworkers[16] discussed previously,

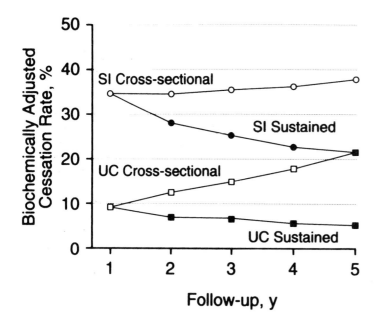

FIGURE 4–4. Biochemically validated smoking cessation rate as a function of years of follow-up. Usual care (UC) participants (*squares*) are compared with smoking intervention (SI) participants (*circles*). Nonattenders at follow-up are counted as smokers. (From Anthonisen NR, Connett JE, Kiley JP, et al: Effects of smoking intervention and the use of an inhaled anticholinergic bronchodilator on the rate of decline of FEV_1: the Lung Health Study. JAMA 272:1497–1505, 1994, with permission.)

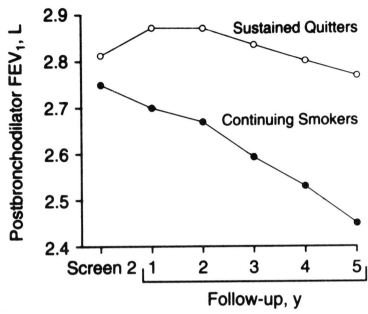

FIGURE 4–5. Mean postbronchodilator forced expiratory volume at 1 second (FEV_1) for participants in the smoking intervention and placebo group who were sustained quitters (*open circles*) and continuous smokers (*closed circles*). (From Anthonisen NR, Connett JE, Kiley JP, et al: Effects of smoking intervention and the use of an inhaled anticholinergic bronchodilator on the rate of decline of FEV_1: the Lung Health Study. JAMA 272:1497–1505, 1994.)

this study found that adverse pulmonary symptoms did not encourage smoking cessation. In fact, cough (for UC participants) and emphysema (for SI participants) were negatively associated with smoking cessation. These associations contradict the notion that health symptoms are an important motivator for achieving health behavior changes. However, anyone who noted these symptoms and immediately quit smoking was not a participant in the LHS. Thus, participants in the LHS with baseline cough or emphysema may reflect the "hardcore" smoker who has greater dependence on cigarettes or less motivation to quit smoking.

Gender Difference in the Lung Health Study

With 1474 women participants, LHS is the largest study reported to date that has examined gender differences in smoking cessation among individuals with pulmonary impairment. At both the 12-month and the 36-month annual visits, significant gender differences were observed in sustained cessation rates, with men having higher cessation rates. The unadjusted odds ratio of sustained cessation for men versus women at 12 and 36 months was 1.22 (P=0.008) and 1.39 (P=0.001). Women who were not married, had less education, had a higher body mass index, had used nicotine gum in a prior quit attempt, had other smokers in the house, drank more than seven alcohol drinks a week, and who

found their first morning cigarette the most difficult to give up were significantly less likely to quit smoking.[4]

Consistent with many other studies,[30] the authors found that both men and women who quit smoking gained weight. Fifty percent of weight gain occurred within the first 4 months after cessation; however, participants who remained nonsmoking continued to gain weight over a 2-year follow-up period. Although men and women gained the same average amount of weight, this gain reflected a significantly greater proportional weight gain for women (6.8% for men, 8.3% for women).

In multivariate analysis, gender was not a significant predictor of cessation at 12 months. At 36 months, however, gender emerged as a significant predictor of sustained cessation, in part because women had a higher relapse rate than men. Overall, demographic and smoking history variables were more powerful than gender as predictors of cessation. Gender differences in observed cessation rates in LHS appeared to be due, in part, to differences in baseline demographic and smoking history characteristics between men and women recruited into LHS. Male participants in LHS were better educated, more likely to be married, and less likely to be living with another smoker. Because of the age of the cohort randomized into LHS (mean age = 48 years), most female smokers who entered the study initiated their smoking behavior at a time when education differences between men and women were more pronounced and the initiation of smoking was more strongly related to socioeconomic status and social class for women than for men.[67]

At baseline, male participants were heavier smokers, with higher cotinine levels and more years of smoking. Female participants had a shorter latency to their first morning cigarette (a measure of nicotine dependence) and claimed greater physical and emotional dependence on cigarettes. Male LHS participants were more likely to have greater than three prior quit attempts and to have quit for over a year in the past, whereas female participants were more likely than men to have tried nicotine gum in the past. Thus, although objective indices such as smoking level and cotinine level might indicate that male LHS participants were more dependent smokers than women, women reported more attitudes and behaviors suggesting emotional and physical dependence and were more likely to have sought out nicotine replacement treatment, suggesting that women perceived their dependence on cigarettes as greater than did men.

Nicotine Gum Use in the Lung Health Study

Nicotine gum use was strongly encouraged as a part of the smoking cessation intervention. Most participants were encouraged to use 10 to 12 pieces per day for the first weeks after smoking cessation. Some participants required 24 pieces or more per day to avoid withdrawal symptoms. As a result of the intensive instruction and supervision, participant acceptance and appropriate use of nicotine gum were high. At the 4-month follow-up, 85.5% of SI participants reported that they had used nicotine gum in the past 4 months, and 64.8% of the nonsmokers were still using nicotine gum. Although gum tapering was initiated by 6 months for most participants, some continued its use for longer periods. At 12 months, 28.9% of the SI participants were using nicotine gum, reflecting both intermittent smokers who were making new attempts to quit as well as those who remained nonsmoking. Although mild side effects such as mouth irritation or dental problems were common (34% of all gum users), rates of significant self-reported side effects were very low (<1%).[5]

This study also found that those who used nicotine gum gained less weight than non–gum users as long as the former continued to use the gum. After discontinuing gum use, however, weight gain was comparable to non–gum users.

Men who were still using nicotine gum at 12 months gained the least weight, followed by non–gum-using men and gum-using women. The greatest proportional increase in body weight was experienced by women who were not using nicotine gum. By the second year of follow-up, nonsmoking men who continued to use gum (more than nine pieces a day) had gained 5.1% of their precessation weight, whereas nonsmoking women using the same level of nicotine gum had gained an average of 9.2% of their body weight. Number of pieces of nicotine gum used per day was also found to be inversely related to the percentage of baseline body weight gained through the first year for men and women.[41]

Recommended Smoking Cessation Strategies in the Pulmonary Care Setting

Tens of thousands of smokers concerned about their lung function and interested in quitting smoking participated in the public recruitment screenings for LHS. Close to 6000 people enrolled in a 5-year trial in which they agreed to be randomly distributed into treatment and control groups. This level of interest underscores the fact that most smokers do want to quit smoking but may lack the skills or confidence necessary to attempt this alone.

Although LHS smoking cessation program was an effective intervention, it was far too costly to be applied to all willing smokers. Therefore, drawing from smoking cessation research, it appears reasonable to recommend that physicians consider a patient-centered, stepped-care approach to smoking cessation counseling beginning with the least intensive and least costly strategies.

RECOMMENDATIONS FOR ALL ADULT SMOKERS

1. Offer smokers 35 years or older pulmonary function testing every 2 years and chart their rate of decline.
2. Use these testing results to encourage smoking cessation.
3. Discuss with the patient his or her readiness to quit smoking, barriers to quitting, and potential coping strategies, and develop a long-range smoking cessation plan. For motivated patients, negotiate a quit date, offer self-help material, and refer interested patients to

existing community or hospital-based programs.

4. Discuss nicotine replacement therapy with all patients motivated to set a quit date.

5. Reassess smoking cessation readiness and redefine smoking cessation goals at each visit for those who fail to quit.

References

1. Anda RF, Remington PL, Sienko DG, et al: Are physicians advising smokers to quit: The patient's perspective. JAMA 257:1916–1919, 1987.

2. Anthonisen NR, Connett JE, Kiley JP, et al: Effects of smoking intervention and the use of an inhaled anticholinergic bronchodilator on the rate of decline of FEV_1: The Lung Health Study. JAMA 272:1497–1505, 1994.

3. Baile WF, Bigelow GE, Gottlieb SH, et al: Rapid resumption of cigarette smoking following myocardial infarction: Inverse relation to MI severity. Addict Behav 7:373–380, 1982.

4. Bjornson W, Rand C, Connett JE, et al: Gender differences and smoking cessation after three years in the Lung Health Study. Am J Pub Health 85:223–230, 1995.

5. Bjornson-Benson W, Nides M, Dolce J, et al: Nicotine gum use in the first year of the Lung Health Study. Addict Behav 18:491–502, 1993.

6. Browner WS, DuChane AG, Hulley SB: Effects of the multiple risk factor intervention trial smoking cessation program on pulmonary function: A randomized controlled trial. West J Med 157:534–538, 1992.

7. Burt A, Thornley P, Illingworth D, et al: Stopping smoking after myocardial infarction. Lancet 1:304–306, 1974.

8. Centers for Disease Control: Smoking-attributable mortality and years of potential life lost: United States 1988. MMWR 40:62–71, 1991.

9. Cohen S, Lichtenstein E: Partner behaviors that support quitting smoking. J Consult Clin Psychol 58:304–315, 1990.

10. Cohen SJ, Stookey GK, Katz BP, et al: Encouraging primary care physicians to help smokers quit: A randomized, controlled trial. Ann Intern Med 110:648–652, 1989.

11. Committee on Environmental Hazards of the American Academy of Pediatrics: Involuntary smoking—a hazard to children. Pediatrics 77:755–757, 1986.

12. Connett JE, Kusek JW, Bailey WC, et al: A randomized clinical trial of early intervention for chronic pulmonary disease. Controlled Clin Trials 14:3S–19S, 1993.

13. Crowley TJ: Any man's death: Presidential Address. Washington, D.C., NIDA Research Monograph 140, NIH Pub. No. 94–3748, 1993, pp 5–10.

14. Daughton DM, Fix AJ, Kass I, et al: Smoking cessation among patients with chronic obstructive pulmonary disease (COPD). Addict Behav 5:125–128, 1980.

15. DiTullio M, Granata D, Taioli E, et al: Early predictors of smoking cessation after myocardial infarction. Clin Cardiol 14:809–812, 1991.

16. Duncan CL, Cummings SR, Hudes ES, et al: Quitting smoking: Reasons for quitting and predictors of cessation among medical patients. J Gen Intern Med 7:398–404, 1992.

17. Edelman NH, Kaplan RM, Buist AS, et al: Chronic obstructive pulmonary disease. Chest 102:243S–256S, 1992.

18. Emmons KM, Weidner G, Foster WM, et al: Improvement in pulmonary function following smoking cessation. Addict Behav 17:301–306, 1992.

19. Fiore MC, Novotny TE, Pierce JP, et al: Trends in cigarette smoking in the United States: The changing influence of gender and race. JAMA 261:49–55, 1989.

20. Fiore MC, Smith SS, Jorenby DE, et al: The effectiveness of the nicotine patch for smoking cessation: A meta-analysis. JAMA 271:1940–1947, 1994.

21. Foxman B, Sloss EM, Lohr KN, et al: Chronic bronchitis: Prevalence, smoking habits, impact, and antismoking advice. Prev Med 15:624–631, 1986.

22. Frank E, Winkleby MA, Altman DG, et al: Predictors of physicians' smoking cessation advise. JAMA 266:3139–3144, 1991.

23. Freund KM, D'Agostino RB, Belanger AJ, et al: Predictors of smoking cessation: The Framingham Study. Am J Epidemiol 135:957–964, 1992.

24. Glynn T, Manley M: How to Help Your Patients Stop Smoking: A National Cancer Institute Manual for Physicians. Bethesda, MD, U.S. Department of Health and Human Services, National Institutes of Health publication 90–3064, 1990.

25. Halpern MT, Gillespie BW, Warner KE: Patterns of absolute risk of lung cancer mortality in former smokers. J Natl Cancer Inst 85:457–464, 1993.

26. Hebert JR, Kristeller J, Ockene JK, et al: Patient characteristics and the effect of three physician-delivered smoking interventions. Prev Med 21:557–573, 1992.

27. Holland WW: Chronic obstructive lung disease prevention. Br J Dis Chest 82:32–44, 1988.

28. Hollis JF, Lichtenstein E, Mount K, et al: Nurse-assisted smoking counseling in medical settings: Minimizing demands on physicians. Prev Med 20:497–507, 1991.

29. Hollis JF, Lichtenstein E, Vogt TM, et al: Nurse-assisted counseling for smokers in primary care. Ann Intern Med 118:521–525, 1993.

30. Klesges RC, Meyers AW, Klesges LM, et al: Smoking, body weight, and their effect on smoking behavior: A comprehensive review of the literature. Psychol Bull 106:204–230, 1989.

31. Koslowski L: Psychosocial influences on cigarette smoking. In Krasnegot NA (ed): The Behavoral Aspects of Smoking. Washington, D.C., NIDA, Research Monograph 26, DHEW publication (ADM) 79–882, 97–125, 1979.

32. Kristeller JL, Merriam PA, Ockene JK, et al: Smoking intervention for cardiac patients: In search of more effective strategies. Prev Cardiol 82:317–324, 1993.

33. Kristeller JL, Rossi JS, Ockene JK, et al: Processes of change in smoking cessation: A cross-validation study in cardiac patients. J Subs Abuse 4:263–276, 1992.

34. Krzyzanowski M, Robbins DR, Lebowitz MD: Smoking cessation and changes in respiratory symptoms in two populations followed for 13 years. Int J Epidemiol 22:666–673, 1993.

35. Lange P, Groth S, Nyboe J, et al: Effects of smoking and changes in smoking habits on the decline of FEV_1. Eur Respir J 2:811–816, 1989.

36. Manley M, Epps RP, Husten C, et al: Clinical interventions in tobacco control: A National Cancer Institute training program for physicians. JAMA 266:3172–3173, 1991.

37. Mattson ME, Pollack ES, Cullen JW: What are the odds that smoking will kill you? Am J Public Health 77:425–431, 1987.

38. Mermelstein R, Cohen S, Lichtenstein E, et al: Social support and smoking cessation and maintenance. J Consult Clin Psychol 54:447–453, 1986.

39. Mulcahy R: Influence of cigarette smoking on morbidity and mortality after myocardial infarction. Br Heart J 49:410–415, 1983.

40. Murray RP, Connett JE, Lauger GG, et al: Error in smoking measures: Effects of intervention on relations of cotinine and carbon monoxide to self-reported smoking. Am J Pub Health 83:1251–1257, 1993.

41. Nides M, Rand C, Dolce J, et al: Weight gain as a function of smoking cessation and 2-mg nicotine gum use among middle-aged smokers with mild lung impairment in the first 2 years of The Lung Health Study. Health Psychol 13:354–361, 1994.

42. O'Hara P, Grill J, Ridgon MA, et al: Design and results of the initial intervention program for the Lung Health Study. Prev Med 22:304–315, 1993.

43. Ockene JK: Smoking intervention: The expanding role of the physician. Am J Pub Health 77:782–787, 1987.

44. Ockene JK, Benfari RC, Nuttall RC, et al: Relationship of psychosocial factors to smoking behavior change in an intervention program. Prev Med 11:13–28, 1982.

45. Ockene JK, Kristeller J, Goldberg R, et al: Smoking cessation and severity of disease: The Coronary Artery Smoking Intervention Study. Health Psychol 11:119–126, 1992.

46. Ockene JK, Kristeller JL, Goldberg R, et al: Increasing the efficacy of physician-delivered smoking interventions: A randomized clinical trial. J Gen Intern Med 6:1–8, 1991.

47. Pederson LL, Baskerville JC: Multivariate prediction of smoking cessation following physician advice to quit smoking: A validation study. Prev Med 12:430–436, 1983.

48. Pederson LL, Baskerville JC, Wanklin JM: Multivariate statistical models for predicting change in smoking behavior following physician advice to quit smoking. Prev Med 11:536–549, 1982.

49. Pederson LL, Wanklin JM, Lefcoe NM: Self-reported long-term smoking cessation in patients with respiratory disease: Prediction of success and perception of health effects. Int J Epidemiol 17:804–809, 1988.

50. Pederson LL, Williams JI, Lefcoe NM: Smoking cessation among pulmonary patients as related to type of respiratory disease and demographic variables. Can J Public Health 71:191–194, 1980.

51. Pierce JP, Fiore MC, Novotny TE, et al: Trends in cigarette smoking in the United States: Educational differences are increasing. JAMA 261:56–60, 1989.

52. Pierce JP, Fiore MC, Novotny TE, et al: Trends in cigarette smoking in the United States: Projections to the year 2000. JAMA 261:61–65, 1989.

53. Prochaska JO, DiClemente CC: Stages and processes of self-change of smoking: Toward an integrative model. J Consult Clin Psychol 51:390–395, 1983.

54. Rigotti NA, McKool KM, Shiffman S: Predictors of smoking cessation after coronary artery bypass graft surgery: Results of a randomized trial with 5-year follow-up. Ann Intern Med 120:287–293, 1994.

55. Rose G, Colwell L: Randomized controlled trial of anti-smoking advice: Final (20 year) results. J Epidemiol Commun Health 46:75–77, 1992.

56. Sansores RH, Pare P, Abboud RT: Effect of smoking cessation on pulmonary carbon monoxide diffusing capacity and capillary blood volume. Am Rev Respir Dis 146:959–964, 1992.

57. Schwartz JL: Review and Evaluation of Smoking Cessation Methods: The United States and Canada, 1978–1985. Bethesda, MD, U.S. Public Health Service, publication 81–2940, 1987.

58. Sköld CM, Forslid J, Eklund A, et al: Metabolic activity in human alveolar macrophages increases after cessation of smoking. Inflammation 17:345–352, 1993.

59. Swan GE, Hodgkin JE, Roby T, et al: Reversibility of airways injury over a 12-month period following smoking cessation. Chest 101:607–612, 1992.

60. Taylor CB, Houston-Miller N, Killen JD, et al: Smoking cessation after acute myocardial infarction: Effects of a nurse-managed intervention. Ann Intern Med 113:118–123, 1990.

61. Thompson SC, Schwankovsky L, Pitts J: Counselling patients to make lifestyle changes: The role of physician self-efficacy, training and beliefs about causes. Fam Pract 10:70–75, 1993.

62. Transdermal Nicotine Study Group: Transdermal nicotine for smoking cessation: Six-month results from two multicenter controlled clinical trials. JAMA 266:3133–3138, 1991.

63. U.S. Department of Health and Human Services: Public Health Service. The health consequences of smoking: Nicotine addiction. A report of the surgeon general. Washington, D.C., U.S. Government Printing Office, DHHS publication no. (CDC) 88–8406, 1988.

64. U.S. Department of Health and Human Services: The Health consequences of smoking: Cancer. A Report of the Surgeon General. Washington, D.C., Department of Health and Human Services, Public Health Service, Office on Smoking and Health, DDHS Publ. No. (PHS) 82–50179, 1982, pp 21–63.

65. U.S. Department of Health and Human Services: Public Health Service. The health benefits of smoking cessation. Washington, D.C., Public Health Service, Centers for Disease Control, Center for Chronic Disease Prevention and Health Promotion, Office on Smoking and Health, DHHS publication no. (CDC) 90–8416, 1990.

66. Visweswaran C, Schmidt FL: A meta-analytic comparison of the effectiveness of smoking cessation methods. J Appl Psychol 77:554–561, 1992.

67. Waldron I: Patterns and causes of gender differences in smoking. Soc Sci Med 32:989–1005, 1991.

68. Wilson DM, Taylor DW, Gilbert JR, et al: A randomized trial of a family physician intervention for smoking cessation. JAMA 260:1570–1574, 1988.

Pharmacologic Interventions

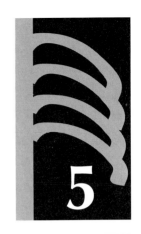

5

Kenneth R. Chapman, MD, MSc, FRCPC, FACP

Rising asthma death rates and rising asthma prevalence have sparked the development of new treatment algorithms for the management of this inflammatory airways disease.[9,35,39,45] Regrettably, less attention has been given to the pharmacologic management of chronic obstructive pulmonary disease (COPD), an obstructive lung disease responsible for considerably more disability and death.[36] Only recently have treatment protocols been discussed and developed for COPD at a national or international level. In the interim, surveys suggest that primary care physicians tend to treat asthma and COPD similarly in practice despite appreciating theoretic differences between these diseases.[40]

The following review of pharmacologic interventions in COPD draws heavily on published guidelines for the management of COPD.[12,26] Although there appears to be a growing international consensus on optimal pharmacologic management of this disorder, one must note that no single guideline should be accepted unthinkingly as a rigid step-care protocol. COPD is presumably a heterogeneous group of disorders with potential differences in care appropriate for each subcategory. Moreover, optimal management of COPD requires patient compliance and therefore must take into account individual patient preferences. Nonetheless, the following management scheme offers a framework around which detailed individual treatment plans can be built.

SECONDARY PREVENTION

Smoking cessation is the most essential first step in secondary prevention of further airway damage. This subject is dealt with in a separate chapter. Although smoking cessation has been shown to slow the rate of forced expiratory volume in 1 second (FEV_1) decline in smokers with COPD,[27] the importance of other secondary preventive measures is less well established. The annual influenza vaccination is recommended for those with chronic cardiopulmonary disease, although its role in COPD specifically has not been assessed in large-scale clinical trials. Nonetheless the rationale for its use is appealing, and the risk-to-benefit ratio is thought to be low. This intervention is unlikely to be subjected to a large-scale clinical trial in the future. A similar intervention, the pneumococcal vaccination, owes its popularity to the observation that *Streptococcus pneumoniae* is one of two common bacterial colonizers in the sputum of patients with COPD. It is not clear, however, that pneumococcal sepsis is more common among COPD patients than among the general population. Attempts to validate use of polyvalent pneumococcal vaccines in COPD have thus far been unsuccessful. Published studies of polyvalent pneumococcal vaccine in COPD have involved small numbers of patients and have failed to show any survival advantage among the vaccinated.[22] Such studies leave considerable room for type II error, and the question must be considered unresolved. For most clinicians, the decision is straightforward, and this low-cost vaccination is offered once every 6 years to elderly patients with COPD. The other common bacterial colonizer in the sputum of patients with COPD is *Haemophilus influenzae*. No commercially available vaccine is currently available for routine clinical use, but clinical trials of oral vaccines have found reduced frequency and severity of exacerbations in chronic bronchitis.[44]

Mucolytic therapy, discussed in greater detail subsequently, has been a popular intervention in Europe where several oral mucolytic agents are widely prescribed. The role of mucolytic therapy has been less popular in North America, perhaps as a consequence of the difficulty posed by studying the properties of sputum. Studies of sputum volume and viscosity are difficult and cumbersome with results that are less easily understood by most pulmonary physicians than spirometric outcomes. Patient benefit is most often quantified not in terms of the rheologic properties of sputum but in terms of subjective symptom scores. Whether or not the thinning of airways secretions is a practical intervention in the day-to-day management of COPD, an alternative rationale has been offered for the use of some currently available mucolytic agents. The use of oral N-acetylcysteine has been described as an antioxidant intervention with *biologic response modifying* properties.[20] That is, the ongoing airway injury of worsening COPD is thought to involve oxidant mechanisms. N-acetylcysteine is purported to act as an antioxidant by acting as a source of glutathione. Placebo-controlled multicenter European studies have reported a decreased frequency of COPD exacerbations among patients receiving oral N-acetylcysteine.[20] The effect appears to be limited to those who smoke cigarettes, perhaps giving credence to the theory of antioxidant mechanisms.

BRONCHODILATORS

Rationale

The literature is replete with descriptions of COPD as an *irreversible* obstructive lung disease. Acute bronchodilator challenges in the pulmonary function laboratory, usually done with small metered-dose inhaler (MDI) doses of adrenergic bronchodilator, often fail to show the marked responsiveness considered characteristic of asthma. This view of little or no bronchodilator responsiveness among COPD patients, however, may be unnecessarily pes-

simistic. First, there is marked day-to-day variability in a given individual's bronchodilator responsiveness in relation to baseline FEV_1 on the day of testing.[4,33] That is, patients who arrive in the laboratory at or near their own optimal FEV_1 show little bronchodilator response on that day, there being little room left for improvement. On another day, perhaps earlier in the morning and after exposure to atmospheric pollution, baseline FEV_1 may be lower and the bronchodilator challenge may produce a greater absolute and percentage increase. Second, it is common to challenge patients with adrenergic bronchodilators in the pulmonary function laboratory. Although patients with asthma respond well to adrenergic compounds, this is not the case for those with COPD. With aging, the sensitivity of the adrenergic nervous system decreases, leaving patients less responsive to this class of agents. The cholinergic nervous system, however, does not *down-regulate* with aging so that antimuscarinic drugs retain their potency. Few laboratories test with a variety of bronchodilator agents, and few wait long enough to measure the peak bronchodilator effect of slower-acting antimuscarinic agents. Third, the goal of bronchodilator therapy is more modest in COPD than in asthma. In those patients suffering from severe obstruction and considerable disability, even a small improvement in airway caliber may make bronchodilator therapy worthwhile. An additional and controversial rationale for the use of bronchodilators in COPD is the nonbronchodilator properties attributed to some agents, in particular, theophylline.

Bronchodilators are customarily prescribed for symptomatic relief of dyspnea. For most patients, dyspnea is not a troublesome symptom until the FEV_1 drops to approximately half of the predicted normal value. The paucity of troublesome symptoms with milder degrees of obstruction means that patients are seldom diagnosed until their illness is at least moderately severe. Presumably, airways obstruction develops slowly and insidiously with patients accommodating the growing pulmonary impairment for many years. Although bronchodilators are generally reserved for the symptomatic phase of the disease, it has been suggested that the early presymptomatic use of bronchodilators may confer longterm benefit. This suggestion arose in part from the multicenter intermittent positive-pressure breathing (IPPB) trial in which patients received bronchodilators regularly for prolonged periods of time. The annual rate of decline in FEV_1 seemed to be reduced in those with greatest bronchodilator responsiveness.[4] The National Institutes of Health (NIH) Lung Health Study was developed to test the hypothesis that early and regular administration of bronchodilators would help to preserve lung function. As noted later, the preliminary results of this study and the simultaneous publication of similar studies suggest that the regular use of bronchodilators does not have a beneficial disease-modifying effect in COPD.

Route of Administration

Inhaled bronchodilators are generally preferred in the management of obstructive airways disease given their relatively rapid onset of response as compared with oral agents. Moreover, delivery of drugs directly to the tracheobronchial tree minimizes systemic side effects. Agents are customarily given by pressurized suspension MDI. This route of administration, however, is not without its problems. Patients with various forms of lung disease have been shown to have difficulty using MDIs effectively.[19,21,25] This should not be surprising; even their caregivers are often unsure of proper MDI technique.[34,42] Estimates of inhaler misuse in the average clinic population range from 14% to 89% with most figures averaging about one-third of patients. It has been suggested that elderly patients may have more difficulty using MDIs (and other inhalation devices) than younger patients.[3,41] One alternative to the pressurized suspension MDI would be a dry powder delivery system. Such systems, however, require high inspiratory flow rates, which may exceed the capacity of patients with severe airflow limitation. Delivery of adequate amounts of drug to the tracheobronchial tree of the COPD patient may therefore be problematic. Another approach has been to use multiple puffs of the MDI format. Drug delivery is also enhanced and coordination problems eased by the use of a spacing chamber with the MDI.[50] A more expensive and more cumbersome approach is to use the wet nebulization of aerosol bronchodilators. There is no evidence that greater bronchodilation is achieved by these means as compared with adequate doses delivered by MDI. Many patients, however, prefer a nebulizer for regular at-home use. This must be complemented with the use of MDIs when the patient is away from home.

Although MDI and nebulizer dosage equivalence can vary widely with patient technique, choice of nebulizer, and specific compound formulations, it is a safe rule of thumb that 4 to 8 MDI puffs approximately equal a nebulizer treatment for a given bronchodilator in its customary therapeutic dosage.

Selection of Agent

The marked day-to-day variability in bronchodilator responsiveness described previously makes it difficult to select specific agents for individual patients based on therapeutic trial. As shown by Guyatt and colleagues,[33] the bronchodilator response of a single day's challenge in the laboratory bears little or no correlation to responses on subsequent days. Presumably the selection of a single agent for a single patient would require a series of drug challenges in the laboratory to the various agents available for use. Such an approach has not been investigated and would seem not only cumbersome, but also prohibitively expensive. Thus, selection of the agent is generally based on the results of clinical trials in which only group mean results are presented.

In most patients who have COPD, inhaled quaternary anticholinergic agents offer bronchodilation at least equal to and often greater than that seen with beta$_2$-agonists.[8,32,56] The greater bronchodilating effect of anticholinergic drugs compared with adrenergic agents in COPD is opposite to the result seen in patients with asthma. This contrast between the obstructive lung diseases may be a consequence of aging.[59] There is a relative decline in the number and sensitivity of adrenergic receptors with age; this leaves the cholinergic system more readily manipulated for purposes of bronchodilation. Ipratropium bromide is the most widely available and extensively studied of the quaternary anticholinergic bronchodilators. Similar to all agents in its class, it is poorly absorbed across biologic membranes, and after inhalation it produces effects largely limited to the airway.[30] It produces no systemic atropinelike side effects. Despite its atropinic heritage, it has no apparent effect on mucociliary transport, sputum volume, or sputum viscosity in customary dosages.[47] Its drying effects appear to be limited to the mouth, where minor drying may occur particularly at higher dosage. The use of a spacing device may minimize oropharyngeal deposition and thereby minimize this minor side effect. Inhalation of even high doses of ipratropium is not accompanied by tachycardia or other atropinelike cardiovascular effects.[17] When compared with inhaled beta$_2$-agonist, quaternary anticholinergic agents offer slightly better peak and apparently better sustained bronchodilator effects. By comparison to the familiar adrenergic agents, however, the onset of bronchodilation is slower with the anticholinergic drugs.

Adrenergic agents appear to be unlike quaternary anticholinergic agents, in that the former are absorbed systemically to a minor degree with mild attendant systemic side effects. Tremor is a common side effect that appears to diminish with continued use of the agent. Less commonly appreciated are the cardiovascular effects of inhaled $beta_2$-agonists. For example, the use of albuterol or fenoterol is accompanied by vasodilation and decreased peripheral vascular resistance. This leads to a reflex increase in stroke volume and heart rate with consequent increase in cardiac output. In normal volunteers, 2 MDI puffs of fenoterol (400 μg) may double cardiac output.[16] Because this occurs by means of an afterload reducing mechanism, the effect may be benign even in elderly patients with COPD. Similar vasodilation, however, occurs in the pulmonary vasculature. The consequences in this vascular bed are less benign. In a patient with COPD, blood begins to perfuse poorly ventilated lung segments with a consequent worsening of the $\dot{V}/\dot{Q}$ matching. At least acutely, the inhalation of selected $beta_2$-agonists is accompanied by a drop in the partial pressure of oxygen in arterial blood.[31]

Theophylline

For almost 50 years, theophylline had been a mainstay of asthma and COPD therapy. Despite long familiarity with this drug, its mechanism of action remains a mystery. Its modest bronchodilator properties were previously attributed to inhibition of phosphodiesterase. Although this mechanism of action appeared plausible, it is now understood that inhibition of phosphodiesterase is unlikely to be achieved by therapeutic doses of theophylline. Pharmaceutical chemists remain mystified by theophylline's bronchodilator properties but have a better appreciation of its side effects. It appears that many side effects seen with theophylline are attributable to its adenosine-blocking properties. Similar to all methylxanthines, which have a substitution at the N_1 position, theophylline blocks adenosine. Adenosine is a naturally occurring autocoid found in many tissues as a response to stress. In the brain, adenosine has mild sedative properties, and of course theophylline may produce mild insomnia. Similarly, adenosine reduces gastric acid secretion, whereas theophylline increases gastric acid secretion. Indeed, most of

theophylline's minor side effects can apparently be attributed to its ability to block adenosine.[5] If approximately 10 to 15% of patients are unable to tolerate long-term theophylline therapy because of headache, insomnia, nausea, tremor, or other troublesome minor side effect, it is plausible that a methylxanthine without adenosine blocking properties would offer considerable clinical advantage in the maintenance treatment of obstructive lung disease. Such compounds have been developed; the best studied is enprofylline. This agent has not been examined in the management of COPD, but in the treatment of asthma it has demonstrable bronchodilator properties.[13] Although not devoid of side effects, it may produce less insomnia than does theophylline.[11,15] Neither enprofylline nor any other similar methylxanthine compound, however, has progressed beyond clinical research. Enprofylline itself may be associated with liver enzyme changes that would prohibit its widespread clinical use.[15]

The clinical application of theophylline has improved with the better understanding of its pharmacokinetic properties. In the past, it was common to titrate serum theophylline levels aggressively with the expectation that bronchodilation was linearly related to serum theophylline levels. Clinicians now appreciate that theophylline dosing obeys a *law of diminishing returns*. That is, there is a plateau effect such that considerable bronchodilation is achieved at serum levels between 5 and 12 mg/L with minimal additional bronchodilator benefit with higher levels.[5] Higher serum levels, however, are clearly associated with increasing side effects and a rising risk of lethal systemic toxicity.

The bronchodilator properties of theophylline are modest, and, in the treatment of COPD, inhaled agents offer greater bronchodilator benefit. As described by Bleecker and colleagues,[7] inhaled ipratropium alone offers greater improvement in FEV_1 than oral theophylline therapy. These investigators, however, also described greater benefit with combination therapy such that the inhaled agent and the oral agent combined afforded greater improvement in FEV_1 than either monotherapy.

Theophylline formulations are widely available for twice-daily or even once-daily administration, thereby simplifying long-term therapy. Compliance with all drugs is inversely related to dosing frequency, and for many patients compliance with an oral agent is simpler than compliance with inhaled agents. Theophylline is also available at relatively low cost when compared with many inhaled bronchodilators.

Theophylline is a modest respiratory stimulant, a property often touted as potentially beneficial in the treatment of patients with COPD. Hypoventilation with CO_2 retention is certainly a feature of severe COPD and at a glance would appear to offer a rationale for the use of respiratory stimulants. It is not clear, however, that COPD patients who hypoventilate are able to respond to such stimulation. CO_2 retention was previously attributed to blunted ventilatory drive in COPD. When ventilatory responses to inhaled CO_2 are measured in physiologic laboratories, patients with COPD show less brisk responses than normal individuals. Such findings, however, are easily explained by the overwhelming mechanical impediment to ventilation faced by such patients. Measurement of occlusion pressure responses in patients with COPD indicate that they are maximally stimulated to breathe at times of exacerbation and respond appropriately to inhaled CO_2 by augmenting their efforts to breathe if not their minute ventilation. Nonetheless, theophylline and other respiratory stimulants have been used clinically in the management of COPD with apparent modest beneficial effect. For example, nocturnal hypoventilation is common in COPD. Fletcher and coworkers[28] have estimated that 25% of patients with COPD who have adequate daytime oxygenation have transient nocturnal desaturation. Berry and colleagues[6] reported that the use of theophylline by such patients improves mean arterial oxygen saturation overnight with a tendency to improve transcutaneous CO_2 level. Benefits may not be confined to blood gas changes; such patients may suffer fewer arousals and have improved quality of overnight sleep.

Schedule of Bronchodilator Administration

In the treatment of asthma, the appropriate schedule for bronchodilator administration has been hotly debated. The once common practice of giving bronchodilators on a scheduled basis (such as albuterol 2 puffs four times daily) has been blamed by some as the cause of worsening airway disease. Evidence for any deleterious effect of regular bronchodilator use in asthma comes from three types of studies. First, epidemiologic studies have associated frequent beta$_2$-agonist use with an excess risk of asthma death.[55] Although such findings are worrisome, they do not prove causality but merely demonstrate an association. It is not difficult to understand that patients with severe life-threatening asthma may require greater amounts of medication more frequently than patients with milder asthma. Second, various laboratories have shown that inhaled beta$_2$-agonist bronchodilators taken regularly for periods of time as short as 1 or 2 weeks may develop heightened airway responsiveness to inhaled bronchoconstrictors such as methacholine.[43] Such changes are small in magnitude and have been demonstrated only in patients with mild asthma who would be unlikely to use regular bronchodilator therapy in a clinical setting. The clinical relevance of such findings has therefore been debated. Finally, one clinical study has suggested that the regular use of fenoterol four times daily is more likely to be associated with loss of asthma control than the as-needed use of the same drug.[53] This 1-year study by Sears and colleagues[53] used a novel approach to assess asthma control and failed to express findings in traditional fashion, such as change in FEV_1 or change in peak flow. Moreover, in this long-term clinical trial, almost one third of the patients initially enrolled had dropped out by the end of the treatment period. The authors have examined the regular versus as-needed use of inhaled albuterol in the treatment of 341 patients with moderate-to-severe asthma.[14] In a 4-week crossover trial, the authors found that patients were less likely to suffer asthma symptoms when they took their drugs on a scheduled basis than when they took their drugs on an intermittent as-needed basis. There was no evidence of deterioration in peak flow as might have been expected given the reasoning of investigators critical of beta$_2$-agonist use. Indeed, by all measures of symptom control, patients demonstrated greater improvement on the regular versus as-needed regimen. The regular use of beta$_2$-agonist bronchodilators has been viewed with some suspicion in asthma, but the existence of significant deleterious clinical effects remains to be proven.

Of what relevance is the regular versus as-needed bronchodilator debate in COPD? Various European investigators have examined the long-term use of inhaled bronchodilators in mixed populations of patients with asthma or COPD. The reported results of these studies appear to be internally contradictory. A major difficulty for the North American reader is distinguishing results obtained for asthma patients from results obtained for COPD patients. An additional difficulty in interpreting the findings of these studies is the repeated post hoc analyses to which they have been subjected. For example, Van Schayck and colleagues[60] first reported 18-month results of a 2-year study in which large groups of patients were treated with either regular or as-needed inhaled bronchodilator. They measured histamine responses of patients before and during regular treatment with albuterol for 1 year crossing over to ipratropium for 6 months or ipratropium for 1 year crossing over to albuterol for 6 months. Their data clearly showed increasing airway irritability in patients treated with albuterol and no effect of regular ipratropium. At the end of the 2-year trial, however, they reported that patients with either asthma or COPD responded adversely to regular treatment with either form of inhaled bronchodilator.[58] Specifically, this second paper reported that annual rates of FEV_1 decline were fastest when patients were treated with regular bronchodilator versus as-needed bronchodilator. Later post hoc subgroup analysis suggested less consistent effects with ipratropium and no consistent effect in COPD patients.[24] In a final editorial comment published in *Thorax* most recently, Van Schayck and Van Herwaarden[61] stated that there was no demonstrated cause for concern regarding regular bronchodilator use and that physicians were unnecessarily fearful of this means of therapy. In short, data describing adverse effects of regular bronchodilator use in COPD have not been consistent and have been repudiated by their own authors.

The debate about regular versus as-needed bronchodilators in the treatment of COPD is nonsensical when applied to severe COPD. Patients with COPD have persistent airflow limitation, which, if sufficiently severe, interferes with activities of daily living. The patient with an FEV_1 of less than 1 L is likely to find that he or she is dyspneic when dressing in the morning, when walking to the grocery store at midday, and when playing with grandchildren in the evening. Asking such a patient to take bronchodilator on an as-needed basis would likely lead to almost regular bronchodilator use. Because it is difficult to anticipate each and every moment of physical exertion, the scheduled use of bronchodilator would seem to afford the best clinical result with the minimum of inconvenience. This is in sharp contrast to asthmatic wheezing episodes, which can be dealt with rapidly by means of inhaled beta$_2$-agonist.

Long-Term Use of Bronchodilators

Bronchodilators given for the treatment of COPD are likely to be administered frequently or regularly over long periods of time. As noted previously, there has been considerable debate about long-term adverse effects of bronchodilators in the management of obstructive lung disease. At present, many previously expressed fears appear to be unfounded. It has long been known that the regular use of adrenergic agents is accompanied by mild tachyphylaxis to the bronchodilating effects of the medication. The literature also suggests a mild tachyphylaxis to the bronchoprotective effects of inhaled short-acting and long-acting adrenergic bronchodilators in the setting of asthma.[18,46] No similar data are available for COPD. Tachyphylaxis has been used to explain the decreased bronchodilator efficacy of adrenergic drugs given over a long period of time. Tachyphylaxis, however, appears to be mild and self-limited. That is, decreased effectiveness of the medication can be obscured during the first few weeks of its use and may not subsequently be progressive. There are no similar data describing decreased effectiveness of inhaled quaternary anticholinergic bronchodilators over time. Indeed the available data appear to suggest that as adrenergic bronchodilators lose their efficacy with repeated use, the anticholinergic bronchodilators retain their efficacy.[52] Such findings suggest that the acute bronchodilator response comparisons between adrenergic and anticholinergic bronchodilators may not be an accurate reflection of their comparative properties in actual clinical practice. There appear to be no long-term trials of theophylline therapy in COPD, and therefore no evidence exists of tachyphylaxis to its bronchodilator or nonbronchodilator properties with regular use. The only trials that describe theophylline therapy over long periods of time are in asthma, in which there appears to be no evidence of decreased effectiveness.[15,57]

Questions of decreased efficacy aside, the regular use of bronchodilators has been thought by some to be a potentially useful strategy for preventing long-term decline in lung function in COPD. The NIH Lung Health Study was developed to test this hypothesis.[38] Although the study confirmed that smoking cessation slows the accelerated decline in lung function seen in the smoker with early COPD, and, therefore, smoking cessation appears to be the most important intervention in this population, it failed to show any benefit from regular bronchodilator therapy. That is, the rate of lung function decline was slightly and statistically slower in the group receiving inhaled bronchodilators, but the difference was so small as to be clinically unimportant. Nonetheless, these data do reassure that regular bronchodilator use is not accompanied by accelerated lung function decline as has been speculated by others. It is also questionable whether or not the Lung Health Study was an adequate trial of long-term regular bronchodilator use. The investigators monitored compliance closely in their study and found that few patients complied with three times daily use of inhaled bronchodilators.[51] This may not be surprising in this minimally symptomatic group and suggests that bronchodilators may be appropriate only for those COPD patients who are symptomatic.

CORTICOSTEROID THERAPY

The role of corticosteroid therapy in COPD remains controversial with significant international differences in approach. The rationale for the use of steroids is appealing in this setting. There is clear evidence of airway inflammation in COPD. Many of the cells lavaged from the airways of smokers are polymorphonuclear leukocytes, suggesting ongoing airway injury. It is less clear, however, that the use of steroids can significantly alter this airway inflammation. Studies that have attempted to address this question were difficult to undertake and interpret. Difficulties included defining the study population so as to exclude asthmatics, detecting effects of steroids on a wide range of baseline lung function, and ensuring that COPD patients were tested when clinically stable. Attempts to compare various steroid intervention studies were made more difficult by the differing dosages and durations of steroid treatment. Many published studies addressing the question of steroid administration in COPD have involved small numbers of patients so that a type II error cannot be excluded. Nonetheless a review of published studies including a recent meta-analysis suggested that few patients with COPD benefit from either systemic or inhaled corticosteroid therapy.

Stable Chronic Obstructive Pulmonary Disease

Callaghan and associates[10] have reviewed published studies in which stable COPD patients received oral steroid therapy. The analysis suggested that only approximately 10% of COPD patients, as defined by currently acceptable criteria, were steroid responsive. Steroid response in this context meant a significant increase in spirometric findings after at least 2 weeks of oral steroid administration. Unfortu-

nately, there appears to be no simple way to predict which COPD patients are likely to be steroid-responsive. Studies have examined blood eosinophilia, sputum eosinophilia, acute bronchodilator responsiveness, and other clinical characteristics thought to be helpful in distinguishing asthma from COPD. No one variable or set of variables has been successful in predicting response to steroids.

Acute Exacerbations of Chronic Obstructive Pulmonary Disease

Despite the lack of steroid responsiveness in most patients with stable COPD, there is one study that suggests a beneficial role of steroids in the treatment of acute exacerbations of COPD. Albert and colleagues[2] reported that patients given intravenous methylprednisolone during their hospitalizations had more rapid improvement in FEV_1 than patients given intravenous saline. In this randomized, double-blind, placebo-controlled trial, the improvement in flow rates was more rapid over the first 3 days of hospitalization but there was no detectable difference in outcome, such as duration of hospital stay or survival attributable to the steroid intervention. This single study has been the rationale for giving corticosteroids aggressively to COPD patients who are sick enough to be hospitalized. The study has not been replicated. It is conceivable that the inadvertent inclusion of asthmatic patients in the study might have skewed the results in favor of steroids. In any event, most clinicians would choose to reconcile the data of this acute intervention study with the lack of long-term effectiveness of steroids by keeping courses of steroid administration short in the COPD exacerbation setting.

Inhaled Corticosteroids

There is as yet no definite evidence that inhaled corticosteroids are of benefit in COPD. Indeed, given the lack of benefit of oral steroids, it would seem unlikely that inhaled steroids offer benefit in this setting. Nonetheless, for those few patients with COPD who appear to be oral-steroid responsive, a trial of inhaled steroids may be reasonable. High-dose inhaled steroids given twice daily may allow the cessation of oral steroids, thereby minimizing systemic side effects. Several large-scale trials are underway to test the effect of inhaled steroids in long-term COPD management. Among them, the Euroscop trial may be best known. This randomized controlled trial will attempt to assess long-term decline in lung function in patients treated with inhaled steroids versus those treated with inhaled placebo.[48] Regrettably the study is limited to smokers with COPD; thus, it is apparently evaluating the use of a medication to protect against the effects of continued smoking.

Oral Steroid Trial

Given that only a few patients respond to oral steroids but that some may do so dramatically, an oral steroid trial is often appropriate when severe COPD is present. If patients remain severely disabled by COPD despite smoking cessation and aggressive bronchodilator therapy, a trial of oral steroids is easily conducted in the ambulatory setting. Such a trial should take place only when the patient is clinically stable. This should be undertaken neither shortly after an exacerbation and hospitalization nor shortly after smoking cessation. When the patient is stable, postbronchodilator spirometry is done to measure the maximal FEV_1 obtainable. The patient is then given prednisone in a dosage of 40 to 50 mg per day, and this therapy is continued for 2 weeks. At the end of the treatment period, spirometric end points are again measured. If the postbronchodilator FEV_1 has risen by at least 20% and 200 mL, the patient might be regarded as steroid responsive. Some pulmonologists would set the threshold for a positive response somewhat higher. They would argue that at least 30% increase and a 300 ml absolute increase are needed before the hazards of long-term oral steroid therapy should be considered. Although oral steroid trials are described as following a period of treatment with bronchodilators,[12,26] some would argue that a trial of oral steroids should occur at the outset of COPD management. A few patients who are remarkably responsive to oral steroids might be termed the *hidden asthmatics*. A return of lung function to normal or nearly normal values would alter the algorithm used to treat the patient.

ANTIBIOTICS

Patients with COPD may cough chronically, and the cough may be productive of purulent sputum. The sputum of such patients is commonly colonized with bacteria. Nonetheless the regular or preventive use of antibiotics is unwarranted. It is impossible to sterilize the sputum of COPD patients with chronic cough. At times of exacerbation, however, the judicious use of antibiotics may hasten the resolution of the episode.[54] Many of the older antibiotics appear to be equally effective to the newer, more expensive agents. Allowing patients with COPD to self-administer antibiotics at times of exacerbation may be a useful self-management strategy analogous to the self-administration of steroids in asthma. Such an approach may keep some COPD patients out of the hospital during their wintertime viral-induced exacerbations; no randomzied, controlled trial has verified this reasonable hyothesis.

MUCOLYTIC THERAPY

As noted previously, mucolytic therapy is widely used in many European nations but is less popular in North America. Clinical trials are made difficult by the lack of easily understood objective end points. One currently available mucolytic, iodinated glycerol, has been shown to offer modest symptomatic benefit in patients with chronic bronchitis.[49] The differences between mucolytics and placebo in this study were small. Nonetheless, for some patients with troublesome sputum production, mucolytic agents may be worth a clinical trial.

Alpha-dornase has been manufactured using recombinant DNA techniques. It works by lysing the DNA bridges naturally found in any sputum. This agent has already been shown to be of significant clinical benefit in the management of cystic fibrosis.[37] The role of this effective mucolytic in COPD remains unknown but is the subject of ongoing clinical trials.

ALPHA₁-ANTITRYPSIN REPLACEMENT THERAPY

For patients with emphysema associated with alpha₁-antitrypsin deficiency, it is possible to administer purified alpha₁-antitrypsin protein. This intravenous preparation, however, is costly and cumbersome, requires either weekly or monthly infusions, and appears useful only for patients with this disorder. Regrettably, no clinical trial has established that the use of this medication actually delays the progression of emphysema. Instead, injections of the drug have been shown to produce blood and alveolar levels of protein that are thought to be protective on theoretic grounds.[29,62] A review of the natural history of alpha₁-antitrypsin deficiency emphysema raises considerable doubt about the need for such replacement therapy. The deficiency state is one of the most common inherited genetic abnormalities with an estimated population prevalence of between 1 in 1600 and 1 in 4000.[1] Despite this, clinicians identify relatively few patients who have emphysema attributable to the deficiency state. It seems likely that patients do not develop clinically important emphysema unless they are both deficient in alpha$_1$-antitrypsin protein and smoke. Nonsmokers may develop little or no clinically significant lung disease during the average life span. Thus a $30,000 per year protein replacement regimen may offer protection only to smokers and may be of no clinical relevance to those who are deficient but have stopped smoking. These important questions clearly deserve further clinical investigation. The protein therapy, however, is currently available for prescription use in North America.

COMPLIANCE

Therapy for COPD is administered regularly and for a period of years, making compliance an important issue. Reports suggest that COPD patient compliance is poor, however, with approximately half of patients underusing the drugs prescribed for maintenance therapy.[23] This is particularly worrisome in the case of theophylline; the same study suggests that at times of exacerbation patients may overuse their medications.

Drugs are often used in combination in the management of COPD, and this may interfere with compliance. Whenever possible, the regimen should be simplified. As noted earlier, the dosage of a single inhaled bronchodilator should be maximized before the addition of a second inhaled agent is considered. Many patients are adequately treated with just a single agent. In addition to simplifying therapy, patients should be educated about the nature of their therapy and the nature of their disease. The role of patient education has received less attention for COPD than for asthma. This is unfortunate because many patients with COPD display anxiety about their disease and would welcome the opportunity to discuss important issues such as treatment and prognosis.

SUMMARY

Modern treatment algorithms for the management of COPD differ greatly from the treatment algorithms for the management of asthma. Asthma management relies on intermittent use of quick relief adrenergic bronchodilators and preventive therapy with inhaled steroids or nonsteroidal drugs. By contrast, patients with COPD do not have intermittent symptoms and therefore receive inhaled bronchodilators on a regular basis. This older patient population is likely to be treated with inhaled quaternary anticholinergic bronchodilators as first-line agents, with beta$_2$-agonists and theophylline given supplementally if necessary. The role of corticosteroids is minimal in COPD. Few patients respond to oral steroids when stable, although a transient benefit may be evident when steroids are given during times of acute exacerbation. There is no well-defined role for inhaled steroids in the management of stable COPD.

References

1. Ad Hoc Committee on Alpha-1-Antitrypsin Replacement Therapy of the Standards Committee, Canadian Thoracic Society: Current status of alpha-1-antitrypsin replacement therapy: Recommendations for the management of patients with severe hereditary deficiency. Can Med Assoc J 146:841–844,1992.
2. Albert RK, Martin TR, Lewis SW: Controlled clinical trial of methylprednisolone in patients with chronic bronchitis and acute respiratory insufficiency. Ann Intern Med 92:753–758, 1980.
3. Allen SC, Prior A: What determines whether an elderly patient can use a metered dose inhaler correctly? Br J Dis Chest 80:45–49, 1986.
4. Anthonisen NR, Wright EC: Response to inhaled bronchodilators in COPD. Chest 91(5 suppl):36S-39S, 1987.
5. Barnes PJ, Pauwels RA: Theophylline in the management of asthma: Time for reappraisal? Eur Respir J 7: 579–591, 1994.
6. Berry RB, Desa MM, Branum JP, Light RW: Effect of theophylline on sleep and sleep-disordered breathing in patients with chronic obstructive pulmonary disease. Am Rev Respir Dis 143:245–250, 1991.
7. Bleecker ER, Johns M, Britt EJ: Greater bronchodilator effects of ipratropium compared to theophylline in chronic airflow obstruction. Chest 94(suppl 1):3S, 1988.
8. Braun SR, McKenzie WN, Copeland C, et al: A comparison of the effect of ipratropium and albuterol in the treatment of chronic obstructive airway disease. Arch Intern Med 149:544–547, 1989.
9. British Thoracic Society, British Paediatric Association, Research Unit of the Royal College of Physicians of London, King's Fund Centre, National Asthma Campaign, Royal College of General Practitioners in Asthma Group, British Association of Accident and Emergency Medicine, and British Paediatric Respiratory Group: Guidelines on the management of asthma. Thorax 48: S1-S24, 1993.
10. Callaghan CM, Dittus RS, Katz BP: Oral corticosteroid therapy for patients with stable chronic obstructive pulmonary disease. Ann Intern Med 114:216–223, 1991.
11. Chapman KR, Boucher S, Hyland RH, et al: A comparison of enprofylline and theophylline in the maintenance therapy of chronic reversible obstructive airway disease. J Allergy Clin Immunol 85:514–521, 1990.
12. Chapman KR, Bowie DM, Goldstein RS, et al: Guide-

lines for the assessment and management of chronic obstructive pulmonary disease. Canadian Thoracic Society Workshop Group. Can Med Assoc J 147:420–428, 1992.

13. Chapman KR, Bryant RD, Marlin GE, et al: A placebo-controlled dose-response study of enprofylline in the maintenance therapy of asthma. Am Rev Respir Dis 139:688–693, 1989.

14. Chapman KR, Kesten S, Szalai JP: Regular vs as-needed inhaled salbutamol in asthma control. Lancet 343:1379–1382, 1994.

15. Chapman KR, Ljungholm K, Kallen A, and International Enprofylline Study Group: Long-term xanthine therapy of asthma: Enprofylline and theophylline compared. Chest 1994, 106:1407–1413, 1994.

16. Chapman KR, Smith DL, Rebuck AS, Leenen FHH: Hemodynamic effects of an inhaled beta-2 agonist. Clin Pharmacol Ther 35:762–767, 1984.

17. Chapman KR, Smith DL, Rebuck AS, Leenen FHH: Hemodynamic effects of inhaled ipratropium bromide, alone and combined with an inhaled beta 2-agonist. Am Rev Respir Dis 132:845–847, 1985.

18. Cheung D, Timmers MC, Zwinderman AH, et al: Long-term effects of a long-acting β_2-adrenoceptor agonist, salmeterol, on airway hyperresponsiveness in patients with mild asthma. N Engl J Med 327:1198–1203, 1992.

19. Coady TJ, Stewart CJ, Davies HJ: Synchronization of bronchodilator release. Practitioner 217:273–275, 1976.

20. Cotgreave I: The in vitro effects and biotransformation of N-acetylcysteine. In Oxidative Stress in the Lung—Intervention with Thiols. Lund, AB Draco, 1986, p 19–20.

21. Crompton GK: The adult patient's difficulties with inhalers. Lung 168 (suppl):658–662, 1990.

22. Davis AL, Aranda CP, Schiffman G, Christianson LC: Pneumococcal infection and immunologic response to pneumococcal vaccine in chronic obstructive pulmonary disease. A pilot study. Chest 92:204–212, 1987.

23. Dolce JJ, Crisp C, Manzella B, et al: Medication adherence patterns in chronic obstructive pulmonary disease. Chest 99:837–841, 1991.

24. Dompeling E, Van Schayck CP, van den Broek PJJA, Van Weel C: The decline in lung function during continuous versus on demand use of salbutamol and ipratropium bromide in asthma and COPD. Am Rev Respir Dis 145:A61,1992.

25. Epstein SW, Manning CP, Ashley MJ, Corey PN: Survey of the clinical use of pressurized aerosol inhalers. Can Med Assoc J 120:813–816, 1979.

26. Ferguson GT, Cherniack RM: Management of chronic obstructive pulmonary disease. N Engl J Med 328:1017–1022, 1993.

27. Fletcher C, Peto R: The natural history of chronic airflow obstruction. BMJ 1:1645–1648, 1977.

28. Fletcher EC, Miller J, Divine GW, et al: Nocturnal oxyhemoglobin desaturation in COPD patients with arterial oxygen tensions above 60 mmHg. Chest 92:604–608, 1987.

29. Gadek JE, Klein HG, Holland PV, Crystal RG: Replacement therapy of alpha 1-antitrypsin deficiency. Reversal of protease-antiprotease imbalance within the alveolar structures of PiZ subjects. J Clin Invest 68:1158–1165, 1981.

30. Gross NJ: Ipratropium bromide. N Engl J Med 319:486–494, 1988.

31. Gross NJ, Bankwala Z: Effects of an anticholinergic bronchodilator on arterial blood gases of hypoxemic patients with chronic obstruction pulmonary disease. Am Rev Respir Dis 136:1091–1094, 1987.

32. Gross NJ, Skorodin MS: Role of the parasympathetic system in airway obstruction. N Engl J Med 311:421–425, 1984.

33. Guyatt GH, Townsend M, Nogradi S, et al: Acute response to bronchodilator. An imperfect guide for bronchodilator therapy in chronic airflow limitation. Arch Intern Med 148:1949–1952, 1988.

34. Hanania NA, Wittman R, Kesten S, Chapman KR: Medical personnel's knowledge of and ability to use inhaling devices: Metered-dose inhalers, spacing chambers, and breath-actuated dry powder inhalers. Chest 105:111–116, 1994.

35. Hargreave FE, Dolovich J, Newhouse MT: The assessment and treatment of asthma: A conference report. J Allergy Clin Immunol 85:1098–1111, 1990.

36. Higgins M: Epidemiology of COPD. State of the art. Chest 85:3S-8S, 1984.

37. Hubbard RC, McElvaney NG, Birrer P, et al: A preliminary study of aerosolized recombinant human deoxyribonuclease I in the treatment of cystic fibrosis. N Engl J Med 326:812–815, 1992.

38. Istvan JA, Nides MA, Buist AS, et al: Salivary cotinine, frequency of cigarette smoking, and body mass index: Findings at baseline in the Lung Health Study. Am J Epidemiol 139:628–636, 1994.

39. Keskinen H, Kalliomaki PL, Alanko K: Occupational asthma due to stainless steel welding fumes. Clin Allergy 10:151–159, 1980.

40. Kesten S, Chapman KR: Physician perceptions and management of COPD. Chest 104:254–258, 1993.

41. Kesten S, Elias M, Cartier A, Chapman KR: Patient handling of a multidose dry powder inhalation device for albuterol. Chest 105:1077–1081, 1994.

42. Kesten S, Zive K, Chapman KR: Pharmacist knowledge and ability to use inhaled medication delivery systems. Chest 104:1737–1742, 1993.

43. Kraan J, Koeter GH, Mark TW, et al: Changes in bronchial hyperreactivity induced by 4 weeks of treatment with antiasthmatic drugs in patients with allergic asthma: A comparison between budesonide and terbutaline. J Allergy Clin Immunol 76:628–636, 1985.

44. Lehmann D, Coakley KJ, Coakley CA, et al: Reduction in the incidence of acute bronchitis by an oral *Haemophilus influenzae* vaccine in patients with chronic bronchitis in the highlands of Papua New Guinea. Am Rev Respir Dis 144:324–330, 1991.

45. Lenfant C, Sheffer AL, Bousquet J, et al: International consensus report on diagnosis and management of asthma. Bethesda, U.S. Department of Health and Human Services, publication no. 92–3091, 1992.

46. O'Connor BJ, Aikman SL, Barnes PJ: Tolerance to the nonbronchodilator effects of inhaled β_2-agonists in asthma. N Engl J Med 327:1204–1208, 1992.

47. Pakes GE, Brogden RN, Heel RC, et al: Ipratropium bromide: A review of its pharmacological properties and therapeutic efficacy in asthma and chronic bronchitis. Drugs 20:237–266, 1980.

48. Pauwels RA, Lofdahl C, Pride NB, et al: European Respiratory Society study on chronic obstructive pulmonary disease (EUROSCOP): Hypothesis and design. Eur Respir J 5:1254–1261, 1992.

49. Petty TL: The National Mucolytic Study. Results of a randomized, double-blind, placebo-controlled study of iodinated glycerol in chronic obstructive bronchitis. Chest 97:75–83, 1990.

50. Pierce RJ, McDonald CF, Landau LI, et al: Nebuhaler versus wet aerosol for domiciliary bronchodilator therapy. A multi-centre clinical comparison. Med J Aust 156:771–774, 1992.

51. Rand CS, Wise RA, Nides M, et al: Metered-dose inhaler adherence in a clinical trial. Am Rev Respir Dis 146:1559–1564, 1992.

52. Rebuck AS, Gent M, Chapman KR: Anticholinergic and

sympathomimetic combination therapy of asthma. J Allergy Clin Immunol 71:317–323, 1983.

53. Sears MR, Taylor DR, Print CG, et al: Regular inhaled beta-agonist treatment in bronchial asthma. Lancet 336: 1391–1396, 1990.

54. Shim C, Williams Jr MH: Comparison of oral aminophylline and aerosol metaproterenol in asthma. Am J Med 71:452–455, 1981.

55. Spitzer WO, Suissa S, Ernst P, et al: The use of β-agonists and the risk of death and near death from asthma. N Engl J Med 326:501–506, 1992.

56. Tashkin DP, Ashutosh K, Bleecker ER, et al: Comparison of the anticholinergic bronchodilator ipratropium bromide with metaproterenol in chronic obstructive pulmonary disease. A 90-day multi-center study. Am J Med 81:81–90, 1986.

57. Tinkelman DG, Moss BA, Bukantz SC, et al: A multicenter trial of the prophylactic effect of ketotifen, theophylline, and placebo in atopic asthma. J Allergy Clin Immunol 76:487–497, 1985.

58. Van Schayck CP, Dompeling E, Van Herwaarden CLA, et al: Bronchodilator treatment in moderate asthma or chronic bronchitis: Continuous or on demand? A randomised controlled study. BMJ 303:1426–1431, 1991.

59. Van Schayck CP, Folgering H, et al: Effects of allergy and age on responses to salbutamol and ipratropium bromide in moderate asthma and chronic bronchitis. Thorax 46:355–359, 1991.

60. Van Schayck CP, Graafsma SJ, Visch MB, et al: Increased bronchial hyperresponsiveness after inhaling salbutamol during 1 year is not caused by subsensitization to salbutamol. J Allergy Clin Immunol 86:793–800, 1990.

61. Van Schayck CP, Van Herwaarden CLA: Bronchodilators and bronchial hyperresponsiveness. Reply. Thorax 49:190–191, 1994.

62. Wewers MD, Casolaro MA, Sellers SE, et al: Replacement therapy for alpha 1-antitrypsin deficiency associated with emphysema. N Engl J Med 316:1055–1062, 1987.

Supplemental Oxygen in Chronic Respiratory Disease

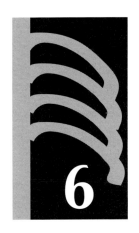

6

Roger S. Goldstein, MB, ChB, FRCP(UK), FRCP(C), FCCP

In the last 20 years, there have been major advances in both basic and applied knowledge of oxygen therapy. At atmospheric pressure, arterial hypoxemia occurs if pulmonary or cardiac conditions alter the ventilation-perfusion distribution within the lung or if alveolar hypoventilation increases the alveolar carbon dioxide tension sufficiently to decrease the alveolar oxygen tension. The extent to which an increase in inspired oxygen concentration improves the PaO_2 varies depending on the magnitude of the mismatch between ventilation and perfusion, with almost no improvement occurring when the shunt fraction reaches 50% of the cardiac output. Increasing alveolar ventilation increases the $PaCO_2$ both by decreasing alveolar $PaCO_2$ and by diminishing regions of low ventilation-perfusion, for example, by expanding atelectatic lung. Tissue oxygen delivery depends not only on the oxyhemoglobin saturation (SaO_2) (determined by the PaO_2 and the oxyhemoglobin dissociation curve), but also on the hemoglobin concentration, the cardiac output, local organ perfusion, and cellular extraction.

Clinical studies have begun to unravel some of the mechanisms of hypoxia and the benefits of treatment with supplemental oxygen. Oxygen delivery systems enable many individuals to benefit from home oxygen therapy. At the same time, the era of cost containment has presented new challenges to those who administer, fund, and deliver health care to use oxygen therapy only when it is likely to be of benefit and to apply it in the most cost-effective way.[19]

Most studies of long-term oxygen therapy (LTOT) have involved subjects with chronic obstructive pulmonary disease (COPD); many clinicians believe that the data obtained from oxygen therapy in COPD can be applied to other situations in which chronic hypoxemia occurs. This chapter focuses on some of the classic studies of oxygen therapy in COPD, some of the outstanding issues in oxygen therapy, and the more frequently used methods of oxygen delivery.

COMPREHENSIVE CARE FOR THE PATIENT WITH CHRONIC RESPIRATORY CONDITIONS

The role of supplemental oxygen must be placed within the context of a continuum of care, which should include cessation of smoking, optimal pharmacologic therapy, appropriate vaccinations, prompt attention to infectious exacerbations, and supervised rehabilitation aimed at improving exercise tolerance and quality of life. Psychosocial factors, such as good coping skills and motivation, optimism, and flexibility, may enhance compliance with oxygen therapy, as does the involvement of a supportive family and suitable home environment. Patient and family education improves the understanding of the technical aspects of oxygen delivery and facilitates realistic goals and expectations.

MULTICENTER TRIALS

This section addresses two of the studies that justify the prescription of supplemental oxygen to reduce mortality and to improve morbidity. Despite optimal treatment of lung impairment, without oxygen therapy, patients with COPD and hypoxemia have a poor prognosis. In a study reported by the Nocturnal Oxygen Therapy Trial Group,[26] 203 subjects were randomly allocated to either a continuous oxygen therapy group or 21 hours of oxygen therapy (nocturnal oxygen therapy [NOT] group) and monitored for at least 12 months. Entry criteria (Table 6–1) included a PaO_2 of less than 55 mm Hg or less than 59 mm Hg if accompanied by edema, an increased hematocrit, or electrocardiographic evidence of pulmonary hypertension. The patients were representative of stable patients with COPD as a whole. Oxygen was administered to maintain the resting PaO_2 above 60 mm Hg with the flow increased by 1 L/minute for exercise and sleep. A variety of delivery systems were used, and patient compliance was monitored. The average patient was 66 years of age and had severe airflow limitation ($FEV_1 < 30\%$ predicted), a limited maximal exercise capacity (37 watts), a resting tachycardia (93 bpm), and modest pulmonary hypertension (mean pulmonary artery pressure 29 mm Hg). The mean PaO_2 was 44 mm Hg. The mean sleep SaO_2 was 84% on room air and 94% on oxygen. After 12 months, 64 patients had died, 41 in the NOT group and

TABLE 6–1
Entry and Exclusion Criteria

Entry criteria
  Clinical diagnosis of chronic obstructive lung
    disease
  Hypoxemia
  $PaO_2 \leq 55$ mm Hg
  $PaO_2 \leq 59$ plus one of the following:
    Edema
    Hematocrit $\geq 55\%$
    P pulmonale on ECG: 3 mm in leads II, III, aVf

Lung function*
  $FEV_1/FVC \leq 70\%$ after inhaled bronchodilator
  TLC $\geq 80\%$ predicted
  Age >35

Exclusion criteria
  Previous O_2 therapy: 12 h/d for 30 d during
    previous 2 mo
  Other disease that might be expected to influence
    mortality, morbidity, compliance with therapy,
    or ability to give informed consent

*FEV_1 = Forced expiratory volume in 1 second; FVC = forced vital capacity; TLC = total lung capacity.
From Kvale PA, Cugell DW, Anthonisen NR, et al: Continuous or nocturnal oxygen therapy in hypoxemic chronic obstructive lung disease. Ann Intern Med 93:391–398, 1980.

23 in the continuous oxygen group; thus, the 12 month mortality was 21% for NOT and 12% for continuous oxygen use. Only the hematocrit and the pulmonary vascular resistance showed changes as a function of the treatment regimen. At 12-month and 18-month treatment intervals, hematocrit values were decreased significantly more in patients using continuous oxygen than in those using only nocturnal oxygen. At 18 months, hematocrit values had decreased by 2% in the former group and by 9% in the latter. The pulmonary vascular resistance measured after 6 months of treatment had increased by a mean of 6.5% in the NOT group, whereas it had decreased by a mean of 11% in the continuous oxygen users. In addition, several measures of quality of life and neuropsychological functioning had improved in both treatment groups. Thus, the treatment was shown to have achieved its short-term goal of reducing mortality and improving quality of life.

In a second classic study, the British Medical Research Council[38] reported the results of a three-center prospective, randomized, controlled trial established to determine whether oxygen given for 15 hours/day over 3 years could reduce mortality among 87 subjects with severe airways obstruction, hypoxia ($PaCO_2$ 51 mm Hg), and moderate pulmonary hypertension (mean pulmonary artery pressure 34 mm Hg). This study differed from the previous one in that subjects were hypercapneic (mean $PaCO_2$ 54 mm Hg). Subjects were randomized to receive oxygen therapy for 15 hours a day or no supplemental oxygen. In those receiving oxygen, the PaO_2 was kept above 60 mm Hg. In the treated group, 19 of the 42 patients died, but in the control group 30 of the 45 patients died. Of note, this study reported different mortality patterns between men and women. In men, the mortalities of the treated and control groups (Fig. 6–1) were similar for the first 500 days, after which the groups diverged with mortalities of 12% per annum in the treated group and 29% per annum in the control group. Women showed an unexpectedly divergent pattern of mortality from the onset of the study (Fig. 6–2), but the smaller number of women (21 out of 87) made more detailed analysis difficult. Of the variables measured, a combination of red cell mass and $PaCO_2$ while breathing room air provided the best discriminant between those men who survived for 500 days and those who died within this period. The subjects in whom the red cell mass plus the $PaCO_2$ exceeded 98 had a higher mortality at 500 days (61% versus 17%). The study failed to confirm that LTOT could reduce

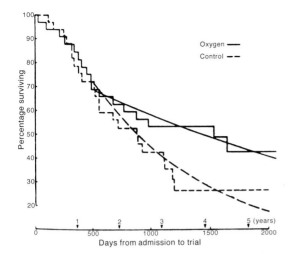

FIGURE 6–1. Mortality in male patients. Smooth curves indicate expected proportions surviving a constant risk of 12%/annum in the treated patients and 29%/annum in the controls. (From Report of the Medical Research Council Working Party: Long term domiciliary oxygen therapy in chronic hypoxic cor pulmonale complicating chronic bronchitis and emphysema. Lancet 1:681–686, 1981)

established pulmonary hypertension, but the treatment did appear to prevent a further rise in total pulmonary vascular resistance in the treated group as compared with the control subjects. The report concluded that further studies were needed to clarify which patients would be most likely to benefit from supplemental oxygen and to establish whether in those who are less hypoxic supplemental oxygen might pre-

vent progression of their disease to cor pulmonale and premature death.

HEMODYNAMIC RESPONSES TO OXYGEN THERAPY

Some clarification of the questions posed in the multicenter trials may have been provided from studies that evaluated the hemodynamic response to oxygen therapy among chronically hypoxemic subjects. The following two studies addressed the influence of supplemental oxygen on pulmonary artery pressure. Ashutosh and coworkers[2] gave 28% supplemental oxygen for 24 hours a day to 28 stable hypoxemic patients with COPD and characterized them as responders (17 subjects) or nonresponders (11 subjects) depending on whether their mean pulmonary artery pressure fell by more than 5 mm Hg. The subjects were then prescribed continuous oxygen for a minimum of 18 hours/day and followed for the next 2 years. At the end of this period, 88% of the responders but only 22% of nonresponders were alive. Thus, there was a 2-year mortality of only 12% in responders but 78% in nonresponders. The authors concluded that a mean pulmonary artery pressure change of greater than 5 mm Hg after 24 hours of breathing supplemental oxygen may predict survival in those eligible for long-term domiciliary oxygen therapy. Weitzenblum and coworkers[43] reported the results of serial right-sided heart catheterizations in 16 subjects with COPD and stable hypoxia. The initial catheterization

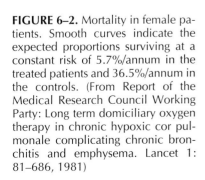

FIGURE 6–2. Mortality in female patients. Smooth curves indicate the expected proportions surviving at a constant risk of 5.7%/annum in the treated patients and 36.5%/annum in the controls. (From Report of the Medical Research Council Working Party: Long term domiciliary oxygen therapy in chronic hypoxic cor pulmonale complicating chronic bronchitis and emphysema. Lancet 1: 81–686, 1981)

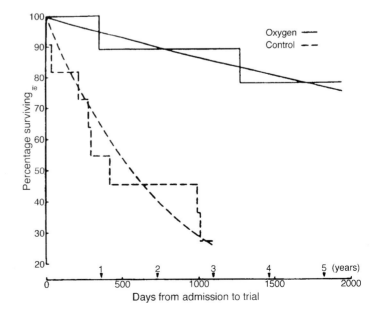

had been performed for diagnostic purposes and occurred 47 ± 28 months before the initiation of oxygen therapy. A second catheterization was performed just before oxygen therapy was started and a third after 31 ± 19 months of oxygen therapy of at least 15 hours/day titrated to achieve a PaO_2 of 65 mm Hg. All subjects continued to receive appropriate pharmacologic therapy and participated in a supervised exercise reconditioning program. In the 4 years before the supplemental oxygen, the PaO_2 for the 16 subjects decreased from 59 ± 9 to 50 ± 7 mm Hg, and the $PaCO_2$ increased from 43 ± 6 to 51 ± 6 mm Hg. The hematocrit increased from 51 ± 7 to 57 ± 6, and the mean pulmonary artery pressure increased from 23 ± 7 to 28 ± 7 mm Hg. Thirty-one months after supplemental oxygen, the hematocrit had fallen to 54 ± 8 and the mean pulmonary artery pressure to 24 ± 7 mm Hg. Thus, there had been an increase in pulmonary artery pressure of 1.5 ± 2 mm Hg before the onset of supplemental oxygen and a decrease of 2.1 ± 4 mm Hg in the period between the second and third catheterization. The mean values of the hemodynamic parameters at the three times (T_0, T_1, T_2) have been summarized (Table 6–2). The aforementioned two studies indicate that supplemental oxygen when administered to patients with COPD who are hypoxemic results in improvements in mean pulmonary artery pressure. Longer longitudinal studies are required to evaluate the influence of this improvement on morbidity and mortality.

CLINICAL STABILITY

The results of multicenter trials plus the technologic improvements in oxygen delivery have stimulated the widespread use of LTOT. It is essential, however, that subjects be clinically stable before the commencement of LTOT. In a study by Levi-Valensi and associates,[28] 77 patients in whom the initial PaO_2 was 41 to 59 mm Hg and who were thought to have been clinically stable for at least 1 month before entry into the study were followed for 3 months to evaluate the stability of their arterial hypoxemia. At the end of 3 months (Table 6–3), 23 subjects (30%) had a PaO_2 of greater than 59 mm Hg and therefore were no longer eligible for LTOT. These subjects could not be distinguished at baseline by their age, pulmonary function, or clinical history. The progressive pattern of improvement in PaO_2 meant that some individuals would have been accepted for LTOT had the follow-up period been limited to 1 or 2 months. The trend to improvement was less marked when the initial

TABLE 6–2
Comparison of the Mean Values of Hemodynamic Parameters at T_0 (47 months before oxygen), T_1 (immediately before oxygen), and T_2 (31 months after oxygen)*

	T_0	T_1	T_2	Difference T_0–T_1	Difference T_1–T_2	Difference T_0–T_2
Ppa, mm Hg	23.3 ± 6.8	28.0 ± 7.4	23.9 ± 6.6	$P < 0.005$	$P < 0.05$	NS
Ppa syst, mm Hg	35.8 ± 13.7	43.1 ± 12.8	37.4 ± 10.8	$P < 0.02$	$P < 0.05$	NS
Ppa, diast, mm Hg	15.7 ± 4.6	18.3 ± 5.9	16.2 ± 4.9	NS	NS	NS
RVEDP, mm Hg	4.1 ± 1.4[†]	5.4 ± 3.2	4.3 ± 2.6	NS	NS	NS
Pcw (mm Hg)	5.9 ± 1.4[†]	5.5 ± 2.7[‡]	5.7 ± 2.4[§]	—	—	—
Ppa-Pcw, mm Hg	17.4 ± 6.2[†]	21.3 ± 7.4[‡]	17.1 ± 4.7[§]	—	—	—
Q, L·in^{-1}·min	3.94 ± 0.79	3.87 ± 0.62	3.35 ± 0.82	NS	NS	NS
PVR, mm Hg·L^{-1}·min	2.41 ± 0.76[†]	3.27 ± 0.71[‡]	2.68 ± 0.51[§]	—	—	—
HR, beats·min^{-1}	82 ± 9	91 ± 14	89 ± 16	NS	NS	NS
SVI, mL/m^2	49 ± 13	44 ± 11	38 ± 11	NS	NS	$P < 0.01$
Mean systemic pressure, mm Hg	100.3 ± 11.1	98.0 ± 6.6	91.0 ± 8.0	NS	$P < 0.02$	$P < 0.02$

*Values are mean $\pm$ SD.
[†] n = 14.
[‡] n = 11.
[§] n = 8.
Ppa syst = Systolic pulmonary artery pressure; Ppa diast = diastolic pulmonary artery pressure; RVEDP = right ventricular end-diastolic pressure; PcW = pulmonary capillary wedge pressure; Q = cardiac index; PVR = pulmonary vascular resistance; HR = heart rate; SVI = stroke volume index.
From Weitzenblum E, Sautegeau A, Ehrhart M, et al: Long term oxygen therapy can reverse the progression of pulmonary hypertension in patients with chronic obstructive pulmonary disease. Am Rev Respir Dis 131:493–498, 1985.

PaO$_2$ was lower. Of those with an initial PaO$_2$ below 50 mm Hg (19 subjects), only one became ineligible for the study at 3 months.

SAFETY OF SUPPLEMENTAL OXYGEN AMONG CLINICALLY STABLE PATIENTS

It has long been appreciated that acute hypercapnia may develop in some patients with obstructive lung disease when treated with supplemental oxygen and that this complication is most apt to occur among patients who have chronic carbon dioxide retention. The issue of carbon dioxide retention was not addressed in the two major prospective studies of supplemental oxygen. The documentation of carbon dioxide retention especially during sleep has been limited by the need to sample arterial blood repeatedly through an indwelling arterial line for measurements of the partial pressure of arterial carbon dioxide (PaCO$_2$). PaCO$_2$ monitored transcutaneously, however, accurately reflects the trends in arterial PaCO$_2$. In a study of 15 patients with severe COPD with a resting daytime PaO$_2$ of 50.7 $\pm$ 1.4 mm Hg and a PaCO$_2$ of 53.1 $\pm$ 1.5 mm Hg, measurements were carried out on two consecutive nights.[21] On the first night, the subjects breathed room air, and on the second, they breathed supplemental oxygen sufficient to keep their SaO$_2$ at or above 90% (Figs. 6–3 and 6–4).[21] There were only small increases in PaCO$_2$ (<6 mm Hg) throughout sleep (Fig. 6–5). These increases occurred early in the

night and were not progressive. Larger increases in PaCO$_2$ were observed during sleep in three subjects (Fig. 6–6). Among these subjects, nighttime polysomnographic measurements showed obstructive sleep apnea in addition to obstructive lung disease. Therefore, it would appear that nocturnal oxygen therapy does not induce clinically important increases in PaCO$_2$ during sleep in patients with stable obstructive lung disease and can safely be used to prevent the consequences of hypoxia. In patients in whom a large PaCO$_2$ increase does develop during sleep or in whom morning headaches are reported, the coexistence of obstructive sleep apnea should be suspected.

SELECTING PATIENTS FOR LONG-TERM OXYGEN THERAPY

In a review of the criteria and indications for home oxygen therapy,[36] it was pointed out that LTOT could be helpful in a number of conditions other than COPD (Table 6–4). Supporting data for LTOT in such conditions, however, are

TABLE 6–3
Evolution of PaO$_2$ and PaCO$_2$ in Patients Who Remained Eligible (Group A) or Who Became Ineligible (Group B) For Long-Term Oxygen Therapy After 3 Months

	Group A (n=54) Mean $\pm$ SD	Group B(n=23) Mean $\pm$ SD
PaO$_2$ mm Hg		
T$_O$	51.3 (5.5)	54.5 (3.8)
T$_1$	52.2 (4.4)	56.0 (6.3)
T$_2$	51.1 (4.5)	61.2 (6.8)
T$_3$	51.6 (5.3)	63.4 (5.7)
PaCO$_2$ mm Hg		
T$_O$	48.5 (7.0)	47.5 (7.6)
T$_1$	47.1 (7.0)	46.2 (5.2)
T$_2$	47.9 (6.8)	47.3 (7.7)
T$_3$	48.9 (7.9)	45.0 (5.6)

T$_O$ = baseline; T$_1$–T$_3$ = 1-3 months after baseline respectively.
From Levi-Valensi P, Weitzenblum E, Pedinielli JL, et al: Three month follow up of arterial blood gas determinations in candidates for long term oxygen therapy.

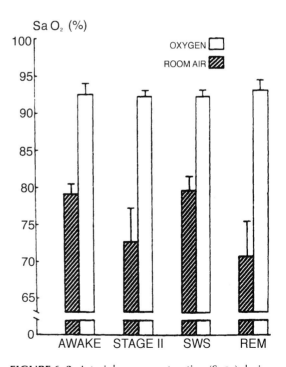

FIGURE 6–3. Arterial oxygen saturation (SaO$_2$) during air and oxygen breathing according to sleep stage. Values represent mean $\pm$ SE. SWS=Slow wave sleep; REM=rapid eye movement sleep. (From Goldstein RS, Ramcharan V, Bowes G, et al: Effect of supplemental nocturnal oxygen on gas exchange in patients with severe obstructive lung disease. N Engl J Med 310: 425–429, 1984.)

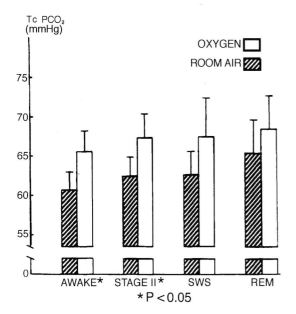

FIGURE 6-4. Transcutaneous carbon dioxide pressure during air and oxygen breathing according to sleep stage. Note the small increase in $PaCO_2$ with oxygen. (From Goldstein RS, Ramcharan V, Bowes G, et al: Effect of supplemental nocturnal oxygen on gas exchange in patients with severe obstructive lung disease. N Engl J Med 310:425–429, 1984.)

generally anecdotal because there is a lack of properly designed clinical trials. The decision to prescribe oxygen is therefore based on the clinician's judgment and experience. In the United States, there have been four conference reports on the prescription and supply of oxygen,[3,29,34] and an international review of the current status and indications for LTOT has been published.[35] A general consensus suggests that the prescription be based on

1. An appropriately documented diagnosis.
2. Concurrent optimal use of other rehabilitative approaches, such as pharmacotherapy, cessation of smoking, and exercise training.
3. Properly documented chronic hypoxemia.

In addition, nonclinical factors may influence the extent to which subjects may benefit from LTOT. These include

1. An acceptable home environment.
2. The ability and willingness of the patient to understand how to use supplemental oxygen in the community setting.
3. Realistic goals shared by the patient, caregivers, and health care team.

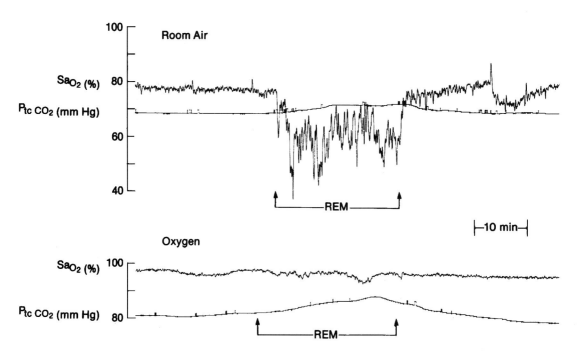

FIGURE 6-5. Tracings in a patient with chronic obstructive lung disease demonstrating the effects of oxygen and room air on arterial oxygen saturation (SaO_2) and transcutaneous carbon dioxide pressure ($P_{tc}CO_2$). Note the transient episodes of oxyhemoglobin desaturation while breathing room air during REM sleep and the relatively small increase in PCO_2 with supplemental oxygen. (From Goldstein RS, Ramcharan V, Bowes G, et al: Effect of supplemental nocturnal oxygen on gas exchange in patients with severe obstructive lung disease. N Engl J Med 310:425–429, 1984.)

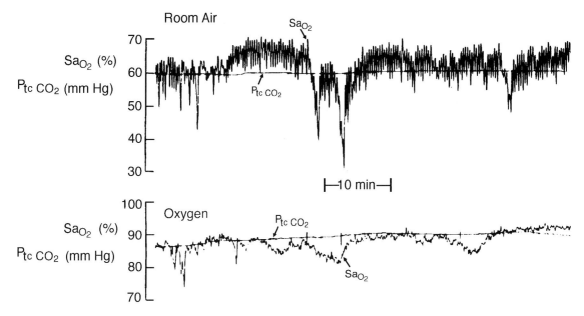

FIGURE 6–6. Tracings in a patient with chronic obstructive lung disease and obstructive sleep apnea demonstrating the effects of breathing room air and breathing supplemental oxygen on arterial oxyhemoglobin saturation (SaO_2) and transcutaneous carbon dioxide pressure ($P_{tc}CO_2$). With room air breathing, the tracing shows a swinging pattern of SaO_2 characteristic of sleep apnea. When breathing supplemental oxygen, SaO_2 rarely fell below 80% and the carbon dioxide level increased appreciably. (From Goldstein RS, Ramcharan V, Bowes G, et al: Effect of supplemental nocturnal oxygen on gas exchange in patients with severe obstructive lung disease. N Engl J Med 310:425–429, 1984.)

Current indications for LTOT in the United States are summarized in Table 6–5.[36] In most centers, although pulse oximetry readings are accepted for ongoing monitoring, arterial blood gas PaO_2 measurements are used to indicate the initiation of LTOT. The need for continued use of LTOT should be verified on an annual basis by the patient's physician, who should be knowledgeable as to the oxygen source (compressed gas cylinder, liquid oxygen, or concentrator), the delivery device (nasal cannulae,

Venturi mask, transtracheal catheter, conserving devices), and the appropriate flow to maintain SaO_2 in excess of 88% for 18 hours/day. The 1990 conference report on the supply, reimbursement, and certification of medical necessity for LTOT[34] suggested that those who receive home oxygen therapy usually fit into one of three groups:

1. Sedentary, bed-bound or home-bound patients or those requiring supplemental oxygen only during sleep—such individuals may require only a large-size cylinder for home use or a concentrator with a backup small cylinder for occasional use.
2. Ambulatory or mobile patients who occasionally leave the home—these patients can usually be managed with an oxygen concentrator and supplemental cylinders on a stroller for portability.
3. Highly mobile, ambulatory patients who leave home several times each week for several hours at a time—these individuals benefit from highly portable systems such as lightweight cylinders or small portable liquid units to which conserving devices can be interfaced.

TABLE 6–4
Conditions Other Than COPD for Which Long-Term Oxygen Therapy Might be of Benefit

Cystic fibrosis	Interstitial lung disease
Sequelae of tuberculosis	Bronchiectasis
Kyphoscoliosis	Sequelae of neuro-muscular disease
Sleep apnea syndromes	Chronic mountain sickness
Pulmonary hypertension	Lung cancer
Congestive heart failure	Sickle cell anemia

Modified from Pierson DJ: Criteria and indications for home oxygen therapy. In Kira S, Petty TL (eds): Progress in Domiciliary Respiratory Care—Current Status and Perspective. New York, Elsevier Science BV, 1994, pp 149–152.

TABLE 6–5
Indications for Long-Term Oxygen Therapy

Diagnosis of chronic obstructive pulmonary disease*,†
Clinical stability
Other aspects of medical management optimized (e.g., bronchodilator therapy, diuretics, reconditioning
    exercises) according to indiviudal needs of patient
Documentation of hypoxemia, while awake, at rest‡
A. PaO_2 <55 mm Hg (<7.3 kPa)§ or
B. PaO_2 55–59 mm Hg (7.3–7.8 kPa)§ *plus* evidence of significant end organ dysfunction due to chronic
    hypoxia, as shown by one or more of the following:
        P pulmonale (P waves 3 mm or more in lead II, III or a Vf of ECG)
        Clinical right-sided heart failure (pedal edema)
        Erythrocytosis (hematocrit over 55%)
Demonstration that hypoxemia is chronic, by follow-up assessment, breathing room air, at least 3–4 wk after
    above criteria are met, by either:
        Persistence of above P_aO_2 findings or
        SaO_2 <89% for condition A above∥
        SaO_2 89% for condition B above∥
Appropriate social and economic resources
Physical/psychological compatability of patient to use apparatus appropriately and safely
Willingness of patient to comply with prescribed regimen

*Diagnosis of COPD assumes appropriate spirometric evidence of obstruction (i.e., reduced FEV_1/FVC ratio), although no
threshold level of severity for FEV_1 or $PaCO_2$ is generally applied in the United States.
†These indications may also apply to patients with other chronic pulmonary conditions (e.g., interstitial pulmonary fibrosis, cystic fibrosis, kyphoscoliosis), although this has not been proved in terms of increased survival and other benefits.
‡If the patient does not meet these arterial oxygenation criteria at rest, while awake, but does so during exercise or sleep,
long-term oxygen therapy is appropriate at those times but not continuously.
§Although arterial oxyhemoglobin saturation measurements using pulse or ear oximetry are currently acceptable for reimbursement purposes in the United States, these do not provide sufficient physiologic assessment for *initiation* of therapy. They
may be used in follow-up, as shown.
∥If criteria are not met according to results of oximetry at follow-up, arterial blood gas measurements should be obtained.
From Pierson DJ: Criteria and indications for home oxygen therapy. *In* Kira S, Petty TL (eds): Progress in Domiciliary Respiratory Care—Current Status and Perspective. New York, Elsevier Science BV, 1994, pp 115–124.

In practice, the decision as to whether an individual receives liquid oxygen, cylinders, or a concentrator is often driven by economics. In the United Kingdom,[37] liquid oxygen is rarely available because it is expensive, so oxygen is mainly supplied in large 1350-L cylinders from contracted chemists. The chemists are responsible for the delivery and removal of the cylinders as well as the provision of adequate reducing valves, tubing, and masks. Oxygen concentrators are used for those not receiving large cylinders. In Japan,[1] more than 80% of patients use oxygen concentrators with liquid oxygen having been officially approved as of 1990. In Italy, liquid oxygen requires only a family practitioner's prescription, which has led to about 75% of patients using liquid oxygen and only 20% using concentrators.[14] In the United States, where approximately 800,000 citizens receive LTOT, all three oxygen delivery systems have been available for many years. Liquid systems used to be the most widespread because they were the most profitable, but in recent years, as a result of adjustments in the reimbursement schedule,

concentrators have become the most prevalent modality. In countries such as Canada and the United States, any licensed physician may prescribe supplemental oxygen, whereas in countries such as Australia and Spain prescription is by specialists only. A home health care survey in Spain[32] carried out over a period of 1 year on 620 patients who received LTOT concluded that only 40% of patients fulfilled the criteria and that two thirds of the patients indicated that they used supplemental oxygen for fewer than 5 hours/day. Subsequently, new regulations were established in 1991 introducing broadly accepted criteria and limiting the number of prescribing centers to those with access to a respiratory specialist and a pulmonary function laboratory. The authors observed that the total number of patients on LTOT decreased and the use of concentrators increased.

PHYSICIAN EDUCATION

In the author's view, entering into a debate as to whether oxygen should continue to be prescribed by any licensed physician or whether its prescription should be limited to those who specialize in respiratory or internal medicine is potentially divisive and broadly irrelevant. More importantly, in the interest of both health and economics, the prescribing physician must understand the indications for oxygen therapy and be familiar with the various systems available for the supply and delivery of oxygen best to provide good health care at a reasonable cost. Education programs with certification, plus monitoring of prescription patterns by peer audit, would alleviate many of the discrepancies currently found among physicians who prescribe oxygen.

TRANSIENT HYPOXEMIA DURING SLEEP AND EXERCISE

This section addresses the prescription of supplemental oxygen for the transient hypoxemia that can occur during sleep or exercise. The clinical benefit of treating transient hypoxemia remains unclear in the absence of long-term controlled trials with clearly defined clinical outcome measures.

Transient Hypoxemia During Sleep

Several studies have demonstrated that during sleep, patients with COPD are prone to episodes of arterial SaO_2, often to a profound degree.[16,30] Such episodes of hypoxemia have been associated with nocturnal cardiac arrhythmias and with acute increases in pulmonary arterial pressure. They have been implicated in the development of chronic pulmonary hypertension and cor pulmonale. Although most reports address patients with COPD, patients with cystic fibrosis and those with nonobstructive ventilatory conditions such as interstitial lung disease, neuromuscular disease, or thoracic restrictive disease may also exhibit nighttime desaturation. Several attempts have been made to predict the presence of nocturnal desaturation from daytime clinical measurements. Although the overall predictive value is low, it appears as though those who desaturate more at night have a lower daytime PaO_2, some evidence of blunted chemosensitivity, and more severe respiratory dysfunction. Managing nocturnal hypoxemia is attractive because it may prevent progression of pulmonary hypertension to cor pulmonale and

premature death. The evidence to support this hypothesis, however, remains equivocal.

In a report of 135 subjects with COPD, Fletcher and associates[17] noted that during sleep 37 subjects desaturated below 90% for 5 minutes or more, reaching a nadir of 85% or lower. Those who would desaturate could not be identified based on their pulmonary function, but it was noted that their awake PaO_2 at rest was lower and that their $PaCO_2$ was higher than those who did not desaturate. In another study of 48 patients with severe but stable COPD (Table 6–6), Bradley and coworkers[6] attempted to develop a clinically relevant model to determine which factors measured in the awake state might predict the degree of nocturnal hypoxemia. Using stepwise multiple linear regression with the mean nocturnal SaO_2 as the dependent variable, it was found that the supine awake SaO_2 and the $PaCO_2$ correlated significantly and independently with the mean nocturnal SaO_2 and together accounted for 68% of its variability (Table 6–7). Although the FEV_1 had an influence on the mean nocturnal SaO_2, the impact of FEV_1 was lost when its effects on the mean awake SaO_2 and the awake $PaCO_2$ were taken into account. Applied prospectively to 26 similar patients (Fig. 6–7), there was a good correlation between the predicted and observed mean nocturnal SaO_2.[6]

In a 3-year trial of oxygen therapy for COPD patients with transient nocturnal hypoxemia,[18] 38 subjects with known desaturation were randomized to receive either supplemental oxygen or sham oxygen. On follow-up, the nocturnal desaturators who received supplemental oxygen showed a decrease in pulmonary artery pressure of 3.7 mm Hg, whereas during the same period, those untreated had an increase in pulmonary artery pressure by 3.9 mm Hg. Thus, it would appear that nighttime supplemental oxygen may halt the progression of pulmonary hypertension, but whether mortality or morbidity is influenced requires a much larger and more prolonged trial.

Nocturnal Desaturation in Nonobstructive Conditions

In 13 subjects with interstitial lung disease, Bye and colleagues[9] identified decreases in SaO_2, especially during rapid eye movement (REM) sleep, which were associated with decreased excursion of the chest wall and abdomen. The mean duration of these transient episodes of desaturation was 28 seconds; the to-

TABLE 6–6
Variables Entered into Statistical Analysis of
Correlates of Mean Nocturnal SaO₂ and Lowest
Nocturnal SaO₂ for 48 COPD Patients

Variables	Value
Anthropomorphic	
Age, yr	64±9
Weight, BMI	22.3±3.6
Respiratory physiologic	
TLC, % predicted	132±24
FRC, % predicted	189±54
RV, % predicted	228±78
ERV, % predicted	104±66
FVC, % predicted	61±21
FEV$_1$, % predicted	32±15
FEV$_1$/FVC, %	39±10
V$_{50}$, % predicted	12±7
V$_{25}$, % predicted	13±7
Raw, L/s/cm H$_2$O	3.7±1.6
DCO, % predicted	41±15
MIP at RV, cm H$_2$O	−54±23
MEP at TLC, cm H$_2$O	141±43
Awake pH	7.43±0.33
Awake PaO$_2$ mm Hg	64±10
Awake PaCO$_2$ mm Hg	42±7
Awake baseline SaO$_2$, %	93±4

BMI = Body mass index; TLC = total lung capacity; FRC = functional residual capacity; RV = residual volume; ERV = expiratory reserve volume; FVC = forced vital capacity; FEV$_1$ = forced expired volume in 1 second; V$_{50}$ = maximal expiratory flow at 50% VC; V$_{25}$ = maximal expiratory flow at 25% VC; Raw = airway resistance, DCO = single breath diffusing capacity for carbon monoxide; MIP = maximum inspiratory pressure; MEP = maximal expiratory pressure.
From Bradley TD, Mateika J, Li D, et al: Daytime hypercapnia in the development of nocturnal hypoxemia in COPD. Chest 97:308–312, 1990.

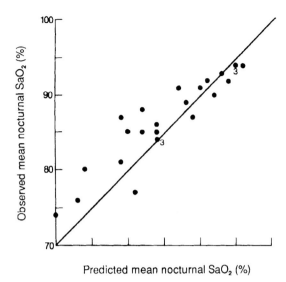

FIGURE 6–7. Predicted versus observed mean nocturnal SaO₂ in patients with COPD. Note that values fall close to the line of identity. The digit 3 indicates that the adjacent point represents three subjects with identical values. (From Bradley TD, Mateika J, Li D, et al: Daytime hypercapnia in the development of nocturnal hypoxemia in COPD. Chest 97:308–312, 1990.)

tal duration of 6.4 minutes represented approximately 60% of REM sleep (Table 6–8).[9] Whether or not treatment of such isolated nocturnal hypoxemia influences morbidity remains unanswered. A number of reports have identified nocturnal desaturation among patients with thoracic restrictive diseases, usually accompanied by an elevation in PaCO₂. Among such individuals, oxygen alone, even at low flow rates, prevents the nocturnal desaturation but frequently results in a marked elevation in PaCO₂. Therefore, although supplemental oxygen may be appropriate initially, mechanical ventilatory support is the preferred therapy (Fig. 6–8).[20]

Transient Hypoxemia During Exercise

Many patients with a resting SaO₂ above 90% exhibit exercise desaturation. Often the decrease in SaO₂ occurs within the first minute, after which the SaO₂ remains constant. Occasionally, there is a progressive decline in SaO₂ with exercise. In a study of 38 subjects in whom the mean resting SaO₂ was 93±3%, a decrease in SaO₂ of 4.7±3.6% (range 1% to 18%) was observed by D'Urzo and colleagues[15] during submaximal exercise. Using stepwise multiple linear regression analysis with mean exercise SaO₂ as the dependent variable, resting SaO₂ and diffusion were found to exert a significant independent effect on the mean exercise SaO₂. A model of mean exercise SaO₂ derived from this statistical analysis was applied to a subsequent group of 19 similar patients and revealed a high degree of correlation (r = 0.85, P±0.001) between the predicted and observed values. Decreases in SaO₂ were noted at physical activity levels comparable to those often encountered during activities of daily living.

The observations of D'Urzo were confirmed in a study by Mak and colleagues.[31] In this study, the mean level of SaO₂ during exercise correlated with the single breath diffusion for carbon monoxide and the baseline mean SaO₂ for 42 patients with severe COPD. In addition, the authors found that the SaO₂ did not correlate with the walk distance (Fig. 6–9) or with the degree of perceived exertion or perceived breathless-

TABLE 6–7
Stepwise Multiple Linear Regression Analyses of Nocturnal SaO_2

Independent Variable	Regression Coefficient	Standard Error	Partial r^2	F	P
Dependent variable: mean nocturnal SaO_2*					
Baseline awake SaO_2	1.140	0.199	0.422	32.890	<0.0001
$PaCO_2$	−0.428	0.107	0.263	16.073	<0.0003
Constant	1.195				

Standard error of the estimate = 4.459
Multiple correlation coefficient (r) = 0.823
$r^2 = 0.679$

Dependent variable: lowest nocturnal SaO_2†					
Baseline awake SaO_2	2.018	0.463	0.296	18.958	<0.0001
$PaCO_2$	−1.147	0.249	0.320	21.214	<0.0001
Constant	−60.760				

Standard error of the estimate = 10.396
Multiple correlation coefficient (r) = 0.798
$r^2 = 0.637$

*Regression equation: predicted mean nocturnal SaO_2 = 1.948 +; baseline awake SaO_2 (1.140) − $PaCO_2$ (0.428).
†Regression equation: predicted lowest nocturnal SaO_2 = −60.760 +; baseline awake SaO_2 (2.018) − $PaCO_2$ (1.148).
From Bradley TD, Mateika J, Li D, et al: Daytime hypercapnia in the development of nocturnal hypoxemia in COPD. Chest 97:308–312, 1990.

TABLE 6–8
Duration of Each Transient Decrease in SaO_2 and Total Duration During Rapid Eye Movement in Nonsnorers

Patient No.	Each Transient Decrease* (s)	Total Duration (min)	Duration as % REM Sleep
1	48 (28)	9.6	30
2	24 (15)	4.0	9
3	23 (7)	8.3	16
4	37 (5)	2.4	7
5	19 (3)	11.7	32
6	16 (3)	2.6	3
Mean (SD)	28 (12)	6.4 (3.9)	16 (12)

*Mean (SD)
From Bye PTP, Anderson SD, Woolcock AJ, et al: Bicycle endurance performance of patients with interstitial lung disease breathing air and oxygen. Am Rev Respir Dis 126:1005–1012, 1982.

ness during 6-minute walks. Fifty percent of the total variance in distance walked, however, could be accounted for by diffusion, age, and peak expiratory flow. The authors concluded that although patients who consider themselves to be the most disabled by breathlessness do have the shortest 6-minute walk distance, they do not necessarily have appreciable desaturation with exercise.

Influence of Oxygen on Exercise Ability

Certainly the response to oxygen cannot be predicted from resting pulmonary function tests, echocardiographic measurements of right ventricular systolic pressure, or other clinical parameters.[13] In a study of 12 subjects with severe COPD, Dean and coworkers[13] noted that four patients more than doubled their duration of exercise while receiving 40% oxygen, but in only two of these was desaturation observed in the absence of oxygen. Bradley and colleagues[5] reported that in subjects with mild hypoxemia and exercise desaturation, supplemental oxygen by nasal prongs did not influence their maximum work rate but did influence their submaximal endurance time. There was no correlation between the degree of desaturation and the subsequent response to oxygen among the 26 subjects

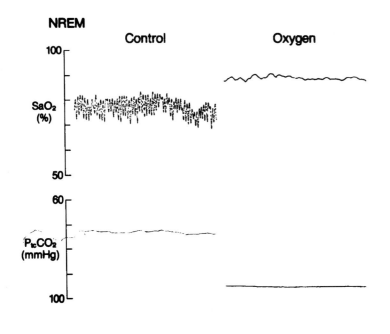

NREM

FIGURE 6–8. Recorder tracing of oxygen saturation and carbon dioxide tension during non-REM sleep in a patient with restrictive respiratory failure accompanied by frequent central apneas and hypopneas. *Left panel,* The patient is breathing room air and the saturation fluctuates between 70% and 80% with the $PaCO_2$ around 72 mm Hg. *Right panel,* sufficient supplemental oxygen has been administered to maintain oxygen saturation at 90%. Note the marked increase in $PaCO_2$ levels in excess of 95 mm Hg. (From Goldstein RS: Hypoventilation, neuromuscular and chest wall disorders. Clin Chest Med 13:507–521, 1992.)

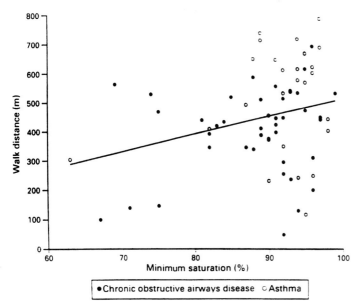

FIGURE 6–9. Scatterplot of 6-minute walk distance correlated with minimum saturation during the walk (r = 0.28, $P<0.05$). (From Mak VHF, Bugler JR, Roberts CM, et al: Effect of arterial oxygen desaturation on six minute walk distance, perceived effort, and perceived breathlessness in patients with airflow limitation. Thorax 48:33–38, 1993.)

studied. Oxygen supplementation might influence dyspnea by influencing chemoreceptor activity, but responses to hypoxia and hypercapnia do not appear to explain either dyspnea or exercise limitation in severe COPD.[39]

The mechanism by which exercise endurance can increase is poorly understood. What has become clear is that during exercise, supplemental oxygen does not uniformly reduce breathlessness or minute ventilation.[12] Davidson and associates[2] noted that oxygen increased the mean walking endurance time by 59% and

the 6-minute walking distance by 17%. Moreover, submaximal cycle time at a constant workload was increased by 51% at a flow rate of 2 L/minute and by 88% at 4 L/minute, suggesting a dose-response curve. Neither the resting SaO_2 nor the abolition of exercise-induced desaturation, however, correlated with the improvement in exercise endurance. In a follow-up paper,[27] the same authors recommended that portable oxygen should be considered only for patients for whom it is shown to improve exercise ability by 50%.

There are still fewer studies that have evaluated the influence of oxygen on exercise among patients with interstitial lung disease. In one such study,[8] maximum working capacity was not influenced, but submaximal endurance improved. The increase in endurance with oxygen correlated with the change in SaO_2 during exercise on room air.

Although a number of studies have suggested that supplemental oxygen may alleviate exercise-induced hypoxemia, reduce dyspnea on exertion, and increase exercise tolerance, the mechanism and influence of supplemental oxygen in the management of transient hypoxemia with exercise remains unclear. This has led to considerable confusion and variety in the prescription of oxygen under such circumstances. Long-term studies are necessary both to clarify the clinical circumstances under which oxygen may be beneficial and to justify its cost to third-party payers. For the present, it is reasonable to recommend that measurements of dyspnea and exercise tolerance be undertaken with and without supplemental oxygen to determine which individuals are less short of breath or walk further when given supplemental oxygen.

METHODS OF OXYGEN DELIVERY

Although a variety of patient interfaces are available (open face masks, Venturi masks, partial rebreathing and nonrebreathing masks), oxygen is most often administered to the stable patient at home, at a predetermined low flow rate via nasal cannulae. In practice, 1 to 2 L/minute at rest and an additional 1 to 2 L/minute during exercise is probably the most common prescription. For patients with no parenchymal disease (thoracic restrictive disease or neuromuscular disease), a lower flow rate is preferred because among these individuals supplemental oxygen may result in marked increases in $PaCO_2$. Although the effective FiO_2 is said to be independent of whether the subject inhales nasally or orally,[22] some authors have noted that during mouth breathing, speaking, and exercising, oxygen delivery may vary. A new applicator with an enlarged outlet area creates additional turbulence that reduces the variance of the effects of oral or nasal breathing on oxygen delivery.[25] It may also minimize the drying effect that supplemental oxygen may have on the mucous membranes. Transtracheal oxygen therapy has been reported as both effective and safe, but despite a variety of reports attesting to its benefits,[23] its overall acceptance has been limited by the expense of the equipment, the procedures relating to insertion of the transtracheal catheter, and the complications of infection and mucous plugs that have been reported. Conventional methods of oxygen supply include cylinders of compressed gas, liquid oxygen, and concentrators. An excellent review of equipment for the supply and delivery of oxygen has been published by Cooper.[11]

Compressed Gas Cylinders

In compressed gas cylinders, oxygen is stored under pressure and down-regulated to approximately 50 PSI proximal to the flowmeter. The cylinders themselves vary in size, weight, and capacity. They are relatively inexpensive. They may be used either as a stationary oxygen source at home or for portability, particularly when they are small and lightweight (Table 6–9).

Liquid Oxygen

Liquid Oxygen may be delivered by a low-pressure system with relatively lightweight units for portability that can be transfilled from larger reservoirs. Liquid oxygen tends to be more expensive than pressurized gas, but it facilitates mobility. Although lightweight portable units can provide flows for several hours only, their duration may be extended if an oxygen conserver is placed in line with the delivery system (Table 6–10).

Oxygen Concentrators

Oxygen concentrators are the cheapest and currently the most popular method of providing supplemental oxygen. The two principal types use either molecular sieves or membrane separators. The servicing requirements are minimal, and an oxygen concentration in excess of 90% can be provided. The performance of oxygen concentrators, however, deteriorates at high flow rates. The disadvantage of concentrators is that they do not offer the portability of small cylinders or of liquid systems because they tend to be large units powered by alternating current. This may change with the technologic advances toward smaller and lighter battery-powered concentrators (Table 6–11).

OXYGEN-CONSERVING DEVICES

There has been increasing interest in reducing the cost of oxygen therapy and extending

TABLE 6–9
Equipment for Oxygen Supply

Apparatus	Weight (lb)	Capacity (L)	Performance
Cylinders			
H-size	150.0	6840	57.0 h at 2 L/min
G-size	—	3600	—
F-size	—	1360	—
E-size	17.0	680	5.0 h at 2 L/min
E-size (aluminum)	13.0	680	5.0 h at 2 L/min
E-size (Oxymatic)	—	680	40.0 h at 2 L/min
D-size	—	420	3.5 h at 2 L/min
D-size (Oxymatic)	—	420	3.5 h at 2 L/min
C-size	—	240	2.0 h at 2 L/min
C-size (Aluminum)	10.0	240	2.0 h at 2 L/min
C-size (Oxymatic)	—	240	14.0 h at 2 L/min
Mini (Oxylite)	4.0	—	9.5 h at 2 L/min

From Cooper CB: Long term oxygen therapy. *In* Casaburi R, Petty T (eds): Principles and Practice of Pulmonary Rehabilitation. Philadelphia, WB Saunders, 1993, pp 183–203.

TABLE 6–10
Equipment for Oxygen Supply

Apparatus	Weight (lb)	Capacity (L)	Performance
Liquid			
Walker (Linde)	6.5	—	4.0 h at 2 L/min
C-1000 (Puritan Bennett)	7.5	—	8.5 h at 2 L/min
C-T (Puritan Bennett)	8.4	—	—
OMS I (Pulsair)	7.5	400	10.0 h at 2 L/min
OMS II (Pulsair)	10.3	824	23.0 h at 2 L/min

From Cooper CB: Long term oxygen therapy. *In* Casaburi R, Petty T (eds): Principles and Practice of Pulmonary Rehabilitation. Philadelphia, WB Saunders, 1993, pp 183–203.

the portability of liquid and cylinder systems. If a patient breathes at 20 breaths/minute and has an inspiratory-to-expiratory ratio of 1:2, the inspiratory tidal volume would be delivered in 1 second. In fact, the last part of the inspiratory flow remains as airway dead space and contributes minimally to gas exchange. Therefore, if oxygen is delivered by continuous flow, much of it is wasted during the latter part of the inspiratory phase and during all of the expiratory phase. For this reason, a number of new conserving devices have become available.

Moustache and Pendant Storage Nasal Cannula :

Tiep and coworkers[41] described an oxygen-conserving nasal cannula with a storage reservoir that fits over the moustache area of the face. The goal of this device was to increase the amount of oxygen flow during early inspiration and thereby achieve adequate SaO_2 while reducing the total oxygen delivered. At flows of 0.5 L/minute, SaO_2 reached levels normally achieved at 2 L/minute with continuous flow cannulae. Patient acceptance was limited because the moustache reservoir was obtrusive. Subsequently the cannula was redesigned with the conservation component displaced to the chest in the form of a pendant. In seven subjects with stable COPD in whom the mean SaO_2 while breathing room air was $88.4 \pm 2.8\%$, the mean SaO_2 when receiving at 0.5 L/minute via a standard cannula was $90 \pm 2.9\%$ and was $93.2 \pm 2.7\%$ with a pendant conserver (Table 6–12). At 1 L/minute, the mean SaO_2 was $91 \pm 3.1\%$ with the standard cannula and $95.3 \pm 2.4\%$ with the pendant. Thus, the pendant oxygen-conserving cannula provided effective oxygen delivery at reduced flow rates when compared with the standard cannula. The estimated oxygen savings

TABLE 6–11
Equipment for Oxygen Supply

Apparatus	Weight (lb)	Performance
Membrane sieves		
PVO2D (DeVilbiss)	46	93% O_2 at 3 L/min
MC44D (DeVilbiss)	48	90% O_2 at 5 L/min
H-300 (Healthdyne)	40	90% O_2 at 3 L/min
BX-5000 (Healthdyne)	53	90% O_2 at 5 L/min
DC-100* (Roman)	29	93% O_2 at 2 L/min
AC-300* (Roman)	34	93% O_2 at 3 L/min
Emperor (Roman)	49	93% O_2 at 5 L/min
Mobilaire III (Invacare)	51	94% O_2 at 3 L/min
Mobilaire V (Invacare)	54	94% O_2 at 5 L/min
Spirit (Kee-Ox)	46	93% O_2 at 3 L/min
Elite (Kee-Ox)	56	90% O_2 at 5 L/min
429a (Puritan Bennett)		92% O_2 at 4 L/min
590 (Puritan Bennett)		90% O_2 at 5 L/min
Membrane separators		
Oxycare	35	45% O_2 at 10 L/min
OE Plus (Gulfstream)	68	40% O_2 at 6 L/min

(Values of % are ± 3%)
*Samsonite suitcase.
From Cooper CB: Long term oxygen therapy. *In* Casaburi R, Petty T (eds): Principles and Practice of Pulmonary Rehabilitation. Philadelphia, WB Saunders, 1993, pp 183–203.

TABLE 6–12
Oxyhemoglobin Saturation Achieved in 7 Patients by Using the Pendant Conserver Nasal Cannula Versus the Steady-Flow Cannula

	O_2 (L/min)	Patient No.							Mean O_2 Saturation
		1	2	3	4	5	6	7	
Steady-flow nasal Cannula									
	0.5	93	92	86.5	86	88.5	92	92	90 (2.9)
	1.0	93.5	94	86.5	87	91	93	93	93 (3.1)
	2.0	95	94.5	92	94.5	95	95	93	93 (1.3)
	3.0	96	96	94	96	97	96	94	95 (1.1)
	4.0	97	97	97	97.5	96	96	95	96 (0.8)
Pendant conserver cannula									
	0.5	94.5	96	88	92	94	95.5	93	93.3 (2.7)
	1.0	96	97	90.5	96	96	97.5	94	95.3 (2.4)
	2.0	97	97	96	97	97	99	95	96.8 (1.2)

From Tiep BL, Belman MJ, Mittman C, et al: A new pendant storage oxygen-conserving nasal cannula. Chest 87:381–383, 1985.

may be as high as 50% for many patients with COPD but only 14% among patients with restrictive lung disorders.[40]

Demand Oxygen-Conserving Devices

Given that in subjects with obstructive lung disease, one third of the respiratory cycle is in the inspiratory phase and only the initial portion of the inspired volume reaches the lungs' gas exchange membranes, demand delivery devices have been designed to deliver a bolus of oxygen only during the early part of inspiration. Oxygen sparing increases at lower respiratory rates. Several such devices are available that can be attached to existing oxygen supply systems and result in substantial savings whether used at rest or during exercise. In nine hypoxemic patients with COPD, an electronic demand oxygen delivery system (DODS) was evaluated.[42] The DODS could sense the beginning of inhalation and direct a solenoid valve to open momentarily to permit the delivery of a 32-mL bolus of oxygen. The delivery pulse was completed within 200 msec after the onset of inhalation. The amount of oxygen delivered to the patient could be adjusted by varying the number of breaths/minute during which oxygen is pulsed to the patient. For example, at a setting of 1, the oxygen pulse occurs only once in four breaths, while at a setting of four, the oxygen pulse occurs with each breath. The authors concluded that oxygen savings with the DODS was in excess of 7:1 both at rest and during exercise when compared to steady flow delivery.

Bower and colleagues[4] evaluated the efficacy of another DODS during rest, sleep, and exercise and noted savings of 45% at rest, 44% during exercise, and 39% during sleep when compared with a standard continuous flow system. The system used a standard nasal cannula to deliver a pulse of oxygen in response to a negative pressure of -0.04 cm H_2O sensed within the cannula. The volume of each oxygen pulse varied continuously in response to the sensed respiratory rate. In a subsequent study, the same device was used by six patients with COPD and six patients with idiopathic pulmonary fibrosis. Again, comparable levels of oxygenation were achieved, and the device triggered appropriately even during exercise at high respiratory rates. In another study, pulsed oxygen flow was alternated with continuous oxygen delivery over 5.5-hour intervals for 100 hospitalized patients. Similar levels of SaO_2 were achieved but with substantial cost savings in the pulsed oxygen group.[24] DODSs are reasonable options for reducing the cost of oxygen therapy and extending the duration of ambulation possible using a portable reservoir. This must be balanced against the initial equipment costs and the bulky appearance of the oxygen-conserving device. When various conserving devices were compared, resting levels of SaO_2 were found to be similar, but there were differences in the mean

TABLE 6–13
Hemodynamic and Ventilatory Effects of Steady-State Submaximal Exercise

	Room Air	30% Oxygen	50% Oxygen
15 Watts			
Ventilation (L/min)	23.0 (4.6)	22.7 (4.8)	21.1 (3.7)
Respiratory rate (br/min)	20.8 (3.2)	20.0 (5.9)	18.6 (4.8)*
Cardiac output (L/min)	6.7 (2.3)	5.9 (2.1)	6.5 1.8)
Tidal volume (L)	1.2 (0.2)	1.3 (0.5)	1.26 (0.57)
Stroke volume (mL)	73 (36)	60 (26)	74 (31)
Heat rate (beats/min)	99 (18)	102 (15)	98 (18)
O_2 delivery (mL/min)	1250 450)	1184 (423)	1308 (390)
30 Watts			
Ventilation (L/min)	29.4 (7.0)	24.9 (4.1)	23.9 (5.9)†
Respiratory rate (br/min)	22.3 (4.4)	20.9 (5.2)	19.0 (5.6)*
Tidal volume (L)	1.4 (0.6)	1.3 (0.5)	1.4 (0.8)
Cardiac output (L/min)	6.6 (2.3)	6.0 (1.6)	6.2 (1.7)
Stroke volume (mL)	68 (35)	59 (20)	65 (31)
Heart rate (beats/min)	105 (19)	108 (16)	101 (20)*
O_2 delivery (mL/min)	1316 (438)	1253 (401)	1263 (378)
40 Watts			
Ventilation (L/min)	36.1 (8.6)	32.9 (5.2)*	28.1 (5.9)‡
Respiratory rate (br/min)	25.6 (7.6)	23.7 (6.7)	21.7 (6.6)*
Tidal volume (L)	1.6 (0.6)	1.6 (0.8)	1.4 (0.6)*
Cardiac output (L/min)	7.3 (2.3)	6.6 (1.8)	6.5 (1.9)*
Stroke volume (mL)	65 (34)	61 (27)	61 (31)
Heart rate (beats/min)	112 (21)	112 (18)	107 (21)*
O_2 deliv ry (mL/min)	1404 (409)	1471 (430)	1440 (388)

Values shown as mean (SD).
*$P <0.05$ vs room air.
†$P <0.01$ vs room air.
‡ <0.001 vs room air.
From Moore DP, Weston AR, Hughes JMB, et al: Effects of increased inspired oxygen concentrations on exercise performance in chronic heart failure. Lancet 339:850–853, 1992.

SaO_2 levels recorded during exercise.[7] In at least one of the subjects, each device was associated with SaO_2 levels that fell to less than 80% during walking. With the variation in individual responses, a conclusion was reached that individuals who receive home oxygen therapy should be tested during exercise with the specific delivery system that is being considered for use during exercise.

OXYGEN CONSERVATION IN INTERSTITIAL LUNG DISEASE

Eight patients with interstitial pulmonary fibrosis[10] were evaluated at rest and during 5 minutes of treadmill exercise at 0.7 to 1 mph using a steady flow of oxygen and a demand delivery system. At rest, the improvements in SaO_2 were similar with both systems, but the amount of oxygen required to produce them was substantially less for the demand system, 216 mL/minute versus 1000 mL/minute, a saving of more than 75%. During exercise, the oxygen requirements were seven times higher for the steady flow system as compared with the demand system. Thus, the DODS can achieve adequate SaO_2 at rest and during exercise in patients with restrictive lung disease while using only a fraction of the oxygen required under steady flow conditions.

EFFECTS OF OXYGEN IN CHRONIC HEART FAILURE

One of the relatively unexplored roles for supplemental oxygen is in patients with chronic heart failure. In a study by Moore and associates,[33] 12 subjects with chronic congestive heart failure underwent serial, submaximal, and maximal exercise tests at inspired oxygen concentrations of 21%, 30%, and 50%. The mean exercise duration during progressive exercise testing was prolonged from 548 ± 276 seconds on room air to 632 ± 285 seconds on 50% oxygen (Table 6–13). During steady-state exercise at 45 watts, 50% oxygen was associated with an increased SaO_2 $97.5 \pm 1.3\%$ versus $94.6 \pm 1.9\%$ and significantly reduced minute ventilation, 28.1 ± 5.9 L/minute versus 36.1 ± 8.6 L/minute. The authors concluded that supplemental oxygen increased exercise efficiency at submaximal workloads with a dose-response relationship between the concentration of inspired oxygen and the change in ventilation and cardiac output (Fig. 6–10). This raises yet another interesting physiologic and clinical challenge. It appears

that the mechanism for improving exercise tolerance with supplemental oxygen is quite unclear because during this study the SaO_2 values were above 92%. Undoubtedly, this will be a rich area of inquiry over the next few years.

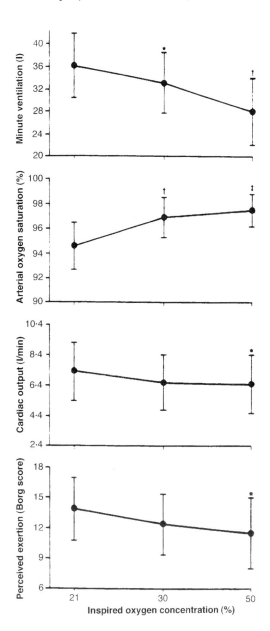

FIGURE 6–10. Effects of steady-state exercise at 45 watts and breathing 21%, 30%, and 50% inspired oxygen concentrations on minute ventilation (*top*), SaO_2 (*upper middle panel*), cardiac output (*lower middle panel*), and Borg score for perceived exertion (*bottom panel*) (*$P<0.05$, $P <0.01$, $P <0.01$). (From Fleetham J, West P, Mezon B, et al: Sleep, arousals and oxygen desaturation in chronic obstructive pulmonary disease: the effect of oxygen therapy. Am Rev Respir Dis 126:429–433, 1982.)

CONCLUSIONS

Although LTOT remains an important part of the continuum of care aimed at improving the quality of life and exercise tolerance of patients with chronic cardiorespiratory conditions, many unanswered questions remain. Optimal dosage and mode of delivery of supplemental oxygen and the indications for the treatment of transient hypoxemia during exercise and sleep remain to be determined. To optimize health care delivery in an era of cost containment, physicians must maintain a current understanding of the indications and expected benefits of oxygen therapy. In addition, they should be actively involved in the prescription of dosage and mode of delivery and regularly evaluate these decisions within the context of the patient's medical and psychosocial situation.

Acknowledgment

Supported in part by West Park Hospital Foundation and the Network of Centres of Excellence–Respiratory Health.

The author is indebted to Diane Peterson for assistance in the preparation of this manuscript.

References

1. Aida M, Takahashi H, Tsutomu S, et al: Current status of home oxygen therapy in Japan. *In* Kira S, Petty TL (eds): Progress in Domiciliary Respiratory Care—Current Status and Perspective. New York, Elsevier Science BV, 1994, pp 41–48.
2. Ashutosh K, Mead G, Dunsky M: Early effects of oxygen administration and prognosis in chronic obstructive pulmonary disease and cor pulmonale. Am Rev Respir Dis 127:399–404, 1983.
3. Block JA, Cherniack RM, Christopher KL: Conference report: Problems in prescribing and supplying oxygen for medicare patients. Am Rev Respir Dis 134:340–341, 1986.
4. Bower JS, Brook CJ, Zimmer K, et al: Performance of a demand oxygen saver system during rest, exercise and sleep in hypoxemic patients. Chest 94:77–80, 1988.
5. Bradley BL, Garner AE, Billiu D, et al: Oxygen assisted exercise in chronic obstructive lung disease: The effect on exercise capacity and arterial blood gas tensions. Am Rev Respir Dis 118:239–243, 1978.
6. Bradley TD, Mateika J, Li D, et al: Daytime hypercapnia in the development of nocturnal hypoxemia in COPD. Chest 97:308–312, 1990.
7. Braun SR, Spratt G, Scott GC, et al: Comparison of six oxygen delivery systems for COPD patients at rest and during exercise. Chest 102:694–698, 1992.
8. Bye PTP, Anderson SD, Woolcock AJ, et al: Bicycle endurance performance of patients with interstitial lung disease breathing air and oxygen. Am Rev Respir Dis 126:1005–1012, 1982.
9. Bye PTP, Issa F, Berthon-Jones M, et al: Studies of oxygenation during sleep in patients with interstitial lung disease. Am Rev Respir Dis 129:27–32, 1984.
10. Carter R, Tashkin D, Djahed B, et al: Demand oxygen delivery for patients with restrictive lung disease. Chest 96:1307–1311, 1989.
11. Cooper CB: Long term oxygen therapy. *In* Casaburi R, Petty T (eds): Principles and Practice of Pulmonary Rehabilitation. Philadelphia, WB Saunders, 1993, pp 183–203.
12. Davidson AC, Leach R, George RJD, et al: Supplemental oxygen and exercise ability in chronic obstructive airways disease. Thorax 43:965–971, 1988.
13. Dean NC, Brown JK, Himelman RB, et al: Oxygen may improve dyspnea and endurance in patients with chronic obstructive pulmonary disease and only mild hypoxemia. Am Rev Respir Dis 146:941–945, 1992.
14. Donner CF, Braghiroli A, Zaccaria S, et al: Current status of home oxygen therapy in Italy. *In* Kira S, Petty TL (eds): Progress in Domiciliary Respiratory Care—Current Status and Perspective. New York, Elsevier Science BV, 1994, pp 35–40.
15. D'Urzo AD, Mateika J, Bradley TD, et al: Correlates of arterial oxygenation during exercise in severe chronic obstructive pulmonary disease. Chest 95:13–17, 1989.
16. Fleetham J, West P, Mezon B, et al: Sleep, arousals and oxygen desaturation in chronic obstructive pulmonary disease: the effect of oxygen therapy. Am Rev Respir Dis 126:429–433, 1982.
17. Fletcher AC, Miller J, Divine GW, et al: Nocturnal oxyhemoglobin desaturation in COPD patients with arterial oxygen tensions above 60 mm Hg. Chest 92:604–608, 1987.
18. Fletcher EC, Luckett RA, Goodnight-White S, et al: A double blind trial of nocturnal supplemental oxygen for sleep desaturation in patients with chronic obstructive pulmonary disease and daytime PaO_2 above 60 mm Hg. Am Rev Respir Dis 145:1070–1076, 1992.
19. Fulmer JD, Snider GL: ACCP-NHLBI National Conference on Oxygen Therapy. Chest 86:234–247, 1984.
20. Goldstein RS: Hypoventilation, neuromuscular and chest wall disorders. Clin Med Chest 13:507–521, 1992.
21. Goldstein RS, Ramcharan V, Bowes G, et al: Effect of supplemental nocturnal oxygen on gas exchange in patients with severe obstructive lung disease. N Engl J Med 310:425–429, 1984.
22. Gould GA, Forsyth IS, Flenley DC: Comparison of two oxygen conserving nasal prong systems and the effects of nose and mouth breathing. Thorax 41:808–809, 1986.
23. Heimlich HJ: Respiratory rehabilitation with transtracheal oxygen system. Ann Otolaryngol Rhinol 91:643–647, 1982.
24. Kerby GR, O'Donohue WJ, Romberger DJ, et al: Clinical efficacy and cost benefit of pulse flow oxygen in hospitalized patients. Chest 97:369–372, 1990.
25. Koehler D, Kanoch M, Sommerfield C, et al: A new oxygen applicator for simultaneous mouth and nose breathing. Chest 103;1157–1160, 1993.
26. Kvale PA, Cugell DW, Anthonisen NR, et al: Continuous or nocturnal oxygen therapy in hypoxemic chronic obstructive lung disease. Ann Intern Med 93:391–398, 1980.
27. Leach RM, Davidson AC, Chinn S, et al: Portable liquid oxygen and exercise ability in severe respiratory disability. Thorax 47:781–789, 1992.
28. Levi-Valensi P, Weitzenblum E, Pedinielli JL, et al: Three month follow up of arterial blood gas determinations in candidates for long term oxygen therapy. Am Rev Respir Dis 133:547–551, 1986.
29. Levin DC, Neff TA, O'Donohue WJ, et al: Conference report: Further recommendations for prescribing and

supplying long term oxygen therapy. Am Rev Respir Dis 138:745–747, 1988.

30. Littner MR, McGinty DJ, Arand DL: Determinants of oxygen desaturation in the course of ventilation during sleep in chronic obstructive pulmonary disease. Am Rev Respir Dis 122:849–857, 1980.

31. Mak VHF, Bugler JR, Roberts CM, et al: Effect of arterial oxygen desaturation on six minute walk distance, perceived effort, and perceived breathlessness in patients with airflow limitation. Thorax 48:33–38, 1993.

32. Manresa F, Escarrabill J: Long term oxygen therapy in Catalonia (Spain). *In* Kira S, Petty TL (eds): Progress in Domiciliary Respiratory Care—Current Status and Perspective. New York, Elsevier Science BV, 1994, pp. 63–69.

33. Moore DP, Weston AR, Hughes JMB, et al: Effects of increased inspired oxygen concentrations on exercise performance in chronic heart failure. Lancet 339:850–853, 1992.

34. Petty TL, O'Donohue WJ, Gracey DR, et al: Conference report: New Problems in supply, reimbursement and certification of medical necessity for long term oxygen therapy. Am Rev Respir Dis 142:721–724, 1990.

35. Pierson DJ: Current status of home oxygen in the U.S.A. *In* Kira S, Petty TL (eds): Progress in Domiciliary Respiratory Care—Current Status and Perspective, New York, Elsevier Science BV, 1994, pp 93–98.

36. Pierson DJ: Criteria and indications for home oxygen therapy. *In* Kira S, Petty TL (eds): Progress in Domic-

iliary Respiratory Care—Current Status and Perspective. New York, Elsevier Science BV, 1994, pp 115–124.

37. Rahman S, Howard P: Cost effectiveness of home oxygen therapy. *In* Kira S, Petty TL (eds): Progress in Domiciliary Respiratory Care—Current Status and Perspective. New York, Elsevier Science BV, 1994, pp 149–152.

38. Report of the Medical Research Council Working Party: Long term domiciliary oxygen therapy in chronic hypoxic cor pulmonale complicating chronic bronchitis and emphysema. Lancet 1:681–686, 1981.

39. Robinson DP, White DP, Zwillich CW: Occlusion pressure responses to hypoxia and hypercapnia do not explain dyspnea or exercise limitation in severe COPD. Am Rev Respir Dis 133:A61, 1986.

40. Soffer AS: Cost effective or quality care. Which shall it be? Chest 88:806–807, 1985.

41. Tiep BL, Belman MJ, Mittman C, et al: A new pendant storage oxygen-conserving nasal cannula. Chest 87:381–383, 1985.

42. Tiep BL, Carter R, Brooke N, et al: Demand oxygen delivery during exercise. Chest 91:15–20, 1987.

43. Weitzenblum E, Sautegeau A, Ehrhart M, et al: Long term oxygen therapy can reverse the progression of pulmonary hypertension in patients with chronic obstructive pulmonary disease. Am Rev Respir Dis 131:493–498, 1985.

Physical Therapy Interventions for Persons with Chronic Obstructive Pulmonary Disease

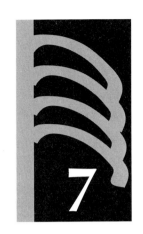

7

Susan Leslie Garritan, MA, PT, CCS

The physical therapist is an important member of the pulmonary rehabilitation team. Depending on the availability of other professional disciplines, the role of the physical therapist may vary somewhat from one setting to another.[4] From acute care, to inpatient or outpatient rehabilitation, to home care, the allied health care professionals who may be involved include nurses, physical therapists, respiratory therapists, occupational therapists, and exercise physiologists.

The physical therapist who specializes in pulmonary rehabilitation must have a sound background in the anatomy and physiology of the cardiopulmonary system as well as an understanding of the pathophysiology of the many pulmonary diseases seen in patients who may benefit from pulmonary rehabilitation. These diagnoses include *obstructive processes*, such as asthma, bronchiectasis, chronic bronchitis, chronic obstructive pulmonary disease (COPD), cystic fibrosis, and emphysema, and *restrictive processes*, such as interstitial and occupational lung diseases, as well as postoperative lung resections.

The purpose of this chapter is to describe the physical therapy evaluation and treatment of patients with COPD. The physical therapist provides instruction in basic skills to be mastered prior to the initiation of any exercise or reconditioning program. Mastery of these skills is important for ensuring that the patient exercises with lungs that are as clear as possible and possesses breathing mechanisms and coping strategies for dealing with shortness of breath. These skills are building blocks in the foundation of any sound pulmonary rehabilitation program.

PHYSICAL THERAPY GOALS

Chest physical therapy interventions are utilized to

1. Optimize pulmonary hygiene;
2. Improve breathing patterns by diaphragmatic breathing, pursed-lip exhalation, muscle reeducation, and paced breathing techniques;
3. Improve chest wall mobility;
4. Improve mechanisms for coping with and recovering from shortness of breath;
5. Coordinate breathing patterns with activities of daily living (ADL); and
6. Recondition individuals with COPD by aerobic training.

Therapeutic Exercise

Therapeutic exercise techniques address flexibility, posture, and strength deficits noted during the initial physical therapy evaluation. Understanding preexisting neuromuscular or orthopedic deficits is important to determine the most appropriate exercise modalities and equipment to be used by individual patients in the physical reconditioning and endurance training phases of the pulmonary rehabilitation program.

Education

Patient and family education is an important component of physical therapy treatment. Preparing the patient and family for living independently with COPD involves helping them to gain confidence in their ability to handle the various situations that may arise as a result of the disease. Instruction in self-treatment or care partner-assisted pulmonary hygiene techniques may reduce doctor visits. Clear guidelines regarding appropriate times to seek medical assistance can reduce worry and uncertainty.

Psychological Support

The importance of psychological support, provided by all members of the pulmonary rehabilitation team as well as the physical therapist, should not be underestimated. The fear and anxiety triggered by shortness of breath often can be incapacitating. Learning to control, alleviate, and become desensitized to shortness of breath, as well as exercising with shortness of breath under direct medical supervision, can play an important role in increasing a patient's confidence in his or her ability to be more physically active.[14]

MEDICAL CHART OR DATA REVIEW

The medical chart or data review identifies the primary and secondary diagnoses and their severity. A variety of data are reviewed prior to evaluation and treatment:

1. The review of symptoms guides the emphasis and priorities of treatment.
2. Past cardiac, orthopedic, neurologic, vascular, or psychological disorders are considered so that they will not be exacerbated by treatment and the most appropriate form of exercise can be determined.
3. Pulmonary function tests indicate the severity of pulmonary disease and whether airway reactivity is present. Patients with airway reactivity may benefit from using bronchodilators prior to using secretion clearance techniques and exercise.
4. Arterial blood gases and pulse oximetry provide information concerning the degree of

respiratory insufficiency present at rest and indicate how well the patient responds to the challenge of exercise. Decisions regarding oxygen use at rest or during exercise are based on these values.

Chest radiographs and computed tomographic (CT) scans provide information concerning the location of suspected mucus plugging by identifying areas of atelectasis or pneumonia. Acute infections, hyperinflation, and blebs or bullae can also be identified. Medication schedules need to be coordinated with the patient's exercise so that medications will have their peak effect at the desired time and so that heart rate and blood pressure responses to exercise can be accurately interpreted (Table 7–1).

PHYSICAL THERAPY EVALUATION

Physical therapy evaluation includes the following components that help to identify the needs of each individual:

1. Assessment of baseline vital signs and oxyhemoblogin saturation
2. Breathing pattern evaluation
3. Range of motion /flexibility evaluation
4. Manual muscle test
5. ADL evaluation
6. 6-minute walk test

GOAL SETTING

The goals of physical therapy are set following the evaluation process. These goals fall into

TABLE 7–1
Commonly Used Cardiopulmonary Medications: Effects on Heart Rate and Blood Pressure

Medication	Heart Rate	Blood Pressure
β-Adrenergic blockers	↓↓	↓
Methylxanthines	↑	↑
Calcium entry blockers	None or ↑	↓
Sympathomimetics	↑ or ↑↑	↑
Parasympatholytics	↑ or ↑↑	↑
Diuretics	None or ↑	↓
Angiotensin inhibitors	None or ↑	↓
Vasodilators	None or ↑	↓
Nitrates	Slight ↑	↓

From Cohen M, Hoskins Michel T: Cardiopulmonary Symptoms in Physical Therapy Practice. New York, Churchill Livingstone, 1988.

general categories but must be specific to address the needs of each patient and disease process. Exploring the patient's own goals for pulmonary rehabilitation encourages the motivation necessary for hard work and compliance with the program.

TREATMENT PROGRAM

Physical therapy treatment is focused on correcting or modifying any deficits identified during evaluation as well as addressing the needs dictated by each individual's pulmonary diagnosis. Treatment also lays the foundation for mastery of techniques and skills that will be used in the aerobic training phase of the pulmonary rehabilitation program.

RELAXATION TECHNIQUES

In the treatment of patients with COPD, relaxation techniques are used to achieve:

1. Reduction in muscular tension in the accessory muscles of breathing;
2. Reduction in the energy cost of breathing;
3. Reduction in anxiety caused by dyspnea; and
4. A generalized sense of well being.

Supported Positioning

Supported positioning in either the sidelying or semi-Fowler's position promotes relaxation. These positions are good choices for the performance of diaphragmatic breathing and basal lung expansion, which, in turn, further promote relaxation.

In the semi-Fowler's position, pillows under the shoulders and upper extremities encourage relaxation of tense muscles of the neck and shoulder girdle which are accessories of respiration. Flexion of the knees with the support of bolsters or pillows and flexion of the trunk encourage relaxation of the abdominal muscles (Fig. 7–1). This position, in addition to the side-lying position, increases an individual's awareness of diaphragmatic excursion.

Gentle Repetitive Movements

Gentle manual stretching of the patient's neck and scapular muscles encourages relaxation of tense musculature. Repetitive shaking of the upper extremities also encourages relaxation. Other relaxation techniques that may be incorporated during postural drainage or instruction in breathing techniques include scapular mobilization and trunk rotation and counter-rotation.

CONTROLLED BREATHING TECHNIQUES

The purposes of controlled breathing include:

1. Controlling respiratory rate and breathing pattern to decrease air trapping[7];
2. Improving use of the diaphragm;
3. Improving rib cage and thoracic mobility;
4. Improving ventilation without increasing the energy cost of breathing;
5. Building confidence in the ability to control breathing and recover from dyspnea; and
6. Helping to restore patients to their highest

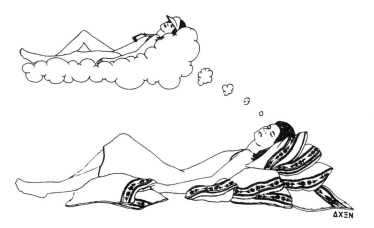

FIGURE 7–1. Supported positioning to facilitate relaxation. (From Haas F, Axen K (eds): Pulmonary Therapy and Rehabilitation: Principles and Practice, 2nd ed. Baltimore, Williams & Wilkins, 1991, p 218; with permission.)

possible functional capacity and quality of life.[8]

While performing controlled breathing techniques, patients are encouraged to breathe in through the nose to ensure maximal filtering, warming, and humidification of the inspired air. Mouth breathing in cold weather or during vigorous exercise can result in bronchospasm in some patients. Most controlled breathing techniques are effective only while they are being used.

Pursed-Lip Breathing (PLB)

Patients are encouraged to exhale through pursed lips during performance of most controlled breathing techniques. It is often the first technique taught and usually the easiest to learn. To perform PLB, the patient inhales through the nose for several seconds with the mouth closed, and then exhales slowly (for roughly twice as long as inhalation) through pursed lips held in a wide, narrow slit. During PLB, no expiratory airflow occurs through the nose due to the involuntary occlusion of the nasopharynx by the soft palate.[27] PLB creates an obstruction to air flow at the mouth that decreases the flow of the exhaled air and increases airway pressure,[34] decreasing the transmural pressure gradient[12] and maintaining patency of collapsible airways during exhalation.[8,29] This process helps to reduce air trapping (Fig. 7–2).

PLB in COPD patients significantly decreases respiratory rate and increases tidal volume.[23,34,35] Improved alveolar ventilation can be demonstrated by decreases in $PaCO_2$[23,34] and increases in PaO_2[23] and SaO_2 measured at rest during PLB.[35] Similar improvements in arterial blood gases were observed without PLB when a slower, deeper breathing pattern was used by patients with severe emphysema.[22]

The effect of PLB on arterial blood gases during exercise has not been studied extensively. In 1970, Mueller and associates evaluated $PaCO_2$, PaO_2, and SaO_2 during exercise and found no change in these parameters.[23] However, some of their patients did claim symptomatic benefit from PLB, and they were noted to use PLB spontaneously with exertion, although they did not always use it at rest. This area is an important one for further research, because maintaining blood gas parameters during exercise through use of PLB would be beneficial for patients whose blood gases would otherwise deteriorate.

PLB relieves dyspnea for some subjects. How-

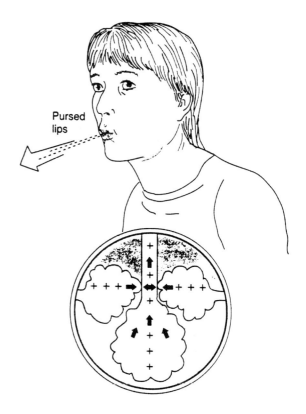

FIGURE 7–2. Demonstration of pursed-lip breathing in patients with COPD and its effects. The weakened bronchial airways are kept open by the effects of positive pressure created by pursed lips during expiration. (From Hillegass EA, Sadowsky HS (eds): Essentials of Cardiopulmonary Physical Therapy. Philadelphia, WB Saunders, 1994.)

ever, the relief from dyspnea is often too immediate to be explained by alterations in blood gases alone.[1] PLB may also have some effect on circulation in the capillary bed of the lung. Barach reported an increase in peripheral venous pressure during PLB and hypothesized that the positive pressure generated in the airways prevented serum from entering the alveoli.[1]

PLB does not significantly decrease functional residual capacity.[12,34] This makes it unlikely that improvement in dyspnea is the result of restoring the diaphragm to a more cranial position in the thorax, where it would be contracting with a more advantageous length-tension relationship.[8] PLB also does not decrease but, rather, increases the work of breathing.[12,26] Using transnasally placed esophageal and gastric balloons to measure pleural, gastric, and transdiaphragmatic pressures during breathing, Roa et al. studied the effects of PLB on ventilatory muscle recruitment in COPD patients at rest.[26] PLB was found to shift a major portion of the inspiratory work of breathing from the diaphragm to the rib cage muscles. The temporary reduction in diaphragmatic work, but not the overall work of breathing, may help to explain why some COPD patients report a reduction in dyspnea with PLB.[8]

PLB has been used spontaneously by some patients to relieve dyspnea, whereas other patients claim they feel no benefit from this technique. Further research is warranted to help identify those patients who will benefit most by PLB. Until this subset of COPD patients is identified, PLB should be recommended to all COPD patients for use during activities that precipitate dyspnea.

Diaphragmatic Breathing

Diaphragmatic breathing has been one of the cornerstones of breathing retraining. COPD patients who present with predominantly upper thoracic expansion and little abdominal movement, or with inward movement of the lower ribs during inspiration may be the best candidates for diaphragmatic breathing. The technique may be difficult to learn, however, for those with very low and flattened diaphragms. Instruction in diaphragmatic breathing usually begins in the semi-Fowler's or side-lying position with pillow support to achieve relaxation. Instructions for performing diaphragmatic breathing are listed in Table 7–2.

Once diaphragmatic breathing is mastered in the semi-Fowler's and side-lying positions, patients learn to perform it when sitting and standing for carryover to more functional activities. Because the correct motion is less obvious in the standing position it is often necessary to facilitate diaphragmatic excursion and cue the patient. Diaphragmatic breathing should also be practiced during walking and stair climbing (Fig. 7–3).

To assess the effectiveness of diaphragmatic breathing for any individual patient, monitoring equipment, such as a pulse oximeter, can provide objective data. Oximetry is particularly helpful in determining whether abdominal muscle contraction during expiration, often used in conjunction with PLB, is improving oxygenation. The use of abdominal muscle contraction during expiration has been advocated by some as a method for helping to achieve a more complete exhalation and to elevate the di-

TABLE 7–2
Instructions for Diaphragmatic Breathing

1. Position the patient comfortably, with flexion at the waist.
2. Place the patient's dominant hand over the mid-abdominal area.
3. Place the patient's nondominant hand over the midsternum.
4. Ask the patient to inhale through the nose, performing several "sniffs" in a row, if necessary, to achieve a slight rise in the midabdominal region during inspiration.
5. Direct the patient's attention to the gradual rise of the dominant hand during the slow inspiration.
6. Direct the patient's attention to the lack of movement of the nondominant hand.
7. Resistance can be applied during inspiration by the therapist's hand to facilitate diaphragmatic excursion.

aphragm to a higher resting position within the thoracic cage.[13] An elevated diaphragm has greater excursion during its next inspiratory effort. However, contraction of the abdominal muscles increases the energy cost of breathing and is difficult to coordinate during complex functional activities or during exercise. Therefore, objective data regarding improvement in oxygenation should be obtained before recommending this technique to any individual patient.

Although some patients report reduced dyspnea and clinical improvements when utilizing diaphragmatic breathing, physiologic studies have been inconclusive and conflicting regarding the effectiveness of the technique.[8] Miller reported that training in diaphragmatic breathing is effective in increasing diaphragmatic excursion, thereby increasing tidal volumes and decreasing respiratory rates.[21] He also noted improvements in blood gases following diaphragmatic breathing. Three other studies were less successful in demonstrating physiologic benefits from the technique.[6,21,31] However, even in these three studies, some subjects did improve considerably. There may be a subset of COPD patients, who we are as yet unable to identify, who benefit from diaphragmatic breathing.[8]

There is no change in regional ventilation or improvement in ventilation/perfusion relationships at the bases of the lungs in COPD patients using diaphragmatic breathing, as compared to using their spontaneous breathing patterns.[5,28] There are also indications that diaphragmatic breathing may be a less mechanically efficient breathing pattern than natural breathing for

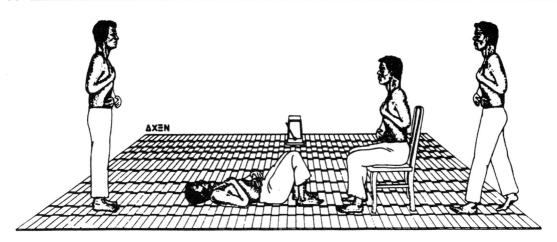

FIGURE 7–3. Positions utilized in training for diaphragmatic breathing. (From Haas F, Sperber Haas S: The Chronic Bronchitis and Emphysema Handbook. New York, John Wiley & Sons, 1990.)

some COPD patients. Willeput et al. studied the effects of diaphragmatic breathing on thoracoabdominal movement in COPD patients.[38] Diaphragmatic breathing was found to increase asynchronous and paradoxical motion of the rib cage and, therefore, may increase the energy cost of breathing.

Thus, the benefits of diaphragmatic breathing are unclear from currently available research. Because diaphragmatic breathing has always been one of the main tools in breathing retraining, and because selected patients do appear to benefit from the technique, it is unlikely that diaphragmatic breathing will be totally abandoned. However, when patients who perform it properly do not feel helped by the technique, clinicians should emphasize other breathing strategies. Hopefully, further research will identify the subset of COPD patients who benefit from diaphragmatic breathing and elucidate the mechanisms of their subjective improvements.

Paced Breathing

Rapid shallow breathing patterns, seen in some patients with COPD, can lend to air trapping if expiratory time is inadequate.[7] The technique of paced breathing attempts to facilitate a more complete exhalation by having the patient exhale roughly twice as long as the inhalation time. Inspiratory:expiratory time counts (seconds) of 2:4, 3:6, and 3:5 are most common. A count of 4:7 may be achieved by a mildly involved individual, but excessively prolonging the count can increase the work of breathing and prolong exhalation to the point where lung

volume falls below the functional residual capacity. This step may be undesirable in patients with early airway closure or very collapsible airways.[38]

A general introduction to the concept of paced breathing is preferable to employing a rigid counting pattern throughout breathing exercises and ADL. Paced breathing is usually used in conjunction with PLB, diaphragmatic breathing, or both.

Segmental Breathing

Segmental breathing or localized expansion exercises are used to direct airflow into a specific area of the thorax. These techniques are useful when a restrictive component is present as part of the patient's respiratory condition. Three segmental expansions are commonly used during chest physical therapy treatment:[10] (1) apical expansion, (2) lateral costal expansion, and (3) posterior basal expansion.

Segmental expansion is often used during postural drainage of a specific segment or in attempting to achieve reexpansion of an atelectatic or collapsed segment or lobe. This condition can be seen in patients with bronchiectasis or cystic fibrosis, in whom central mucus plugging and distal lung collapse can contribute to recurrent pneumonias. In lobar collapse, the right middle lobe is particularly vulnerable,[11] and both the right middle lobe and lingula appear to have less collateral ventilation than other lobes.[19] Localized thoracic expansion exercises, combined with a deep breath and an inhalation-hold maneuver, can help to move air into alveolar units distal to airways blocked by mucus plugs or secretions. This distal air movement is accomplished by collateral ventilation from adjacent alveoli or bronchioles. Collateral ventilation is possible through the pores of Kohn (alveolus to alveolus) and the channels of Lambert (bronchiole to alveolus). If air can be moved distal to mucus obstruction, postural drainage techniques will be more successful.[37] Thoracic expansion exercises with a deep inspiration or inspiration-hold may cause lengthening and widening of the airways, which facilitates movement of secretions on the bronchial walls.[36]

Another use for localized expansion exercises is in hypoventilation syndromes, such as pickwickian syndrome, or restrictive thoracic conditions, such as scoliosis, kyphoscoliosis, tetraplegia, or hemiplegia. Thoracic expansion exercises are performed by using the accessory muscles of respiration or by the external intercostals. The diaphragm may also participate in lateral costal and posterior basal expansions. One method of instructing patients in segmental expansions is outlined in Table 7–3.

Positions for Recovery from Shortness of Breath

An important part of teaching controlled breathing techniques is to instruct COPD patients in optimal positioning and breathing patterns to assist in recovery from shortness of breath. The knowledge that one has strategies to employ to regain control of breathing once the

---

TABLE 7–3
Instructions for Thoracic Expansion Exercises

1. Position the patient comfortably, with slight flexion at the knees and waist.
2. Place the therapist's hands on the thoracic cage over the segments to be expanded.
3. Apply firm pressure at the end of the patient's exhalation to the area to be expanded.
4. Instruct the patient to inspire in through the nose and attempt to direct the inspired air into the therapist's hand.
5. Pressure is gradually released as the patient inspires so that the motion is not resisted.
6. Quick stretches may be applied throughout the inspiration to recruit more muscle fibers.
7. Ask the patient for an inhalation-hold maneuver, if the goal is to move air behind an atelectatic area or mucus plugs.
8. Ask the patient to exhale.
9. Teach self-monitored thoracic expansions when appropriate.

---

dyspnea threshold has been exceeded helps to avoid the addition of panic and anxiety to the picture. Most patients already know that sitting more upright and especially bending forward at the waist will help them to regain control of their breathing. The bending-forward posture causes the abdominal viscera to push the diaphragm up into a higher resting position within the thorax. The diaphragm becomes more effective because of its more favorable length-tension relationship, and decreased use of the accessory muscles is observed. Dyspnea is most reduced by bending forward for COPD patients, who demonstrate inspiratory paradoxical movements of the upper abdominal wall in the upright position.[30]

The upper extremities should be stabilized by resting the elbows or hands on the knees or leaning with the forearms on a table or ledge. In these positions, the serratus anterior, latissimus dorsi, and pectoral muscle insertions are fixed, and their actions assist in thoracic expansion.

PLB should also be used, and the rate of breathing should be one that feels comfortable to the patient. PLB is often initially done at a too rapid rate. Gradually expiration is prolonged in a 1:2 inspiratory:expiratory ratio. As control of breathing is regained, the rate is gradually decreased and the depth of inspiration is increased. Positions for recovery from shortness of breath that are used when sitting can also be used when standing. Flexion at the waist is important, as well as stabilizing the upper extremities against a firm surface or on the legs (Fig. 7–4).

During physical therapy sessions, recreating and managing situations that typically produce shortness of breath help the patient to gain confidence in his or her ability to cope successfully with these occurrences. Some activities that may be helpful to practice include walking up inclines, climbing stairs, rushing to answer the phone, lifting objects, and grooming activities that require repetitive upper extremity movements.

PULMONARY CARE

The need for instruction in secretion clearance techniques depends on the patient's diagnosis. Patients with cystic fibrosis, bronchiectasis, and chronic bronchitis, as well as any other patients who produce large quantities of mucus, require assistance with clearance of secretions. The mucociliary transport system may be abnormal in these patients, causing retention or

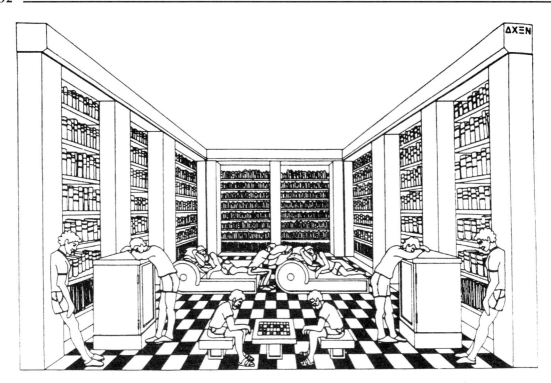

FIGURE 7–4. Positions utilized for recovery from shortness of breath. (From Haas F, Sperber Haas S: The Chronic Bronchitis and Emphysema Handbook. New York, John Wiley & Sons, 1990.)

even stasis of pulmonary secretions. Some causes include increased mucus production, alterations in the physical properties of mucus, impairment of ciliary function, and the loss of ciliated epithelial cells. Mucus impaction and impairments in gas exchange can result from these changes.[8]

The quantity of mucus produced should not be the only criterion for utilizing postural drainage or other secretion clearance techniques. Mucus plugs located in critical airways, such as the right middle lobe or lingula, may cause atelectasis and recurrent pneumonias. When secretions are thick or tenacious, several approaches may be used to help thin them prior to applying clearance techniques. Methods for thinning secretions include:

1. Increasing fluid intake to 6 to 8 glasses of water daily, unless the patient is on fluid restrictions for cardiac or renal disorders;
2. Using ultrasonic nebulizer or aerosol treatments;
3. Prescribing hot, steamy showers;
4. Drinking hot liquids, such as tea; and
5. Using prescribed metered-dose bronchodilators 20 to 30 minutes prior to treatment.

Postural Drainage

Postural drainage uses gravity to help move mucus through the tracheobronchial tree to larger airways. The patient is positioned with the lung segment to be drained uppermost, so that the segmental bronchus is vertical and drainage of secretions is facilitated. There are 12 basic postural drainage positions. Most are mirror images of each other, but there are some important variations in positions for the right and left upper lobe posterior segments (Figs. 7–5, 7–6, and 7–7).

Although only selected positions are usually used, postural drainage treatment for diseases that affect the entire lung, such as cystic fibrosis, may require the use of all 12 positions. The positions are chosen by considering chest CT scans, chest radiographs, auscultatory findings of rhonchi, wheezing, or decreased breath sounds due to mucus plugging and atelectasis, and the patient's subjective observations. Statements such as "I always cough when I lie flat on my back" may provide useful clues as to which lobes contain retained secretions. Some patients may report thoracic pain in areas where they are experiencing mucus plugging.

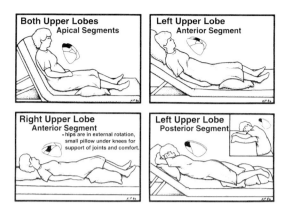

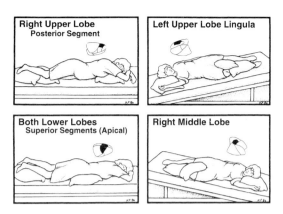

FIGURE 7–5. Postural drainage positions for the upper lobes. (From Frownfelter D: Chest Physical Therapy and Pulmonary Rehabilitation, 2nd ed. Chicago, Year Book Medical Publishers, 1987.)

FIGURE 7–6. Postural drainage positions for the upper, middle, and lower lobes. (From Frownfelter D: Chest Physical Therapy and Pulmonary Rehabilitation, 2nd ed. Chicago, Year Book Medical Publishers, 1987.)

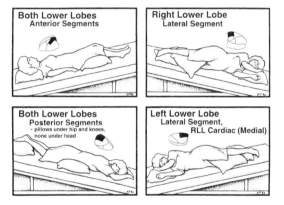

FIGURE 7–7. Postural drainage positions for the lower lobes. (From Frownfelter D: Chest Physical Therapy and Pulmonary Rehabilitation, 2nd ed. Chicago, Year Book Medical Publishers, 1987.)

Postural drainage positioning is usually well tolerated, although some patients are unable to lie flat without experiencing dyspnea. In these cases, modified drainage positions are used with gradual attempts to lower the head. Theoretically, postural drainage for unilateral pulmonary diseases has the potential to improve blood gas exchange, because the more abnormal lung will be uppermost throughout the entire treatment and the majority of ventilation and perfusion will be shifted to the dependent, or more normal, lung.

Manual Techniques

Other techniques may be added to postural drainage positioning to facilitate the drainage of secretions and speed their removal. The lack of cilia in the distal regions of the tracheobron-chial tree makes it impossible to mobilize secretions via the mucociliary escalator from the lung periphery.[15] The addition of manual techniques, such as percussion, vibration, and shaking, can be effective in helping to dislodge retained secretions.

Percussion is performed by tapping the chest wall with cupped hands, alternating between right and left hands. A hollow sound is produced as the chest wall is struck by the cushion of air under the therapist's hand. The mechanical force generated helps to dislodge mucus plugs and move mucus toward larger airways. Percussion is performed throughout the inspiratory and expiratory cycles, with a thin layer of cloth covering the patient's thorax (Fig. 7–8). The intensity of percussion varies depending on the integrity of the bony thorax. Patients with severe osteoporosis or long-term steroid use are treated more gently.

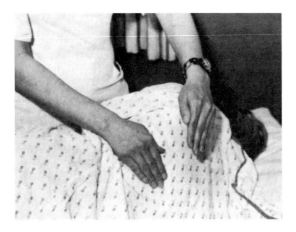

FIGURE 7–8. Hand position for chest percussion. (From Frownfelter D: Chest Physical Therapy and Pulmonary Rehabilitation, 2nd ed. Chicago, Year Book Medical Publishers, 1987.)

Shaking and *vibration* are performed only during expiration. Shaking is a rhythmic downward motion of the rib cage caused by gentle pressure from the therapist's hands. Shaking increases mobility of the rib cage and is often used in combination with localized expansion exercises. It is frequently used to improve aeration to a specific area. Quick stretches, or rib springing, may also be used to facilitate the actions of the external intercostal muscles and to further increase rib cage excursion.

Vibration is a finer oscillating movement of the therapist's hands on the patient's thoracic cage combined with a light downward pressure. It is usually the best technique to use for patients who are experiencing pain.

Active Cycle of Breathing (Self-treatment)

Active cycle of breathing has been helpful in treating patients with bronchospasm, in whom gentle treatment is required, and is especially helpful in a home program for independent facilitation of secretion clearance.[37] The active cycle of breathing consists of three techniques: relaxed breathing, thoracic expansion exercises, and the forced expiratory technique. The *relaxed breathing* is continued for 2 to 3 minutes in a comfortable position, focusing on expanding the basal segments of the lung, breathing in through the nose and out through the mouth in a shallow breathing pattern. This is followed by three to four deeper *thoracic expansions* that the patient monitors with his or her hands. Percussion, vibration, or shaking techniques may be performed either by the patient or an assistant

during the thoracic expansions. These two steps are repeated until the patient feels ready to clear secretions. The final step is to perform the *forced expiratory technique* to raise secretions. The forced expiratory technique is a combination of one or two forced expirations (huffs) and periods of breathing control. The forced expiratory technique, huffing from middle to low lung volumes with an open glottis, helps to maintain stability of the airways and to prevent premature collapse. The periods of breathing control are important to prevent any increase in airway obstruction. A huff performed to a low lung volume moves more peripherally located secretions and a huff from a high lung volume clears secretions from the proximal airways.[37]

Effectiveness of Techniques

Studies utilizing inhaled radioaerosol particles have shown that manual techniques of chest physical therapy significantly increase clearance of secretions from central, intermediate, and peripheral lung regions in COPD[2] and in cystic fibrosis[17,18] patients with profuse secretions. Coughing and chest physical therapy are complementary in improving central lung clearance, but only chest physical therapy produces a significant increase in peripheral lung clearance when mucociliary action is impaired.[3]

The routine use of postural drainage with manual techniques on all patients with COPD is not indicated, but the techniques are generally taught to enable patients to clear secretions if they develop a cold or more serious respiratory infection. The use of these treatment skills is especially indicated in treating cystic fibrosis and bronchiectasis. In a study by Sutton et al., both the forced expiratory technique and the combination of postural drainage with the forced expiratory technique produced more sputum than directed coughing alone.[33] In a study by Pryor et al., the forced expiratory technique was shown to clear more sputum in less time than conventional therapy in patients with cystic fibrosis.[25]

Timing of Postural Drainage

Patients with large quantities of mucus generally have the best results by performing postural drainage in the morning. This helps to reduce coughing during the day. For patients with multiple areas of involvement who require many different postural drainage positions, sessions may be done several times throughout the day, with emphasis on different areas in each session.

Patients who report being awakened by cough during the night should perform secretion clearance techniques 1 to 2 hours before sleep.

Precautions for Postural Drainage and Manual Treatment Techniques

1. During positioning for and performance of postural drainage, blood gases may deteriorate when diseased lung, such as lobes affected by pneumonia, are in the most dependent position or when mobilized secretions temporarily block small airways. In some instances, supplemental oxygen may be needed during postural drainage.
2. When lung abscesses or necrotizing pneumonias are present, it is important to avoid spillage of virulent organisms into healthy lung tissue. This is accomplished by treating the affected areas first, then prophylactically draining unaffected lobes.
3. Vigorous manual applications should not be used on patients with severe osteoporosis or rib fractures.
4. Frank hemoptysis in patients with bronchiectasis is a contraindication to treatment with vigorous manual techniques or excessive coughing.
5. Asthmatic patients should receive adequate bronchodilation prior to attempts to clear excessive secretions and should be treated with more gentle treatment techniques, such as during the active cycle of breathing. They should be monitored closely by auscultation to ensure that they do not develop, or have an increase in, wheezing during treatment.
6. Trendelenburg positions should not be used following meals.

FUNCTIONAL TRAINING

Performance of ADL is evaluated by physical and occupational therapists. Monitoring of pulse oximetry during these activities can help to document difficulties. Severely involved COPD patients may need to learn to modify their breathing with even simple position changes, such as rolling over in bed or coming to sitting. The patient should breathe in prior to the activity and blow themselves into the new position.[9] Coordination of breathing techniques with the following activities is also taught: reaching, bending, carrying items, level walking, inclined walking, and stair climbing.

Generally, movements that expand the thorax are coordinated with inspiration, and movements that compress the thorax are coordinated with expiration. Particular attention is directed toward avoiding the breath-holding that may be seen with exertion and avoiding rushing through activities. Stair climbing is made easier by pausing during inspiration and climbing only during expiration. This accomplishes two goals: slowing performance of the activity and allowing optimal conditions for a full inspiration.

It is often helpful to have the patient keep a diary of activities that increase shortness of breath. These activities can then be analyzed and suggestions made to help the patient perform them with greater ease. It is also important to look at how COPD patients move in general. Often, they may be observed to move rapidly, to hold their bodies and extremities stiffly, and to move their bodies as a whole when performing activities. These habits utilize more energy than movements that are performed in a smoother, slower, more relaxed way and when moving the extremities individually.

Three energy conservation approaches typically used by COPD patients are[24]:

1. Increasing awareness of how ADLs are performed;
2. Modifying activities or using assistive devices; and
3. Compensating by using other methods or by increasing reliance on others to perform activities.

EXERCISE

Flexibility, Stretching, and Posture

Accessory muscles of inspiration are often shortened by overuse in COPD patients. These muscles may benefit from exercises to stretch them to their more normal lengths. Commonly shortened muscles include the sternocleidomastoids, external intercostals, upper trapezii, pectoralis major and minor, latissimus dorsi, serratus anterior, and hip flexors. Trunk mobility exercises increase flexibility of the thoracic spine and rib cage (Figs. 7–9 and 7–10). Posture and neck alignment exercises can help to reinforce the proper length and alignment of these often shortened muscle groups as well.

Strengthening

Strengthening exercises to the over-lengthened antagonists of chronically shortened mus-

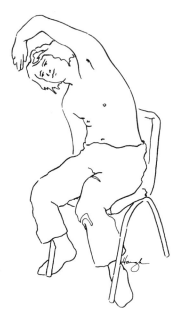

FIGURE 7–9. Chest mobilization with lateral flexion, while the patient exhales during lateral bending. (From Frownfelter D: Chest Physical Therapy and Pulmonary Rehabilitation, 2nd ed. Chicago, Year Book Medical Publishers, 1987.)

cles can help to restore better postural alignment. Muscles to be strengthened include the lower and middle trapezii, rhomboids, and hip and back extensors.

Weight training for COPD patients, as part of a general conditioning program, can be initi-

ated with light weights or an elastic resistive material such as Theraband (Hygenic Corporation, Akron, OH). Gradual progression to the heavier weights necessary for a true strengthening effect can be done with patients who can tolerate more resistance without undue shortness of breath. It is important to coordinate breathing patterns with weight lifting and to avoid breath-holding.

General Conditioning Exercise

For severely involved or hospitalized COPD patients, general conditioning exercises without resistance are used initially to preserve strength and to prepare them for more advanced exercise. Unilateral upper or lower extremity exercise coordinated with breathing is usually best tolerated, with progression to bilateral or combined upper and lower extremity and trunk exercise (Fig. 7–11). Positions for exercise may also progress in difficulty, from semi-Fowler's position to sitting and finally to standing. The number of repetitions of each exercise, initially limited to three or four, may be gradually increased.

Endurance Training

Different types of aerobic exercise utilizing large muscle groups are used by COPD patients to achieve repetitive movements of the arms and legs. Types of aerobic exercise include:

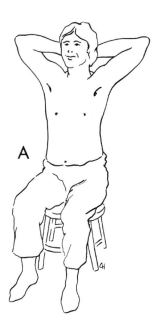

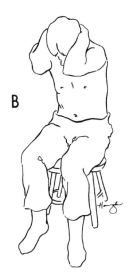

FIGURE 7–10. Chest mobilization exercises. *A,* Inspiration with extension. *B,* Expiration during flexion. (From Frownfelter D: Chest Physical Therapy and Pulmonary Rehabilitation, 2nd ed. Chicago, Year Book Medical Publishers, 1987.)

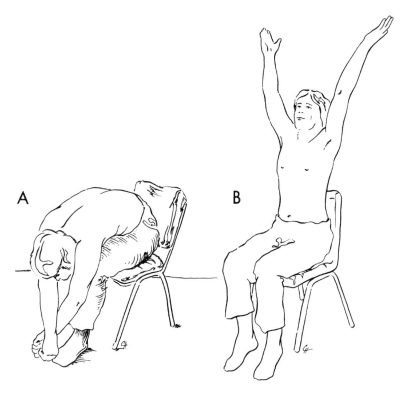

FIGURE 7–11. Chest mobilization, proprioceptive neuromuscular facilitation patterns: *A,* Patient exhales during flexion. *B,* Patient stretches and breathes in during extension. (From Frownfelter D: Chest Physical Therapy and Pulmonary Rehabilitation, 2nd ed. Chicago, Year Book Medical Publishers, 1987.)

1. Bicycling for lower extremities;
2. Upper extremity ergometry;
3. Use of a Schwinn Airdyne for reciprocal upper and lower extremity exercise (Schwinn Cycling and Fitness, West Chicago, IL);
4. Use of rowing machines;
5. Treadmill walking, level or with an incline;
6. Distance or lap walking;
7. Cross-country skiing simulators;
8. Stair climbing, stepping, or Stair Master; and
9. Swimming.

All aerobic exercise is preceded by a warm-up period of at least 5 minutes, a continuous peak exercise target of 20 to 30 minutes, and a cool-down period of at least 5 minutes. Supplemental oxygen is used during exercise as needed to maintain oxyhemoglobin saturation levels >90%. Very debilitated individuals may not be able to exercise continuously during their initial sessions.

Respiratory Muscle Exercise

The inspiratory muscles can be exercised directly by having the patient breathe in and out through a narrowed orifice, increasing the workload of breathing. Inspiratory muscle trainers, such as the P-flex trainer (Health Scan Inc., Cedar Grove, NJ), can be used for this purpose. There is a choice of six different settings for resistance, depending of the diameter of the opening selected for the patient to breathe through. Resistive inspiratory muscle exercise is recommended for 15 minutes, twice a day. It has been shown to increase both the strength and endurance of inspiratory muscles.[16,32]

CONCLUSION

The physical therapist makes a unique contribution to pulmonary rehabilitation programs because of expertise in breathing retraining and secretion clearance techniques, evaluation and treatment of musculoskeletal problems, therapeutic and aerobic exercise, motivation enhancement, and modifying ADL. Therapists' contributions depend on the organization of any particular pulmonary rehabilitation team. As a patient with COPD gains confidence in coping with COPD, new horizons may be opened to them, which will hopefully include increased physical activity and travel away from the home environment.

References

1. Barach AL: Physiological advantages of grunting, groaning and pursed-lip breathing: Adaptive symptoms related to the development of continuous positive pressure breathing. N Y Acad Med Bull 49:666–673, 1973.
2. Bateman JR, Newman SP, Daunt KM, et al: Regional clearance of excessive bronchial secretions during chest physiotherapy. Lancet 1:294–297, 1979.
3. Bateman JR, Newman SP, Daunt KM, et al: Is cough as effective as chest physiotherapy in the removal of excessive bronchial secretions? Thorax 36:683–687, 1981.
4. Borkgren MW: Diversity in pulmonary rehabilitation: A geographic survey study. J Cardiopulm Rehabil 9:63–71, 1989.
5. Brach BB, Chao RP, Sgroi VL, et al: Xenon washout patterns during diaphragmatic breathing. Chest 71:735–739, 1977.
6. Campbell EJM, Friend J: Action of breathing exercises in pulmonary emphysema. Lancet 1:325–329, 1955.
7. Failing LJ: Pulmonary rehabilitation—Physical modalities. Clin Chest Med 7:599–618, 1986.
8. Failing LJ: Controlled breathing techniques and chest physical therapy in chronic obstructive pulmonary disease and allied conditions. In Casaburi R, Petty T (eds): Principles and Practice of Pulmonary Rehabilitation. Philadelphia, WB Saunders, 1993, pp 167–182.
9. Frownfelter D: Chest Physical Therapy and Pulmonary Rehabilitation, 2nd ed. Chicago, Year Book Medical Publishers, 1987.
10. Gaskell DV, Webber BA: Breathing exercises and postural drainage. In The Brompton Hospital Guide to Chest Physiotherapy, 2nd ed. Oxford, Blackwell Scientific Publications, 1973, pp 5–15.
11. Hinshaw HC, Murray JF: Bronchial obstruction, atelectasis, and broncholithiasis. In Diseases of the Chest, 4th ed. Philadelphia, WB Saunders, 1980, pp 606–625.
12. Ingram RH, Schilder DP: Effect of pursed lips expiration on the pulmonary pressure-flow relationship in obstructive lung disease. Am Rev Respir Dis 96:381–388, 1967.
13. Kigin CM: Breathing exercises for the medical patient: The art and the science. Phys Ther 70:707–706, 1990.
14. Kohlman-Carrieri V, Janson-Bjerklie S: Coping and self-care strategies. In Mahler DA (ed): Dyspnea. Mt. Kisco, NY, Futura Publishing Co., 1990, pp 201–230.
15. Leith DE: Cough. Phys Ther 48:439–447, 1968.
16. Leith DE, Bradley M: Ventilatory muscle strength and endurance training. J Appl Physiol 41:508–516, 1976.
17. Lorin MI, Denning CR: Evaluation of postural drainage by measurement of sputum volume and consistency. Am J Phys Med 50:215–219, 1971.
18. May DB, Munt PW: Physiologic effects of chest percussion and postural drainage in patients with stable chronic bronchitis. Chest 75:29–31, 1979.
19. McKenzie CF: Chest Physiotherapy in the Intensive Care Unit, 2nd ed. Baltimore, Williams & Wilkins, 1989.
20. McNeill RS, McKenzie JM: An assessment of the value of breathing exercises in chronic bronchitis and asthma. Thorax 10:250–252, 1955.
21. Miller WF: A physiologic evaluation of the effects of diaphragmatic breathing training in patients with chronic pulmonary emphysema. Am J Med 17:471–477, 1954.
22. Motley HL: The effects of slow deep breathing on the blood gas exchange in emphysema. Am Rev Respir Dis 88:485–492, 1963.
23. Mueller RE, Petty TL, Filley GF: Ventilation and arterial blood gas changes induced by pursed lips breathing. J Appl Physiol 28:784–789, 1970.
24. Ogden LM, deRenne C: Chronic Obstructive Pulmonary Disease: Program Guidelines for Occupational Therapists and Other Health Professionals. Laurel, MD, RAMSCO Publishing, 1985.
25. Pryor JA, Webber BA, Hodson ME, Batten JC: Evaluation of the forced expiration technique as an adjunct to postural drainage in treatment of cystic fibrosis. BMJ 2:417–418, 1979.
26. Roa J, Epstein S, Breslin E, et al: Work of breathing and ventilatory muscle recruitment during pursed lip breathing in patients with chronic airway obstruction. Am Rev Respir Dis 143:A77, 1991.
27. Rodenstein DO, Stanescu DC: Absence of nasal air flow during pursed lips breathing. Am Rev Respir Dis 128:716–718, 1983.
28. Sackner MA, Silva G, Banks JM, et al: Distribution of ventilation during diaphragmatic breathing in obstructive lung disease. Am Rev Respir Dis 109:331–337, 1974.
29. Schmidt RW, Wasserman K, Lillington GA: The effect of air flow and oral pressure on the mechanics of breathing in patients with asthma and emphysema. Am Rev Respir Dis 90:564–571, 1964.
30. Sharp JT, Drutz WS, Moisan T, et al: Postural relief of dyspnea in severe chronic obstructive pulmonary disease. Am Rev Respir Dis 122:201–211, 1980.
31. Sinclair JD: The effect of breathing exercises in pulmonary emphysema. Thorax 10:246–249, 1955.
32. Sonne LJ, Davis JA: Increased exercise performance in patients with severe COPD following inspiratory resistive training. Chest 81:436–439, 1982.
33. Sutton PP, Parker RA, Webber BA, et al: Assessment of the forced expiration technique, postural drainage and directed coughing in chest physiotherapy. Eur J Respir Dis 64:62–68, 1983.
34. Thoman RL, Stoker GL, Ross JC: The efficacy of pursed-lips breathing in patients with chronic obstructive pulmonary disease. Am Rev Respir Dis 93:100–106, 1966.
35. Tiep BL, Burns M, Kao D, et al: Pursed lips breathing training using ear oximetry. Chest 90:218–221, 1986.
36. Webber B, Parker R, Hofmeyr J, Hodson M: Evaluation of self-percussion during postural drainage using the forced expiration technique. Physiother Pract 1:42–45, 1985.
37. Webber B, Pryor JA: Physiotherapy Skills: Techniques and Adjuncts. Edinburgh, Churchill Livingstone, 1993, p 116.
38. Willeput R, Vachaudez JP, Lenders D, et al: Thoracoabdominal motion during chest physiotherapy in patients affected by chronic obstructive lung disease. Respiration 44:204–214, 1983.

Exercise Training in Patients with Chronic Obstructive Pulmonary Disease

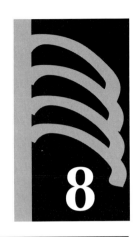

8

Michael J. Belman, MD

Exercise is widely promoted as a means of improving physical endurance. Exercise is recommended not only for the healthy, but also for individuals with various disabilities and disease. In respiratory medicine, several decades of investigation have been directed not only at the pathophysiology of exercise in patients with chronic obstructive pulmonary disease (COPD), but also at the effects of exercise training in improving function. As was initially the case with coronary artery disease, many physicians of the mid-20th century adopted a conservative approach and generally discouraged exercise in patients with significant COPD. Despite the pleas for greater physical exercise for patients with chronic lung disease by Barach, a pioneer of pulmonary medicine,[2] it was only in the late 1960s and early 1970s that his ideas were aggressively pursued. In the United States, widespread support exists for pulmonary rehabilitation programs, which, almost without exception, include a liberal dose of exercise training. The transference of the standard recommendations for exercise training from healthy subjects and even from cardiac patients has not been easy. The pattern of exercise response in COPD presents some unusual, and in some cases unique, features that require radical rethinking of the traditional advice given to the normal subject and the subject with heart disease. This chapter will highlight key features of the exercise pattern in COPD and review the evidence on exercise training.

EXERCISE TRAINING IN CHRONIC OBSTRUCTIVE PULMONARY DISEASE

COPD is the fifth leading cause of death in the United States and is second only to coronary heart disease as a cause of disability among Social Security disability recipients.[38] Of considerable concern is the fact that in contrast to heart disease, there has been a rapid increase in death and disability from COPD in recent years. Smoking cessation is clearly of critical importance in reducing the incidence of COPD. In established cases, the only therapy that increases survival is long-term oxygen therapy in hypoxemic patients.[38] Many different approaches and techniques, however, have been advocated as a means of improving function and reducing symptoms in these patients.[16,38] Thus, pulmonary rehabilitation programs vary in their complexity and can include a number of therapeutic components. These are:

1. Patient and family education.
2. Treatment of bronchospasm by means of bronchodilators or reduction in bronchial secretions.
3. Treatment of bronchial infections.
4. Treatment of congestive heart failure.
5. Oxygen therapy.
6. Chest physical therapy, including breathing technique training.
7. Exercise reconditioning.

8. Psychosocial therapy and vocational rehabilitation.

Although exercise reconditioning has long been considered an essential component of the rehabilitation process, only recently have randomized studies confirmed this belief.[34,43] In the study by Toshima and Ries,[43] 119 patients with COPD were randomized either to a comprehensive rehabilitation program including exercise reconditioning or to a control educational program. The investigators provided education, physical and respiratory therapy, psychosocial support, and supervised exercise training to the treated group, whereas the control group received twice-weekly classroom instruction in respiratory therapy, lung disease, parmacology, and diet but did not exercise. Before and after the 8-week treatment and after an additional 6 months, both groups underwent extensive physiologic and psychosocial tests. The major finding of this study was that at 8 weeks the improvement in exercise endurance as measured by treadmill walking showed a mean increase in treadmill time from 12.5 minutes to 23 minutes in the treated group as compared with an insignificant change from 12 to 13 minutes in the control group. At 6 months, the treated group still maintained a comparable advantage with a treadmill endurance of approximately 21 minutes as compared with 12 minutes in the control group. No difference in the quality of well-being scale, a measure of health-related quality of life, was noted. This well-designed, randomized, controlled study provides strong support for exercise therapy as an essential component of the pulmonary rehabilitation process. The study of O'Donnell and colleagues[34] used fewer patients but also showed significant reductions in breathlessness and increased exercise capacity in the treated group as compared with controls.

Relatively few other studies have compared treated and control groups. In the study by Cockcroft and Berry,[15] a treated group (19 patients) was compared with a control group (20 patients). During training, the patients used cycle exercise, rowing machines, and swimming. In addition, free range walking was performed. This treatment was carried out for 6 weeks in a rehabilitation center; patients were subsequently discharged and encouraged to continue walking and stair climbing. The control group was given no special instructions to exercise. The findings showed an increase in 12-minute walk distance and peak exercise oxygen consumption ($\dot{V}O_2$) and minute ventilation ($\dot{V}E$) in the treated group at 2 months, and these differences were significantly greater than those in the control group. The treated group also showed improvement in general well-being and dyspnea. In a study by McGavin and McHardy,[31] training was done by means of stair climbing at home, but the patients were tested with a 12-minute walk. In this study of 24 patients (12 in the exercise and 12 in a control group), a significant improvement in the 12-minute walk distance, albeit small, was noted. Other notable findings were an increase in stride length in the exercise group but no change in peak $\dot{V}O_2$, heart rate, or minute ventilation as measured during an incremental cycle ergometer test. Additional studies comparing treated and control groups are summarized elsewhere.[38]

STUDIES OF PULMONARY EXERCISE TRAINING

Numerous studies of exercise training have been performed during the past three decades. The results have been summarized in other publications.[3,9,16,35,38] Here, several of the more recent studies are discussed in detail. Apart from the study of Casaburi and coworkers,[12] the findings are similar to previous work. These studies, however, do effectively highlight the methods of testing and training and raise important questions regarding mode and intensity of exercise training. The interpretation of these studies has particular importance in deciding whether strict control of exercise intensities is required or whether a less structured approach is adequate.

EXERCISE TRAINING (HIGHLY STRUCTURED APPROACH)

In an editorial published in 1986, Casaburi and Wasserman[13] emphasized the role of carbon dioxide output as the major drive to ventilation during exercise. Recognizing the well-known relationships between $\dot{V}E$ on the one hand and $\dot{V}CO_2$, arterial PCO_2 and VD/VT ratio on the other, they suggested that aerobic training in patients with COPD would reduce carbon dioxide output and the ventilatory stimulus. The interrelationship of these variables is expressed in the following equation:

$$\dot{V}E = \frac{k \cdot \dot{V}CO_2}{PaCO_2 \, (1 - VD/VT)}$$

where $\dot{V}E$ is expired minute ventilation, $\dot{V}CO_2$ is carbon dioxide output, $PaCO_2$ is partial pressure of arterial CO_2, VD/VT is the physiologic dead space-to-tidal volume ratio, and k is a constant.

The lactic acid produced during exercise is buffered mainly by bicarbonate with the generation of carbonic acid, which dissociates to CO_2 and H_2O. The CO_2 produced by the buffering of lactic acid must be excreted by the lungs in addition to the CO_2 produced by muscle metabolism during exercise. Exercise training delays the rise in blood lactate. Thus, any delay in lactic acid production, by reducing the CO_2 load, decreases the ventilatory requirements during exercise. The effect of aerobic training and reduction in $\dot{V}E$ during exercise has been well documented in normal subjects by these investigators. At high levels of work near peak $\dot{V}O_2$, large reductions of 30 to 40 L/minute in $\dot{V}E$ can be achieved in normal individuals.[12]

With this rationale in mind, Casaburi and Wasserman from the United States, in conjunction with a group of Italian investigators,[12] performed a study in which high- and low-intensity training were performed in patients with COPD and examined in detail the effects on lactate production. Before and after the training, exercise testing was performed on a cycle ergometer with breath-by-breath measurements of gas exchange. In addition, arterial blood gas measurements and arterial lactate measurements were made. The anaerobic threshold (AT) was determined by means of the modified V-slope technique.[42] Training was performed on a calibrated cycle ergometer 5 days a week for 8 weeks. A high-intensity group performed exercise at 45 minutes per day at an intensity 60% of the difference between the AT and the $\dot{V}O_2$max. The low-intensity group exercised at 90% of the AT level, but the duration was increased so that total work performed in the two groups was similar.

The major results of Casaburi's study were reduction in the peak $\dot{V}CO_2$ and the maximal ventilatory equivalent for oxygen ($\dot{V}E/\dot{V}O_2$) in the high-intensity group. In a high work rate, constant load test, the high intensity–trained group showed significant reductions in blood lactate, $\dot{V}E$, $\dot{V}CO_2$, $\dot{V}O_2$, and $\dot{V}E/\dot{V}O_2$. In addition, heart rate at comparable work rates was reduced. All these findings confirm the development of a true aerobic training effect (Fig. 8–1). The group that trained at the low intensity, even though the total work performed was similar, showed smaller changes in these variables. In this latter group, although the lactate decrease was significant (10%), the decreases in $\dot{V}E$, $\dot{V}CO_2$,

and $\dot{V}O_2$ were not statistically significant. Furthermore, the significant increase in endurance for exercise at the higher work rate seen in the high intensity–trained group (6.6 to 11.4 minutes) was not seen in the low intensity–trained group (6.9 to 7.5 minutes).

There was a significant relationship between the decrease in minute ventilation during exercise and the decrease in blood lactate (r = 0.73, $\dot{V}E$ = 2.46 L/minute per mEq lactate). The slope of the relationship $\dot{V}E$/lactate in these patients (Fig. 8–2) was considerably lower than that recorded in a previous study in normal subjects in whom the $\dot{V}E$ decreased by 7.2 L/minute for each mEq of decrease in lactate. This study clearly showed that (1) significant lactic acidemia occurs in patients with mild-to-moderate chronic airflow obstruction, and in some cases this may develop at low work rates (pedalling at 0 watts); (2) both high and low intensity training reduce the rise in lactate, but the effect with high-intensity training is considerably greater; and (3) although lactate levels and $\dot{V}E$ are lower after training in patients with COPD, the reduction in ventilation in patients is only about a third as large as that seen in normal subjects. The explanation for this difference is related to the fact that these patients show a reduced ventilatory response to the lactic acidosis of exercise, and therefore a decrease in lactic acid after training produces a comparably smaller decrease in $\dot{V}E$.

Although this study clearly shows the generation of a true aerobic training response, this was accomplished in a group of relatively young (49 years on average) patients with rather mild disease (FEV_1 percentage predicted 56% and FEV_1/FVC ratio 58%). These patients may not be representative of most commonly found in rehabilitation programs. The majority of studies performed in the past examined patients in whom the FEV_1 was considerably lower. In the United States, it is not unusual to find patients with FEV_1 less than 1.0 L participating in exercise programs.[38] Moreover, before the training, these patients were relatively unfit, as shown by the AT that occurred at oxygen consumptions below 1 L/minute. It is not surprising, therefore, that they responded dramatically to the exercise programs. The fact that the ventilatory response to exercise acidosis is blunted in patients with COPD further detracts from the practical benefit of lactate reduction. As noted, Casaburi and coworkers' study[12] documented a $\dot{V}E$/lactate change only one third that of normals in mildly affected patients. In severely affected patients, one would anticipate an even smaller re-

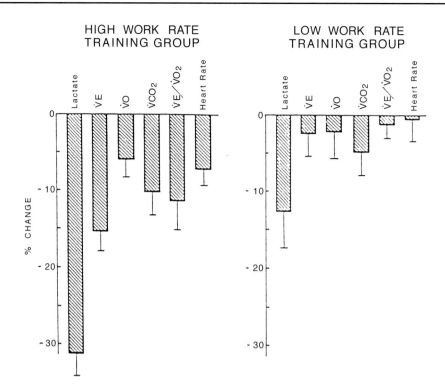

FIGURE 8–1. Changes in physiologic responses to identical exercise tasks. *Left panel,* High work rate trained group. *Right panel,* Low work rate trained group. (From Casaburi R, et al: Reductions in exercise lactic acidosis and ventilation as a result of exercise training in patients with obstructive lung disease. Am Rev Respir Dis 143:9–18, 1991.)

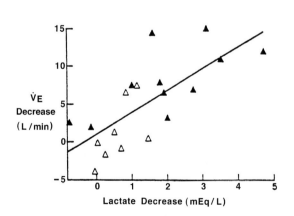

FIGURE 8–2. Relation between the decrease in ventilation and the decrease in arterial lactate in response to a high constant work rate test as a result of a program of exercise training. *Closed triangles* = High work rate trained group. *Open triangles* = Low work rate trained group. Solid line is obtained by linear regression. $\dot{V}E$ = 2.84 lactate + 1.19 (From Casaburi R, Patessio A, Ioli F, et al: Reductions in exercise lactic acidosis and ventilation as a result of exercise training in patients with obstructive lung disease. Am Rev Respir Dis 143:9–18, 1991.)

duction in lactate and consequently a smaller decrease in ventilation during exercise. The vast majority of studies[38] other than Casaburi et al have treated patients with moderate-to-severe disease and FEV_1s to generally 1 L and in some cases less. Similar results in a more severely affected group of patients would be helpful before the following exercise recommendations could be generalized.[8]

EXERCISE TRAINING TO TOLERANCE (UNSTRUCTURED APPROACH)

Exercise testing and training directed at manipulation of blood lactate involve complex measurements. This can be contrasted with the more unstructured approach of exercising to tolerance, an approach that has been used in a large number of studies.[38] These studies, despite the fact that they have not necessarily documented reductions in lactate, have shown that even severely obstructed patients, some of them with extreme hypercapnia,[21] can be exercised safely and show impressive gains in submaximal exercise endurance. This is particularly striking in the study of Niederman and coworkers,[33] in whom the greatest percentage improvements was seen in those patients with the lowest FEV_1 and low pretraining exercise endurances. In that study, the training was done without emphasis on intensity, patients being allowed to choose their own exercise level. Exercise sessions were conducted three times a week for 2 hours for a total of 9 weeks. During each session, the time was divided among cycling, treadmill walking, and lifting weights. The most impressive gains were in cycle endurance, which increased from 129.5 to 726.1 watts/minute. The increase in cycle endurance was comparable to that of patients in the study of Casaburi et al,[12] despite unregulated exercise training intensity. Similar results also were obtained by Holle and Schoene,[23] who showed large increases in treadmill endurance.

In two studies, large gains in endurance were achieved using high-intensity training, and patients were encouraged to reach maximal levels of ventilation during training.[10,37] In one study,[37] patients were initially separated into two groups based on whether an AT was reached. In those unable to reach an AT, training was done at the maximal work load achieved on the treadmill. In the patients who passed the AT, training intensity was initially aimed at the AT level itself. In both groups, intensity and duration were increased as tolerated. Of interest was the finding that these patients could train at exercise ventilations close to or even exceeding the maximum level reached on initial testing. In contrast to the work of Casaburi and coworkers,[12] both groups showed significant and comparable improvements in endurance on the treadmill. The investigators were quick to point out that this does not mean that a high-intensity training regimen

is therefore desirable for patients with COPD. In fact, gains in endurance were similar to those described by Casaburi et al. Clearly, both approaches are successful in the moderately to severely affected patient; there does not appear to be an intrinsic benefit in demanding that training be performed at almost maximal ventilatory capacity. Moreover, high-intensity exercise may also be disadvantageous because of higher risk of injury and because the discomfort of extreme exercise may reduce compliance with exercise programs.[5] The results of these studies are summarized in Table 8–1.

UPPER LIMB EXERCISE TRAINING

Upper extremity activities can[14,18] hamper diaphragmatic function. During arm work, the stabilizing effect of the shoulder girdle on the thorax is lost, and the inspiratory load is shifted onto the diaphragm and muscles of expiration. In these circumstances, the diaphragm is required to assume a greater load and, as noted, is ill prepared to do so (Fig. 8–3). The net result is a greater limitation of arm than of leg exercise associated with the earlier onset of dyspnea in many patients with severe airflow obstruction. Because performance of most activities of daily living requires repetitive upper extremity movements, this phenomenon has important implications for patients with COPD.

Two studies[17,30] have confirmed the value of specific arm training. In both studies, specific arm training resulted in an increased arm exercise endurance and a reduction in the metabolic cost for arm exercise. In the latter study, the improvements in unsupported arm activity were

TABLE 8–1
Exercise Training in Chronic Obstructive Pulmonary Disease

	Casaburi et al,[12] 1991	Punzal et al,[37] 1991	Niederman et al,[33] 1991
Number of Patients	9	57	24
FEV_1/FVC	58%	44%	50%
Intensity	High—90% $\dot{V}O_2$max	$\dot{V}Emax$	Unstructured
		At anaerobic threshold	Laissez faire
Frequency	5/week	Daily TM	3/week
Duration and method	8 weeks IP	Supervised 2/week × 4,	9 weeks
	45-min cycle	and then 1/week × 4 of free	20-min cycle,
		daily unsupervised walking	TM, UE
Test	Cycle endurance	Treadmill endurance	Cycle endurance
	6.6–11.4* min	12.1–22.0 min	5.0–12.0 min
	Anaerobic threshold ↑	12 min walk ↑	
Peak $\dot{V}O_2$	10% ↑	10% ↑	19% ↑
Psychosocial	Not measured	Breathlessness ↓	Depression ↓
	Fatigue ↓	Disability ↓	

UE, upper extremity; IP-inpatient; TM-treadmill.

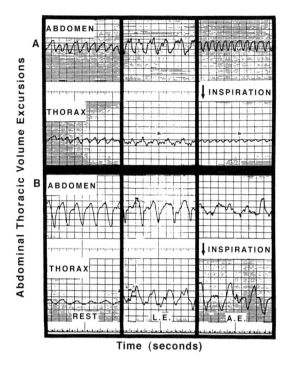

Time (seconds)

FIGURE 8–3. Tracings of abdominal and thoracic excursions. *A,* Excursions in a patient with synchronous thoracoabdominal movements at rest, during leg exercise (LE), and during arm exercise (AE). *B,* Synchronous pattern observed at rest and during LE becomes dyssynchronous during AE. Full inward retraction during inspection is seen in the last two breaths of the arm exercise tracing. (From Celli BR: Dyssynchronous breathing during arm but not leg exercise in patients with chronic airflow obstruction. N Engl J Med 314:1485–1490, 1986.)

seen only in the group that performed unsupported arm exercise and not in the group using supported arm exercise. The improved endurance in conjunction with the reduced metabolic cost are indicative of improved mechanics of arm muscles and possibly breathing muscles during arm activity. The specificity of limb training is emphasized by the findings of Lake and associates,[26] who randomized patients to one of three groups. The first group was a control group that received no training; the second group received upper limb training only; and the third group performed combined upper and lower limb training. Upper limb training included cycle ergometry with varying resistances, throwing a ball against a wall with the arms above the horizontal, passing a bean bag over the head, and arm exercise with ropes and pulleys. Lower limb exercise was tested by cycle er-

gometry and a 6-minute walk distance. Training was continued for 1 hour, three times a week, for 8 weeks. The results showed that limb training was limb specific. Thus, it was only in the group that trained with the upper extremities that upper extremity endurance increased, while walk distance improved in the lower limb–trained group. The combination-trained group showed improvements in both upper and lower limb muscle endurance. A modified quality of life questionnaire was also used but produced significant changes only in the group that received combined upper and lower limb training.

The study of Dolmage and coworkers[19] has stressed the value of support of the arms during exercise. In their study, the patients' arms were supported by means of a specially designed sling while they performed leg exercise. This situation was compared with unsupported elevated arms and with the arms in the control position (arms down). The results showed that the metabolic cost of leg work and dyspnea were both reduced during arm support and arms down as compared with arms elevated without support. The authors emphasized the importance of arm support as a means of reducing work and breathlessness during activity.

Ries and coworkers[39] performed a randomized study that compared a control group with two groups that used two different forms of upper arm training. Testing was done by means of cycle ergometry and unsupported arm exercise. In addition, three tests of activities of daily living were used; these included dishwashing, dusting a blackboard, and placing grocery items on shelves. Training was performed for at least 6 weeks and showed that although the patients who underwent the upper extremity training improved their performance on an arm cycle ergometer, it was disappointing to find that they did not improve performance in arm activities of daily living.

Early work by Keens and associates[25] on patients with cystic fibrosis suggested that upper extremity exercise may have a cross-over effect and improve respiratory muscle endurance. This was not confirmed, however, in a study of patients with COPD by Belman and Kendregan,[7] in which a group of patients who performed upper extremity cycle ergometry did not improve their ventilatory muscle endurance. Similarly, in both studies of upper extremity training described previously,[26,39] no significant change in ventilatory muscle function was found.

MECHANISMS OF IMPROVEMENT

Improvements in exercise tolerance may be ascribed to one or more of the following factors: improved aerobic capacity, improved muscle strength, increased motivation, desensitization to the sensation of dyspnea, improved ventilatory muscle function, or improved technique of performance. Despite the multiplicity of studies performed, there is as yet no clear consensus on the predominant mechanism of improvement.

IMPROVED AEROBIC CAPACITY

In normal subjects, increased endurance has largely been ascribed to changes in the trained muscles.[24] These changes, which mainly consist of increased capillary and mitochondrial density, plus increased concentrations of oxidative enzymes, occur concomitantly with training-induced decreases in the exercise heart rate and constitute the major components of the aerobic training response in normal subjects. Apart from the study by Casaburi and coworkers,[12] this pattern has not been observed in patients with COPD, and so it is not possible to ascribe improved exercise endurance to improved aerobic performance. A striking feature of the results of exercise training in COPD is the fact that almost without exception investigators have claimed success for their respective programs. This is true despite the fact that training modes, intensity, and frequency have varied widely.[11,38] Moreover, in a study in which aerobic training effects were specifically examined by means of muscle biopsies from the trained limbs, no significant improvement in oxidative enzymes was found.[6] These authors concluded that COPD patients were unable to exercise at the threshold intensity necessary to elicit a true aerobic response.

Although the emphasis on training has concentrated on endurance activities, evidence supports an important role for peripheral muscle strength. A third of patients with COPD implicated muscle fatigue as the limiting factor during exercise. A subsequent randomized study evaluated the effect of a weightlifting program in these patients.[40] The patients performed weight training three times a week for 8 weeks. Both arm and leg strengthening exercises were done. The results showed an increase in cycle endurance and reduction in symptoms as assessed by a questionnaire. This study certainly reinforces the need not to neglect strength training as an important component of the training regimen.

INCREASED MOTIVATION

Increased motivation might easily account for the improvement seen in some studies. This could be evaluated by noting an increase in the maximal $\dot{V}E$ or heart rate. Neither of these variables, however, has increased consistently in cases in which there has been an increase in endurance. In submaximal steady-state exercise tests in which exercise endurance time is the measure of improvement, motivation may certainly play an important role.

REDUCTION IN DYSPNEA

Research into the mechanisms of dyspnea is complicated by the inherent problems with measurement of intensity of a symptom. This topic has been reviewed in a monograph by Mahler and Harver.[29] Various scales and questionnaires are in use, including the Borg Scale for perceived exertion, the baseline and transitional dyspnea indices, and the chronic respiratory disease questionnaire.[22] Moreover, techniques are available that allow measurement of quality of life. Improved measurement in these areas is essential to gauge the impact of pulmonary rehabilitation programs in general and exercise training in particular.

Dudley and associates[20] have reviewed the psychosocial aspects of pulmonary rehabilitation and cited several studies that have found correlations between improved exercise endurance and improved feeling of well-being. One study found that psychological improvement resulted from either pulmonary rehabilitation including exercises or psychotherapy alone. Furthermore, it has been shown that there is a better correlation between mood and motivation and exercise endurance as compared with pulmonary function and exercise endurance.[32] Several other studies of exercise training have also shown improvements in the sense of well-being and reduction in breathlessness.[1,16,38] In the Agle and coworkers study,[1] the authors speculated that the process of graduated exercise training in the presence of trained medical personnel "inadvertently functioned as a desensitizing form of behavior therapy." They believed, therefore, that progressive exercise led to a decrease in the unrealistic fear of activity and dyspnea. A study by Belman and coworkers[4] showed that four repetitive episodes of treadmill walking over 10 days at a relatively high intensity resulted in a decrease in the perceived level of breathlessness over this short period of exercise. They speculated that *desensitization* may have played a role in this study as well. In a study of ventilatory muscle training,[27] a control group showed significant increases in exercise after participating in the testing sequence only. This evidence has given rise to the speculation that when patients with dyspnea experience their symptoms in a medically controlled environment while simultaneously receiving support and encouragement, they learn to overcome the anxiety and apprehension associated with dyspnea. This desensitization to dyspnea may be a key component to improved endurance after exercise, but further investigation is necessary to prove this point.

VENTILATORY MUSCLE TRAINING

Ventilatory muscle training is dealt with in a separate chapter. Its role in improving endurance is as yet unclear. A meta-analysis of ventilatory muscle training concluded that any effect if present is small and unlikely to contribute significantly to improved exercise tolerance in these patients.[41]

IMPROVED MECHANICAL SKILL

Improved skill in performance has been found in several studies. Good examples of this are in the early studies by Paez and coworkers,[36] which showed that skill in treadmill walking improved with repeated attempts. Clearly, skillful performance of the task decreases both the oxygen cost and the ventilatory requirements of work, although the actual work rate is unchanged.[28] This effect constitutes training of technique and can be used to advantage in that these patients can be trained to perform specific tasks more efficiently. Although the technique of treadmill walking has been shown to improve in some studies, it is not known if this is indeed a component of improvement seen in walking other than on a treadmill.

From the large number of studies performed to date, it is striking that there is no appreciable benefit on pulmonary function and gas exchange.[3,16,38] As noted earlier, with the exception of the work of Casaburi et al,[12] no true aerobic training effect has been demonstrated.

Even in the absence of a training effect, it is impressive that there is almost universal success shown for studies of exercise training when the outcome measure is increased exercise endurance. This includes studies in which the training intensity is low. The precise mechanism responsible for the improvement is not clear, but the absence of objective cardiopulmonary improvements raises the possibility that a reduction in dyspnea perception and increased motivation are important. Further research to evaluate these mechanisms is indicated. Moreover, additional research that combines measurements of exercise as well as valid measures of breathlessness and quality of life is indicated. The transference of the improved walking endurance to increase endurance for carrying out activities of daily living also requires improved documentation.

SUMMARY

Sporadic office visits to the local physician followed sometimes with changes in oral and inhaled bronchodilators, and on occasion the addition of steroids, frequently does little to improve symptoms and function in the disabled patient with COPD. As in other chronic diseases, the management of these patients is facilitated by a team approach and using general rehabilitation principles.[16] The rationale and practical implementation of such programs has been outlined by the American Association of Cardiopulmonary Rehabilitation. These are multifaceted programs, but a key component as outlined in this chapter is exercise training. In this brief chapter, the various approaches available have been described. Controversy still reigns regarding the optimal modes of training, and there are important differences among the several approaches. Two main groups can be delineated. One emphasizes the detailed definition of the impaired physiology with therapeutic measures targeted to specific defects.[12] There is good documentation that, conversely, unstructured programs that use treadmill and free range walking and cycling also improve endurance for exercise.[33,37] Upper extremity training is of benefit for improving endurance of the arms and reducing metabolic cost of arm elevation. Less well documented, however, is the carryover effect of laboratory exercise training to activities of daily living. In cases in which weakness of arms or leg fatigue is especially prominent, attention can be directed to strength training programs rather than endurance only.

Programs with as little as three sessions per week of 1 to 2 hours of low intensity activity have achieved success. Thus, we know that simple programs can be helpful. Moreover, without the necessity for complex testing and training methods, these programs can be implemented with relatively low costs. Future investigation to examine the relationship between improved exercise capacity for walking and arm exercise on the one hand and the ease of performance of activities of daily living on the other will help reinforce the effectiveness of exercise programs.

References

1. Agle DP, Baum GL, Chester EH, et al: Multi-discipline treatment of chronic pulmonary insufficiency: Function status at one year follow-up. In Johnston RF (ed): Pulmonary Medicine: A Hahnemann Symposium. New York, Grune & Stratton, 1973, p 355.
2. Barach AL, Bickerman HA, Beck G: Advance in the treatment of non tuberculous pulmonary disease. Bull NY Acad Med 28:353–384, 1952.
3. Belman MJ: Exercise in chronic obstructive pulmonary disease. Clin Chest Med 7:585–597, 1986.
4. Belman MJ, Brooks LR, Ross DJ, Mohsenifar Z: Variability of breathlessness measurement in patients with chronic obstructive pulmonary disease. Chest 99:566–571, 1991.
5. Belman MJ, Gaesser GA: Exercise training below and above the lactate threshold in the elderly. Med Sci Sports Exerc 23:562–568, 1991.
6. Belman MJ, Kendregan BK: Exercise training fails to increase skeletal muscle enzymes in subjects with chronic obstructive pulmonary disease. Am Rev Respir Dis 123:256–261, 1981.
7. Belman MJ, Kendregan BK: Physical training fails to improve ventilatory muscle endurance in patients with chronic obstructive pulmonary disease. Chest 81:440–443, 1982.
8. Belman MJ, Mohsenifar Z: Reductions in exercise lactic acidosis and ventilation as a result of exercise training in patients with obstructive lung disease [letter; comment]. Am Rev Respir Dis 144:1220–1221, 1991.
9. Carter R, Coast JR, Idell S: Exercise training in patients with chronic obstructive pulmonary disease. Med Sci Sports Exerc 24:281–291, 1992.
10. Carter R, Nicotra B, Clark L, et al: Exercise conditioning in the rehabilitation of patients with chronic obstructive pulmonary disease. Arch Phys Med Rehabil 69:118–122, 1988.
11. Casaburi R: Exercise Training in chronic obstructive lung disease. In Casaburi R, Petty TL (eds): Principles and Practice of Pulmonary Rehabilitation. Philadelphia, WB Saunders, 1993, p 204–224.
12. Casaburi R, Patessio A, Ioli F, et al: Reductions in exercise lactic acidosis and ventilation as a result of exercise training in patients with obstructive lung disease [see comments]. Am Rev Respir Dis 143:9–18, 1991.
13. Casaburi R, Wasserman K: Exercise training in pulmonary rehabilitation. N Engl J Med 314:1509–1511, 1986.
14. Celli BR, Make BJ: Dyssynchronous breathing during arm but not leg exercise in patients with chronic airflow obstruction. N Engl J Med 314:1485–1490, 1986.
15. Cockcroft AE, Berry G: Randomized controlled trial of rehabilitation in chronic respiratory disability. Thorax 36:200–203, 1981.
16. Connors G, Hilling L: Human Kinetics. In Guidelines for Pulmonary Rehabilitation Programs. Champaign, IL, American Association of Cardiopulmonary Rehabilitation, 1992.
17. Couser JL, Martinez FJ, Celli BR: Pulmonary rehabilitation that includes arm exercise reduces metabolic and ventilatory requirements for simple arm elevation. Chest 103:37–41, 1993.
18. Criner GJ, Celli BR: Effect of unsupported arm exercise on ventilatory muscle recruitment in patients with severe chronic airflow obstruction. Am Rev Respir Dis 138:856–861, 1988.
19. Dolmage TE, Maestro L, Avendano MA, Goldstein RS: The ventilatory response to arm elevation of patients with chronic obstructive pulmonary disease. Chest 104:1097–1100, 1993.
20. Dudley DL, Glaser EM, Jorganson PN: Psychosocial concomitants to rehabilitation in chronic obstructive pulmonary disease. Chest 77:413–420, 1980.
21. Foster S, Thomas HM: Pulmonary rehabilitation in COPD patients with elevated PCO_2. Am Rev Respir Dis 138:1519–1523, 1988.
22. Guyatt GH, Chambers LW: A measure of quality of life for clinical trials in chronic lung disease. Thorax 42:773–778, 1987.
23. Holle RHO, Schoene RB: Increased muscle efficiency and sustained benefit in an outpatient community hospital based pulmonary rehabilitation program. Chest 94:1161–1168, 1988.
24. Holloszy JO, Coyle EF: Adaptations of skeletal muscle to endurance exercise and their metabolic consequences. J Appl Physiol 56:831–838, 1984.
25. Keens TG, Krastins IRB, Wanamaker EM: Ventilatory muscle endurance training in normal subjects and patients with cystic fibrosis. Am Rev Respir Dis 116:853–860, 1977.
26. Lake FR, Henderson K, Briffa T, et al: Upper-limb and lower-limb exercise training in patients with chronic airflow obstruction. Chest 97:1077–1082, 1990.
27. Levine S, Weiser P, Gillen J: Evaluation of a ventilatory muscle endurance training program in the rehabilitation of patients with COPD. Am Rev Respir Dis 133:400–406, 1986.
28. Lustig FM, Maas A, Castillo R: Clinical and rehabilitation regime in patients with COPD. Arch Phys Med Rehabil 53:315–322, 1972.
29. Mahler DA, Harver A: Dyspnea. Mount Kisco, NY, Futura Publishing, 1990, pp 75–126.
30. Martinez FJ, Vogel PD, Dupont DN, et al: Supported arm exercise vs unsupported arm exercise in the rehabilitation of patients with severe chronic airflow obstruction. Chest 103:1397–1402, 1993.
31. McGavin CR, McHardy GJR: Physical rehabilitation for the chronic bronchitic: Results of a controlled trial of exercises in the home. Thorax 32:307–311, 1977.
32. Morgan AD, Peck DF, Buchanan DR: Effects of attitudes and beliefs on exercise tolerance in chronic bronchitis. BMJ 286:171–173, 1983.
33. Niederman MS, Clemente PH, Fein AM, et al: Benefits of a multidisciplinary pulmonary rehabilitation program. Improvements are independent of lung function. Chest 99:798–804, 1991.
34. O'Donnell DE, Webb KA, McGuire MA: Older patients with COPD: Benefits of exercise training. Geriatrics 48:59–66, 1993.
35. Olopade CO, Beck KC, Viggiano RW, Staats BA: Exer-

cise limitation and pulmonary rehabilitation in chronic obstructive pulmonary disease. Mayo Clin Proc 67:144–157, 1992.

36. Paez PN, Phillipson EA, Mosangkay M: The physiologic basis of training patients with emphysema. Am Rev Respir Dis 95:944–953, 1967.

37. Punzal PA, Ries AL, Kaplan RM, Prewitt LM: Maximum intensity exercise training in patients with chronic obstructive pulmonary disease. Chest 100:618–623, 1991.

38. Ries AL: Position paper of the American Association of Cardiovascular and Pulmonary Rehabilitation. Scientific basis of pulmonary rehabilitation. J Cardiopulmonary Rehabil 10:418–441, 1990.

39. Ries AL, Ellis BE, Hawkins RW: Upper extremity exercise training in chronic obstructive pulmonary disease. Chest 93:688–692, 1988.

40. Simpson K, Killian K, McCartney N, et al: Randomized controlled trial of weightlifting exercise in patients with chronic airflow limitation. Thorax 47:70–75, 1992.

41. Smith K, Cook D, Guyatt GH, et al: Respiratory muscle training in chronic airflow limitation: A meta-analysis. Am Rev Respir Dis 145:533–539, 1992.

42. Sue DY, Casaburi R: Metabolic acidosis during exercise in patients with chronic obstructive pulmonary disease. Chest 94:931–938, 1988.

43. Toshima MT, Ries AL: Experimental evaluation of rehabilitation in chronic obstructive pulmonary disease: Short-term effects on exercise endurance and health status. Health Psychol 9:237–252, 1990.

Biofeedback and Upper Extremity Exercise in Chronic Obstructive Pulmonary Disease

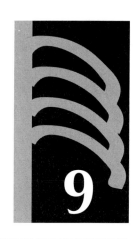

9

Bartolome Celli, MD
Seth Gottlieb, MD

The changes in the lungs of patients with chronic obstructive pulmonary disease (COPD) include progressive airflow obstruction, hyperinflation, and an increase in the dead space-to-tidal volume ratio (VD/VT). There also are changes in blood gases and increased energy demand. The way in which the respiratory system adapts to these changes is extremely important in planning therapeutic strategies for symptomatic patients.

VENTILATORY DRIVE AND BREATHING PATTERN

The simplest way to measure the increased drive is to analyze the final product of the effort. This is done in terms of the final output, the minute ventilation ($\dot{V}E$) and its components, the respiratory rate and the tidal volume (VT). Patients with COPD have an absolute increase in $\dot{V}E$ and in the respiratory rate component of that $\dot{V}E$. The VT changes depend on the severity of the obstruction. In moderate and severe (but not decompensated) COPD, the VT increases so the patient is breathing deeper and faster; but as obstruction progresses, the VT decreases until it reaches values below normal and the patient breathes with a rapid, shallow pattern. Unfortunately the obstruction to expiratory flow makes any increase in ventilation an unwise compensatory choice because it favors

further hyperinflation, with worsening in chest wall mechanics.

The evidence from studies of central drive in COPD patients with normal $PaCO_2$ indicates an increased value that almost doubles that seen in normal volunteers.[11,51,66,99] As would be expected, the drive increases as the level of $PaCO_2$ increases. Further, patients on assisted ventilation have the highest recorded values.[87] The increased respiratory drive is manifest when mouth occlusion pressure (P O.1) is measured, whereas the mean inspiratory flow (VT/Ti) shows less of a change, owing to airflow impedance. The duration of inspiration (the active phase of work for the inspiratory muscles) is slightly shortened in COPD, resulting in a duty cycle (Ti/Ttot) that is lower than normal in these patients.

RESPIRATORY MUSCLE FUNCTION

The hyperinflation of the thorax in patients with COPD places the inspiratory muscles at a mechanical disadvantage because it decreases the radius of curvature of the diaphragm and the length of its fibers.[86] The other inspiratory muscles are also shortened, but the evidence is that they are less affected than the diaphragm. As is reviewed later, with COPD progression, patients change their breathing pattern from one of predominantly diaphragm action to one in which accessory muscle activity predominates.[20,71] Another compensatory mechanism is alternating use of the different respiratory muscles at different times and different intensities (respiratory alternans). This is a pattern that has been documented in patients in ventilatory failure but that can also occur in patients with increased inspiratory loads and less severe disease.[71,99]

To complicate the problem further, many patients with COPD develop malnutrition. This has been implicated in the genesis of decreased respiratory muscle pressure generating capacity. The combination of mechanical and nutritional factors at a time when the drive and the load are increased places the respiratory muscles at risk for fatigue.[86] To prevent this from happening, the respiratory system adopts a breathing pattern that is characterized by a progressive decrease in V_T and a faster breathing rate (rapid shallow breathing). As a result, as shown by Begin and Grassino,[11] $PaCO_2$ can increase, and it tends to increase the most in the most severe patients. Theoretic considerations suggest that, at this stage, patients with COPD would benefit from breathing at a slower rate. Why do they maintain this rapid pattern? Although there are no specific answers, some of the therapeutic techniques used in patients with symptomatic severe COPD aim to reduce the breathing rate and to encourage deeper breathing.

In this chapter, first the use of biofeedback in patients with respiratory diseases in general is reviewed, then its use in COPD is summarized. The relationship between upper extremity exercise and ventilation in patients with COPD is then reviewed.

BIOFEEDBACK

Biofeedback is a technique that allows human beings to become aware of and influence internal physiologic functions that are normally not considered to be under voluntary control. The feedback signals are usually audio or visual and can be derived from many sources, including electromyographic (EMG) electrodes, strain gauges, flowmeters, temperature gauges, and pressure transducers. Other forms of biofeedback that rely on internal perception rather than specific sensorial response include yoga training and postural changes. Likewise, the simple use of pursed lip breathing represents a feedback maneuver that induces decreases in respiratory rate and deeper breathing.

Biofeedback has been applied clinically since the late 1960s. Examples of disorders that have been treated with the assistance of biofeedback include anxiety, hypertension, headaches, muscle spasticity, neuromuscular derangements, and movement disorders.[10] Although biofeedback has not yet had widespread clinical use in the treatment of respiratory disorders, there has been a significant body of literature investigating its potential usefulness. These investigations have focused on techniques that maximize ventilatory function by optimizing respiratory muscle strength and coordination, decreasing respiratory rate, decreasing airway resistance, or achieving some combination of the aforementioned. Although most of the biofeedback investigations in pulmonary diseases have concentrated on asthma, some have focused on weaning from mechanical ventilation and in the rehabilitation of the patient with COPD.

Biofeedback and Asthma

In asthma, biofeedback has primarily been evaluated for its ability to aid subjects in decreasing their airway resistance. In 1973, Davis and colleagues[32] combined general relaxation techniques with EMG biofeedback of the frontalis (scalp) muscle to help induce relaxation in asthmatic children. Frontalis tension was believed to be a reliable marker of the general level of relaxation. They used as their outcome variable the peak expiratory flow rate (PEFR), which they assumed was an indirect measure of airway resistance. Among the group of children with nonsevere asthma, the PEFR increased more in the group taught relaxation compared with the controls. The increase in PEFR was even greater in those subjects who combined relaxation with frontalis EMG biofeedback to lower frontalis tension, compared with those who used biofeedback alone. Despite the increased PEFRs, the relationship between frontalis tension and relaxation was unclear because the lowest level of EMG did not correlate with the highest observed PEFR.

In a further analysis of the significance of the electrical activity of the frontalis, Kotses and associates[59] measured PEFR in asthmatic children who, with the aid of EMG biofeedback, decreased frontalis muscle tension. In contrast to their previous study, this one did not include general relaxation techniques. The group of children receiving accurate (contingent) feedback were able to lower frontalis electrical activity and had increased PEFR when compared with groups who either had no treatment or had inaccurate (noncontingent) frontalis EMG. This study suggested a link between frontalis muscle tension and airway resistance, although the mechanism was not known.

Glaus and Kotses[50] extended this relationship to nonasthmatic subjects. They found that not only was biofeedback-assisted frontalis tension decrease associated with increased PEFRs, but also that frontalis muscle tension increases were associated with decreased flow rates compared with controls. In the second phase of this study, the authors also demonstrated that changes in brachioradialis tension were not associated with PEFR changes, thereby strengthening the argument that specific frontalis tension and not general muscular tension had a unique relationship with airway resistance. The authors explained their finding by the possible presence of a neural reflex composed of a trigeminal nerve afferent pathway and a vagal nerve efferent pathway. The trigeminal afferent would then be capable of altering airway resistance through its effects on vagal output. Despite this apparent relationship, there is concern regarding the validity of the PEFR as a measure of airway resistance. It is an effort-dependent maneuver that is significantly influenced by the motivation and coaching of the subject. Additionally the maneuver itself can lead to an increase in airway resistance.

Another reliable measure of airway resistance is the total respiratory resistance (TRR), which is measured by a forced oscillation technique as originally described by Dubois and colleagues.[40] This method employs a pulsation at a known low frequency and pressure that is applied to the airways. Feldman[48] was one of the first to use TRR in biofeedback training to lower airway resistance. In this study, four patients with severe asthma had TRR feedback that was interpreted with an audio output. The patients were told to lower the tone that corresponded to decreasing the TRR. Interestingly the decreased TRR values were associated with increased midmaximum expiratory flows (MMEF), but there was no significant change in PEFR. Vachon and Rich,[100] in a study controlled for contingent and noncontingent TRR biofeedback, were also able to demonstrate an ability of asthmatic patients receiving accurate (contingent) biofeedback to lower TRR. Subsequent studies of biofeedback and TRR, however, have not been as successful in demonstrating an ability of subjects to lower respiratory resistance.[42,54,95]

Although some reports have demonstrated increased flow rates and decreased respiratory resistance, biofeedback has not been shown to reduce asthma severity reliably in long-term follow-up. Kotses and associates[61] studied 29 asthmatic children who were assigned either to a group that maintained baseline facial tension or to a group that decreased it with the use of frontalis EMG biofeedback. In a follow-up, 5 months after the first biofeedback session, the subjects in the facial relaxation group had higher pulmonary flow rates, decreased chronic anxiety, and more positive attitudes toward asthma. They did not, however, differ from the control group on self-rated asthma severity, frequency of attacks, self-concept, or medication usage.

Biofeedback and Chronic Obstructive Pulmonary Disease

Little has been published on the use of biofeedback in patients with COPD. Casciari and associates[20] studied 22 patients with severe COPD who exercised on a treadmill three times a week for 6 weeks. Twelve of the patients (controls) continued to exercise for 3 more weeks, and the other 10 received breathing retraining for an additional 3 weeks. The breathing retraining included instruction in pursed lip breathing as well as biofeedback-assisted synchronization of abdominal and thoracic respiratory movements and biofeedback-assisted relaxation of accessory muscles. The subjects receiving biofeedback-assisted breathing retraining demonstrated significant improvement in exercise tolerance as measured by increased V_T, decreased respiratory rate, and increased maximum oxygen uptake ($\dot{V}O_2max$). This study was provocative because it indicated that biofeedback with breathing retraining could add to the already well-accepted practice of exercise conditioning for patients with any degree of COPD.

Yoga

Other ways exist to alter ventilatory patterns that must be considered. Yoga is a philosophical doctrine that includes voluntary control of posture and breathing. The latter includes slow deep breaths with apnea at end of inspiration and expiration with or without use of rapid abdominal maneuvers. The breathing rate may be brought down to 4 to 6 breaths per minute. Stanescu and coworkers[93] compared the breathing pattern of eight well-trained yoga practitioners with eight controls matched for sex, age, and height. The yoga group had a pattern of breathing characterized by ample V_T and slow breathing frequency. They also had a lower ventilatory response to CO_2 rebreathing. The mechanisms by which this seems to occur are not clear, but they may include habituation to chronic overstimulation of stretch receptors. Again, it is possible that because ventilation is automatically controlled by structures in the upper medulla and brain stem and voluntarily by the cortex, sustained slow deep breathing may become a *learned* reflex. Whatever the mechanism, this may have applications. Tandon[97] studied patients with COPD trained in yoga breathing and compared them with controls. The patients better controlled dyspnea and improved their exercise tolerance when compared with controls.

Postural Changes

It is known that musculoskeletal tone and contraction may be influenced by habitual positioning. Over the last few years, increasing attention has been given to the voluntary inhibition of undesirable postural patterns. This has been particularly useful for artists.[2,57] Austin and Asubel[5] demonstrated improved PEFR, maximal voluntary ventilation, and maximal inspiratory and expiratory pressures in normal subjects who underwent lessons in proprioceptive musculoskeletal education compared with controls. These lessons per se have not been systematically evaluated in patients with lung disease, but breathing retraining (pursed lip and diaphragmatic breathing) constitutes forms of therapy that resemble the above-discussed techniques.

Pursed Lip Breathing

Pursed lip breathing results in slowing of the breathing rate with increases in V_T. As Roa and colleagues showed,[84a] pursed lip breathing results in a shift in the pattern of recruitment of the ventilatory muscles from one that is predominantly diaphragmatic to one that recruits more the accessory muscles of the ribcage and abdominal muscles of exhalation. Perhaps this shift may contribute to the relief of dyspnea that has been reported by patients when this breathing technique is adopted. Patients using ventilatory assistance with an indwelling endotracheal tube cannot pursed lip breathe, but it has been

shown that the administration of respiratory retard or positive end-expiratory pressure (PEEP) improves oxygenation, decreases respiratory rate, augments ventilation, and decreases work of breathing in weaning patients. Pursed lip breathing and PEEP may have similar physiologic effects and make the former therapy indicated once the latter has been discontinued.

Biofeedback and Mechanical Ventilation

There have been several case reports[1,29,64] of biofeedback-assisted weaning from mechanical ventilation. Corson and associates[29] published two case reports. The first was a 60-year-old man with a history of poliomyelites who had suffered a respiratory arrest and was unable to wean for 3 months. Feedback was formed by a pneumotachygraph inserted between the tracheostomy and ventilator tubing. The signals were relayed to an oscilloscope, which traced respiratory volumes. The patient was given target volumes to achieve on the oscilloscope. The volumes were increased in subsequent sessions. A target decrease in respiratory rate was also given. The patient was extubated after 3.5 months of biofeedback sessions. The second patient was a 54-year-old man with C-6 transverse myelitis who was depressed about recent family matters and was not interested in weaning. Chest wall electrodes were placed to measure impedance with transmission to an oscilloscope. This patient was able to increase V_T and respiratory rate progressively and was eventually extubated.

The most extensive and scientifically valid study was by Holliday and Hyers.[52] They published a controlled trial of 40 patients requiring ventilation for at least 7 days. On the eighth day of weaning, the patients were divided into two groups: a control group and a biofeedback group. Biofeedback included V_T tracings using respiratory inductance plethysmography (RIP) and frontalis EMG. Those in the experimental group were encouraged to increase V_T thresholds and to decrease the frontalis EMG readings from the previous session. Those patients receiving biofeedback had a decrease in mean ventilator use days (20.6 versus 32.6) as well as improved measures of respiratory drive (V_T/Ti) and respiratory muscle efficiency (V_T/diaphragm EMG).

Although in its infancy for use in respiratory diseases, biofeedback is gaining ground. Given the intimate relationship between cortical function, control of breathing, and ventilatory pump output, it is likely that carefully planned and executed studies may help clinicians to use this less conventional, albeit exciting therapeutic tool.

ARM EXERCISE

Arm exercise and ventilation are the focus in the second part of this chapter. Emphasis is made on those aspects of arm anatomy and physiology that are important in the role of arm exercise in the training and rehabilitation of patients with symptomatic lung diseases.

Homo sapiens are best described by three characteristics: large brain size, upright biped position, and highly developed use of the upper extremities and hands. The change from the quadruped stance of most mammals to the biped one, which then allows full expression of dexterity, is associated with important adaptations of the musculoskeletal system. Much has been learned about the physiologic response to activities that involve the lower extremities. In contrast, surprisingly little is known about arm exercise, even though the accomplishment of manual tasks, an activity known to characterize high brain development, requires the use of not only the hand muscles, but also the concerted action of other muscle groups that participate in upper torso and arm positioning. The rest of this chapter reviews what is known about arm exercise, its complex interaction with the rest of the respiratory system, and, importantly, its use as a therapeutic modality to improve activities of daily living in patients limited by respiratory diseases.

Anatomic and Mechanical Considerations

To understand fully the relationship between arm exercise and respiration, some understanding of the respiratory muscles is necessary. The diaphragm is the best studied respiratory muscle. It is thought to exert its inflating action on the ribcage by three mechanisms: (1) by using the abdomen as a fulcrum against which it leans, exerting an expanding action on the ribcage; (2) by the vertical and downward orientation of its fibers and the curvature of its shape; and (3) by the transmission of the increase in abdominal pressure during contraction to the ribcage through its zone of apposition.[86,89] As stated previously, with the hyperinflation of COPD, as the fibers become more horizontal, the curvature of the diaphragm decreases, and this decreases its capacity to generate pressures.[89,99] Evidence obtained from animal[46,96] and human studies[91] suggests that the diaphragm adapts to the chronic changes of COPD by shortening the optimal length of its fibers, so that each bundle generates its maximal tension for that new length. If this is correct, the decreased diaphragmatic pressure generating capacity of patients with COPD is due to mechanical derangement or to contractile dysfunction and not to simple length tension changes. The external intercostals, the parasternal part of the internal intercostals and the scalenes are essential muscles of respiration, because they are active even during quiet breathing in normals.[35,47] Their functional importance increases with the hyperinflation of COPD because they appear to undergo less marked shortening and are at less of a mechanical disadvantage than the diaphragm.[78,81]

Other important muscles are called *accessory* inspiratory muscles because although they are inactive during quiet breathing in normal subjects, owing to their anatomic arrangement, they may be inspiratory in action under certain circumstances.[39,76] The sternomastoid, subclavian, pectoralis minor and major, serratus anterior, upper and lower trapezius, and latissimus dorsi share a common anatomic arrangement. They have an extrathoracic anchoring point (shown for some of them in Fig. 9–1) and a ribcage insertion. If they are fixed on their extrathoracic anchoring points, they can exert a pulling force on the ribcage. Except for the sternomastoid and pectoralis, the respiratory function of these muscles has not been fully studied.[39,76,82] They are probably inactive during quiet breathing in normal subjects but may be called to partake in ventilation during strenuous circumstances. This may explain the common observation that normal subjects after fatiguing exercise brace their arms, thereby anchoring the shoulder girdle accessory muscles and allowing them to pull the ribcage during inspiration. Three studies confirm this observation. Banzett and colleagues showed that normal volunteers could sustain a higher ventilatory target if their arms were braced on a table than if they were unsupported at the sides. Maestro and coworkers[67] and Dolmage and coworkers[38] showed that normal volunteers would manifest higher $\dot{V}E$ at similar work loads when cycling with the arms elevated versus supported on the ergometer handle.

The authors have shown that unsupported arm exercise may be more limiting than leg exercise and have hypothesized that this is due to derecruitment of the shoulder girdle muscles from their ventilatory contribution during un-

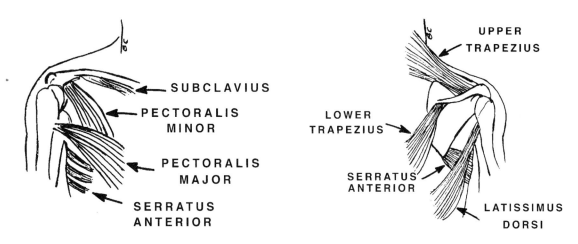

FIGURE 9–1. *A* and *B,* Anterior and posterior views of some of the muscles of the shoulder girdle that may share a ventilatory and a positional function.

supported arm activity.[25,30] As is discussed later, these muscles become most important in patients with poorly functioning diaphragms as is the case with severe COPD. The understanding of their function opens new therapeutic avenues. Techniques aimed at either decreasing ventilatory requirements during arm exercise or improving the function of these muscles should prove beneficial to patients with ventilatory limitations specifically when performing upper extremity activities.

The abdominal muscles are considered muscles of expiration.[17] Inasmuch as they oppose diaphragmatic contraction by helping generate abdominal pressure, they are also inspiratory.[24] It is also thought that by contracting during expiration, they tend to decrease end-expiratory lung volume, a position in which the chest wall stores elastic energy to assist in the subsequent inspiratory effort.[37] The authors have shown that, with worsening of airflow obstruction, there is progressive recruitment of the abdominal muscles of exhalation.[71] This finding was confirmed by Ninane and coworkers,[78] who showed EMG evidence of transverse abdomini contraction during tidal breathing in patients with COPD and that this contraction increases as the obstruction worsens. It is unclear why patients with the most severe COPD would choose a breathing strategy that tends to further close already compromised airways. The best explanation is that by recruiting accessory muscles during inspiration and the abdominal muscles during expiration, the patients may shift work away from an overworked and inefficient diaphragm. This has been observed to be the case during pursed lip breathing, whereby using this

strategy, the patients are capable of breathing larger inspiratory volumes at similar transdiaphragmatic pressures.[18]

Metabolism, Blood Flow, and Coordination of the Respiratory Muscles

Important in training is the state of blood flow and energy supply because it is believed that imbalances in energy supply and demand may result in fatigue. Most of what is known about blood supply and energetics concerns the diaphragm and, more recently, muscles of the ribcage. Similar to the heart, diaphragmatic perfusion occurs preferentially during relaxation and decreases during contraction, even though the diaphragm is supplied by a well-developed system that is arranged to minimize the decrease in blood flow during inspiration.[26,85,90]

Two factors determine compromise of diaphragmatic contraction during breathing. They are the duration of contraction or duty cycle, which can be expressed as the ratio of inspiratory time to total cycle time ($Ti/Ttot$), and the load, which can be inferred by relating the pressure needed to perform the ventilatory effort as a function of the maximal pressure that the muscle can generate. The latter relationship has been defined as Pdi/Pdi_{max} for the diaphragm or Pi/Pi_{max} for the inspiratory pressures measured at the mouth. The product of both ratios has been termed tension time index (TTi) and has been shown to relate to EMG and other signals of muscle fatigue both in normal individuals[12] and in patients with COPD.[13] It follows that arm exercise testing and training should take this into account to maximize results. This is most important for patients with COPD, for whom it has been shown that increased ventilation can be the limiting factor during exercise.[36,88] The best theoretic training would combine optimal load over a sufficient period of time while avoiding fatigue.

Neural Control and Coordination

The diaphragm and other respiratory muscles are innervated by a wide array of motor neurons that range from cranial nerve 11 to lumbar roots L-2 and L-3. The respiratory cycle is regulated by a complex series of centrally organized neurons. This complex arrangement maintains rhythmic breathing that usually goes unnoticed. This central control can be voluntarily overridden by cortical connections. Because individuals use primarily the diaphragm, the scalene, and some intercostals to breathe quietly, the system usually functions at a low cost of energy and efficiently, making respiration an unnoticed physiologic function.

As previously noted, however, some of the respiratory muscles serve other purposes. Upper torso and shoulder girdle muscles are involved in positioning the upper chest and upper extremity, and the diaphragm and muscles of the abdomen facilitate the generation of sound (speech, singing), coughing, defecation, and parturition. It has been postulated that the autonomic and voluntary ventilatory pathways are different.[45] Along the same line, studies in humans and animals show that the respiratory and tonic functions of these muscles are driven from different central nervous system areas, and input is integrated at the spinal level.[75] When some of these muscles are actively participating in breathing, their activity must be highly coordinated for them to be able to perform concurrent nonventilatory work. Either because of the load or because of competing central integration, muscle function may become dyscoordinated or dysfunctional and result in the perception of dyspnea. From this review, it is clear that a simplistic approach to arm exercise in terms of testing and training is inappropriate.

ARM EXERCISE TESTING

Lower extremity muscle function is evaluated in part by examining rhythmic continuous motion such as walking, using a treadmill, or using a cycle ergometer.[92,101] Of these modalities, ergometry appeared to be the best modality to test the upper extremities because it was an already validated form of exercise for the lower extremities. Thus, it seemed logical to exercise the arms in a similar way as the legs. Unfortunately, leg ergometry bears little resemblance to the way in which the upper extremities are normally used by humans. Nevertheless, because it is widely used and some validity has been established, it remains the gold standard for upper extremity testing.

Arm Cycle Ergometry (Arm Cranking)

Testing is performed with an arm ergometer mounted on an adjustable table so that the axis of the crank can be kept in line with the glenohumeral joint.[15] Subjects or patients crank at a fixed rate (60 to 80 rpm), and resistance is added at regular intervals (2 to 3 minutes). Most laboratories start with no resistance and then increase it, with the increases ranging from 7 to 30 watts. When studying normal subjects, the upper range is preferred. Patients, however, seldom tolerate high loads, and increases are limited to 10 watts. The exercise may be terminated by symptoms (maximal), by reaching a defined end point such as the inability to maintain a cranking rate, or by reaching a targeted submaximal load, such as 60% to 80% of maximal. The measurements obtained are the same as those described for leg exercise and are summarized in Table 9–1. For patients, we strongly recommend the evaluation of dyspnea using either the Visual Analog Scale or a modified Borg Scale because this may help guide subsequent training or, more importantly, provide an important outcome parameter that then allows evaluation of training response.

TABLE 9–1
Method for Arm Cranking Testing

1. Cycle at 60–80 rpm
2. Increase resistance (7–30 watts every 2–3 min)
3. Measure:
   Endurance time (seconds or minutes)
   Heart rate
   Blood pressure
   Minute ventilation
   Oxygen uptake ($\dot{V}O_2$)
   CO_2 production ($\dot{V}CO_2$)
   Respiratory frequency (respiratory rate)
   Oxygen saturation
   Blood gases
   Dyspnea rating

Cardiac and Metabolic Response

In contrast to leg exercise, information regarding response of arm cranking is relatively scarce. Fortunately, the published results are uniform, and there is agreement in their overall interpretation.* Maximal $\dot{V}O_2$, $\dot{V}CO_2$ and $\dot{V}E$ are lower for arm than for leg exercise.[4,16,31,69,94] Stated differently, maximal arm cranking represents a submaximal cardiopulmonary exercise test. Table 9–2 shows the results from several selected series, all of which have found maximal values to range between 65% and 80% of those observed for leg ergometry.[4,31,69] At similar $\dot{V}O_2$ (normalized work), $\dot{V}CO_2$, $\dot{V}E$, and lactate production are higher during arm work. Where it has been measured, anaerobic threshold occurs earlier during arm cranking.[31] These overall changes are best explained by the fact that the smaller muscle mass involved in arm cranking has to "work" more to achieve the same $\dot{V}O_2$. The response of the cardiovascular system is also different with arm versus leg cycling, and the changes described parallel those seen in the metabolic parameters. At similar $\dot{V}O_2$ (normalized work), heart rate, blood pressure, and peripheral vascular resistance are higher during arm cranking, but overall cardiac output and stroke volume are lower for this exercise.[4,31] From such findings, it has been said that upper extremity exercise is of some danger to patients with heart disease. The practical experience on these patients is different, perhaps because peak exercise for them occurs at much lower loads than that achieved by normal individuals doing leg exercise.[6,8,18,79] With appropriate monitoring, there is little danger in evaluating exercise performance with the use of arm ergometry, and arm cranking remains a good option for the testing of cardiopulmonary reserve of patients who cannot complete leg exercise.

Gas Exchange Response

Arm cranking modifies gas exchange. Martin and coworkers[69] have shown that arm cranking induces a higher PaO_2, SaO_2, and VD/VT and a lower PAO_2–PaO_2 at the same $\dot{V}O_2$ compared with leg cycling. The explanation for these changes remains elusive and may include differences in alveolar ventilation, CO_2 production, ventilation-perfusion inequality, diffusion, and control of breathing. Studying patients with dyspnea,[70] the same authors have established criteria for the normal gas exchange response to maximal arm cranking. The criteria are (1) PAO_2–PaO_2 equal to or less than 13 torr, (2) PaO_2 equal to or greater than 85 torr, and (3) VD/VT equal to or less than 0.26. Interestingly the findings for patients with COPD are similar, although not as well characterized. It has been shown that with arm exercise SaO_2 falls, but the decrease is of a lesser magnitude than that observed during leg exercise.[25,30] Although not proven for arm exercise, the data from lower extremity exercise indicate that with advancing age, there is worsening in gas exchange with an increase in the A-a O_2 gradient and a decrease in *efficiency*, that is, less power at the same $\dot{V}O_2$.[101] Because testing is often performed in elderly individuals, the values mentioned should be used with caution.

Training Upper Extremities with Arm Cranking

Many groups have included arm cranking as a therapeutic tool that may improve upper extremity function. The most important concept that has promoted its inclusion is the one of specificity of training, that is to say that only those muscles that are trained manifest a response to the training. The best example of this is the study of Belman and Kendregan.[14] They studied 15 patients with COPD before and after 6 weeks of training. The patients were divided into two groups; eight underwent training of the upper extremities using arm cranking, and seven exercised using leg ergometry. The ses-

TABLE 9–2
Effect of Arm Cranking on Cardiopulmonary and Metabolic Function in Normal Individuals

	Maximum $\dot{V}O_2$, L/min		Maximum Heart Rate		Maximum $\dot{V}E$, L/min	
	LC	AC	LC	AC	LC	AC
Astrand et al,[4] 1968	4.7	3.3	190	177	173	122
Reybrock et al,[83] 1975	3.7	2.4	168	150	178	73
Martin et al,[69] 1991	3.3	2.2	189	168	144	101
Mean	3.9	2.6	182	165	165	99

LC = Leg cycling; AC = arm cycling.

*References 3, 6, 15, 44, 53, 56, 63, 61, 65, 74, 77, 80, 88, 94, 102 and 103.

sions lasted 20 minutes four times weekly. The study demonstrated a significant increase in arm cycle endurance for the arm-trained group and in leg cycle endurance for the leg-trained group, without cross-over effect. Since then, several other studies have shown beneficial effects when arm cranking is added to leg exercise as part of comprehensive programs of rehabilitation.[28,62]

The training protocols vary greatly from group to group. The authors train patients at 60% of maximal $\dot{V}O_2$, as determined by a baseline test (Table 9–3). For many patients who stop exercising even without added resistance, such as patients with severe COPD using ventilators, exercise time is progressively increased until reaching a total of 20 minutes daily. For those patients capable of completing 20 minutes, resistance is increased on a regular basis (every three sessions). The results of several studies indicate that a minimum of 12 sessions may be required to obtain improvement in endurance.[17] It also must be emphasized that once started, regular exercise must be maintained because deconditioning occurs rather quickly. Arm cranking is well tolerated and liked but requires an ergometer, which may not be available in sufficient numbers even in large centers and is rarely available at home. Unsupported arm exercise (UAE) is another form of training, requires no apparatus, is easy to perform, and offers a valid alternative to arm ergometry.

Unsupported Arm Exercise

The arms are used much differently than the legs. The latter are used to support individuals (posture and locomotion), whereas the former require considerable action against gravity (without support). The unsupported activities of the arms range from work (typing, painting) to sports (karate, baseball) but most importantly include personal care (eating, grooming, cleaning). It is surprising that clinicians have persisted in testing the upper extremities with the same tool used to test the lower extremities

---

TABLE 9–3
Arm Cranking Training

1. Train at 60% of maximal work capacity*
2. Increase load every 3rd–5th session as tolerated
3. Monitor heart, dyspnea
4. Train for as long as tolerated, up to 30 min
5. Aim for 24 sessions

*Work capacity as determined by an arm ergometer test.

---

when in humans arm function is so different. As a matter of fact, it was not until 1973 that it was reported that patients with COPD complained of severe dyspnea while performing simple activities of daily living with upper extremities.[98] In this study, Tangri and Wolf[98] studied the breathing patterns of seven patients while they tied their shoes or combed their hair. The patients developed an irregular, shallow, rapid pattern of breathing while performing the activities. After the exercise, the patients breathed faster and deeper. The authors postulated that this pattern was best explained by rapid ineffective shallow breathing during arm exercise with compensatory hyperventilation after the tasks were completed.[98]

The authors have explored the respiratory and metabolic responses to UAE and compared them with those seen with leg and arm ergometry in normal subjects and in patients with COPD.[22,23,25,30] It was shown that UAE results in dyssynchronous thoracoabdominal excursion and dyspnea at an earlier time and at lower $\dot{V}O_2$ than the more metabolically demanding leg exercise.[25] In that study, the thoracoabdominal dyssynchrony was not solely due to diaphragmatic fatigue because the postexercise maximal transdiaphragmatic pressure decreased by the same magnitude in both groups. The authors postulated that UAE shifts work to the diaphragm as some of the shoulder girdle muscles decrease their participation in ventilation and have to increase their participation in arm positioning.[21] These changes may have led to earlier fatigue of the involved muscles. To test this hypothesis, the authors have used gastric-pleural pressure (Pg-Ppl) plots (using gastric and esophageal balloons) while patients and normal subjects performed UAE and arm and leg cycle ergometry. Lower peak $\dot{V}O_2$, $\dot{V}CO_2$, and heart rates were documented during UAE than during the other forms of exercise. There are, however, increased gastric pressure swings during UAE, which can be explained by a greater contribution to ventilatory pressure generation by the diaphragm and abdominal muscles and a lesser contribution by the inspiratory muscles of the ribcage.[22,30]

To perform and quantitate UAE, a pegboard with pegs separated 10 cm vertically is used. The patient sits with a straight back and has to shift rings with the extended arms at the shoulder level. In the authors' experience with patients, exercise time is a good indicator of exercise endurance. In normal subjects, weights are added to the arms.

The authors have evaluated a simple test that

is useful for patients with severe COPD. The test consists of simple anterior elevation of the arms. The authors studied 22 normal subjects and noted that arm elevation significantly increased $\dot{V}O_2$, $\dot{V}CO_2$, $\dot{V}E$, VT, and Pg without changes in respiratory rate. The change in Pg with arm elevation and the sudden drop immediately after lowering the arms indicate a mechanical rather than a metabolic or ventilatory cause for the changes in respiratory muscle recruitment.[27] The changes observed may be of limited significance in normals, but they may become more important in patients with COPD. To test this hypothesis, the same parameters in 20 patients with COPD were evaluated. Arm elevation resulted in significant increases in $\dot{V}O_2$ and $\dot{V}CO_2$ for these patients. In contrast to normals, and likely owing to the inability to increase VT at a low mechanical cost, patients increased $\dot{V}E$ by increasing the respiratory rate and, less so, the VT. The respira-

tory muscle recruitment pattern indicated that arm elevation not only increased diaphragmatic recruitment during inspiration, but also generated a more vigorous recruitment of the abdominal muscles.[71,72] These data support the hypothesis that simple arm elevation can be used as a submaximal arm exercise test, especially in patients with COPD, because it is simple and well tolerated. As is discussed later, it may be used as a test of intervention outcome because a lower rise in $\dot{V}O_2$, $\dot{V}E$, or $\dot{V}CO_2$ after therapy would support a beneficial effect from the exercise.

Unsupported Arm Training

There are few studies of the effects of unsupported arm training in the rehabilitation of patients with COPD. They are summarized in Table 9–4. Perhaps the oldest one is by Keens

TABLE 9–4
Controlled Studies of Arm Exercise in Patients with Chronic Obstructive Lung Disease

Study	Number Pts., Exercise	Duration	Course	Type	Results
Keens et al,[58] 1977	7 Arm exercise	1.5 hour/day	4 weeks	Swimming Canoeing	↑VME (56%)
	4 VMT	15 min/day	4 weeks	VMT	↑VME (52%)
	4 Controls	—	—	None	↑VME (22%)
Ries et al,[84] 1988	8 Gravity resistance Arm exercise	15 min/day	6 weeks	Low resistance/ endurance High repetition	↑Arm endurance ↓Dyspnea
	9 Neuromuscular facilitation Arm exercise	15 min/day	6 weeks	Weight lifts endurance	↑Arm strength, endurance ↓Dyspnea
	11 Controls	—	6 weeks	Walk	No change
Epstein et al,[41] 1991	13 Arm exercise	30 min/day	8 weeks	Upper arm exercise	↓$\dot{V}O_2$ and ↑$\dot{V}_E$ for arm elevation ↑PI$_{max}$
	10 VMT	30 min/day	8 weeks	VMT	↑PI$_{max}$ and VME

VMT = Ventilatory muscle training;
VME = ventilatory muscle endurance;
PI_{max} = maximal inspiratory pressure.

and coworkers,[58] who studied a group of patients with cystic fibrosis before and after a training period of 6 weeks. Arm training consisted of swimming and canoeing for 1.5 hours daily. After training, the authors observed an increase in upper extremity endurance, but, perhaps more importantly, there was an increase in maximal sustainable ventilatory capacity that was similar in magnitude to the increase observed in another group of patients treated with ventilatory muscle training. Ries and coworkers[84] studied the effects of two forms of arm exercise, gravity resistance and modified proprioceptive neuromuscular facilitation, on a group of patients with COPD. They compared the results with those obtained in another group who did not complete arm exercise.[84] All of the 45 COPD patients were involved in a comprehensive, multidisciplinary pulmonary rehabilitation program. Even though only 20 patients completed the program, they showed improved performance on the tests that were specific for the training. In that study, the patients reported a decrease in fatigue in all tests performed.

Because the authors had shown that simple arm elevation results in a significant increase in $\dot{V}E$ and $\dot{V}O_2$, they reasoned that if they trained the arms to perform more work or decreased the ventilatory requirement for the same work, they should improve the capacity of the patient to perform arm activity. The authors first studied 14 patients with COPD before and after 8 weeks of three times weekly, 30-minute sessions of UAE, as part of a comprehensive rehabilitation program that included leg exercise. The arm exercise consisted of intermittent vertical and oblique lifting of a dowel[28] as described in Table 9–5. After training, there was a 35% decrease in the pretreatment rise in $\dot{V}O_2$ and $\dot{V}CO_2$ seen with arm elevation. There was a small but significant drop in the rise of $\dot{V}E$ during arm elevation. The authors have completed a study of 26 patients with COPD, randomized to either unsupported arm training (11 patients) or threshold resistance breathing training (14 patients).[41] Arm training increased arm exercise endurance and decreased the $\dot{V}E$, $\dot{V}O_2$ and $\dot{V}CO_2$ during arm elevation, whereas ventilatory muscle trainees did not show any change in those values. Interestingly, maximum inspiratory pressure increased significantly for both groups, indicating that arm training may induce increases in force generation by those muscles of the ribcage that hinge on the shoulder girdle.

Martinez and colleagues[73] compared training using arm ergometry with training using UAE as part of a rehabilitation program for patients with COPD. They found that unsupported arm training decreased the metabolic requirement for exercise that more closely resembled that which is performed during daily living activities and concluded that simple repeated arm elevation may help more than arm ergometry.[73] More work is needed to select those patients who may benefit most from arm training. Training programs should also be developed for the different muscles of the shoulder girdle that may exert ventilatory force. This concept has already been explored for the pectoralis muscle.[35] Estenne and associates[43] trained the pectoralis muscle of six tetraplegic patients with negative isometric exercise and evaluated their strength and pulmonary function after 6 weeks. The results were compared with those obtained in six patients who underwent conventional pulmonary rehabilitation. Trained patients significantly increased their expiratory muscle strength and expiratory reserve volume. Taken together, these results indicate a possible role for the training of shoulder girdle muscles as a way to improve respiratory muscle function.

Certainly, arm exercise training results in improved performance for arm activities and in a decrease in the ventilatory requirement for upper extremity activity, such as elevating the arms. Whether this results in decreased symptoms for similar work remains to be determined.

TABLE 9–5
Method for Unsupported Arm Training

1. Dowl (weight 500–750 g)
2. Lift to shoulder level for 2 min at a frequency equal to breathing rate
3. Rest for 2 min
4. Repeat sequence as tolerated up to 7–8 times (28–32 min)
5. Monitor dyspnea, heart rate
6. Increase weight (250 g) every 5th session, as tolerated
7. Aim for 24 sessions

CONCLUSIONS

As with biofeedback, there has been a revival of interest in the interaction between arm exercise and ventilation. Although arm ergometry continues to be the gold standard for the testing and training of the upper extremities, an increasingly larger body of evidence indicates a more important role for the testing and training of the upper extremities in forms that more closely resemble their physiologic adaptation in humans. As knowledge of the functional anatomy of shoulder girdle muscles improves, so will the capacity to apply this knowledge in more rational and effective exercise regimens.

References

1. Acosta F: Biofeedback and progressive relaxation in weaning the anxious patient from the ventilator: A brief report. Heart Lung 17:299–301, 1988.
2. Alexander FM: The resurrection of the body: The essential writings of F. Mathias Alexander. New York, Dell Publishing, 1974.
3. Astrand I: ST depression, heart rate and blood pressure during arm and leg work. Scand J Clin Lab Invest 30:4114, 1972.
4. Astrand I, Guhray A, Wahren J: Circulatory responses to arm exercise with different arm positions. J Appl Physiol 25:528–532, 1968.
5. Austin JH, Asubel P: Enhanced respiratory muscular functions in normal adults after lessons in proprioceptive musculoskeletal education without exercise. Chest 102:486–490, 1992.
6. Balady GJ, Weiner DA, McCabe CH, Ryan TJ: Value of arm exercise testing in detecting coronary artery disease. Am J Cardiol 55:37–39, 1985.
7. Balady GJ, Weiner DA, Rose L, Ryan TJ: Physiologic responses to arm ergometry exercise relative to age and gender. J Am Coll Cardiol 16:30–35, 1990.
8. Balady GJ, Weiner DA, Rothendicr JA, Ryan TJ: Arm exercise-thallium imaging testing for the detection of coronary artery disease. J Am Coll Cardiol 9:84–88, 1987.
9. Banzett R, Topulos G, Leith D, Natios C: Bracing arms increases the capacity for sustained hyperpnea. Am Rev Respir Dis 133:106–09, 1983.
10. Basmajian JV: Introduction: Principles and background. In Basmajian JV (ed): Biofeedback—Principles and Practice for Clinicians. Baltimore, Williams & Wilkins, 1979, pp 1–4.
11. Begin P, Grassino A: Inspiratory muscle dysfunction and chronic hypercapnia in chronic obstructive pulmonary disease. Am Rev Respir Dis 143:905–912, 1991.
12. Bellemare F, Grassino A: Evaluation of diaphragmatic fatigue. J Appl Physiol 53:1196–206, 1982.
13. Bellemare F, Grassino A: Force reserve of the diaphragm in patients with chronic obstructive pulmonary disease. J Appl Physiol 35:8–15, 1983.
14. Belman M, Kendregan BA: Exercise training fails to increase skeletal muscle enzymes in patients with chronic obstructive pulmonary disease. Am Rev Respir Dis, 36:256–261, 1981.
15. Blomqvist CG: Upper extremity exercise testing and training. Cardiovasc Clin 15:175–183, 1985.
16. Bobbert AC: Physiological comparison of three types of ergometry. J Appl Physiol 15:1007–1014, 1960.
17. Bohanon RW: Adapting a bicycle ergometer for arm crank ergometry. Suggestions from the field. Phys Ther 66:362–363, 1986.
18. Breslin E: The pattern of respiratory muscle recruitment during pursed lip breathing Chest 101:75–78, 1991.
19. Campbell EJM, Agostoni E, Newsom-Davis J: The Respiratory Muscles. Mechanics and Neural Control, ed 2. London, Lloyd-luke, 1970.
20. Casciari RJ, Fairbuster RD, Harrison A, et al: Effects of breathing retraining in patients with chronic obstructive pulmonary disease. Chest 79:393–398, 1981.
21. Celli BR: Arm exercise and ventilation [editorial]. Chest 93:673–674, 1988.
22. Celli BR, Criner G, Rassulo J: Ventilatory muscle recruitment during unsupported arm exercise in normal subjects. J Appl Physiol 64:1936–1941, 1988.
23. Celli BR, Martinez F, Couser J, Rassulo J: Factors determining the pattern of ventilatory muscle recruitment (VMR) in patients with chronic obstructive pulmonary disease (COPD). Chest 97:68S, 1990.
24. Celli BR, Rassulo J, Berman JS, Make B: Respiratory consequences of abdominal hernia in a patient with severe chronic obstructive pulmonary disease. Am Rev Respir Dis 131:178–180, 1985.
25. Celli BR, Rassulo J, Make BJ: Dyssynchronous breathing during arm but not leg exercise in patients with chronic airflow obstruction. N Eng J Med 314:1486–1490, 1986.
26. Comtois A, Gorczyca A, Grassino A: Anatomy of diaphragmatic circulation. J Appl Physiol 58:238–244, 1987.
27. Couser JI Jr, Martinez FJ, Celli BR: Respiratory response and ventilatory muscle recruitment during arm elevation in normal subjects. Chest 101:336–40, 1992.
28. Couser J, Martinez F, Celli, BR: Pulmonary rehabilitation that includes arm exercise reduces metabolic and ventilatory requirements for simple arm elevation. Chest 103:37–41, 1993.
29. Corson JA, Grant JL, Moulton DP, et al: Use of biofeedback in weaning paralyzed patients from respirators. Chest 76:543–545, 1979.
30. Criner GJ, Celli BR: Effect of unsupported arm exercise on ventilatory muscle recruitment in patients with severe chronic airflow obstruction. Am Rev Respir Dis 138:856–861, 1988.
31. Davis JA, Vodak P, Wilmore JH, et al: Anaerobic threshold and maximal aerobic power for three modes of exercise. J Appl Physiol 41:544–550, 1976.
32. Davis MH, Saunder DR, Creer TL, Chai H: Relaxation training facilitated by biofeedback apparatus as a supplemental treatment in bronchial asthma. J Psychosom Res 17:121–128, 1973.
33. Delk KK, Gervitz R, Hicks DA, et al: The effects of biofeedback assisted breathing retraining on lung functions in patients with cystic fibrosis. Chest 105:23–28, 1994.
34. DeTroyer A, Estenne M: Coordination between ribcage muscles and diaphragm during quiet breathing in humans. J Appl Physiol 57:899–906, 1984.
35. DeTroyer A, Estenne M, Heilporn A: Mechanism of active expiration in tetraplegic subjects. N Engl J Med 314:740–744, 1986.
36. Dillard T: Ventilatory limitation of exercise: Prediction in COPD. Chest 92:195–196, 1987.
37. Dodd DS, Brancatisano T, Engle LA: Chest wall mechanics during exercise in patients with severe chronic airflow obstruction. Am Rev Respir Dis 129:33–38, 1984.
38. Dolmage TE, Maestro L, Avendano MA, Goldstein RS: The ventilatory response to arm elevation of patients with chronic obstructive pulmonary disease. Chest 104:1097–1100, 1993.
39. Druz WS, Sharp JT: Activity of the respiratory muscles in upright and recumbent humans. J Appl Physiol 51:1552–1561, 1981.
40. Dubois AB, et al: Oscillation mechanics of lung and chest in man. J Appl Physiol 8:587, 1956.
41. Epstein S, Breslin E, Roa J, Celli BR: Impact of unsupported arm training (AT) and ventilatory muscle training (VMT) on metabolic and ventilatory consequences of unsupported arm elevation (UE) and exercise

(UAEX) in patients with chronic airflow obstruction (CAO). Am Rev Respir Dis 143:A-81, 1991.

42. Erskine-Millis JM, Cleary PJ: Respiratory resistance feedback in the treatment of bronchial asthma in adults. J Psychosom Res 31:765–775, 1987.

43. Estenne M, Knoop C, Janvaerenbergh, J, et al: The effect of pectoralis muscle training in tetraplegic subjects. Am Rev Respir Dis 139:1218–1222, 1989.

44. Eston RG, Brodie DA: Responses to arm and leg ergometry. Br J Sports Med 20:4–6, 1986.

45. von Euler C: On the central pattern generator for the basic breathing. J Appl Physiol 55:1647–1659, 1983.

46. Farkas G, Roussos CH: Adaptability of the hamster's diaphragm to emphysema and/or exercise. J Appl Physiol 53:1263–1271, 1982.

47. Farkas GA, Decramer M, Rochester DF, et al: Contractile properties of intercostal muscles and their functional significance. J Appl Physiol 59:528–535, 1985.

48. Feldman GM: The effect of biofeedback training on respiratory resistance of asthmatic children. J Psychosom Med 38:27–34, 1976.

49. Gallego J, et al: Electromyographic feedback for learning to activate thoracic inspiratory muscles. Am J Phys Med Rehab 70:186–190, 1983.

50. Glaus KD, and Kotses H: Facial muscle tension influences lung airway resistance: Limb muscle tension does not. Biol Psychol 17:105–120, 1983.

51. Gorini M, Spinelli A, Ginanni R, et al: Neural respiratory drive and neuromuscular coupling in patients with chronic obstructive pulmonary disease (COPD). Chest 98:1179–1186, 1990.

52. Holliday JE, Hyers TM: The reduction of weaning time from mechanical ventilation using tidal volume and relaxation biofeedback. Am Rev Respir Dis 141:1214–1230, 1990.

53. Ishi M, Ogawa T, Ushiyama K, et al: Cardiorespiratory responses to standing arm ergometry in patients with ischemic heart disease. Comparison with the results of treadmill exercise. Jpn Heart J 32:425–433, 1991.

54. Janson-Bjerklie S, Clarke E: The effects of biofeedback training on bronchial diameter in asthma. Heart Lung 11:200–207, 1982.

55. Javahari S, Blum J, Kazemi H: Patterns of breathing and carbon dioxide retention in chronic obstructive lung disease. Am J Med 71:228–234, 1981.

56. Jensen J: Neural ventilatory drive during arm and leg exercise. Scand J Clin Lab Invest 29:177–184, 1972.

57. Jones F: Voice production as a function of head balance in singers. J Physiol 82:209–215, 1983.

58. Keens TG, Krastins B, Wannamaker EM, et al: Ventilatory muscle endurance training in normal subjects and patients with cystic fibrosis. Am Rev Respir Dis 116:853–860, 1977.

59. Kotses H, Glaus KD, Crawford PL, et al: Operant reduction of frontalis EMG activity in the treatment of asthma in children. Psychosom Res 20:453–459, 1976.

60. Kotses H, Miller DJ: The effect of changes in facial muscle tension on respiratory resistance. Biol Psychol 25:211–219, 1987.

61. Kotses H, Harver A, Segretto J, et al: Long term effects of biofeedback-inducted facial relaxation on measures of asthma severity in children. Biofeedback Self-Regulation 16:1–21, 1991.

62. Lake FR, Herndersen K, Briffa T, et al: Upper limb and lower limb exercise training in patients with chronic airflow obstruction. Chest 97:1077–1082, 1990.

63. Lamont LS, Finkelhor RS, Rupert SJ, et al: Combined arm-leg ergometry exercise test. Am Heart J 124:1102–1104, 1992.

64. LaRiccia RJ, Katz RH, Peters JW, et al: Biofeedback and hypnosis in weaning from mechanical ventilators. Chest 87:267–269, 1985.

65. Louhevaara V, Sojijarvi A, Llmarinen J, Teraslinna P: Differences in cardio-respiratory responses during and after arm and crank and cycle exercise. Acta Physiol Scand 138:133–143, 1990.

66. Loveridge B, West P, Kryger MH. Anthonisen NK: Alternation in breathing pattern with progression of chronic obstructive pulmonary disease. Am Rev Respir Dis 134:930–934, 1986.

67. Maestro L, Dolnage T, Avendano MA, Goldstein R: Influence of arm position in ventilation during incremental exercise in healthy individuals. Chest 98:113S, 1990.

68. Make BJ, Buckolz J: Exercise training in COPD patients improves cardiac function. Am Rev Respir Dis 143:80A, 1991.

69. Martin TW, Zeballos RJ, Weisman IM: Gas exchange during maximal upper extremity exercise. Chest 99:420–425, 1991.

70. Martin TW, Zeballos RJ, Weisman IM: Use of arm crank exercise in the detection of abnormal pulmonary gas exchange in patients at low altitude. Chest 102:169–175, 1991.

71. Martinez FJ, Couser JI, Celli BR: Factors influencing ventilatory muscle recruitment in patients with chronic airflow obstruction. Am Rev Respir Dis 142:276–282, 1990.

72. Martinez FJ, Couser JI, Celli BR: Respiratory response to arm elevation in patients with chronic airflow obstruction. Am Rev Respir Dis 143:476–480, 1991.

73. Martinez FJ, Vogel PD, Dupont DN, et al: Supported arm exercise vs. unsupported arm exercise in the rehabilitation of patients with chronic airflow obstruction. Chest 103:1397–1402, 1993.

74. Moldover JR, Downey JA: Cardiac response to exercise: Comparison of 3 ergometers. Arch Phys Med Rehabil 64:155–159, 1983.

75. Moltke E, Skouby AP: The influence of tonic neck reflexes on the activity of some muscles of the trunk in patients with asthma. Acta Med Scand 173:299–305, 1963.

76. Moxham J, Wiles CM, Newham D, et al: Sternomastoid function and fatigue in man. Clin Sci Mol Med 59:463–468, 1980.

77. Nagle FJ, Richie JP, Giese MD: VO_{2max} responses in combined arm and leg air-braked ergometer exercise. Med Sci Sports Exerc 16:563–566, 1984.

78. Ninane V, Rypens F, Yernault JC, DeTroyer A: Abdominal muscle use during breathing inpatients with chronic airflow obstruction. Am Rev Respir Dis 146:16–21, 1992.

79. Osmundson PJ: Noninvasive tests in the diagnosis of peripheral vascular disease. Cardiovasc Clin 10:271–277, 1980.

80. Owens GR, Thompson FE, Sciurba FC, et al: Comparison of arm and leg ergometry in patients with moderate chronic obstructive lung disease. Thorax 43:911–914, 1988.

81. Raper AJ, Tagliaferro-Thompson W, Shapiro W, et al: Scalene and sternomastoid muscle function. J Appl Physiol 21:497–502, 1966.

82. Reid DC, Bowden J, Lynne-Davies P: Role of selected muscles of respiration as influenced by position and tidal volume. Chest 70:636–640, 1976.

83. Reybrock T, Heigenhouser GF, Faulkner JA: Limitations to maximum oxygen uptake in arms, leg and combined arm-leg ergometry. J Appl Physiol 38:774–779, 1975.

84. Ries AL, Ellis B, Hawkins RW: Upper extremity exercise training in chronic obstructive pulmonary disease.

Chest 93:688–692, 1988.
84a. Roa J, Epstein S, Breslin E, et al: Work of breathing and ventilatory muscle recruitment during pursed-lip breathing in patients with chronic airways obstruction. Am Rev Respir Dis 143(4):A-77, 1991.
85. Rochester DF: Measurement of diaphragmatic blood flow and oxygen consumption in the dog by the Key-Schmidt technique. J Clin Invest 53:1216–1225, 1974.
86. Roussos CH, Macklem PT: The respiratory muscles. N Engl J Med 307:786–797, 1974.
87. Sassoon C, Te TT, Mahutte CK, Light R: Airway occlusion pressure. An important indicator for successful weaning in patients with chronic obstructive pulmonary disease. Am Rev Respir Dis 135:107–113, 1987.
88. Swanka MN: Physiology of upper body exercise. Exerc Sport Sci Rev 14:175–211, 1986.
89. Sharp JT: Therapeutic considerations in respiratory muscle function. Chest 88:118–123, 1985.
90. Sieck GC: Diaphragm muscle: Structural and functional organization. Clin Chest Med 9:195–210, 1988.
91. Simolowski T, Yan S, Gauthier AP, et al: Contractile properties of the human diaphragm during chronic hyperinflation. N Engl J Med 325:917–923, 1991.
92. Spiro SG: Exercise testing in clinical medicine. Br J Dis Chest 71:145–172, 1977.
93. Stanescu D, Nemery B, Veriter C, Marechal C: Pattern of breathing and ventilatory response to CO_2 in subjects practicing Hatha-Yoga. J Appl Physio 151:1625–1630, 1991.
94. Stenberg J, Astrand PO, Ekblom B, et al: Hemodynamic response to work with different muscle groups, sitting and supine. J Appl Physiol 22:61–70, 1967.
95. Steptoe A, Phillips J, Harlin J: Biofeedback and instructions in the modification of total respiratory resistance: An experimental study of asthmatic and non-asthmatic volunteers. J Psychosom Res 25:541–551, 1981.
96. Supinsky GS, Kelsen SG: Effects of elastase-induced emphysema on the force generating ability of the diaphragm. J Clin Invest 70:978–980, 1982.
97. Tandon M: Adjunct treatment with yoga in chronic severe airways obstruction. Thorax 33:514–517, 1973.
98. Tangri S, Wolf CR: The breathing pattern in chronic obstructive lung disease during the performance of some common daily activities. Chest 63:126–127, 1973.
99. Tobin M: Respiratory muscles in disease. Clin Chest Med 9:263–286, 1979.
100. Vachon L, Rich ES: Visceral learning in asthma. Psychosom Med 38:122–130, 1976.
101. Wasserman K: Principles of Exercise Testing and Interpretation, ed 3. Philadelphia, Lea & Febiger, 1987.
102. Wetherbee S, Franklin BA, Hollingsworth V, et al: Relationship between arm and leg training work loads in men with heart disease, implications for exercise prescription. Chest 99:1271–1273, 1991.
103. Williams JR, Armstrong N, Kirby BJ: The influence of the site of sampling and assay medium upon the measurements and interpretation of blood lactate responses to exercise. J Sports Sci 10:95–107, 1991.

Inspiratory Muscle Training in Chronic Obstructive Pulmonary Disease

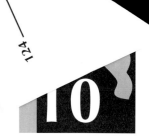

Thomas K. Aldrich, MD

The increasingly more common syndrome known as chronic obstructive pulmonary disease (COPD) or chronic airways obstruction (CAO) is characterized by cough, wheezing, dyspnea, exercise intolerance, pulmonary hyperinflation, and persistent expiratory flow limitation. It can be caused by one or more of several different conditions, including chronic bronchitis, emphysema, and bronchiectasis. Many patients have features of more than one of these conditions, and many also have elements of asthma or asthmatic bronchitis.

Most patients, those with mild-to-moderate disease, have shortness of breath on exertion. They may also have attacks of shortness of breath at rest that may interfere with activities of daily living from time to time but do not cause chronic disability. Patients with severe COPD have unremitting shortness of breath and exercise intolerance compounded by frequent exacerbations that require hospital treatment and sometimes mechanical ventilation.

PATHOPHYSIOLOGY

The major cause of shortness of breath and exercise intolerance in COPD is a much higher than normal energy cost of breathing. Even in COPD, with its prolonged expiratory phase of breathing, almost all of the energy cost of breathing is inspiratory.[37] The energy required for expiratory airflow is largely accomplished by pressure gradients set up by elastic recoil of lung and chest wall. The high inspiratory cost of breathing is due to abnormally high resistive and often elastic and threshold loads (Fig. 10–1).

Resistive loads are produced by broncoconstriction, mucus, and airway edema. In COPD, inspiratory resistive loads may be several times normal, but they do not approach the severity of the expiratory resistive loads, which are responsible for the characteristic wheezing and prolonged expiratory phase of breathing. Although emphysematous lungs typically show higher than normal compliance, which might be expected to be associated with lower than normal elastic loads, the pulmonary hyperinflation that is characteristic of COPD leads to increased elastic loads because the tidal volume occurs over a relatively steep portion of the pressure-volume curves of lung and particularly chest wall. The hyperinflation of COPD is largely a dynamic process, brought about because the severely limited expiratory airflow at low lung volumes does not permit enough expiratory time to allow complete exhalation down to the normal resting volume of the respiratory system. Under conditions of dynamic hyperinflation, the inspiratory muscles must work against an increased level of elastic recoil of both lung and chest wall; effectively, they contend with an abnormal inspiratory threshold load that may be quite severe.[3] In addition to the increased energy cost of breathing brought about by increases in resistive, elastic, and threshold loads, patients with COPD must usually breathe at higher than normal levels of minute ventilation, even at rest, be-

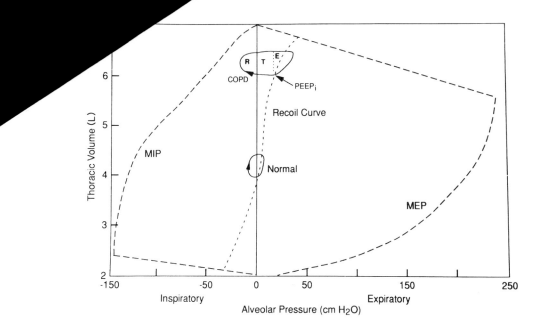

FIGURE 10–1. The decreased respiratory reserve in severe COPD. The *inner dashed line* represents respiratory system recoil pressure. The *outer dashed lines* represent maximal inspiratory and expiratory pressures. The *loops* trace typical tidal breaths. Inspiratory work of breathing is represented by the area bounded on the left by the tidal breathing loop and on the right by the recoil curve. R = Resistive work; E = elastic work; and T = the work required to overcome the threshold load. In addition to the increased work of breathing, COPD patients must contend with shortened inspiratory muscles and consequent reduced inspiratory strength, causing tidal inspiratory pressure to approach the maximal inspiratory pressure curve (*leftmost dashed line*). Malnutrition, cachexia, detraining, or fatigue can further reduce reserve. (From Aldrich TK: Acute and chronic respiratory failure. In Casaburi R, Petty TL [eds]: Principles and Practice of Pulmonary Rehabilitation. Philadelphia, WB Saunders, 1993, pp 124–137.)

cause of their excessive dead space-to-tidal volume ratios.

To compound the problem, many patients with COPD have impaired strength and endurance of the respiratory muscles, owing to some combination of malnutrition, electrolyte imbalances, cytokines produced in response to acute or chronic infections, an unfavorable position on the inspiratory muscles' length-tension curves, the need to contract the inspiratory muscles at an excessively high velocity of shortening (because of the shortened inspiratory time), and the side effects of one or more drugs such as adrenocorticosteroids and calcium channel blocking agents.[5] Furthermore, it has been suggested that the chronically high energy cost of breathing in COPD may predispose such patients to chronic inspiratory muscle fatigue, which may further impair inspiratory muscle performance.[19] Finally, despite COPD patients' chronically high energy cost of breathing, their often sedentary lifestyle may lead to detraining of inspiratory and other skeletal muscles.

Both abnormally high inspiratory loads and

inspiratory muscle weakness function to increase the fraction of maximum breathing capacity that a COPD patient must use for ordinary activities (Fig. 10–2). This may result in symptoms of dyspnea at rest or on minimal exertion, the inability to do more than minimal exertion, or, in severe cases, the development of ventilatory insufficiency.

Treatment for COPD usually focuses on measures to reduce the severity of airway obstruction, using bronchodilators, mucolytics, antibiotics when purulent sputum is present, and corticosteroids when an element of asthmatic bronchitis is suspected. In many cases, such treatment is only marginally effective, and symptoms and disability persist despite optimal medical management. Because ventilatory function depends not only on load, but also is influenced by inspiratory muscle function,[8] an improvement in inspiratory muscle strength and endurance might reduce symptoms and improve the functional capabilities of patients with severe COPD, even if there can be no further improvement in airways obstruction. Inspiratory

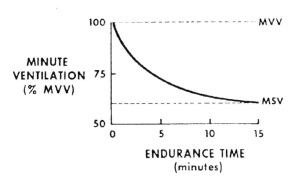

FIGURE 10–2. The limits of tolerance of various levels of minute ventilation. The maximal sustainable ventilation (MSV), as a percentage of maximum voluntary ventilation (MVV), is plotted as a function of time. High percentages of MVV can be tolerated for short periods only, regardless of whether the MVV is low because of load or because of inspiratory muscle weakness. (From Rochester DF, Braun NMT: The respiratory muscles. Basics of RD American Lung Association 6:1–6, 1978.

muscle training is one method that has been recommended. This chapter reviews the theory, methods, and results that have been achieved in training inspiratory muscles of COPD patients for improved strength and endurance.

THEORY

If a patient with COPD could train the inspiratory muscles for increased strength and endurance, the result would be improved tolerance of the excessive respiratory loads, even if there were no improvement in the underlying disease. Strength and endurance are related but different properties of skeletal muscles.[22] Strength depends on the number and size of nonmyopathic muscle fibers, the adequacy of their innervation, the efficiency of neuromuscular transmission, and the ability of the subject to recruit motor units and to activate motor nerves with adequate firing frequencies. The fiber type distribution is also important. Type I muscle fibers are high in oxidative enzymes and low in myosin ATPase activity, indicating that they are slow-twitch fibers resistant to fatigue. Type IIB fibers are high in glycolytic enzymes and myosin ATPase, indicating that they are fast-twitch fibers and easily fatigued. Type IIA fibers are an intermediate group high in both oxidative and glycolytic enzymes and are relatively fatigue-resistant. People who inherit a high number of fast-twitch fibers are considered more likely to be speed and power athletes, whereas those with more slow-twitch fibers tend toward more endurance activities.[31]

Endurance can be relative or absolute. Relative endurance measures the ability of a muscle or group of muscles to sustain repeated contractions at a specific fraction of their maximal strength. It depends on fiber type distribution, mitochondrial density, myoglobin content, delivery of oxygen and other nutrients to the contracting muscle, and removal of byproducts of

energy metabolism; it is independent of absolute strength. Absolute endurance measures the ability of a muscle or group of muscles to sustain contractions of a specific tension. It depends on strength and on all the factors that determine relative endurance. Because breathing is primarily an endurance task, requiring repeated generation of inspiratory muscle forces that are mainly determined by workload, absolute endurance is the most important requirement for inspiratory muscles.

The principles of training for improving performance of strength and endurance tasks have been developed primarily for athletic training: a situation involving highly motivated individuals, usually without acute or chronic illness, with a normal state of nutrition, and with the ability to rest the training muscles between training bouts. For COPD patients, not all of these conditions always apply; consequently the results of training and perhaps the optimal training methods may be quite different. Nevertheless the general principles of athletic training provide a useful starting point for designing appropriate training techniques for inspiratory muscles.

Training can be divided into three types: cardiovascular conditioning, endurance training of specific muscle groups, and strength training for specific muscle groups (Table 10–1). The goal of cardiovascular fitness training is to increase aerobic capacity of as much skeletal muscle as possible, possibly by increasing capillary and mitochondrial density. Generally, optimal cardiovascular conditioning (aerobic training) requires relatively long periods (> 30 minutes per day) of more or less continuous moderate exertion of many large muscle groups, by walking, cycling, jogging, or the like. It is thought that exercise at or near the anaerobic threshold is required for successful cardiovascular fitness training. A major benefit for COPD patients is that increasing aerobic capacity translates into less exertion-induced lactic acid production, which, in turn, translates into lower CO_2 pro-

TABLE 10–1
Techniques of Training

Type of Training	Cardiovascular conditioning	Strength training of specific muscle groups	Endurance training of specific muscle groups
Frequency and Duration	> 30 min/day	3 sets of 5–7 repetitions, 3–5 times/week	> 30 min, 3–7 times/week
Load	Continuous moderate exertion	Near maximal contractions	Submaximal, but fatiguing contractions
Target Muscle(s)	Many large muscle groups	Specific muscle(s) to be trained	Specific muscle(s) to be trained

duction and therefore a lower minute ventilation requirement for any given level of exercise.[15] Because the primary goal of any muscle training for COPD patients is to improve symptoms, cardiovascular fitness training is probably the most appropriate selection for those who can do it. Unfortunately, many patients with COPD are too short of breath on exertion to accomplish enough exertion to produce a cardiovascular training effect; they often stop exercising well below their anaerobic threshold. For such patients, specific respiratory muscle training may be worth considering.

Strength training is based on the overload principle: Training is carried out with repetitive, brief, near-maximal contractions of the target muscles. The optimal duration and frequency of training are not known with certainty, but three sets per session of five to seven repetitions per set, with three to five sessions per week, is a reasonable training regimen.[7,23,45] The concern with more frequent training is that muscle or joint injury becomes more likely when fatigued muscle is being exerted. For respiratory muscles, strength training can be carried out by repetitive maximal inspiratory contractions against a closed mouthpiece or (for the diaphragm) by maximal expulsive efforts, the Valsalva maneuver. In normal subjects, approximately 50% improvements in maximal inspiratory pressure can be achieved after 4 to 5 weeks of daily strength training.[35] Strength training is usually accompanied by improvements in endurance. Because breathing is primarily an endurance task, endurance training is generally considered most desirable for COPD patients.

Endurance training is carried out with repetitive contractions of the target muscle or muscles over a relatively long period of time. Each contraction is individually submaximal, but the load is adjusted to be the maximum that can be repetitively sustained over the course of training. Thus, as with strength training, endurance training for any skeletal muscle includes brief periods of fatiguing exertion alternating with rest.[21,31] In a study of quadriceps training in normals, Delateur and coworkers[21] compared the results of training by two methods. For each subject, one leg underwent daily repetitive weight lifting to the point of acute fatigue, while the contralateral leg performed the same number of repetitions but was allowed rest periods to prevent fatigue. After 30 days of training, the legs trained with fatigue showed 15% to 100% higher endurance than those trained without fatigue.

As with strength training, the optimal duration and frequency of endurance training are unknown, but, to avoid fatigue-related injury, an every-other-day regimen is usually recommended. There is evidence, however, that endurance gains continue as the frequency of training increases. Acker and associates[1] have shown that continuous stimulation of the canine diaphragm at 2 to 4 Hz for 1 year resulted in a transformation of the muscle from a mixed fiber–type muscle to a purely type I fiber muscle, with the associated high endurance characteristics. Similarly, in a study of inspiratory flow resistance training in COPD, Pardy and coworkers[41] showed that patients made significantly better gains in endurance if they were subjected to fatiguing loads than if they were trained without apparent respiratory muscle fatigue. Although periods of acute fatigue promote training, severe or chronic fatigue may prevent an effective training response.[14]

RESULTS OF INSPIRATORY MUSCLE TRAINING IN CHRONIC OBSTRUCTIVE PULMONARY DISEASE

Two types of respiratory muscle endurance training have been used: repeated bouts of isocapnic hyperpnea[11,32,36] and repeated bouts of resistance breathing, either with flow resistors or with threshold resistors (See later) (Fig. 10–3). Levine and associates[36] conducted a careful evaluation of the isocapnic hyperpnea method and determined that no more benefits could be derived from it than could be achieved using periodic intermittent positive-pressure breathing treatments, a regimen that was considered equivalent to a placebo.

Resistive training has been more successful. More than three dozen publications have reported the results of inspiratory flow resistive training (or its close relative, inspiratory threshold resistance training) in patients with COPD, asthma, kyphoscoliosis, and neuromuscular diseases. Among patients with COPD, 21 reports have documented results of controlled studies in a total of 259 patients (Table 10–2). Of the 15 studies in which it was measured, inspiratory muscle strength (as reflected by maximal inspiratory pressure [MIP])[13] increased more in the experimental than in the control groups in 8. In several other studies, MIP improved in both experimental and control groups, and in no cases did average MIP decline after training. The mean change in MIP (weighted by the numbers of subjects in each study) was a 19% increase. Inspiratory muscle endurance (measured as sus-

tainable inspiratory pressure [SIP]) increased significantly more than for control subjects in all four studies in which it was measured, with a weighted average increase of 68%. In several studies, inspiratory muscle endurance was measured by the less easily quantifiable technique of determining the highest level of inspiratory resistance eventually tolerated during the endurance training regimen. In most such cases, higher resistances were tolerated after training.

Most studies demonstrated significant improvements in exercise tolerance, but most also showed improvements among the control subjects. In 7 of 15 studies in which it was measured, exercise tolerance was significantly better for the trained group as compared with a control group; in 6 of the other 8, exercise tolerance improved in both groups, and the improvements were comparable. The weighted average improvement in exercise tolerance among trained subjects was 17%.

The pressure drop across a simple flow resistor increases approximately as the square of the flow rate through the resistor. Consequently, inspiratory flow rate has a major effect on the level of load imposed by the resistor. It became apparent that many of the subjects of inspiratory resistive training consciously or unconsciously

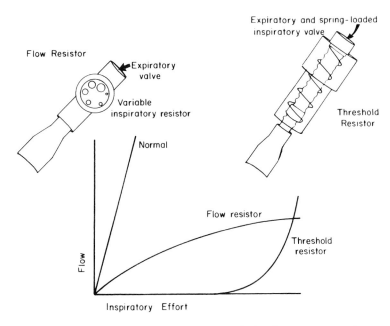

FIGURE 10–3. Comparison of flow and threshold resistors. With the flow resistor, airflow can be produced by relatively weak efforts; the flow is small but not absent. With the threshold resistor, no flow occurs until the pressure threshold is exceeded.

TABLE 10–2
Summary of Results of Controlled Trials of Inspiratory Resistive Training
in Chronic Obstructive Pulmonary Disease

Study	n*	Duration (min)	Frequency (per week)	Course (weeks)	Change in Maximal Inspiratory Pressure	in Sustainable Inspiratory Pressure	in Exercise Tolerance
Flow Resistors							
Without Feedback							
Pardy et al, 1981	9	15	14	8	—	—	+12%[Y]
Bjerre-Jepson et al,[12] 1981	14	15	21	6	—	—	+23%[N]
Sonne and Davis,[49] 1982	6	30	7	6	—	—	+15%[Y]
Reid and Warren,[46] 1984	5	5	30	6	+13%	—	—
Chen et al,[17] 1985	7	15	14	4	+6%[N]	+59%[Y]	+10%[N]
Falk et al,[24] 1985	12	10	21	13	—	—	+60%[Y]
Jones et al,[20] 1985	7	15	14	10	—	—	+22%[N]
Renzi and Renzi,[47] 1985	9	15	14	18–26	+20%[Y]	—	+19%[Y]
McKeon et al,[38] 1986	10	15	21	6	+5%[N]	—	+4%[N]
Noseda et al,[40] 1987	10	15	14	8	—	—	+6%[N]
Patessio et al,[42] 1989	8	—	—	8	+23%[Y]	—	—
Guyatt et al,[28] 1992	43	10	35	26	0[N]	—	+2%[N]
Totals and weighted averages	140				+5.9%	+59%	+14.2%
Flow-Targeted or							
Threshold Resistors							
Clanton et al,[18] 1985	4	7.5	3	10	+33%[Y]	—	—
Larson et al,[33] 1988	10	30	7	9	+20%[Y]	+81[Y]	+8%[Y]
Belman and Shadmehr,[10] 1988	8	15	14	6	+29%[Y]	+32%[Y]	—
Flynn et al,[26] 1989	8	15	14	6	+65%[Y]	+95%[Y]	+9%[N]
Harver et al,[29] 1989	10	15	14	8	+13%[N]	—	—
Goldstein et al,[27] 1989	6	10–20	10	4	+6%[N]	—	+24%[N]
Dekhuijzen et al,[20] 1990	20	15	14	10	+34%[Y]	—	+25%[Y]
Weiner et al,[50] 1992	12	—	—	13	+17%[Y]	—	+91%[Y]
Kim et al,[33] 1993	41	30	7	25	+30%[N]	—	+3%[N]
Totals and weighted averages	119				+28.3%	+70.2%	+21.1%
Overall totals and weighted averages	259				+19.4%	+67.8%	+17.3%

*Sample sizes of the experimental (resistive training) groups; the control groups had similar sample sizes.
[Y]Result that was significantly better than for the control group.
[N]Result that did not differ significantly from that of the control group.

reduced their inspiratory flow rates and lengthened their inspiratory time to reduce the severity of the imposed loads. For subjects breathing tidal volumes at rest, the resulting shortening of the expiratory phase was generally well tolerated, especially because there was no added expiratory resistance. In many cases, the result was to prevent the imposition of a severe enough increase in inspiratory load to result in a training effect. Consequently, targeted[10,20,29] or threshold[18,26,27,33,34,50] inspiratory muscle training has been recommended over the simpler flow-resis-

tive training, to ensure adequate intensity of inspiratory muscle activity during training.

With targeted training, the subject is provided feedback regarding the inspiratory flow rates through the resistor or the inspiratory pressure generated by flow through the resistor; with threshold training, the subject is unable to generate flow through the device until a predetermined pressure is achieved. Six of the nine controlled evaluations of the use of targeted or threshold resistor devices in COPD have documented significantly better improvements in inspiratory muscle function in the treated than in the control subjects (see Table 10–2). In three of the six studies in which it was assessed, exercise tolerance was greater for trained subjects than for controls. In general, improvements in inspiratory muscle function and in exercise tolerance were greater for the targeted and threshold studies than for the flow resistor studies (see Table 10–2).

A problem with interpretation of the results of inspiratory resistive training is that the outcome variables may not be objective. For example, the standard index of inspiratory muscle strength, the maximal static inspiratory pressure (MIP or $P_i$max),[13] is effort dependent and, therefore, not necessarily reliable. It is clear that the MIP can be a reliable index of inspiratory muscle strength only if the subject's effort is truly maximal. In practice, it is often assumed that reproducibility of multiple MIP efforts indicates that the efforts are maximal. In a study of patients on mechanical ventilation, however, the authors showed that MIP could not be relied on as an index of strength, despite relatively good reproducibility of triplicate efforts.[39] It has also been shown in normals that the reproducibility of deliberately submaximal efforts can be equal to the reproducibility of MIP efforts, indicating that reproducibility cannot be relied on to document maximal effort in spontaneously breathing ambulatory subjects.[6] Thus, unless a more objective test is used, such as the superimposed twitch test developed by Bellemare and Bigland-Ritchie,[9] there remains considerable doubt whether the generally demonstrated improvements in MIP after inspiratory muscle training reflect improvements in inspiratory muscle strength or improvements in effort after weeks of repetitive testing. Because true blinding is not practical, it is quite possible that subjects assigned to the experimental (training) groups may have shown more improvement in MIP than did the control groups simply because of higher expectations. Similar problems limit the confidence with which improvements in maximum voluntary ventilation (MVV), exercise tolerance, or dyspnea ratings can be interpreted.

In 1992, a meta-analysis of 17 controlled studies of inspiratory muscle training in COPD (15 resistive training and 2 isocapnic hyperpnea) demonstrated no significant improvement in standard pulmonary function tests, exercise capacity, or quality of life but did demonstrate a significant improvement in MVV.[48] In an analysis of the five studies in which targeted or threshold training was used, results were marginally

better, with significant improvements demonstrated in MIP and severity of dyspnea. The authors concluded that there was little evidence that inspiratory muscle training resulted in major improvements in clinical status of COPD patients, but that any small benefits were much more likely to occur when targeted or threshold training was used than when flow rates and pressures were left uncontrolled.

Despite these disappointing results, on theoretic grounds and at least for highly motivated normal subjects,[35] it appears that inspiratory muscle training can improve inspiratory muscle strength and endurance if undertaken with enough energy, commitment, and perseverance. As demonstrated by the general lack of exciting results in COPD, however, it appears that patients with COPD are not always, or even usually, willing and able to undertake the necessary training, or their inspiratory muscles may not be capable of responding to training.

REASONS FOR DISAPPOINTING RESULTS OF INSPIRATORY MUSCLE TRAINING

There are a number of reasons why many COPD patients fail to demonstrate significantly better improvements from inspiratory muscle training than do untrained or sham-trained subjects (Table 10–3). It is clear that improvements in strength and endurance of any muscle require a relatively high work intensity. Because breathing through an inspiratory muscle trainer is tedious and uncomfortable, many COPD patients are simply unwilling to use a trainer consistently. In other cases, the presence of chronic inspiratory muscle fatigue may prevent patients from progressing to higher levels of resistance. Also, as previously noted, when a flow-resistive type of inspiratory muscle trainer is used, patients may consciously or unconsciously reduce their inspiratory flow rates to the point that the trainer provides an inadequate stimulus for training.

TABLE 10–3
Reasons for Poor Responses to Training

Inadequate intensity of training
    Lack of commitment by subject
    Fatigue
    Inadequate severity of load
Malnutrition
Cachexia
Drugs
Training not specific for desired outcome

It is also clear that training-induced improvements in inspiratory muscle strength and endurance require a minimum level of nutrition. Patients with advanced COPD are often cachexic, either because they cannot take in adequate nutrition or because of cytokine-associated cachexia. Such patients may be unable to respond to regular exercise with increases in mass or oxidative capacity of inspiratory muscles.

In some cases, drug therapy for other aspects of disease may impair a COPD patient's ability to respond appropriately to a training regimen. Beta-adrenergic blocking agents are the best example of drugs that impair responses to endurance training regimens,[2] but few COPD patients are treated with beta-blockers. Adrenocorticosteroids, which are commonly used by patients with COPD, can promote atrophy of nonrespiratory and respiratory muscles,[44] but their effect on endurance is unclear. Steroids appear to promote atrophy preferentially of the high-strength but low-endurance type II muscle fibers, causing major decrements in strength but minimal if any decrements in endurance.[44] There are no available data on the effect of steroids on training. Beta-adrenergic agonists are also commonly used by COPD patients, most often by the inhalational route. There is emerging evidence that at least one beta-agonist, clenbuterol, dramatically impairs endurance of inspiratory muscles, at least when given by a systemic route.[43] There is no information on the effect of beta-agonists on training.

In many of the reported studies, inspiratory muscle training was added to a comprehensive program of rehabilitation including exercise training, and the experimental group, treated with rehabilitation plus inspiratory muscle training, was compared with a group that received all of the benefits of rehabilitation except inspiratory muscle training. Because, in general, the most appropriate method of rehabilitation is specific to the activity in which improvement is desired, it may not be surprising that exercise training is as good as the combination of exercise and inspiratory muscle training at improving exercise tolerance.

Casaburi and Wasserman[16] have pointed out that for most patients with COPD, exercise training would be the most appropriate way to improve quality of life, but that for those whose exercise tolerance is too limited to allow them to perform exercise training, inspiratory muscle training provides a reasonable hope for reduced symptoms and perhaps for improved functional status. In a study of patients in chronic ventilator-dependent respiratory failure, some with COPD and some without, it was found that many such patients who could not be weaned from mechanical ventilation by standard means could use inspiratory muscle training to improve their inspiratory muscle strength and endurance sufficiently to resume spontaneous breathing.[4] Despite the dyspnea that they experienced during training sessions, such patients generally preferred inspiratory muscle training, with its relatively brief periods of exertion, to the often open-ended weaning trials of standard approaches. Thus, these most severely affected COPD patients, in whom the desired outcome is improved respiratory muscle strength and endurance and in whom adequate inspiratory muscle loading can be enforced, may well be the optimal target group for inspiratory muscle training.

CONCLUSIONS

The goal of improving inspiratory muscle strength and endurance is an appropriate one for a patient with severe COPD in whom symptoms persist despite optimal nutrition, bronchodilation, and infection control. In theory, inspiratory muscle training offers a means to accomplish the goal. Unfortunately, controlled trials of inspiratory muscle training in a total of more than 200 patients have thus far failed to demonstrate convincing evidence that inspiratory muscle training can make a major difference in a broad range of patients. Nevertheless, there is reason to believe that individual highly motivated and adequately nourished patients who are free of cachexia can benefit from training. The challenges for the future are to find means of identifying good candidates for training, to design less tedious training techniques, and perhaps to define metabolic and pharmacologic treatments to enhance the training effect.

References

1. Acker MA, Mannon JD, Brown WE, et al: Canine diaphragm muscle after 1 year of continuous electrical stimulation: Its potential as a myocardial substitute. J Appl Physiol 62:1264–1270, 1987.
2. Ades PA, Gunther PG, Meyer WL, et al: Cardiac and skeletal muscle adaptations to training in systemic hypertension and effect of beta blockade (metaprolol or propranolol). Am J Cardiol 66:591–596, 1990.
3. Aldrich TK, Hendler JM, Vizioli LD, et al: Intrinsic positive end-expiratory pressure in stable patients with airways obstruction. Am Rev Respir Dis 147:845–849, 1993.

4. Aldrich TK, Karpel JP, Uhrlass R, et al: Weaning from mechanical ventilation: Adjunctive use of inspiratory muscle resistive training. Crit Care Med 17:143–147, 1989.

5. Aldrich TK, Rochester DF: The lung in neuromuscular disease. In Murray JF, Nadal JA (eds): Textbook of Respiratory Medicine. Philadelphia, WB Saunders, 1993, pp 2492–2523.

6. Aldrich TK, Spiro P: Maximum inspiratory pressure: Does reproducibility indicate full effort? [abstract]. Am Rev Respir Dis 145:A159, 1992.

7. Atha J: Strengthening muscle. Exerc Sport Sci Rev 9:1–73, 1981.

8. Begin P, Grassino A: Inspiratory muscle dysfunction and chronic hypercapnia in chronic obstructive pulmonary disease. Am Rev Respir Dis 143:905–912, 1992.

9. Bellemare F, Bigland-Ritchie B: Assessment of human diaphragm strength and activation using phrenic nerve stimulation. Respir Physiol 58:263–277, 1984.

10. Belman MJ, Shadmehr R: Targeted resistive ventilatory muscle training in chronic obstructive pulmonary disease. J Appl Physiol 65:2726–2735, 1988.

11. Belman MJ, Mittman C: Ventilatory muscle training improves exercise capacity in chronic obstructive pulmonary disease patients. Am Rev Respir Dis 121:273–280, 1980.

12. Bjerre-Jepson K, Secher NH, Kok-Jensen A: Inspiratory resistance training in severe chronic obstructive pulmonary disease. Eur J Respir Dis 62:405–411, 1981.

13. Black LF, Hyatt RE: Maximal respiratory pressures. Am Rev Respir Dis 99:696–702, 1969.

14. Braun NMT, Faulkner J, Hughes RL, et al: When should respiratory muscles be exercised? Chest 84:76–84, 1983.

15. Casaburi R, Patessio A, Ioli F, et al: Reductions in exercise lactic acidosis and ventilation as a result of exercise training in patients with obstructive lung disease. Am Rev Respir Dis 143:9–18, 1991.

16. Casaburi R, Wasserman K: Exercise training in pulmonary rehabilitation. Engl J Med 314:1509–1510, 1986.

17. Chen H-I, Dukes R, Martin BJ: Inspiratory muscle training in patients with chronic obstructive pulmonary disease. Am Rev Respir Dis 131:251–255, 1985.

18. Clanton TL, Dixon G, Drake J, Gadek J: Inspiratory muscle conditioning using a threshold loading device. Chest 87:62–66, 1985.

19. Cohen CA, Zagelbaum G, Gross D, et al: Clinical manifestations of inspiratory muscle fatigue. Am J Med 73:308–316, 1982.

20. Dekhuijzen PRN, Folgering HTM, Van Herwaarden CLA: Target-flow inspiratory muscle training at home and during pulmonary rehabilitation in COPD patients with a ventilatory limitation on exercise. Lung 168 (suppl):502–528, 1990.

21. Delateur BJ, Lehmann JF, Giaconi R: Mechanical work and fatigue: Their roles in the development of muscle work capacity. Arch Phys Med Rehabil 57:319–324, 1975.

22. Edwards RHT, Faulkner JA: Structure and function of the respiratory muscles. In Roussos C, Macklem PT (eds.): The Thorax. New York, Marcel Dekker, 1985, pp 297–326.

23. Enoka RM: Muscle strength and its development: New perspectives. Sports Med 6:146–168, 1988.

24. Falk P, Eriksen A-M, Kolliker K, Andersen JB: Relieving dyspnea with an inexpensive and simple method in patients with severe airflow limitation. Eur J Respir Dis 66:181–186, 1985.

25. Feinlieb M, Rosenberg HM, Collins JG, et al: Trends in COPD morbidity and mortality in the United States. Am Rev Respir Dis 140(suppl):S9–S18, 1989.

26. Flynn MG, Barter CE, Noworthy JC, et al: Threshold pressure training, breathing pattern, and exercise performance in chronic airflow obstruction. Chest 95:535–540, 1989.

27. Goldstein R, DeRosie J, Long S, et al: Applicability of a threshold loading device for inspiratory muscle testing and training in patients with COPD. Chest 96:564–571, 1989.

28. Guyatt G, Keller J, Singer J, et al: Controlled trial of respiratory muscle training in chronic airflow limitation. Thorax 47:598–602, 1992.

29. Harver A, Mahler DA, Daubenspeck JA: Targeted inspiratory muscle training improves respiratory muscle function and reduces dyspnea in patients with chronic obstructive pulmonary disease. Ann Intern Med 111:117–124, 1989.

30. Jones DT, Thomson RJ, Sears MR: Physical exercise and resistive breathing training in severe chronic airways obstruction—are they effective? Eur J Respir Dis 67:159–166, 1985.

31. Joynt RL, Findley TW, Boda W, Daum MC: Therapeutic exercise. In DeLisa JA (ed): Rehabilitation Medicine: Principles and Practice. Philadelphia, JB Lippincott, 1993, p 526–554.

32. Keens TG, Krastins IRB, Wannamaker EM, et al: Ventilatory muscle endurance training in normal subjects and patients with cystic fibrosis. Am Rev Respir Dis 116:853–860, 1977.

33. Kim MJ, Larson JL, Covey MK, et al: Inspiratory muscle training in patients with chronic obstructive pulmonary disease. Nursing Res 42:356–362, 1993.

34. Larson JL, Kim MJ, Sharp JT, Larson DA: Inspiratory muscle training with a pressure threshold breathing device in patients with chronic obstructive pulmonary disease. Am Rev Respir Dis 138:689–696, 1988.

35. Leith DE, Bradley M: Ventilatory muscle strength and endurance training. J Appl Physiol 41:508–516, 1976.

36. Levine S, Weiser P, Gillen J: Evaluation of a ventilatory muscle endurance training program in the rehabilitation of patients with chronic obstructive pulmonary disease. Am Rev Respir Dis 133:400–406, 1986.

37. Loring SH, DeTroyer A: Actions of the respiratory muscles. In Roussos C, Macklem PT (eds.): The Thorax. New York, Marcel Dekker, 1985, pp 327–349.

38. McKeon JL, Turner J, Kelly C, et al: The effect of inspiratory resistive training on exercise capacity in optimally treated patients with severe chronic airflow limitation. Aust NZ J Med 16:648–652, 1986.

39. Multz AS, Aldrich TK, Prezant DJ, et al: Maximal inspiratory pressure is not a reliable test of inspiratory muscle strength in mechanically ventilated patients. Am Rev Respir Dis 142:529–532, 1990.

40. Noseda A, Carpiaux JP, Vandeput W, et al: Resistive inspiratory muscle training and exercise performance in COPD patients. Bull Eur Physiopathol Respir 23:457–463, 1987.

41. Pardy RL, Rivington RN, Despas PJ, Macklem PT: Inspiratory muscle training compared with physiotherapy in patients with chronic airflow limitation. Am Rev Respir Dis 123:421–425, 1981.

42. Patessio A, Rampulla C, Fracchia C, et al: Relationship between the perception of breathlessness and inspiratory resistive loading. Eur Respir J 7:587S–591S, 1989.

43. Prezant DJ, Chung V, Kim H, et al: Long term beta-2 agonist (clenbuterol) therapy produces diaphragm hypertrophy and dysfunction [abstract]. Am Rev Respir Dis 147:A959, 1993.

44. Prezant DJ, Richner B, Aldrich TK, et al: The effect of short and long term corticosteroid treatment on rat diaphragm contractility and fatigue. Chest 97:104S, 1990.

45. Rasch PJ, Burke RK: Principles of training and development. In Kinesiology and Applied Anatomy: The Science of Human Movement; ed 6. Philadelphia, Lea & Febiger, 1978, pp 349–360.

46. Reid WD, Warren CPW: Ventilatory muscle strength and endurance training in elderly subjects and patients with chronic airflow limitation: A pilot study. Physiother Can 36:302–311, 1984.

47. Renzi G, Renzi P: Role de l'entrainement des muscles respiratoires dans un programme de rehabilitation des patients souffrant de maladie obstructive pulmonaire chronique. Union Medicale du Canada 114:897–901, 1985.

48. Smith K, Cook D, Guyatt GH, et al: Respiratory muscle training in chronic airflow limitation: A meta-analysis. Am Rev Respir Dis 145:533–539, 1992.

49. Sonne LJ, Davis JA: Increased exercise performance in patients with severe COPD following exercise resistive training. Chest 81:436–439, 1982.

50. Weiner P, Azgad Y, Ganam R: Inspiratory muscle training compared with general exercise conditioning in patients with COPD. Chest 102:1351–1356, 1992.

Cognitive-Behavioral Interventions and the Quality of Life of Patients with Chronic Obstructive Pulmonary Disease

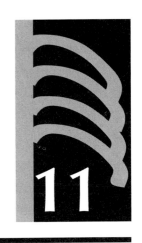

11

Robert M. Kaplan, PhD
Andrew L. Ries, MD, MPH

Chronic obstructive pulmonary disease (COPD) has a profound effect on functioning and everyday life. Current estimates suggest that COPD affects nearly 11% of the adult population, and the incidence is increasing. Trends that indicate that the rate of COPD is increasing among women reflect the increase in tobacco use among women in the later part of this century.[61] Reviews of the medical management of COPD justify the use of symptomatic measures, including prescription of bronchodilators, corticosteroids, and antibiotic therapy. In addition, long-term oxygen therapy has been shown to be beneficial for patients with severe hypoxemia.[24] It is widely recognized, however, that these measures cannot cure COPD and that much of the effort in the management of this condition must be directed toward improving symptoms, patient functioning, and quality of life.

To achieve these outcomes, behavioral interventions are necessary and often include smoking cessation as part of a comprehensive pulmonary rehabilitation program. Many of the chapters in this book provide evidence for the value of behavioral interventions for smoking cessation,[56] exercise training,[15] upper extremity reconditioning exercise,[20] respiratory muscle training,[2] and diet.[45] In this chapter, evidence for the benefits of behavioral intervention is reviewed, and some of the work in the authors' research program is described.

Cognitive-behavior modification methods have been shown to be useful for changing a wide variety of human behaviors.[42] These methods are based on modern learning theory and are supported by a substantial literature on human and animal learning. Most current behavioral intervention methods rely on specific behavioral techniques. These methods, which include self-monitoring, goal specification, stimulus control, self-reinforcement, behavioral reversal, and other techniques, have been shown to be efficacious. Mazzuca[48] reviewed studies that used interventions based on either didactic knowledge-based interventions or behavioral skill-based programs. Using meta-analysis methods, he found that didactic interventions had a relatively small and statistically nonsignificant effect on health behavior (0.26 Z units), whereas behavioral interventions had a significant positive influence on health behaviors (0.64 Z units). In other words, programs based on behavioral intervention are more than twice as effective as those based solely on knowledge. Mazzuca also reviewed physiologic outcomes (blood pressure, blood glucose, weight, and blood cholesterol).[9] In addition to effects on behavior change, behaviorally based programs, averaged across studies, had a strong and significant effect on physiologic outcomes, whereas didactic knowledge-based programs had a nonsignificant effect. Thus, behaviorally based programs can be extremely important for the optimal management of COPD.

BEHAVIORAL INTERVENTION: COST-EFFECTIVENESS AND QUALITY OF LIFE

Over the last 15 years, the authors have conducted and reviewed a variety of studies that evaluate behavioral interventions for patients with COPD. Most of these studies evaluated the benefits of treatment using outcome measures that focused on dyspnea[23] and health-related quality of life.[34] To date, there is little consensus on which measures should be applied. The measure used most frequently is the Chronic Respiratory Questionnaire (CRQ), which was developed by Guyatt and colleagues.[28] Work by the authors has focused on a general outcome measure known as the Quality of Well-Being Scale (QWB), which can be used to quantify outcomes and to assess the cost-utility of treatment.

Within the last few years, there has been growing interest in using quality of life data to help evaluate the cost/utility or cost-effectiveness of health care programs. Cost studies have gained in popularity because health care costs have grown rapidly. Not all health care interventions are equally efficient in returning benefit for the expended dollar. Objective cost studies might guide policymakers toward an optimal and equitable distribution of resources. Cost-effectiveness analysis typically quantifies the benefits of a health care intervention in terms of years of life or quality adjusted life years (QALYs). Cost/utility is a special use of cost-effectiveness that weights observable health states by preferences or utility judgments of quality.[38] In cost/utility analysis, the benefits of medical care, behavioral interventions, and preventive programs are expressed in terms of well-years. These outcomes have also been described as QALYs,[65] discounted life years,[40] or healthy years of life.[34] Because the term QALYs has become most popular, it is used in this chapter. QALYs integrate mortality and morbidity to express health status in terms of equivalents of well-years of life.

If an adult dies of COPD at age 60 and he would have been expected to live to age 75, it might be concluded that the disease was associated with 15 lost life years. If 100 adults with a life expectancy of 75 years died at age 60, it might be concluded that 1500 (100 adults $\times$ 15 years) life years had been lost. Death is not the only outcome of concern in COPD. Many adults may be disabled over long periods of time. Because of respiratory problems, the quality of their lives has diminished. QALYs take into consideration the quality-of-life consequences of illnesses. For example, a disease that reduces qual-

ity of life by one half takes away 0.5 QALYs over the course of each year. If it affects two people, it takes away 1.0 year (equal 2×0.5) over each year period. A medical treatment that improves quality of life by 0.2 for each of five individuals results in the equivalent of 1 QALY if the benefit is maintained over a 1-year period. This system has the advantage of considering both benefits and side effects of programs in terms of the common QALY units. The general measurement system is also capable of quantifying toxic effects of new treatments. Further, it can be used to evaluate the relative importance of side effects so that a net assessment of the treatment can subtract side effects from benefits.

Although there are several different approaches for quantifying QALYs, most of them are similar.[32] The approach preferred by the authors involves several steps. First, patients are classified according to objective levels of functioning. These levels are represented by scales of mobility, physical activity, and social activity. The dimensions and steps for these levels of functioning are shown in Table 11–1. The reader is cautioned that these steps are not actually the scale, only listings of labels representing the scale steps. Standardized questionnaires have been developed to classify individuals into one of each of these scale steps.[6,7] In addition to classification into these observable levels of function, individuals are classified by the one symptom or problem that was reported to be the most undesirable (Table 11–2). About half of the population reports at least one symptom or problem on any day. These may be severe, such as serious chest pain, or minor, such as the inconvenience of taking medication or a prescribed diet for health reasons. The functional classification (see Table 11–1) and the accompanying list of symptoms or problems (see Table 11–2) were created after extensive reviews of the medical and public health literature.[38] Over the last decade, the function classification system and symptom list were repeatedly shortened until the current versions were arrived at. Various methodologic studies on the questionnaire have been conducted.[8,9,37,39] With structured questionnaires, an interviewer can obtain classifications on these dimensions in 7 to 12 minutes.

Once observable-behavioral levels of functioning have been classified, a second step is required to place each individual on the 0-to-1.0 scale of wellness. To accomplish this, the observable health states are weighted by *quality* ratings for the desirability of these conditions. Human value studies have been conducted to place the observable states onto a preference contin-

TABLE 11–1
Quality of Well-Being/General Health Policy Model: Elements and Calculating Formulas (Function Scales, with Step Definitions and Calculating Weights)

Step No.	Step Definition	Weight
	Mobility Scale (MOB)	
5	No limitations for health reasons	−0.000
4	Did not drive a car, health related; did not ride in a car as usual for age (younger than 15 yr), health related, *and/or* did not use public transportation, health related; *or* had or would have used more help than usual for age to use public transportation, health related	−0.062
2	In hospital, health related	−0.090
	Physical Activity Scale (PAC)	
4	No limitations for health reasons	−0.000
3	In wheelchair, moved or controlled movement of wheelchair without help from someone else; *or* had trouble or did not try to lift, stoop, bend over, or use stairs or inclines, health related; *and/or* limped, used a cane, crutches, or walker, health related; *and/or* had any other physical limitation in walking, or did not try to walk as far as or as fast as others the same age are able, health related	−0.060
1	In wheelchair, did not move or control the movement of wheelchair without help from someone else, *or* in bed, chair, or couch for most of all of the day, health related	−0.077
	Social Activity Scale (SAC)	
5	No limitations for health reasons	−0.000
4	Limited in other (e.g., recreational) role activity, health related	−0.061
3	Limited in major (primary) role activity, health related	−0.061
2	Performed no major role activity, health related, but did perform self-care activities	−0.061
1	Performed no major role activity, health related, *and* did not perform or had more help than usual in performance of one or more self-care activities, health related	−0.106

Calculating Formulas
Formula 1. Point-in-time well-being score for an individual (W):

$$W = 1 + (CPXwt) + (MOBwt) + (PACwt) + (SACwt)$$

where "wt" is the preference-weighted measure for each factor and CPX is Symptom/Problem complex. For example, the W score for a person with the following description profile may be calculated for one day as:

CPX-11	Cough, wheezing or shortness of breath, with or without fever, chills, or aching all over	−0.257
MOB-5	No limitations	−0.000
PAC-1	In bed, chair, or couch for most or all of the day, health related	−0.077
SAC-2	Performed no major role activity, health related, but did perform self-care	−0.061

$$W = 1 + (−0.257) + (−0.000) + (−0.077) + (−0.061) = 0.605$$

Formula 2. Well-years (WY) as an output measure:

$$WY = [\text{No. of persons} \times (CPXwt + MOBwt + PACwt + SACwt) \times Time]$$

uum with an anchor of 0 for death and 1.0 for completely well. In several studies, random samples of citizens from a metropolitan community evaluated the desirability of more than 400 case descriptions. Using these ratings, a preference structure that assigned the weights to each combination of an observable state and a symptom/problem has been developed.[39] Cross-validation studies have shown that the model can be used to assign weights to other states of functioning with a high degree of accuracy (R^2 =

0.96). The regression weights obtained in these studies are given in Tables 1 and 2. Studies have shown that the weights are highly stable over a 1-year period and they are consistent across diverse groups of raters.[39] Finally, it is necessary to consider the duration of stay in various health states. For example, 1 year in a state that has been assigned the weight of 0.5 is equivalent to 0.5 of a QALY. Table 1 provides an illustrative example of a calculation. Both reliability[39] and validity studies have been published.[37]

TABLE 11–2
Quality of Well-Being/General Health Policy Model: Symptom/Problem Complexes (CPX) with Calculating Weights

CPX No. Weights	CPX Description	
1	Death (not on respondent's card)	−0.727*
2	Loss of consciousness such as seizure (fits), fainting, or coma (out cold or knocked out)	−0.407
3	Burn over large areas of face, body, arms, or legs	−0.387
4	Pain, bleeding, itching, or discharge (drainage) from sexual organs—does not include normal menstrual (monthly) bleeding	−0.349
5	Trouble learning, remembering, or thinking clearly	−0.340
6	Any combination of one or more hands, feet, arms, or legs either missing, deformed (crooked), paralyzed (unable to move), or broken—includes wearing artificial limbs or braces	−0.333
7	Pain, stiffness, weakness, numbness, or other discomfort in chest, stomach (including hernia or rupture), side, neck, back, hips, or any joints or hands, feet, arms, or legs	−0.299
8	Pain, burning, bleeding, itching, or other difficulty with rectum, bowel movements, or urination (passing water)	−0.292
9	Sick or upset stomach, vomiting or loose bowel movement, with or without chills, or aching all over	−0.290
10	General tiredness, weakness, or weight loss	−0.259
11	Cough, wheezing, or shortness of breath, *with* or *without* fever, chills, or aching all over	−0.257
12	Spells of feeling upset, being depressed, or of crying	−0.257
13	Headache, or dizziness, or ringing in ears, or spells of feeling hot, nervous, or shaky	−0.244
14	Burning or itching rash on large areas of face, body, arms, or legs	−0.240
15	Trouble talking, such as lisp, stuttering, hoarseness, or being unable to speak	−0.237
16	Pain or discomfort in one or both eyes (such as burning or itching) or any trouble seeing after correction	−0.230
17	Overweight for age and height or skin defect of face, body, arms, or legs, such as scars, pimples, warts, bruises, or changes in color	−0.188
18	Pain in ear, tooth, jaw, throat, lips, tongue; several missing or crooked permanent teeth—includes wearing bridges or false teeth; stuffy, runny nose; or any trouble hearing—including wearing a hearing aid	−0.170
19	Taking medication or staying on a prescribed diet for health reasons	−0.144
20	Wore eyeglasses or contact lenses	−0.101
21	Breathing smog or unpleasant air	−0.101
22	No symptoms or problem (not on respondent's card)	−0.000
23	Standard symptom/problem	−0.257
X24	Trouble sleeping	−0.257
X25	Intoxication	−0.257
X26	Problems with sexual interest or performance	−0.257
X27	Excessive worry or anxiety	−0.257

*Note: −0.727 for death becomes 0 when adjustments for mobility, physical activity, and social activity for death are included. A standard weight is used for symptoms 24-27 because specific scores are not available.

The well life expectancy is the current life expectancy adjusted for diminished quality of life associated with dysfunctional states and duration of stay in each state. Using the system, it is possible to consider simultaneously mortality, morbidity, and the preference weights for these observable behavioral states of function. When the proper steps have been followed, the model quantifies the health activity or treatment program in terms of the QALYs that it produces or saves. A QALY is defined conceptually as the equivalent of a completely well year of life, or a year of life free of any symptoms, problems, or health-related disabilities.

The QWB system is currently in use in several multisite clinical trials. For example, it was demonstrated to be sensitive to minor changes in health status in the multicenter clinical trial of Auranafin (oral gold) for patients with rheumatoid arthritis.[18] Among many clinical trials that have used the QWB system are the 15-center Modification of Diet in Renal Disease (MDRD),[43] trials evaluating the benefits of exercise in patients with noninsulin-dependent diabetes mellitus,[41] and a trial of exercise in cystic fibrosis.[52, 53] The measure has also been used in clinical trials evaluating Zidovudine for human immunodeficiency virus (HIV)–infected men,[35] and specific validity data are available for HIV-infected patients. The National Center for Health Statistics estimates QWB scores based on similar questions in their National Health Interview and Health and Nutrition Examination Surveys.[33]

Studies using the QWB system suggest that psychosocial interventions may produce benefits for COPD patients at a cost comparable to many widely advocated surgical and medical programs in other domains of medical care.[62] The authors encourage more cost/utility studies in the future.

BEHAVIORAL INTERVENTIONS TO IMPROVE COMPLIANCE

Comprehensive pulmonary rehabilitation programs have been developed to provide a multidisciplinary therapeutic regimen tailored to the needs of the individual patient. As suggested in this book and elsewhere,[5, 29] rehabilitation efforts are well justified. Such programs may include several components, including individual assessment, education, instruction in respiratory and chest physiotherapy techniques, psychosocial support, and supervised exercise training. The primary goal of pulmonary rehabilitation is to restore the patient to the highest possible level of independent function. Successful programs can help patients to become better educated and more involved in their own care. In addition, patients may experience reduced symptoms,[27] improved exercise tolerance,[16] fewer hospitalizations and physician visits, and more gainful employment.[54] Pulmonary rehabilitation programs have expanded substantially in the last two decades and are now an accepted form of comprehensive therapy for patients with COPD. In 1981, the American Thoracic Society published a position statement supporting the use of pulmonary rehabilitation programs.[5] The American Association of Cardiovascular and Pulmonary Rehabilitation has published guidelines for practice and a review of evidence establishing the scientific basis of these programs.[4]

An important component of most pulmonary rehabilitation programs has been the establishment of a regular exercise regimen. Specific physical conditioning exercises, such as walking, can be undertaken by the patient to help to maintain physical functioning.[14,16] Improvements in patients with COPD following exercise training have been documented in several studies.[17,19,57,60] Specifically, appropriate physical conditioning exercises can improve maximum exercise tolerance and endurance, reduce exertional breathlessness, and improve ventilatory and mechanical efficiency for exercise.[16]

There have been few controlled studies evaluating COPD rehabilitation programs or their components. Reports from nonrandomized studies typically suggest that rehabilitation objectives can be achieved.[19,57] A few controlled trials have documented the benefits of exercise programs for patients with COPD. Cockcroft and associates[21] randomly assigned 39 patients to a 6-week exercise training program or to a no-treatment control group. In comparison to the control group, patients in the exercise group experienced subjective benefits and increased the amount of distance they could walk in 12 minutes. The length of follow-up, however, was only 2 months. McGavin and coworkers[49] randomly allocated 24 patients with COPD to a 3-month unsupervised stair-climbing home exercise program or to a nonexercise control group. The 12 patients in the exercise group noted subjective improvements and an increased sense of well-being and decreased breathlessness. They also reported an objective increase in 12-minute walk distance and maximal level of exercise on a cycle ergometer. These changes did not occur in the control group. The length of follow-up, however, was limited to 3 months. Ambrosino and coworkers[3] randomly assigned 23 patients to a 1-month medical and rehabilitative therapy group and 28 patients to medical therapy alone (without exercise training). The experimental group improved in exercise tolerance and ventilatory pattern as evidenced by decrease in respiratory rate and increase in tidal volume. Again, these changes were not present in the control group.

BEHAVIORAL MODIFICATIONS TO IMPROVE COMPLIANCE WITH REHABILITATION

Developing exercise programs for patients with COPD is difficult for several reasons. First, principles of training that have been well studied for normals or for cardiac patients do not necessarily apply to patients with COPD.[60] Adherence is often a major problem for the patient with COPD. Some studies suggest that the degree of benefits is associated with compliance to the exercise regimen.[50] Although patients can benefit from exercise, the routine is typically uncomfortable for them. Many participants in rehabilitation programs had become physically deconditioned over a long period of time. Exertion may be not only uncomfortable, but also it commonly leads to the frightening symptom of breathlessness (dyspnea). Because of these problems, discontinuation of the exercise regimen is common.

Remarkably few studies have evaluated methods to improve adherence to an exercise regimen. In one experimental trial, patients with COPD underwent exercise testing and were given an exercise prescription. They were then randomly assigned to one of five experimental or control groups. The experimental groups were based on the principles of behavior modification or a variant of behavior modification known as *cognitive behavior modification*. These methods involve setting goals, analyzing the reinforcers, and using behavioral contracts. The experimental programs included six weekly walking sessions in the patient's home. One control group received attention but did not have the behaviorally based sessions, whereas the other control group received no treatment. After 3 months, there was greater compliance with the exercise program for the experimental groups by comparison with the two control groups (Fig. 11–1). These changes were reflected in improvements in exercise tolerance measured 1 month after the treatment (Fig. 11–2) despite an absence of significant changes in spirometric parameters.[11]

Several additional analyses were performed using a general quality-of-life measure[30] and a general health policy model.[31] Over the course of 18 months, the experimental and control groups showed significant differences on a quality-of-life index (Fig. 11–3). These analyses pooled together the three experimental groups and the two control groups. The differences were used to calculate QALYs and perform cost-effectiveness studies. There is considerable debate about the economic value of behavioral and rehabilitation programs. The cost-effectiveness analyses suggested that behavioral programs designed to increase adherence for patients with COPD produce an equivalent of a well-year for approximately $23,000. This is comparable to other widely advocated health care programs.[62]

These same patients were studied again 3 years after the beginning of the program. At this time, observed differences between the experimental and control groups remained for the quality of well-being measure,[10] yet substantial increases in variability precluded statistically significant effects. Analysis of the data using concepts derived from social learning theory[12] sug-

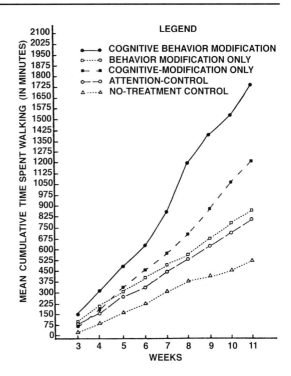

FIGURE 11–1. Cumulative self-reported walking in five groups. The three behavioral modification groups exceeded the two control groups. (From Atkins CJ, Kaplan RM, Timms RM, et al: Behavioral programs for exercise compliance in COPD. J Consult Clin Psychol 52:591–603, 1984.)

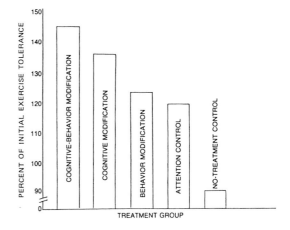

FIGURE 11–2. Percent of initial exercise endurance for five groups at three months. (From Atkins CJ, Kaplan RM, Timms RM, et al: Behavioral programs for exercise compliance in COPD. J Consult Clin Psychol 52:591–603, 1984.)

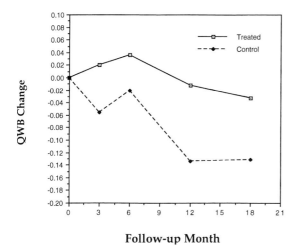

FIGURE 11–3. Change in quality of well-being (QWB) for three treatment groups (combined into treated line) and two control groups (combined into control line). (From Toevs CD, Kaplan RM, Atkins CJ: The costs and effects of behavioral programs in chronic obstructive pulmonary disease. Med Care 22:1088–1100, 1984.)

gested that perceived self-efficacy mediated changes in behavior and function.[36]

LONG-TERM REHABILITATION OUTCOMES

Although comprehensive rehabilitation is believed to improve functional and psychosocial outcomes in COPD patients, studies have not typically monitored patients for longer than 6 months. This has been problematic because the effects of behavioral intervention are often short-lived. A treatment effect that lasts only 1 year, for example, may be of limited value because behavior modification does not cure the condition. Instead, there must be continuing behavior change.

In one of the authors' studies, 119 COPD patients were randomly assigned to either comprehensive pulmonary rehabilitation or to an education control group. Pulmonary rehabilitation consisted of 12 4-hour sessions distributed over an 8-week period. The content of the sessions was education, physical and respiratory care, psychosocial support, and supervised exercise. The education control group attended four 2-hour sessions that were scheduled twice per month but did not include any individual instruction or exercise training. Topics included medical aspects of COPD, pulmonary medicine, pharmacology, nutrition, and respiratory ther-

apy including breathing techniques, and there were a variety of interviews about smoking, life events, and social support. Outcome measures included lung function, maximum and endurance exercise tolerance, perceived breathlessness, subjective fatigue, self-efficacy for walking, Centers for Epidemiologic Studies Depression (CES-D), and the QWB.

In comparison to the educational group, the pulmonary rehabilitation group showed greater improvements in maximum level and endurance measures of exercise performance (Fig. 11–4). In addition, the rehabilitation groups showed greater improvements for resolving breathlessness and in self-efficacy (Fig. 11–5). There were no differences between groups for measures of lung function, depression, or general quality of life. Both groups, however, experienced reductions in quality of life. For exercise variables, benefits tended to relapse toward baseline after 18 months of follow-up.[58]

The effects for pulmonary function were not unanticipated. Nearly all previous studies have also failed to show significant changes in lung function.[3,13,21,26,49,51,55,60] Failure to demonstrate benefits of pulmonary rehabilitation on measures of quality of life and depression was somewhat unexpected. Long-term benefits beyond 12 months were observed only for measures of exercise endurance and perceived breathlessness.

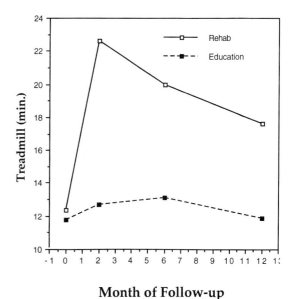

FIGURE 11–4. Exercise endurance by group during follow-up period.

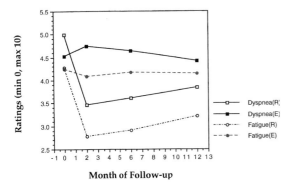

FIGURE 11–5. Perceived dyspnea and perceived fatigue by group (R = rehabilitation, E = education control) during follow-up period.

There are several possible explanations for the failure to demonstrate long-term benefits from comprehensive pulmonary rehabilitation. Behavioral interventions, such as rehabilitation, may be inadequate to produce long-term change. Long-term maintenance of behavioral changes has also been difficult to demonstrate in research on smoking cessation,[25] weight loss,[64] and exercise adherence.[47] The finding that patients experience behavioral changes that are not maintained after treatment has also been seen with a variety of other behavioral interventions.[44] The failure to obtain significant differences on quality-of-life outcomes may be explained by the insensitivities of these measures to small changes in general health status from interventions of this type. The QWB measure, however, has been used in a variety of outcome studies and has correlated significantly with clinical parameters for patients with lung diseases.[23,37,52,53] It is possible that questionnaires that are more specific to COPD may need to be developed.

FOCUS ON DYSPNEA

Dyspnea is the symptom most commonly associated with disability for patients with COPD. One hypothesis is that treatment that focuses on dyspnea results in improved functional outcomes. In one study, the authors evaluated patients for dyspnea and examined the effectiveness of a treatment program designed to train patients to cope with this one symptom. Eighty-nine patients with COPD were randomly assigned to either 6 weeks of treatment or to a general health education program. The treatment was specifically designed to help patients cope with dyspnea. Patients assigned to the treatment

protocol were given instruction in progressive muscle relaxation, breathing exercises, pacing, self-talk, and panic control.

To evaluate the effectiveness of the treatment, all patients were evaluated by a 6-minute walk test, the QWB, and a series of psychological measures. In addition, they completed six different measures of dyspnea. The measures were administered before the treatment, after the treatment, and 6 months later.

Following the 6-week intervention, there were no differences between the treatment and control groups on any outcome measure. At the 6-month follow-up, there was a significant difference for only one variable: the dyspnea index.[46] The results of this study suggest that management of dyspnea alone is not enough to produce significant outcome changes for patients with COPD. Although the program may have had some small effect on dyspnea, it did not have an effect on exercise tolerance, quality of life, or any measure of anxiety or depression. As a result of this experience, the authors now believe that programs must include other behavioral components. In particular, exercise training is probably one of the most important components of any program.[59]

ISSUES

Often, behavioral intervention strategies assume that all or most patients respond in the same way. Clearly, that is not the case. In designing behavioral programs, several individual variables must be considered. In the next sections, three issues that may be of importance are reviewed: compliance, depression, and self-efficacy.

Compliance

The rehabilitation programs prescribed for COPD patients are often difficult to follow. Typically, patients are asked to participate in education, physical and respiratory therapy, and often uncomfortable and anxiety-provoking exercise training. In a controlled study, COPD outpatients participated in 12 exercise training sessions. During these sessions, they walked on a treadmill and performed upper body exercises. The speed of the treadmill was individually determined based on a maximum exercise tolerance test. Patients were individually instructed to translate the treadmill walking into a free walking regimen that included a number of minutes to be walked and steps per minute. The patients were then asked to walk twice daily at the prescribed pace and duration for the 2 months' duration of the program. In addition, they were asked to keep a daily log of the time and distance they had walked for at least 8 weeks.

Each week the logs were reviewed by program staff. A compliance score of the average minutes per day walked was calculated for each patient by dividing the total number of recorded minutes walked during the 8-week period by the total number of days that the patient could have walked. To determine whether compliance was related to outcome, an exercise endurance walk was performed before the program and after 12 weeks. During this test, the patients were urged to walk on the treadmill as long as possible up to a maximum of 20 minutes at the target work load and an additional 10 minutes at a higher work load.

The results of the study indicated a dose-response relationship between compliance with walking prescriptions and improvements in exercise endurance (Fig. 11–6). Thus, compliance with the exercise program was a significant predictor of improved exercise endurance. A variety of analyses were conducted to determine if other variables explained these improvements. The relationship was not diminished by statistical controls for initial levels of disease severity or any other patient characteristic. Thus, it appears that volitional behavior is an important factor for achieving improvements in exercise endurance for patients undergoing pulmonary rehabilitation. In other words, patients' choices to

comply with daily exercise prescriptions may have a significant effect on health outcome.[47]

Depression

A variety of studies demonstrate that patients with chronic illness experience more psychological distress than nondisabled populations. This has clearly been shown in a variety of studies involving patients with COPD.[22] One explanation of the high levels of depression in patients with COPD is that disability prevents patients from obtaining the reinforcers of everyday life. Abramson and colleagues[1] defined hopeless depression as an individual expectation that highly desired outcomes will not occur or highly aversive outcomes will. This definition emphasizes that depression results when people have no control over important events. If this theory is correct, behavioral interventions that give patients more control and improve their activities of daily living might result in reduced depression.

This hypothesis was evaluated in the authors' experimental trial of rehabilitation. Depression was measured using the CES-D Scale. This is a 20-item scale that assesses dimensions of depressed mood, feelings of guilt and worthlessness, appetite loss, sleep disturbance, and energy level.[66]

Although patients randomly assigned to rehabilitation improved on functional outcomes, they did not demonstrate lower levels of depression. Differences between the education and rehabilitation groups were not significant. Within each treatment group, however, other comparisons were made. The patients were subdivided into two groups: One included those who had increased depression (50 patients), and the other included those whose depression had decreased between the baseline and the posttreatment follow-up (52 patients). The data were reanalyzed as a function of treatment circumstances with depression (increased versus decreased) serving as a categorical independent variable. In the rehabilitation group, the patients who had decreases in depression levels showed a significant increase in exercise endurance performance. For those in the education group, increasing or decreasing depression was unrelated to improved exercise endurance (Fig. 11–7).

Another series of analyses separated the patients who were depressed at baseline (N = 25) from those who were not (N = 74). The frequency of depression at baseline was approximately equal in the rehabilitation and the education-only groups. Depression was defined as a

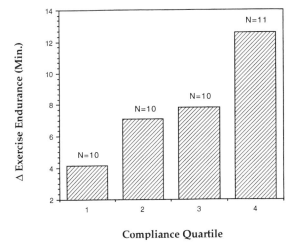

FIGURE 11–6. Change in exercise endurance by quartile of compliance. (From J Cardiopulmon Rehabil 12:108, 1992.)

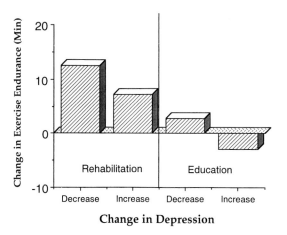

FIGURE 11–7. Changes in exercise endurance among rehabilitation and education patients who increased or decreased in depression. (From Toshima MT, Blumberg E, Ries AL, Kaplan RM: Does rehabilitation reduce depression in patients with chronic obstructive pulmonary disease? J Cardiopulmon Rehabil 12: 261–269, 1992.)

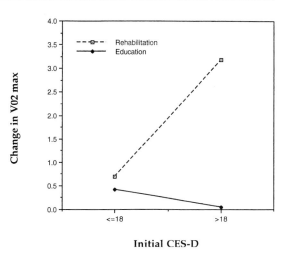

FIGURE 11–8. Changes in $\dot{V}O_2$ max as a function of initial depression for rehabilitation and education patients. (From Toshima MT, Blumberg E, Ries AL, Kaplan RM: Does rehabilitation reduce depression in patients with chronic obstructive pulmonary disease? J Cardiopulmon Rehabil 12:261–269, 1992.)

CES-D score greater than or equal to 18. Eight patients had to be eliminated from the analysis because of missing data. The analyses demonstrated that, for some variables, there was a differential response to treatment as a function of baseline depression. This was most apparent for changes in exercise tolerance ($\dot{V}O_2$ max) for which there were no differences between the education-only and rehabilitation programs for those who initially had low depression scores. For patients who were initially depressed and assigned to the rehabilitation program, however, there were significant improvements in exercise tolerance. In other words, the rehabilitation program was particularly useful for patients who were initially depressed (Fig. 11–8). This finding is particularly interesting because several authors have suggested that depressed patients be screened out of rehabilitation programs. These data suggest that depressed patients may, indeed, gain even more from the rehabilitation interventions.

Depression is likely to be a comorbidity for patients with any chronic illness. Although it is difficult to make comparisons across studies, it appears that about 40% of patients with COPD experience depression. In the authors' work, 29% of patients had clinically significant levels of depression at their initial assessment as determined by CES-D scores greater than 18. The measurement of depression for patients with COPD is difficult because most assessments are based on the general population. For example,

items on the CES-D and other depression measures assess decreased sleep, poor appetite, decreased energy, and so on. These are often symptomatic experiences of lung disease. It is not uncommon for patients with COPD to have trouble sleeping or decreased energy because of dyspnea. Further, many patients with COPD report decreased appetite because of the discomfort associated with a full stomach pressing on the diaphragm. Therefore, scores on depression measures may not accurately reflect the level of clinical depression in patients suffering from chronic diseases such as COPD. Currently, no data are available concerning disease-appropriate depression associated variables, so it is impossible to determine how many patients who report depressionlike symptoms actually have the affective disorder. Considerably more work on the importance of depression and the role of behavioral intervention is needed.[63]

SUMMARY AND CONCLUSION

Traditional models of medical care are challenged by the growing number of older adults with chronic illnesses. COPD, similar to other chronic illnesses, has no cure and typically results in progressive loss of physiologic function over the course of time. Cognitive-behavioral interventions may help patients adapt to loss of function and, when successfully used in a comprehensive rehabilitation program that includes training in energy conservation and the use of assistive devices, may even help to increase function. As a result, behavioral interventions can improve quality of life for patients with chronic pulmonary disease.

Relatively few controlled studies have evaluated behavioral and rehabilitation interventions. The authors' studies suggest that comprehensive pulmonary rehabilitation can enhance exercise endurance and improve self-efficacy. Programs that focus only on the symptom of dyspnea and that do not include exercise training do not result in significant functional gains. Likewise, compliance with the exercise regimen correlates with better outcomes. Further, patients who are initially depressed have been shown to experience significant gains in rehabilitation programs. Thus, outcomes research tends to support the use of more comprehensive programs. To date, however, few systematic outcome studies have appeared. The authors encourage additional systematic outcome studies to evaluate behavioral interventions in comprehensive rehabilitation programs.

Acknowledgments

Supported by Grant HL 34732 from the Lung Division of the National Heart, Lung, and Blood Institute, Grant HD/HL 30912, National Center for Rehabilitation Research, National Institute of Child Health and Human Development, Grant 2RT0268 from the University of California, Tobacco Related Disease Program, and Grant RR 00827 from the NIH Division of Research Resources for the Clinical Research Center.

References

1. Abramson LY, Metalsky GI, Alloy LB: Hopelessness depression: A theory-based subtype of depression. Psychol Rev 96:358–372, 1989.
2. Aldrich T: Respiratory muscle training in COPD. In Bach JR (ed): Pulmonary Rehabilitation: The Obstructive and Paralytic/Restrictive Syndromes. Philadelphia, Hanley & Belfus, 1996.
3. Ambrosino N, Paggiaro PL, Macchi M, et al: A study of short-term effect of rehabilitative therapy in chronic obstructive pulmonary disease. Respiration 41:40–44, 1981.
4. American Association of Cardiovascular and Pulmonary Rehabilitation, Connors G, Hilling L (eds): Guidelines for Pulmonary Rehabilitation Programs. Champaign, IL, Human Kinetics, 1993.
5. American Thoracic Society: Standards for the diagnosis and care of patients with chronic obstructive pulmonary disease (COPD) and asthma. Am Rev Respir Dis 136:225–244, 1987.
6. Anderson JP, Bush JW, Berry CC: Classifying function for health outcome and quality-of-life evaluation: Self-versus interviewer modes. Med Care 24:454–469, 1988.
7. Anderson JP, Bush JW, Berry CC: Internal consistency analysis: A method for studying the accuracy of function assessment for health outcome and quality-of-life evaluation. J Clin Epidemiol 41:127–138, 1988.
8. Anderson JP, Kaplan RM, Berry CC, et al: Interday reliability of function assessment for a health status measure: the quality of well-being scale. Med Care 27:1076–1084, 1989.
9. Anderson JP, Kaplan RM, DeBon M: Comparison of responses to similar questions in health surveys. In Fowler F (ed): Health Survey Research Methods. Washington, National Center For Health Statistics, 1989, pp 13–21.
10. Atkins CJ, Hayes J, Kaplan RM: Four year follow-up of behavioral programs in COPD. University of California Health Psychology Conference. Lake Arrowhead, CA, 1984.
11. Atkins CJ, Kaplan RM, et al: Behavioral programs for exercise compliance in COPD. J Consult Clin Psychol 52:591-603, 1984.
12. Bandura A: Self-efficacy: Toward a unifying theory of behavior change. Psychol Rev 84:191–215, 1977.
13. Bass H, Whitcomb JF, Forman R: Exercise training: Therapy for patients with chronic obstructive pulmonary disease. Chest 57:116–120, 1970.
14. Bell CW, Jensen RH: Physical conditioning. In Jensen RH, Kass I (eds): Pulmonary Rehabilitation Home Programs. Omaha, University of Nebraska Medical Center, 1977.
15. Belman MJ: Exercise training in COPD. In Bach JR (ed): Pulmonary Rehabilitation: The Obstructive and Paralytic/Restrictive Syndromes. Philadelphia, Hanley & Belfus, 1996.
16. Belman MJ: Exercise in chronic obstructive pulmonary disease. Clin Chest Med 7:585–597, 1986.
17. Belman MJ, Wasserman K: Exercise training and testing in patients with chronic obstructive pulmonary disease. Basics Respir Dis 10:1–6, 1981.
18. Bombardier C, Ware J, Russell IJ, et al: Auranofin therapy and quality of life for patients with rheumatoid arthritis: Results of a multi-center trial. Am J Med 81:565–578, 1986.
19. Casaburi R, Petty TL (eds): Principles and Practice of Pulmonary Rehabilitation. Philadelphia, WB Saunders, 1993.
20. Celli BR: Biofeedback and upper extremity exercise in COPD. In Bach JR (ed): Pulmonary Rehabilitation: The Obstructive and Paralytic/Restrictive Syndromes. Philadelphia, Hanley & Belfus, 1996.
21. Cockcroft AE, Saunders MT, Berry G: Randomized controlled trial of rehabilitation in chronic respiratory disability. Thorax 36:200–203, 1981.
22. Dudley DL, Glaser EM, Jorgenson BN, Logan DL: Psychosocial concomitants to rehabilitation in chronic obstructive pulmonary disease: Part 1. Psychosocial and psychological considerations. Chest 77:413–420, 1980.
23. Eakin EG, Kaplan RM, Ries AL: Measurement of dyspnea in chronic obstructive pulmonary disease. Quality of Life Research 2:181–191, 1993.
24. Edelman NH, Kaplan RM, Buist S, et al: Chronic obstructive pulmonary disease. Chest 102:234S-256S, 1992.
25. Fisher EB, Lichtenstein E, Haire-Joshu D, et al: Methods, successes, and failures of smoking cessation programs. Ann Rev Med 44:481–513 1993.
26. Fishmen DB, Petty TL: Physical, symptomatic and psychological improvement in patients receiving comprehensive care for chronic airway obstruction. J Chronic Dis 24:775–785, 1971.
27. Guyatt GH, Berman LB, Townsend M: Long-term outcome after respiratory rehabilitation. Can Med Assoc J 137:1089–1095, 1987.
28. Guyatt GH, Berman LB, Townsend M, et al: A measure of quality of life for clinical trials in chronic lung disease. Thorax 42:773–778, 1987.
29. Hodgkin JE, Connors GL, Bell CW (eds): Pulmonary

Rehabilitation: Guidelines to Success, ed 2. Philadelphia, JB Lippincott, 1993.

30. Kaplan RM: Quality-of-life measurement. In Karoly P (ed): Measurement Strategies in Health Psychology. New York, Wiley-Interscience, 1985, p 115.

31. Kaplan RM, Anderson JP: The general health policy model: an integrated approach. In Spilker B (ed): Quality of Life Assessment in Clinical Trials. New York, Raven Press, 1990, p 131.

32. Kaplan RM, Anderson JP: The quality of well-being scale: Rationale for a single quality of life index. In Walker SR, Rosser RR (eds): Quality of Life: Assessment and Application. London, MTP Press, 1988, pp 51–77.

33. Kaplan RM, Anderson JP, Erickson P: Estimating well-years of life for a new public health indicator. Proceedings of the 1989 Public Health Conference on Records and Statistics. HDDS, National Center for Health Statistics, DHHS Publication Number (PHS) 90–1214, 1989, pp. 298–303.

34. Kaplan RM, Anderson JP, Ganiats TG: The quality of well-being scale: Rationale for a single quality of life index. In Walker SR, Rosser RM (eds): Quality of Life Assessment: Key Issues in the 1990s. London, Kluwer Academic Publishers, 1993, pp 65–94.

35. Kaplan RM, Anderson JP, Wu AW, et al: The quality of well-being scale: Applications in AIDS, cystic fibrosis, and arthritis. Med Care 27(suppl 3):S27-S43, 1989.

36. Kaplan RM, Atkins CJ, Reinsch S: Specific efficacy expectations mediate exercise compliance in patients with COPD. Health Psychol 3:223–242, 1984.

37. Kaplan RM, Atkins CJ, Timms R: Validity of a quality of well-being scale as an outcome measure in chronic obstructive pulmonary disease. J Chronic Dis 37:85–95, 1984.

38. Kaplan RM, Bush JW: Health-related quality of life measurement for evaluation research and policy analysis. Health Psychol 1:61–80, 1982.

39. Kaplan RM, Bush JW, Berry CC: The reliability, stability and generalizability of a health status index. American Statistics Association. Proceedings of the Social Statistics Section 26:415–418, 1978.

40. Kaplan RM, Bush JW, Berry CC: Health status: Types of validity for an index of well-being. Health Services Research 11:478–507, 1976.

41. Kaplan RM, Hartwell SL, Wilson DK, Wallace JP: Effects of diet and exercise interventions on control and quality of life in non-insulin-dependent diabetes mellitus. J Gen Intern Med 2:220–228, 1987.

42. Kaplan RM, Sallis J, Patterson TL: Health and Human Behavior. New York, McGraw-Hill, 1993.

43. Klahr S, Levey AS, Beck GJ, et al: The effects of dietary protein restriction and blood-pressure control on the progression of chronic renal disease. Modification of Diet in Renal Disease Study Group. N Engl J Med 330: 877–884, 1994.

44. Larimer ME, Marlatt GA: Addictive behaviors. In Craighead LW, Craighead WE, Kazdin AE, Mahoney MJ (eds): Cognitive and Behavioral Interventions: An Empirical Approach to Mental Health Problems. Boston, Allyn & Bacon, 1994, pp 157–168.

45. Lewis MI: Nutrition, anabolic steroids and growth hormone. In Bach JR (ed): Pulmonary Rehabilitation: The Obstructive and Paralytic/Restrictive Syndromes. Philadelphia, Hanley & Belfus, in press.

46. Mahler DA, Wells CK: Evaluation of clinical methods for rating dyspnea. Chest 93:580–586, 1988.

47. Martin JE, Dubbert PM: Exercise applications and promotion in behavioral medicine: Current status and future directions. J Consult Clin Psychol 30:1004–1017, 1982.

48. Mazzucca SA: Does patient education in chronic disease have therapeutic value? J Chronic Dis 35:521–529, 1982.

49. McGavin CR, Gupta SP, Lloyd EL, McHardy JR: Physical rehabilitation of chronic bronchitis: Results of a controlled trial of exercises in the home. Thorax 32:307–311, 1977.

50. Mertens DJ, Shephard RJ, Kavanagh T: Long-term exercise therapy for chronic obstructive lung disease. Respiration 35:96–107, 1978.

51. Moser KM, Bokinsky GE, Savage RT, et al: Results of a comprehensive rehabilitation program: Physiologic and functional effects on patients with chronic obstructive pulmonary disease. Arch Intern Med 140:1596–1601, 1980.

52. Orenstein DM, Nixon PA, Ross EA, Kaplan RM: The quality of well-being in cystic fibrosis. Chest 5:344–347, 1989.

53. Orenstein DM, Pattishall EN, Ross EA, Kaplan RM: Quality of well-being before and after antibiotic treatment of pulmonary exacerbation in cystic fibrosis. Chest 98:1081–1084, 1990.

54. Petty TL, Nett LM, Finigan MM, et al: A comprehensive care program for chronic airway obstruction: Methods and preliminary evaluation of symptomatic and functional improvement. Ann Intern Med 70:1109–1120, 1969.

55. Pierce AK, Paez PN, Miller WF: Exercise training with the aid of a portable oxygen supply in patients with emphysema. Am Rev Respir Dis 91:653–659, 1965.

56. Rand C: Smoking cessation. In Bach JR (ed): Pulmonary Rehabilitation: The Obstructive and Paralytic/Restrictive Syndromes. Philadelphia, Hanley & Belfus, 1996.

57. Ries AL: Position paper of the American Association of Cardiovascular and Pulmonary Rehabilitation: Scientific basis of pulmonary rehabilitation. J Cardiopulmon Rehabil 10:418–441, 1990.

58. Ries AL, Kaplan RM, Limberg TM, Prewitt L: Effects of pulmonary rehabilitation on physiologic and psychosocial outcomes in patients with chronic obstructive pulmonary disease. Ann Intern Med 122:823–832, 1995.

59. Sassi-Dambron DE, Eakin L, Ries AL, Kaplan RM: The effect of compliance on exercise training in pulmonary rehabilitation. Rehabil Nurs Res 3:3–10, 1994.

60. Shephard RJ: On the design and effectiveness of training regimens in chronic obstructive lung disease. Bull Eur Physiopathol Respir 13:457–469, 1977.

61. Spiezer R: Overview and summary: The rise in chronic obstructive pulmonary disease mortality. Am Rev Respir Dis 140:5106–5107, 1989.

62. Toevs CD, Kaplan RM, Atkins CJ: The costs and effects of behavioral programs in chronic obstructive pulmonary disease. Med Care 22:1088–1100, 1984.

63. Toshima MT, Blumberg E, Ries AL, Kaplan RM: Does rehabilitation reduce depression in patients with chronic obstructive pulmonary disease? J Cardiopulmon Rehabil 12:261–269, 1992.

64. Wadden TA, Brownell KD: The development and modification of dietary practices in individuals, groups, and large populations. In Matarazzo JD, Weiss SM, Herd JA, et al (eds): Behavioral Health: A Handbook of Health Enhancement and Disease Prevention. New York, Wiley, 1984, pp 608–631.

65. Weinstein MC, Stason WB: Foundations of cost-effectiveness analysis for health and medical practice. N Engl J Med 296:716–721, 1977.

66. Weissman MM, Sholomskas D, Pottenger M, et al: Assessing depressive symptoms in five psychiatric populations: A validation study. Am J Epidemiol 106:203–214, 1977.

Neurocognitive and Psychological Considerations in Chronic Obstructive Pulmonary Disease

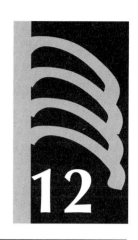

12

Michael Dealy, PhD

Many people are healthier and live longer because of advances in medicine and health education. This increased longevity can be a mixed blessing, however, for individuals with chronic illnesses, many of whom pose a challenge for health care providers. Patients with chronic obstructive pulmonary disease (COPD) experience stress when performing the most basic of functions—breathing. Although medical interventions reduce breathlessness, airway congestion, and the severity of acute exacerbations, the patient must adjust to a world of treatments, assistive devices, and altered quality of life.

Steadily more confining restrictions in everyday life result in a concordant increase in psychosocial stress. A resulting depression can be as debilitating as the COPD itself. The prevalence of depression in COPD is higher than in many other chronic illnesses and approaches 50%.[37] In the United States, this totals about 8 million COPD patients with depression,[35] including many with concomitant anxiety, panic disorders, and feelings of alienation.

Although symptom reduction has been achieved in many cases by adherence to medical regimens and pulmonary rehabilitation, because of the progressive nature of the disease, long-term benefits are not possible. The limited nature of the medical goals is mirrored in patients' poor sense of self-efficacy in coping with the related psychological stresses.

The patient may undergo role changes in the family, as well as in society at large. Wage earning ability may decline, and the patient may become more dependent on others for financial support. Spousal roles and parenting functions may shift. These changes can create miscommunication in the home. As family members become more involved in direct care, the patient may play an obstructive role in the family's social functioning. With the eventual need for ongoing oxygen therapy, the patient may feel that his or her life as an independent, worthwhile adult is over.[39] Because there is a relationship between the patient's psychological response to COPD and medical intervention outcomes,[30] rehabilitation programs must tailor treatments to the psychodynamics of each patient.

Many questions remain to be answered about the neurobehavioral abnormalities associated with COPD and about possible interventions. The effects of chronic lung disease are pervasive and complex, spanning a wide range of psychosocial issues, coping skills, and neurocognitive factors that must be considered in planning treatment. In addition to considering these factors separately, this chapter offers some suggestions for treatment strategies and future research.

PSYCHOSOCIAL ASPECTS

COPD patients are vulnerable to clinical depression. The Beck Depression Inventory[3] and Zung Self-Rating Scale[53] have been especially useful in quantitating and monitoring depression associated with COPD. When untreated, depression tends to amplify the effects of the disease symptoms on daily activities. COPD patients also tend to experience sleep disturbances, reduced appetite, a lower energy level, sexual dysfunction, helplessness, low self-esteem, as well as feelings of guilt and ambivalence toward others.[46] Poor coping is characterized by feelings of hopelessness and failure. This can result in withdrawal, difficulty concentrating, and, at times, suicidal ideation.[12]

Anxiety often accompanies depression,[29] and dyspnea can lead to episodes of panic. The patient may not seek medical attention until long after a cycle of dyspnea, anxiety, panic, and more dyspnea has become established.[25] In a study relating respiratory function and anxiety, one-third of COPD patients reported experiencing panic attacks.[17] They then experienced agoraphobic reactions and serious bodily concerns. The resulting disordered self-concept left many feeling isolated and compelled to fend for themselves psychologically. With the interactive effects of dyspnea, hypersecretion, need for assistive devices, dependency, feelings of alienation, poor self-esteem, and lowered sense of self-efficacy, the COPD patient can be in an emotional straightjacket,[12] which can result in chronic anxiety, irritability, and pseudodementia.

Psychologically, the COPD patient is vulnerable to what Seligman and Maier called "learned helplessness."[47] In their study, animals were placed on grids that could be electrified. When the animals felt the shock, they escaped to another grid. When signals were introduced, the animals were able to avoid the pain by escaping to a nonelectrified grid before theirs was charged. When the experimenter electrified all the grids, the animals gradually resigned themselves to the pain, and remained huddled on one of the grids in constant pain, making no more effort to explore the environment. They had given up hope of changing their condition. At first, medical interventions help patients escape the consequences of COPD. However, the inevitable decline in health leads to more episodes of painful living from which escape becomes minimal, and hopeless resignation is the ultimate result. This is manifested as a labyrinth of psychological defense mechanisms.

Quality of Life

The impact of chronic illness gradually becomes increasingly intrusive on the patient's social functioning, modifying social roles in the work, friendship, and family environments. In a study of the quality of life of COPD patients, Clough et al. described five key social issues.[8]

1. If the patient was the wage earner, he or she might experience a decrease in social status in the family.
2. A change in spousal roles can result in confusion and conflict.
3. Increasing dependence can result in the patient's becoming unable to maintain social contacts, restricting the family's social and recreational life.
4. The oxygen concentrator can become a permanent fixture in the home, accentuating the patient's dependent profile.
5. Increasing dependence raises family tension and increases the patient's feelings of helplessness, loss of control, anger, and uselessness.[41]

Members of the immediate social environment are often enlisted, at least by default, as caregivers, but they may eventually be overwhelmed under the weight of chronicity.[34] The frustrations of family members because of social losses, job changes, and shifting household responsibilities can lead to divisive friction, marked by silence and secretive collaboration.[46] These additional family tensions can accentuate the prevailing sentiments of overdependency, resentment, and ambivalence. Sandhu described a cycle of resentment, harm, and guilt.[46] The family members' resentment can awaken preexisting negative feelings, which can lead to expressions of anger, then guilt, and finally overprotection. The destructive effects of undoing the overprotectiveness can result in further arousing the patient's feelings of helplessness and resentment.

Family members may even project their own frustration and anger to the patient, describing the patient as being oppositional to assistive efforts, when, in fact, they themselves are feeling the resentment. In a study by McSweeny et al., relatives reported strong oppositional patient behavior, when, in actuality, significant levels of anger did not exist in the patients.[37] Sandhu warns of the potential for protracted struggles, an eventual breakdown in communication, and possible avoidance of the patient by family members in retaliation for perceived transgressions as the disease itself continues on an irreversible path of debilitation.[46]

All members of the family must struggle to adjust to the stresses of chronic illness. McSweeny and colleagues, in a recent review, outlined some of the physical, emotional, and financial pressures on family members when they accept the roles of caregivers in the home. They reported that support programs are now becoming more available for families in community health care settings.[36] A supportive environment is important because it is essential that at least one significant member of the household be able to relate to the patient in a psychosocially supportive way.[1] Without a therapeutic ally, the family may become polarized between healthy members and the identified sick person, restricting the patient's role and impeding the attainment of treatment goals. With support, the COPD patient may not only avoid infantilization, but family dynamics and physical functioning can be improved. Mood and self-esteem are related to functional status and the ability to perform activities of daily living (ADL),[51] rather than simple exercise performance or gross motor abilities.

The COPD patient's sociofamilial milieu is prone to the same pattern of emotional changes and dysfunction that the patient undergoes, including depression, anxiety, sleep and appetite disturbances, fatigue, and loss of motivation.[14] The only difference may be that COPD patients tend not to express strong emotions in order not to provoke dyspnea.[13] They seem to develop either difficulty labeling their emotions in an effort to avoid the physiological consequences,[34] or they present with little distress indicative of strong denial.[32] This effort to remain calm under duress is emotionally energy-consuming and leaves them vulnerable to volatile family dynamics.

Likewise, spouses, who may have been accustomed to sharing their emotional reactions to everyday difficulties before the onset of the disease, might now refrain from such communication. In a study by Sexton and Munro, approximately two-thirds of the wives of COPD patients reported that they refrained from sharing their problems with their husbands because they were afraid of causing attacks of dyspnea.[49] Further study is required before extrapolating this finding to other family members.

The intimate life of the COPD patient is also modified by effects of the disease. Some patients experience sexual dysfunction, ranging from impotence[31] to reduced frequency or even cessation of intercourse.[16] Males appear to experience more sexual difficulties than females.[40] Intercourse can be interrupted by dyspnea and bronchospasms.[9] In addition, hypoxemia can affect hormonal levels.[48] Depression and so many physical and psychological obstacles have a neg-

ative effect on sexual activity. Recognizing the need for intervention, rehabilitation programs often disseminate information and practical suggestions for alleviating some of the difficulties.[36] Simple suggestions, like repositioning and intermission taking, can do wonders for both motivation and performance. Thus, the psychosocial variables are myriad and complex, and addressing them requires a multidimensional approach.

Patient Compliance

The patient is expected to take medications on a specific schedule and to engage in prescribed exercise routines. Although physicians generally believe that their recommendations are adhered to,[38] studies fail to support this belief.[7] Patients, in general, tend to have more than a 30% rate of noncompliance with any medical regimen,[29] and patients with chronic disease comply even less.[45] For the COPD patient, the regimen demands can be complex, with many medications to address dyspnea, infection, inflammation, bronchospasm, and other cardiopulmonary symptoms. Complexity can result in an avoidant response. Simple reminders and individual appointments, as opposed to group treatments, tend to improve compliance.[15]

Kaplan et al. suggested that patients do not deliberately try to harm themselves by poor compliance because of some flaw in their personalities, but they merely have difficulty understanding the instructions.[29] Environmental variables, such as family influence and ineffective memory queues, can also lead to noncompliance. They concluded that the patient-physician relationship plays a significant role in compliance because of critical information exchange. In general, patients exhibit poor comprehension of the physicians' instructions, and physicians have a distorted perception of their patients' responses to the prescribed medications. With a basis of poor communication, the patient rationalizes a course of noncompliance because the expected benefits do not seem to materialize.[4] Moreover, even if the patient understands that there will be meaningful benefits after some delay, present discomfort may be considered too great a cost. Kaplan et al. suggested that immediate benefits from such interventions as inhalers might be related to greater compliance than the possible future benefits of medical interventions for hypertension.[29]

This sense of immediacy also applies to compliance with exercise regimens. Although the value of exercise for patients with COPD has been established,[50] compliance can be a problem.[29] The COPD patient is prone to avoid exercise because of the fear of dyspnea and may have been deconditioned for a long time before beginning rehabilitation. Although the patient is cognitively aware of the benefits of exercise, the physical discomfort and emotional distress associated with exercise tend to demotivate. Immediacy of benefits is important. Consequently, the COPD patient is best served by a combination of medical and exercise prescriptions that provide both immediate relief from discomfort and long-term benefit despite initial discomfort.

In general, prescriptions should involve goal-setting with self-monitoring to identify adverse situational variables and self-reward to maintain optimal levels of responding. To maintain optimally low anxiety levels, patients can benefit from systematic desensitization, relaxation therapies, and biofeedback. For these methods to have lasting effects, social intervention is necessary to optimize the network of social support. All of these factors interactively potentiate the patient's ability to cope with the overwhelming stress of chronic disease.

Further complicating the treatment paradigm is the effect of COPD on neuropsychological functioning. As the disease progresses, the effects of hypoxemia become more noticeable. Indeed, there is a direct relationship between hypoxemia and neuropsychological impairment.[21] Patients begin to experience altered concentration on tasks at hand, perceptual-motor dysfunction, and impaired sensation and abstraction of input information. There is also a neuropsychiatric component involving mood changes and occasionally delusions.[10] These, too, must be addressed when considering patient compliance.

NEUROPSYCHOLOGICAL ASPECTS OF COPD

Long-term oxygen deprivation is common in COPD. In 1973, Krop and associates administered the Bender-Gestalt Visual Motor Test and other tests of neurocognitive function to 10 hypoxic COPD patients.[33] They found that cognitive and emotional functioning were impaired and suggested that the decrements were due to oxygen deprivation. After 1 month of continuous oxygen therapy, both cognitive and emotional functioning improved.

Subsequently, in 1993, Rourke et al. reviewed two multicenter studies on the effects of hypoxemia on neurocognitive performance.[44] The Nocturnal Oxygen Therapy Trial in 1980 included 203 hypoxemic COPD patients, and in 1983, the Intermittent Positive Pressure Breathing Trial studied 100 hypoxemic patients; these were the first controlled studies on the neuropsychological functioning of mildly hypoxemic COPD patients. Comparable assessment procedures allowed for a combined analysis by stratification of subjects into groups based on severity of hypoxemia. The instruments used to evaluate the neuropsychological functioning of these patients included the well-validated Halstead-Reitan Neuropsychological Battery (HRB).[43] The HRB subtests measure a variety of neurocognitive functions, including general intellectual ability, attention, concentration, memory, verbal and performance abstraction ability, receptive and expressive language, sensation, and perceptual-motor functioning. The results of the multicenter trial analysis indicated that as hypoxemia increases, neuropsychological functioning steadily and broadly declines, especially in perceptual processing and psychomotor skills. Verbal intelligence seems to be spared.

Oxygen therapy appeared to remediate some neuropsychological deficits, including language and sensorimotor skills. Although continuous oxygen therapy was more effective than nocturnal-only oxygen therapy, it remains unclear how the quantity and duration of oxygen supplementation impact on neuropsychological gains. Furthermore, the effects of oxygen therapy may have been related to interactive processes responsible for gains in cognitive expression. The short-term effects of oxygen supplementation may be dependent on its effects on central nervous system neurotransmitters involved in information processing.[24] Grant et al. suggested that acetylcholine is one such neurotransmitter.[21] They pointed out that because acetylcholine appears to be related to cognitive skills,[2] reductions in the biosynthesis of acetylcholine in hypoxemic patients might contribute to neurocognitive deficits. Neurotransmitter inhibition appears to be presynaptic, with the postsynaptic receptors functioning normally. Therefore, it was suggested that the precursors of cholinergic transmission are normalized by oxygen supplementation. Consistent with this, Grant and Adams noted that pretreatment of laboratory animals with physostigmine delayed the adverse effects of hypoxia, presumably by increasing the availability of acetylcholine.[20] The use of cholinergic precursors may be beneficial for some COPD patients.

Further investigation is needed to examine the relationship between oxygen therapy and neurocognitive gains, as well as the relationship between neurocognitive improvements and psychosocial variables. Neurocognitive skills are utilized in everyday life and directly influence social interactions. McSweeny et al. suggested that because hypoxemia affects neurocognitive skills, some of which have social value, hypoxemia therefore can adversely affect quality of life.[36] Thus, oxygen therapy can enhance quality of life.

Improvements in quality of life were not demonstrated to result from oxygen therapy in the COPD patients in the previously noted multicenter trials. However, Rourke et al. pointed out that these patients did not decline either.[44] In addition, for patients who were previously declining steadily, this plateau may be indicative of positive results. Further exploration of this possible benefit would require controlling for the asynchronous pattern of psychosocial decline in relation to the more predictable hypoxemia-related schedule of neurocognitive deterioration which tends to parallel physical decline.

Psychosocial impairment appears to occur early in the COPD process. In the Intermittent Positive Pressure Breathing Trial, which used the Minnesota Multiphasic Personality Inventory to test personality characteristics, impairment in quality of life, and especially depression, did not appear to be directly related to disease severity or evolution. Psychosocial disturbances appeared both before significant physical limitation and before neuropsychological decline. An in-depth sociomedical history helps to identify periods of decline early in the disease process.

Although oxygen therapy can have positive effects on neurocognitive functioning and may also benefit psychosocial functioning, there are other factors that contribute to overall neuropsychological well-being. Age and education are associated with performance. McSweeny et al., in their heuristic model of the relationship between COPD and quality of life, found that the variable "age" directly influenced not only the disease process but also neuropsychological ability and social functioning.[36] Grant and Adams found that education also accounted for some of the variance in neuropsychological performance, with lower education as a predictor of impairment.[20] Better understanding of the relationships among hypoxemia, age, education, and neurotransmitter synthesis may improve treatment efforts to control the effects of COPD on neuropsychological functioning.

COPING SKILLS DEVELOPMENT

COPD patients experience physiological and psychological stresses in daily living. Dyspnea can be caused by physical activity, environmental conditions such as poor air quality and changes in temperature and humidity, and suboptimal medical management, often because of confusion about complex medical treatment regimens. In addition, stress is produced by the subjective interpretation or the personal meaning of a compromised existence. While the physician employs vigorous medical interventions, there must also be a spirited and carefully formatted approach to psychosocial needs. Management success does not depend on knowledge of symptom-treatment fit relative to some hypothetically normal COPD patient population, but hinges upon an individually tailored approach with physician adherence to some basic psychological rules of thumb. The physician must be a trusted, caring member of the patient's social support network and make every effort to be available on a regular basis, especially in times other than crises, to reinforce positive medical progress and to reaffirm the therapeutic relationship. The physician must be able to listen, not passively accepting the often convoluted ideas of chronic patients who retreat behind self-injurious defenses, but listening assertively, supporting the defenses that help the patient retain a positive self-image in social interaction. The physician must also reassure the patient and relieve anxiety so that the patient can dispense with more negative defenses and broaden horizons for new directions in self-help.

Patient Evaluation

To plan an individualized approach, careful assessment includes a complete medical and socioeducational history, including highlights of childhood. It is important to know positive as well as negative aspects of early experiences, because the positive highlights can be used as resources for psychological healing and growth in a therapeutic context. The social history includes a detailed analysis of the patient's present living situation, including family interaction patterns, social and work relationships, and the patient's baseline coping strategies. One important area to explore is that of close personal relationships. If one such relationship is or can become strongly supportive, this person can have a significant impact on the patient's well-being and social adaptation. In a study on the effects of spousal support on adaptation to stress, Burke and Weir found that men with supportive wives who were suffering from high levels of stress were able to cope far better than those whose wives were nonsupportive.[6] Even if the spouse is nonsupportive, the COPD patient shows better adaptation with at least one strongly supportive member in the household.

Family predispositions to conflict must be examined if members are enlisted as caregivers. The stress of chronic illness affects everyone in the living environment. Frustrations tend to be exacerbated under the pressure, demanding vigilance in monitoring family dynamics so that family members do not do more harm than good. Sandhu recommends observation of family interactions over time and a careful review of the results to understand the changing patterns of strength and weakness in the family support network.[46]

A psychological evaluation includes intellectual, perceptual, projective, and adaptive measures, as well as achievement and neuropsychological assessment if warranted. The results are integrated into a comprehensive profile of the patient's social, cognitive, affective, and adaptive coping styles. For the elderly, psychological dysfunction must not be considered a function of aging. It must be examined with the same care given to the young. The first consideration of the examiner must be that COPD is the catalyst for the dysfunction, causing anxiety, depression, and changes in adaptation. Such an assessment approach can provide an environment of respect and mature concern much needed by the COPD patient. This evaluation leads to a psychosocial treatment plan that can include individual or group psychotherapy, psychopharmacology, family crisis intervention, marital or relationships counseling, vocational guidance, and coping skills training. As needed, appropriate referrals are made to the psychologist for standardized evaluation and psychotherapy, to the psychiatrist for consultation and psychopharmacologic treatment, to the social worker for outreach, clinical family intervention, and marriage counseling, and to a vocational counselor.

COPING STRATEGIES

The need for coping strategies is universal in all people experiencing stress. Coping skills training is beneficial for all health care professionals involved in treatment. In order to cope with the dyspnea-stress-dyspnea cycle, stress reduction is the prime concern. The foundation for this approach is relaxation training, which can lessen tension and reduce the emotional response to discomfort. In addition, for the COPD patient, relaxation can facilitate breathing. According to Frownfelter, there appears to be a neurologic response to relaxation in the hypothalamus, causing reduction in sympathetic and increases in parasympathetic activity.[19] This response to relaxation can improve ability to cope with stress. Relaxation can be achieved in a variety of ways using imagery, music or soothing sound recordings, meditation, or relaxation tapes. Basic to most approaches is a form of progressive muscle relaxation,[26] which has proven successful in reducing dyspnea and anxiety in COPD.[42]

Muscle Relaxation

Muscle relaxation provides a frame of reference for comfort by contracting and subsequently relaxing specific muscle groups. During this procedure, other techniques can be used to enable the patient to cope with stress. Once relaxed, the patient might be able to utilize cognitive and affective modalities to solve problems and facilitate broadening of social interactions. Because much information will be conveyed nonverbally in the interaction with the patient, the health care provider must be a well-schooled practitioner of the relaxation technique and must explain the technique and its ramifications to the patient.

It initially may be difficult for COPD patients to recognize muscular cues of comfort, because avoidance and denial of bodily sensations have been used for pain management. The threshold for recognizing stimulation along the comfort-discomfort continuum has probably risen with the increase of chronic symptoms. Patients need more prompting than normal subjects. They may view muscle relaxation as a letting down of the guard against discomfort, and the attentiveness to bodily sensations is seen as a loss of distraction as a coping mechanism. Such a patient cannot be expected to follow the normal course of progress and may have considerable difficulty in recognizing the cues of physical comfort, which they may experience as weakness and vulnerability. Resistance to the intervention should, therefore, not be interpreted as noncompliance or poor comprehension, but as a cautious reservation about relinquishing defenses that have been of value. The patient should be assured that this technique can provide some immediate results and has no adverse side effects. If the patient is still resistant (because control is always an issue in the care of COPD patients), then following a description of the technique, the patient is asked to try it privately and to give the clinician some feedback on its efficacy. In my experience as well as that of others, this has always had positive results.[27]

For patients who fear loss of control, experiencing new sensations can be frightening and debilitating for their coping repertoire. Kaplan et al. recommended reassuring the patient that the mind is always alert and ready to respond to feared emergencies, even during episodes of deep relaxation.[29]

Usually, the patient is placed supine, but when this position is not possible, the COPD patient should assume a comfortable sitting position. The arms and legs are not crossed, the hands are open, and if necessary, head support can be used.

The patient is typically asked to tighten muscle groups successively in the hands, feet, arms, and legs, and then to relax them respectively and to learn to discriminate between tension and the comfort associated with relaxation. As the patient becomes more familiar with these basic discriminations, the sessions focus on muscles in the chest, shoulders, and abdomen that are more specifically related to respiratory function. Each contraction-relaxation step must be repeated in order to reinforce learning. The patient will eventually be able to discriminate between a state of rest and the slightest contractions within a muscle group.

If, at any time, the patient complains of inability to comply with directions, the directions are modified to maintain the momentum of the session. For instance, if the patient does not feel ready to lift a leg or raise an arm for flexing, then the focus can be reverted to the toes and fingers. When returning to the arm or leg muscles during a repetition, the patient is not asked to actually move the leg but just to flex it in place. If the patient is sensitive to the idea of flexing muscles in the chest or neck area because of illness-related fears, then these areas are avoided during the initial sessions until the patient experiences positive feedback with extremity muscle relaxation. To desensitize the patient to chest muscle activity, he or she is initially instructed to flex these muscles only slightly and then relax briefly. Immediately thereafter, the patient is instructed to contract and relax muscles whose cues are well known and have come to be associated with rewarding sensations. This pairing of stimuli expedites the patient's utilization of the relaxation technique for more psychologically sensitive areas.

The health care provider should be flexible in wording the instructions and note any adverse reactions to particular words. For example, the provider might give the instruction, "Relax, allow any tension to flow out of your hand." The patient may respond anxiously, saying, "I just can't relax." Such absolute statements are not uncommon in high stress situations. The provider need not respond to the absolute quality of the statement but merely repeat the instruction. Attention to detail and nonverbal cues and verbal flexibility will maintain the quality of the session. Sessions should be brief, positive, and regular, with the goal of teaching the patient to practice this technique at home. Kaplan et al. recommended making a tape recording of an office session and allowing the patient to use the recording privately to reduce any performance or evaluation anxiety.[29] Relaxation can be enhanced by performing proper breathing techniques during the training sessions as well as during everyday activities involving sitting, standing, walking, stair climbing, and running or engaging in sports.

Breathing Exercise

Paralleling the dyspnea-stress cycle is the relationship between controlled breathing and relaxation. Proper breathing tends to increase exercise tolerance and enhance relaxation. However, many feel that relaxation training is necessary to prepare the patient for training in proper breathing.[18] Subsequently, proper breathing technique is enhanced further by relaxation training. Normally breathing involves the use of the diaphragm and external intercostal muscles. Undesirable breathing technique involves using the accessory muscles of inspiration. The patient is taught to optimize diaphragm excursion during inspiration, while at the same time using relaxation techniques to relax the accessory muscles. Some patients may need to experience separate relaxation of the shoulders before the breathing exercise begins.

The patient should be in a comfortable position, optimally at a 45° angle, with the knees flexed and hips externally rotated. The knees are supported by pillows. The therapist demonstrates the technique and then shows the patient how to place a hand on the abdomen at the costophrenic angle to feel the action of the diaphragm. The patient takes a deep breath, and the shoulders rise and fall. With succeeding breaths, expansion of the abdomen (diaphragm excursion) is felt and the shoulders are maintained in a relaxed position. Expiration is through pursed-lips to prolong the expiratory phase and to regularize the breathing rate.

Before the patient is instructed to use diaphragmatic breathing in stressful circumstances, such as during travel or while at work, he or she is instructed to use it in conjunction with pleasant activities, such as sitting in a favorite reading chair, walking in the garden, or listening to pleasant music. After the technique has become associated with pleasant, relaxing stimuli, it can then be used to help the patient reinterpret some of the less pleasant events of daily living, such as waiting in line for service at a store check-out or sitting in a doctor's waiting room. Habits that once were annoying could become behaviors from which comfort is derived.

Other Coping Techniques

The effects of progressive relaxation and diaphragmatic breathing can be enhanced by biofeedback, visualization, guided imagery in music, hypnosis, behavioral desensitization, and cognitive-behavioral therapy. *Biofeedback* is the utilization of auditory or visual signals to enable the patient to recognize changes in physiologic processes, such as muscle tension. Although the merits of biofeedback in the treatment of patients with breathing problems are uncertain,[27] it does facilitate relaxation training. It tends to make the patient feel engaged in a legitimate rehabilitation exercise when relaxing. Instead of a decrease in motivation because relaxation appears to be a passive experience, the biofeedback patient feels a sense of accomplishment in that learning is taking place.[10] It also affects the patient's uncertainty about control and tends to change the patient's focus from futile efforts to reduce stress to successful attempts to control and regulate relaxation responses. Merely the attentional shift from indiscernible internal parameters to observable external stimuli can make tension more manageable.

Biofeedback can be beneficial for learning diaphragmatic breathing. By receiving visual or auditory signals from accessory muscle groups such as those in the neck, the patient can maintain decreases in muscular responses while engaging in proper breathing. After discrimination has been achieved, the process can assist in facilitating activity for muscle reeducation.[19]

Visualization is the manipulation of imaginative visual imagery for symbolic accomplishment of controlling and minimizing feelings of distress stemming from physical discomfort. For instance, if the patient is experiencing frustration or anger about some recent setback, he or she is asked to give that anger a mental representation, such as the color red. Using relaxation and proper breathing, the patient is asked to see the red change gradually to a color the patient identifies with more peaceful feelings.

Visualization can be enhanced by the use of music[22] and art. Music can cause the right hemisphere of the brain to release endorphins, which produce a natural opiate soothing effect on the body.[5] There has been promising work in the area of integrating the soothing effects of music with training of proper breathing and progressive relaxation.[17]

For the patient who requires more tangible feedback, thematic artwork, such as animal or cartoon drawing sequences, can be used as an interactive format for modification of visual images. By translating visual symbols into animal or fantasy characters, the action of modification can be brought to life. The process can be synchronized with the schedule of relaxation training sessions to provide a richer, soothing experience.

Hypnotherapy can contribute to the relaxation response as well as be applied to daily living. The patient is provided with suggestions during states of guided relaxation that enable the formulation of selected responses to distress. Attention is paid to the patient's pace of mental and physical activity, including his or her movement and direction of thoughts as well as the movements of the chest during breathing. The patient may be encouraged to find a safe place somewhere in memory or imagination where there is no distress. The patient's description of that safe place provides the therapist with clues to the patient's primary cognitive and affective modalities. One visually oriented patient might describe a safe place as having beautiful colors and striking images, whereas another describes the safe place as warm and breezy with soft sand, because this patient tends to be more tactile in receiving environmental communication. This knowledge is utilized by the therapist to assist the patient in reframing daily experience (medical, work, social, or family) in a more positive way, especially when the experience is reevaluated through a more comfortable modality. Milton Erikson did extensive work in the area of hypnotherapy, and his works provide a comprehensive basis for both theory and practice.[23]

Systematic desensitization was introduced by Joseph Wolpe in the early 1950s.[52] The underlying principle of Wolpe's method is reciprocal inhibition. This involves the pairing of inhibitory responses with anxiety-producing stimuli, thereby weakening the connection between anxiety responses and these stimuli. For the COPD patient, the inhibitory response is the relaxation technique and the anxiety-provoking stimuli can be any of a variety of possibilities including exercise, travel, and going out to dinner. The patient is assisted in prioritizing a hierarchy of stressful stimuli. Starting with the least stressful, the patient is asked to achieve a relaxed state by using progressive relaxation or one of the other methods. While in a state of relaxation, the patient is directed to concentrate on the anxiety-provoking stimulus. After several sessions, when the patient is able to feel relaxed in the presence, at least mentally, of the distressing event, the patient will be asked to perform the same task with the next highest distressing element on the hierarchy, and so forth. Fear reduction is complete when the patient is able to imagine the most anxiety-evoking stimuli clearly and vividly while remaining in a state of relaxation. Desensitization, therefore, can utilize relaxation as an active instrument against the debilitating effects of chronic illness. It can help the patient recover personal, social, and familial ground that had been lost to the intense anxiety created by dyspnea, loss of control, and the need to resort to the use of assistive devices.

Cognitive-behavioral approaches attempt to identify and modify distortions in thinking that impede normal behavior. The patient is encouraged to change his or her self-statements from negative to positive. For example, as opposed to "I can probably not walk without experiencing panic due to breathlessness," the self-statement "I can take a 5-minute walk and relax" is used. In 1988, Kaplan and Atkins reported significant increases in both exercise tolerance and quality of life for COPD patients who had experienced cognitive-behavioral interventions.[28] The patients were taught to identify negative perceptions and change their outlooks with the help of self-reinforcement and behavioral planning. When such patients were able to endure more exercise and engage in more everyday activities, they gained in confidence and in their sense of control. Survival and certain aspects of physiologic functioning also correlated with the resulting improvement in self-efficacy.[36]

In summary, as the numbers of chronically ill increase and patients live longer, the demand for effective coping skills training is increasing. The COPD patient lives with anxiety and depression. Simple ADLs, such as meeting a friend, taking a walk, and, sometimes, just breathing, can cause severe stress. Relaxation techniques, and proper breathing are essential to help the patient feel more in control of basic behaviors. The patient can also learn other techniques, such as systematic desensitization, to recover behavioral territory previously lost to the disease. Intervention strategies have broadened to include the exercise regimens of yoga to improve tolerance, recovery, and control of dyspnea during exercise.[36] Likewise, meditation and even ancient martial arts training can facilitate relaxation and create an enriched sense of self-efficacy.[11] With such a wide range of possible coping strategies, COPD patients can broaden their perspectives and take back some control of their lives.

CONCLUSIONS

It is clear that psychosocial impairments are associated with the COPD process and are even more salient than physical symptoms early on. Thus, along with physical deterioration, the will to live and the potential to enjoy life with others are seriously threatened by depression, anxiety, loss of control, poor sense of self-efficacy, and, at times, neuropsychological deficits that affect everyday interactions. COPD, therefore, affects not only the lungs but the biochemistry of the brain and often results in people losing the desire to carry on with life.

Pulmonary rehabilitation must therefore utilize a multimodal approach that incorporates applied principles of medical, psychological, neurological, physical, and social science research. Such an approach is a change from the priorities of usual patient care. For instance, during a medical crisis that might require intensive care, the COPD patient may also require continuous intensive interpersonal intervention to stave off depression and relieve anxiety. This intervention should be from caregivers who are trained to understand the psychological idiosyncrasies and neuropsychological sequelae inherent to the disease. Awareness of the patient's strengths and coping skills can be invaluable.

Appropriate communication is essential in patient care. Understanding a patient's ability to listen, process, and express ideas and feelings certainly promotes better communication. For example, if a patient with moderate to severe

COPD appears to be having perceptual-motor difficulties and seems slow to respond to questions or instructions, the untrained care provider might assume that the patient does not have the verbal skills necessary for such communication. However, with greater understanding of the patient's neuropsychological impairments, conscientious care providers reduce the number of messages to be delivered and allow more time for responses. There is a good chance that the COPD patient has adequate verbal abilities, but these abilities often hide difficulties in other neurocognitive areas and permit the patient to present a picture that underestimates overall impairments. Imagine the frustration of the patient when it is obvious that the care provider has no idea of the patient's potential for understanding a situation. For the COPD patient, this could be depressing and can trigger the dyspnea-stress cycle, a very real relationship between psychological and physical illness.

In conclusion, the psychological concomitants to COPD, such as depression, are not a direct function of the severity of the disease process. Neuropsychological deficits, however, do appear to be related to aspects of the disease, such as hypoxemia. They tend to be variable and affect perceptual-motor skills more than verbal abilities. Coping strategies include focusing on relaxation and providing social support. These, however, can only be successful when the care providers are educated concerning the neurocognitive manifestations of the illness. Furthermore, because the patient's loved ones share in the frustration, ambivalence, and loneliness that accompany chronic debilitating illness, comprehensive rehabilitation must also provide mechanisms for the care providers themselves to receive psychosocial support.

References

1. Barstow RE: Coping with emphysema. Nurs Clin North Am 9:137–145, 1974.
2. Bartus RT: Effects of cholinergic agents on learning and memory in animal models of aging. Aging 19:271–280, 1982.
3. Beck AT, Ward CH, Mendelson M, et al: An inventory for measuring depression. Arch Gen Psychiatry 4:561–571, 1961.
4. Becker MH: Patient adherence to prescribed therapies. Med Care 23:539–555, 1985.
5. Brody R: Music medicine/mind. Omni 6:24,110, 1984.
6. Burke RJ, Weir R: Marital helping relationships: The moderators between stress and well-being. J Psychol 95: 121–130, 1977.
7. Caron HS, Roth HP: Objective assessment of cooperation with an ulcer diet: Relation to chronic obstructive pulmonary disease antacid intake and to assigned physician. Am J Med Sci 261:61–66, 1971.
8. Clough P, Harnisch L, Cebulski P, Ross D: Method for individualizing patient care for obstructive pulmonary disease patients. Health Soc Work 12:127–133, 1987.
9. Conine TA, Evans JH: Sexual adjustment in chronic obstructive pulmonary disease. Respir Care 26:871–874, 1981.
10. Cugell D, Grant I, Heaton RK, et al: Chronic obstructive pulmonary disease: Socio-emotional adjustment and life quality. Chest 77:308–309, 1980.
11. Dealy MT: Martial Arts Therapy. Brooklyn, Hopeful Press, 1993.
12. Dudley DL, Glaser EM, Jorgenson BN, Logan DL: Psychosocial concomitants to rehabilitation in chronic obstructive pulmonary disease. Chest 77:413–420, 1980.
13. Dudley DL, Wermuth C, Hague W: Psychosocial aspects of care in the chronic obstructive pulmonary disease patient. Heart Lung 2:289–303, 1973.
14. Emery CF: Psychosocial considerations among pulmonary patients. In Hodgkin JE, Connors GL, Bell CW (eds): Pulmonary Rehabilitation, 2nd ed. Philadelphia, JB Lippincott Company, 1984, pp. 279–292.
15. Finnegan DL, Suler JR: Psychological factors associated with maintenance of improved health behaviors in postcoronary patients. J Psychol 119:87–94, 1984.
16. Fletcher EC, Martin RJ: Sexual dysfunction and erectile impotence in chronic obstructive pulmonary disease. Chest 81:413–421, 1982.
17. Fried R: Integrating music in breathing training and relaxation. Biofeedback Self Regul 15:161–169, 1990.
18. Frownfelter D: Breathing exercise and retraining, chest mobilization exercises. In Frownfelter D (ed): Chest Physical Therapy and Pulmonary Rehabilitation. Chicago, Year Book Medical Publishers, 1978, p 153.
19. Frownfelter D: Relaxation principles and techniques. In Frownfelter D (ed): Chest Physical Therapy and Pulmonary Rehabilitation. Chicago, Year Book Medical Publishers, 1978, p 119.
20. Grant I, Adams KM: Neuropsychological Assessment of Neuropsychiatric Disorders. New York, Oxford University Press, 1986.
21. Grant I, Heaton RK, McSweeny AJ, et al: Brain dysfunction in COPD. Chest 77:308–309, 1980.
22. Hanson SB: Music therapy and stress reduction research. J Music Ther 22:193–206, 1985.
23. Havens RA: The Wisdom of Milton Erickson: Vol 1. Hypnosis and Hypnotherapy; Vol. 2. Human Behavior and Psychotherapy. New York, Irvington Publishers, 1992.
24. Heaton RK, Grant I, McSweeny AJ: Psychologic effects of continuous and nocturnal oxygen therapy in hypoxemic chronic obstructive pulmonary disease. Arch Intern Med 143:1941–1947, 1983.
25. Hoffman LA, Berg J, Rogers RM: Daily living with COPD: Self-help skills to improve functional ability. Postgrad Med 86:153–166, 1989.
26. Jacobson E: Progressive Relaxation, 2nd ed. Chicago, University of Chicago Press, 1938.
27. Jerman A, Haggerty MC: Relaxation and biofeedback: Coping skills training. In Casaburi R, Petty TL (eds): Principles and Practice of Pulmonary Rehabilitation. Philadelphia, WB Saunders Co., 1993, p 366.
28. Kaplan RM, Atkins CJ: Behavioral interventions for patients with COPD. In McSweeny AJ, Grant I (eds): Chronic Obstructive Pulmonary Disease: A Behavioral Perspective. New York, Marcel Dekker, 1988, p 123.
29. Kaplan RM, Eakin EG, Ries AL: Psychosocial issues in the rehabilitation of patients with chronic obstructive pulmonary disease. In Casaburi R, Petty TL (eds): Principles and Practice of Pulmonary Rehabilitation. Philadelphia, WB Saunders Co., 1993, p 351.
30. Kaptein AA, Brand PL, Dekker FW, et al: Quality-of-life

in a long-term multicentre trial in chronic nonspecific lung disease: Assessment at baseline. Eur Respir J 6: 1479–1484, 1993.

31. Kass I, Updegraph K, Muffly RB: Sex in chronic obstructive pulmonary disease. Med Aspects Hum Sex 6:33–42, 1972.

32. Kleiger JH, Dirks JF: Psychomaintenance aspects of alexithymia: Relationship to medical outcome variables in a chronic respiratory illness population. Psychother Psychosom 34:25–32, 1980.

33. Krop HD, Block AJ, Cohen E: Neuropsychologic effects of continuous oxygen therapy in chronic obstructive pulmonary disease. Chest 64:317–322, 1973.

34. Livsey CG: Physical illness and family dynamics. In Lysowski ZJ (ed): Psychosocial Aspects of Physical Illness. Basel, Karger, 1972, p 231.

35. McKinney B: COPD and depression: Treat them both. RN 48–50, 1994.

36. McSweeny AJ, Czajkowski S, Labuhn KT: Psychosocial factors in rehabilitation with chronic respiratory disease patients. In Fishman AP (ed): Pulmonary Rehabilitation. New York, Marcel Dekker, in press.

37. McSweeny AJ, Grant I, Heaton RK, et al: Life quality of patients with chronic obstructive pulmonary disease. Arch Intern Med 142:473–478, 1982.

38. Norell SE: Accuracy of patient interviews and estimates by clinical staff determining medication compliance. Soc Sci Med 15:57–61, 1981.

39. Petty T: Home oxygen in advanced obstructive pulmonary disease. Med Clin North Am 65:615–627, 1981.

40. Pietropinto A, Arora A: Chronic pulmonary disease and sexual functioning. Med Aspect Hum Sex 23:78–82, 1989.

41. Rabinowitz B, Florian V: Chronic obstructive pulmonary disease—Psychosocial issues and treatment goals. Soc Work Health Care 16:69–86, 1992.

42. Refroe KL: Effect of progressive relaxation on dyspnea and anxiety state in patients with chronic obstructive pulmonary disease. Heart Lung 17:408–413, 1988.

43. Reitan RM, Wolfson D: The Halstead-Reitan Neuropsychological Test Battery: Theory and Clinical Interpretation. Tucson, AZ, Neuropsychology Press, 1985.

44. Rourke SB, Grant I, Heaton RK: Neurocognitive aspects of chronic obstructive pulmonary disease. In Casaburi R, Petty TL (eds): Principles and Practice of Pulmonary Rehabilitation. Philadelphia, WB Saunders Co., 1993, p 79.

45. Sackett DL, Snow JC: The magnitude and measurement of compliance. In Hayes RB, Taylor DW, Sackett DL (eds): Compliance in Health Care. Baltimore, John Hopkins Press, 1979.

46. Sandhu HS: Psychosocial issues in chronic obstructive pulmonary disease. Chest 7:629–642, 1986.

47. Seligman ME, Maier SF: Failure to escape traumatic shock. J Exp Psychol 74:1–9, 1967.

48. Semple PDA, Beastall GH, Watson WS, Hume R: Serum testosterone depression associated with hypoxia in respiratory failure. Clin Sci 58:105–106, 1980.

49. Sexton DL, Munro BH: Living with a chronic illness: The experience of women with chronic obstructive pulmonary disease. West J Nurs Res 10:26–44, 1988.

50. Unger K, Moser K, Hansen P: Selection of an exercise program for patients with chronic obstructive pulmonary disease. Heart Lung 9:68–76, 1980.

51. Weaver TE, Narsavage GL: Physiological and psychological variables related to functional status in chronic obstructive pulmonary disease. Nurs Res 41:286–291, 1992.

52. Wolpe J: Psychotherapy by Reciprocal Inhibition. Stanford, Stanford University Press, 1958.

53. Zung WW: A self-rating depression scale. Arch Gen Psychiatry 12:63–70, 1965.

Nutrition and Chronic Obstructive Pulmonary Disease: A Clinical Overview

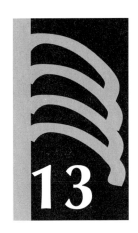

Michael I. Lewis, MD

PREVALENCE OF UNDERNUTRITION AND RATIONALE FOR INTERVENTION

Significant weight loss has been reported to occur in 19% to 71% of patients with chronic obstructive pulmonary disease (COPD).[11,40,79,94,98] Generally, about a quarter to a third of ambulatory outpatients with COPD show some evidence of compromised nutritional status. Of interest, Schols and coworkers[79] reported a greater prevalence of impaired nutritional parameters in ambulatory hypoxemic COPD patients admitted to a rehabilitation center (PaO$_2$ <7.3 kPa/~55 mmHg) compared with patients in whom PaO$_2$ was greater than 7.3 kPa. In hospitalized patients with COPD, the prevalence of undernutrition is higher.[21,49] Labaan and coworkers[49] evaluated 50 consecutive patients with COPD presenting with acute respiratory failure and observed evidence of significant undernutrition in 60% using a multiparameter nutritional index. Impaired nutritional status was more prevalent in those patients requiring mechanical ventilation (74% versus 43%).[49]

Malnutrition complicating COPD has been associated with increased morbidity as well as an increased rate of mortality. Malnutrition in these patients has been associated with an increased susceptibility to infection, owing in part to impaired cell-mediated immunity, reduced secretory IgA, depressed pulmonary alveolar macrophage function, and increased colonization and adherence of bacteria in the upper and lower airways.[30,64,65,91] In addition, malnutrition

occurring in patients with COPD has been associated with decreased exercise capacity,[80,98] cor pulmonale,[94] increased rate of hospitalization for pulmonary-related problems,[38] and a predisposition to acute respiratory failure.[21,49]

Wilson and colleagues[98] analyzed retrospective data on the relationship between body weight, pulmonary function, and survival in 779 male patients with COPD who had been entered into an intermittent positive-pressure breathing trial. They reported that mortality appeared to be influenced by body weight, independent of forced expired volume in 1 second (FEV$_1$) (Fig. 13–1). Criticisms of this study include retrospective nature of the analysis, unclear data on the precise cause of death, exclusion of hypoxemic patients, and relatively short follow-up (3 years). Previous studies have suggested that when a patient with COPD begins to lose weight progressively, life expectancy is less than 2.9 years.[59] Following an episode of acute respiratory failure, life expectancy may be reduced even further.[21]

EFFECTS OF UNDERNUTRITION ON RESPIRATORY MUSCLE STRUCTURE AND FUNCTION

Animal Studies

Prolonged periods of undernutrition have been reported to result in significant atrophy of both respiratory and nonrespiratory muscle fibers. For example, in malnourished adult rats,

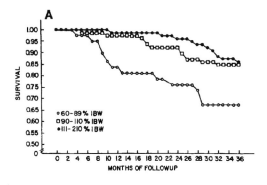

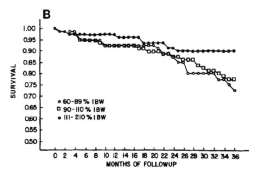

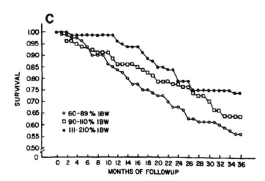

FIGURE 13–1. Survival curves for patients with mild (*A*), moderate (*B*), and severe (*C*) airflow obstruction. (From Wilson DO, Rogers RM, Wright EC, Anthonisen NR: Body weight in chronic obstructive pulmonary disease: The National Institutes of Health intermittent positive pressure breathing trial. Am Rev Respir Dis 139:1435–1438, 1989.)

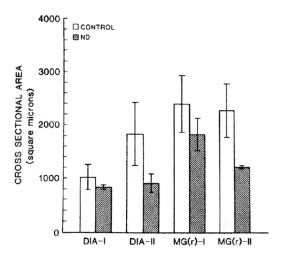

FIGURE 13–2. Bar graphs depicting cross-sectional areas of type I and II muscle fibers in both diaphragm (*DIA*) and deep portion of medial gastrocnemius (*MGr*) for controls and nutritionally deprived. Values of means ± SD. (From Sieck GC, Lewis MI, Blanco CE: Effects of undernutrition on diaphragm fiber size, SDH activity and fatigue resistance. J Appl Physiol 66:2196–2205, 1989.

type I (slow twitch) and type II (fast twitch) diaphragm muscle fiber cross-sectional areas (quantified on histochemical sections using a computer-based image processing system) were significantly reduced, compared with well-nourished controls (Fig. 13–2).[59,87] The fiber atrophy, however, was selective in that type II fibers exhibited a greater degree of atrophy compared with type I fibers (47% to 50% reduction in cross-sectional area in type II versus 18% to 23% reduction in type I diaphragm muscle fibers;

Fig. 13–2). Type II fibers lowest in oxidative capacity were most affected.[87] A similar pattern of selective atrophy of type II diaphragm fibers was evident in a study of malnourished adult hamsters[46]; however, in that study, type I fibers were unaffected.

With regard to nonrespiratory muscles, prolonged undernutrition in the rat produced a similar pattern of selective atrophy of predominantly type II fibers in the deep (red) portion of the medial gastrocnemius, a limb muscle (see Fig. 13–2). Despite atrophy of fibers in the diaphragm and limb muscles in animal models of undernutrition, the proportions of fiber types in these muscles (i.e., percentage of type I versus type II) or their number are unaffected.[59,70,87] It is postulated that with prolonged nutritional deprivation, type I fibers may be *protected* from catabolic influences because these fibers belong to slow twitch (type S) motor units, which are more frequently recruited during normal ventilatory efforts. The fibers most affected most likely belong to fast-twitch fatigable motor units (type FF) that are rarely recruited for ventilatory purposes.[85,86] Thus, protein turnover in type II fibers may be shifted toward net catabolism during prolonged undernutrition. In support of this hypothesis, prior studies have reported enhanced amino acid uptake and protein synthesis with muscle activity.[32,45] Thus the activation history of a muscle is important in determining the impact of a nutritional insult.

Although oxidative enzymes and myofibrillar proteins are clearly under different genetic control, it is of interest that following prolonged undernutrition in the rat, significant reductions in oxidative enzymes were observed in limb muscles[52,63,87] (e.g., medial gastrocnemius, a muscle that is at rest for relatively long periods of time), whereas oxidative enzyme activity (e.g., succinate dehydrogenase) was preserved in the diaphragm, a muscle in which a proportion of its constituent fibers is rhythmically active throughout life.[87] In keeping with their observation, Fuge and coworkers[31] reported reduced oxidative capacity in the gastrocnemius muscle of malnourished sedentary rats. With exercise, however, oxidative capacity increased even in malnourished animals.

In vitro studies of diaphragm contractile properties in undernourished rats revealed a significant reduction in both peak twitch and maximum tetanic force.[46,59,87] When the forces were normalized for either the weight of the muscle strip or its calculated cross-sectional area (i.e., specific force), however, the forces were similar to control diaphragms.[46,59] This suggests that loss of muscle mass is the major factor con-

tributing to the reduction in diaphragm muscle force in the malnourished animals.

The author evaluated the impact of 6 weeks of nutritional deprivation on diaphragm structure and function in malnourished emphysematous hamsters.[54] In well-nourished emphysematous hamsters, hypertrophy of type II diaphragm fibers was noted. This was interpreted as an adaptive response to the chronic persistent loads imposed on the diaphragm by the emphysematous state (Fig. 13–3).[56] Significant atrophy of both type I and II diaphragm fibers was noted, following nutritional deprivation in emphysematous hamsters. As for the nonemphysematous malnourished animal,[46] the atrophy of type II fibers was proportionately greater than that of type I fibers in the malnourished emphysematous diaphragm muscle compared with well-nourished emphysematous animals.[54] Thus, any positive impact offered by the morphometric adaptation of the diaphragm in emphysema was lost following prolonged undernutrition. Preliminary studies evaluating transdiaphragmatic pressure (Pdi; an indirect measure of diaphragm force in vivo) in malnourished emphysematous hamsters showed a significant reduction in Pdi compared with well-nourished emphysematous animals.[55]

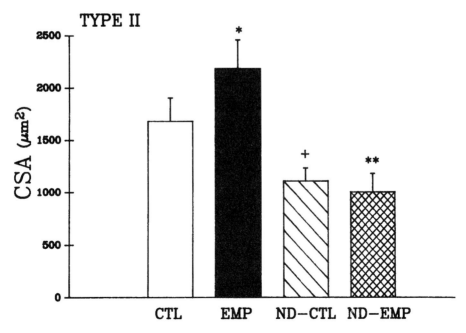

FIGURE 13–3. Bar graphs depicting cross-sectional areas (*CSA*) of type II diaphragm fibers in control (*CTL*), emphysematous (EMP) and nutritionally deprived (ND), CTL and EMP hamsters. Values are means ± SD. (From Lewis M, Monn S, Sieck G: Interactive effects of emphysema and malnutrition on diaphragm structure and function. J Appl Physiol 77:947–955, 1994 [adapted from Table 2].)

The functional impact of prolonged undernutrition on respiratory muscle performance may be considerable. The force-generating ability of the whole diaphragm, for example, is reduced because of reduced contractile mass but preserved contractility (i.e., force/unit cross-sectional area; specific force). The impaired total force–generating capacity of the malnourished diaphragm is likely to limit its endurance capacity and diminish its functional force reserve. It has been reported in a number of classic studies that muscle endurance during various levels of activity is inversely related to the ratio of the force being generated to the maximum force generating capacity of the muscle. For example, Roussos and Macklem[74] found that the critical ratio of Pdi to maximum Pdi (Pdi max) in subjects breathing through inspiratory resistances was 40%. With severe malnutrition, the forces generated during basal conditions are probably preserved. The ability to meet the forces required under conditions of increased load, however, becomes progressively impaired, as one more readily approaches or exceeds the critical force and recruits more fatigable motor units (the constituent fibers of which are most affected by the nutritional stress). With sustained effort, muscle fatigue and task (ventilatory) failure may ensue.

Human Studies

Diaphragm muscle mass was evaluated by Arora and Rochester[2] in a necropsy study. In significantly undernourished patients without chronic lung disease (71% of ideal body weight [IBW]), diaphragm muscle mass was reduced by 43% compared with normal. A similar reduction in diaphragm muscle mass was noted in another necropsy study performed on patients with COPD whose body weight was approximately 73% of IBW.[1] In living patients with COPD, the thickness of the sternomastoid muscle, determined anthropometrically, was reduced in underweight (75% IBW) patients (sternomastoid thickness was approximately 52% that of controls and 77% that of well-nourished patients with COPD).[3] Studies of respiratory muscle performance in well-nourished and poorly nourished patients (71% IBW) without underlying lung disease revealed a significant reduction in respiratory muscle strength (Table 13–1).[4] Mouth pressures, maximum voluntary ventilation, and vital capacity were evaluated as indices of global respiratory muscle strength. As noted in Table 1, respiratory muscle strength (mean of maximum inspiratory and expiratory mouth pressures) was reduced 63% in the undernourished patients. This reduction is proportionately greater than one would have expected from the reduction in diaphragm muscle mass in similarly undernourished patients. Because 12 of the 16 undernourished patients had nonthoracic malignancies, the possibility of a paraneoplastic myopathy cannot be excluded.

Abnormalities of limb skeletal muscle function have also been noted in undernourished patients. These rather elaborate tests may be sensitive indices of undernutrition and the response to nutritional repletion measures. Lopes and colleagues,[61] for example, evaluated the function of the adductor pollicis muscle in underweight patients with gastrointestinal disorders and noted a higher relative force production at 10 pps stimulation as well as a slower maximum relaxation rate. Similar results have been reported for undernourished patients with COPD in whom diaphragm and adductor polli-

---

TABLE 13–1
Respiratory Muscle Performance in Well and Poorly Nourished Patients*

Variable	Well-Nourished Group (n = 16)	Poorly Nourished Group (n = 16)
Maximal static inspiratory pressure (-cm H$_2$O)	95 ± 31	35 ± 14
Maximal static expiratory pressure (cm H$_2$O)	151 ± 52	59 ± 24
Respiratory muscle strength (% predicted)	96 ± 19	37 ± 13
Vital capacity (% predicted)	101 ± 14	63 ± 19
FEV$_1$/FVC (%)	82 ± 10	83 ± 9
Maximal voluntary ventilation (% predicted)	80 ± 24	41 ± 13

*Data represented as mean ± standard deviation.
From Arora NS, Rochester DF: Respiratory muscle strength and maximal ventilation in undernourished patients. Am Rev Respir Dis 126:5–8, 1982.

cis function were evaluated.[29] Likewise, abnormal contractile properties of the adductor pollicis muscle have been reported in patients with anorexia nervosa[77] and following hypocaloric fasting in obese patients.[76]

In patients with COPD, electrolyte abnormalities, derangements in arterial blood gases, and hyperinflation of the lungs may complicate the interpretation of the impact of undernutrition on respiratory muscle performance. Hypophosphatemia may be prevalent in hospitalized patients as well as in critically ill patients.[25,35] Significant improvement of respiratory muscle weakness (as reflected by Pdi measurements) has been well documented in patients on mechanical ventilation for respiratory failure following correction of hypophosphatemia.[5] Fiaccadori and associates[25] reported hypophosphatemia in 21.5% of 158 patients with COPD presenting with an acute exacerbation. A decreased renal threshold for phosphate reabsorption was noted in the majority. The latter may be influenced by the drugs administered (methylxanthines, beta-agonists, diuretics). In addition, intracellular shifts may occur with correction of acute respiratory acidosis.[50] Hypomagnesemia may cause respiratory muscle weakness, which is reversible following magnesium replacement.[62] In patients with COPD admitted to an intensive care unit, hypomagnesemia was present in only 9.4%, whereas low muscle levels of magnesium were evident in 47%.[26] Hypocalcemia[6] and hypokalemia[9] may also cause respiratory muscle weakness. With regard to arterial blood gas derangements, both hypoxia and hypercapnic acidosis have been shown to decrease respiratory muscle contractility and endurance in humans.[41,43]

Hyperinflation, particularly dynamic hyperinflation, may place the diaphragm of patients with COPD at a serious mechanical disadvantage and impair force-generating capacity.[99] With hyperinflation, diaphragm muscle fibers are shortened, appositional and insertional actions may be impaired, and the radius of curvature increases, resulting in a decrement in Pdi for any given tangential tension produced by the diaphragm (law of LaPlace). There may also be uncoupling between the costal and crural portions of the diaphragm.[84] Loss of respiratory muscle bulk, as may occur with severe undernutrition, may thus compound the impaired force-generating capacity of the diaphragm. Rochester and Braun[71] reported that diaphragm length accounted for 41% of the variance in maximal inspiratory mouth pressures observed in patients with COPD, whereas maximum expiratory mouth pressures accounted for 53% of the variance. Thus, inspiratory muscle dysfunction in patients with COPD appeared to be determined by the mechanical inefficiency imposed on the respiratory muscles by hyperinflation and by varying degrees of muscle weakness (as reflected by the maximum expiratory mouth pressures).

Studies in well-nourished stable patients with COPD suggest that adaptations to the state of chronic hyperinflation occur so that the pressure-generating potential of the diaphragm is preserved, particularly at high lung volumes.[89] The authors postulate that *work hypertrophy* and length adaptation (i.e., loss of sarcomeres to readjust force-length relationships) of the diaphragm may underlie the adaptation as suggested in animal models.[24,56] Autopsy studies in COPD have, however, failed to demonstrate diaphragm shortening in COPD.[1] It is likely, however, that respiratory muscle weakness induced by malnutrition in patients with COPD may significantly impair functional force reserve and augment the sense of inspiratory effort, particularly during exacerbations of the condition, when increased loads and dynamic hyperinflation may ensue.[99] In this regard, a strong correlation between inspiratory effort sensation and esophageal pressure (Pes) (expressed as Pes/Pes max) has been described by Bradley and coworkers.[10]

MECHANISMS OF PROGRESSIVE WEIGHT LOSS IN CHRONIC OBSTRUCTIVE PULMONARY DISEASE

Although the exact mechanisms underlying progressive weight loss in patients with COPD are not fully understood, a number of postulates have been put forward.

Inadequate Dietary Intake

There may be a variety of reasons accounting for reduced dietary intake in patients with COPD, including anorexia, dyspnea and arterial oxyhemoglobin desaturation in preparing and consuming food,[13] physical disabilities that limit access to shop for food items, and psychological depression.[60] A number of earlier studies, however, reported that caloric intake in patients with COPD was not less than the recommended standard for healthy adults.[11,40,67] The question of dietary intake is reviewed again when dealing with the concept of energy balance.

Diet-Induced Thermogenesis

This term (formally referred to as the specific dynamic action of food) refers to the obligatory energy expenditure and increase in metabolic rate that ensues during the processing of ingested food nutrients. The increased metabolic rate is reflected by an increase in oxygen consumption ($\dot{V}O_2$) and carbon dixoide production ($\dot{V}CO_2$). The latter may further stimulate ventilation in undernourished patients with COPD resulting in a higher postprandial energy expenditure because of an enhanced oxygen cost of ventilation.[19] Thus, enhanced diet-induced thermogenesis in these circumstances would mean that the amount of energy available from food nutrients is commensurately reduced.

Two studies have suggested enhanced diet-induced thermogenesis in undernourished patients with COPD.[33,36] Both studies, however, have been criticized for methodologic problems in defining the change in energy expenditure following the caloric intake as well as differences in the total caloric content between the groups being tested. A study by Hugli and coworkers[39] evaluated a group of stable patients with COPD and normal controls. A balanced liquid meal with a caloric content equal to 0.3 times their resting energy expenditure (REE) extrapolated

to 24 hours was assessed over a period of 130 minutes. The increment in REE was expressed as a percentage change of the baseline values. No significant differences were noted between the groups.[39] In addition, if the data of Goldstein and associates[33] and Green and Muers[36] are recalculated in an identical fashion to that used by Hugli and colleagues, no apparent differences were noted.[39] Thus, it appears that the contribution of enhanced diet-induced thermogenesis to weight loss in COPD is likely to be small or negligible from the clinical standpoint.[39]

Energy Balance

Schols and coworkers[82] evaluated energy intake and expenditure in a group of weight-losing and weight-stable patients with COPD (Table 13–2). With regard to energy intake, absolute values were significantly lower in weight-losing patients with COPD. These values, however, were still within or above predicted requirements. Normalized values of energy intake were similar across the groups. With regard to energy expenditure (REE), the REE expressed as a percentage of the predicted basal metabolic rate as determined by the Harris

TABLE 13–2
Energy Balance in Weight-Losing and Weight-Stable Patients with Chronic Obstructive Pulmonary Disease

Energy Balance	Weight Losing (n = 39)	Stable Body Weight (n = 41)
Energy intake (E intake)		
E intake, kcal/24 h	1786 (84)*	1995 (65)[†]
E intake/BWt, kcal/kg/24 h	31.7 (1.5)	30.7 (1.2)
E intake/FFM-B1, kcal/kg/24 h	42.0 (1.9)	43.0 (1.7)
E intake/FFM-ANTHER, kcal/kg/24 h	38.1 (1.7)	38.4 (1.7)
E intake/HB, %	141 (6)	146 (5)
Resting energy expenditure (REE)		
REE, kcal/24 h	1492 (36)	1494 (31)
REE/BWt, kcal/kg/24 h	26.4 (0.6)	22.7 (0.5)[††]
REE/FFM-B1, kcal/kg/24 h	35.0 (0.8)	31.8 (0.6)[§]
REE/FFM-ANTHR, kcal/kg/24 h	31.9 (0.8)	28.3 (0.6)[††]
REE/HB, %	117 (3)	108 (2)[§]
E intake/REE, %	119 (5)	134 (5)[†]

*Mean (SEM).
[†]$P<0.05$.
[‡]$P<0.001$.
[§]$P<0.005$

BWt = Body weight; FFM-BI = fat free mass determined by bioelectric impedance; FFM-ANTHR = FFM determined by anthropometric measures; HB = Harris Benedict equation to predict basal metabolic rate;
From Schols AMWJ, Soeters PB, Mostert R, et al: Energy balance in chronic obstructive pulmonary disease. Am Rev Respir Dis 143:1248–52, 1991.

Benedict equation (REE/HB) was significantly elevated in the weight-losing group. This increased REE relative to predicted energy needs has been well described in a number of other reports and is often referred to as a *hypermetabolic* state.[11,19,27,33,96]

In studying the hypermetabolic state in undernourished patients with COPD, Goldstein and colleagues[34] reported that these patients exhibited high carbohydrate oxidation, which contrasts with other hypermetabolic states (e.g., trauma, sepsis) in which fat oxidation is increased. In addition, the patients were not hypercatabolic (i.e., larger nitrogen breakdown than would be expected for a given energy expenditure), which, again, contrasts with other states of hypermetabolism (e.g., sepsis).

Adaptive Response to Undernutrition

Weight loss is usually associated with a decrease in metabolic rate, which has been viewed as an *adaptive response*.[12,47] In Figure 4, data adapted from the Minnesota Study are depicted in which the metabolic response to semistarvation was assessed in normal volunteers. In that study, a 25% reduction in body weight was associated with a 40% reduction in metabolic rate.[47]

This sharply contrasts with the metabolic rate expressed as a percentage of predicted in equally malnourished patients with COPD ($115 \pm 2\%$) reported by Wilson and associates[96] (Fig. 13–4). The elevated REE normalized for body weight or fat free mass in weight-losing patients with COPD reported by Schols and coworkers[82] (see Table 13–2) tends also to contradict the notion that weight loss in COPD might be an adaptive process aimed at conserving $\dot{V}O_2$ as described in other undernourished patients or subjects.[12,47]

Unifying Hypothesis

It is likely that some form of energy imbalance underlies weight loss in patients with COPD. In the study of Schols and coworkers,[82] elevated REE in weight-stable patients was met by an increment in energy intake. With severe airflow obstruction, a further increment in REE was not met by a further increase in energy intake, resulting in a negative energy balance and weight loss. Thus, weight loss in COPD may occur, as a result of insufficient energy intake for the level of energy expenditure and "failure of the normal adaptive response to undernutrition."[82] Further energy imbalance may occur during acute exacerbations of the condition re-

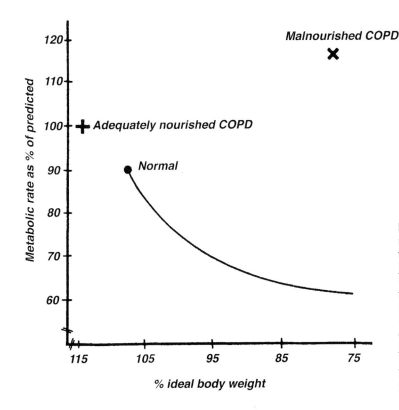

FIGURE 13–4. Graph depicting metabolic rate as a function of body weight in normal volunteers subjected to semistarvation and well-nourished and undernourished patients with COPD. (From Wilson DO, Donahoe M, Rogers RM, Pennock BE: Metabolic rate and weight loss in chronic obstructive lung disease. J Parent Ent Nutr 14:7–11, 1990. [Note: Normal volunteers adapted by Wilson et al from The Minnesota Study[47]].)

sulting in further weight loss. A *stepped* reduction in weight associated with acute exacerbations has been reported as an aggravating factor further compromising baseline nutritional status.[7]

Mechanisms Underlying Relative Increase in Metabolic Rate

The increased energy expenditure relative to predicted values in undernourished patients with COPD may relate to an increased work and oxygen cost of ventilation. Donahoe and co-workers[19] evaluated the oxygen cost of augmented ventilation in patients with COPD and normal controls. The oxygen cost of augmented ventilation was increased 2.1-fold in well-nourished patients with COPD (2.61 ± 1.07 $mL/O_2/L$) compared with controls (1.23 ± 0.51 $mL/O_2/L$). In malnourished patients with COPD, the O_2 cost was even higher (4.28 ± 0.98 $mL/O_2/L$; 3.5-fold that of controls). The estimated resting $\dot{V}O_2$ of the respiratory muscles ($\dot{V}O_2$ resp), expressed as a percentage of total $\dot{V}O_2$, was increased in the malnourished patients with COPD to approximately 21% compared with about 12% for well-nourished patients and about 4% for normal controls (Fig. 13–5).[19] An increased oxygen cost of ventilation and an increased estimated contribution of $\dot{V}O_2$ resp has also been reported during exercise in patients with COPD.[53] The contribution of beta-agonists and theophylline to elevated REE is controversial but probably plays a negligible role.[33,82] Thus, failure to meet the increased energy demands with an appropriate increment in energy intake may result in energy imbalance and weight loss.

NUTRITIONAL REPLETION IN CHRONIC OBSTRUCTIVE PULMONARY DISEASE

Variable results have been reported regarding attempts at nutritional supplementation and repletion in underweight patients with COPD. In unsuccessful trials conducted in the outpatient setting, no significant improvement in nutritional status (weight change -1.8 to 1.5 kg) or improvement in respiratory muscle performance was observed.[48,57,67,68,90] On further analysis, it appears that the total caloric intake during these trials was less than 1.5 times REE. Table 13–3 summarizes the results of six studies that demonstrate a positive impact of nutritional supplementation on some or all of the following: nutritional status, respiratory muscle strength, peripheral muscle strength, and exercise capacity.[20,22,34,73,75,97] Significant increment in absolute lymphocyte counts and improved skin reactivity to common recall antigens have also been reported following refeeding and weight gain over a 3-week period in undernourished patients with COPD.[30]

In reviewing the various studies cited previously, a number of important points can be highlighted. It would appear that significant weight gain can be achieved only if energy intake is increased greater than 1.5 times REE (i.e., about 1.6 to 1.7 times REE)[34,73,97] or by augmenting usual intake by at least 30% (i.e., >45 kcal/kg/day).[28] It should be noted, however,

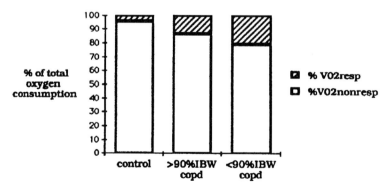

FIGURE 13–5. Bar graphs comparing respiratory muscle and nonrespiratory muscle oxygen consumption ($\dot{V}O_2$ resp and $\dot{V}O_2$ nonresp) during dead space–induced ventilation in control subjects and well (>90% IBW) and undernourished (<90% IBW) patients with COPD. The measurements are expressed as a percentage of the subject's total $\dot{V}O_2$. (From Donahoe M, Roger RM, Wilson DO, Pennock B: Oxygen consumption of the respiratory muscles in normal and malnourished patients with chronic obstructive pulmonary disease. Am Rev Respir Dis 140:385–391, 1989.)

TABLE 13–3
Nutritional Repletion in Chronic Obstructive Pulmonary Disease: Positive Studies*

Study	Setting	Number	Duration	Weight gain (kg)	Results
Wilson et al,[97] 1986	Inpatient	6	3 weeks	3.1	MIP: +43% Pdi max: +37% HD: +11%
Efthimiou et al,[22] 1988	Outpatient	14	12 weeks	4.2	MIP: +16% SM: +9% HD: +8%
Goldstein et al,[34] 1988	Inpatient	10	2 weeks	2.0	MIP: +13% HD: +15%
Donahoe et al,[20] 1989	Inpatient + outpatient	17	12 weeks	2.1	MIP: +32% Pm: +15%
Whittaker et al,[95] 1990	Inpatient	10	16 days	2.4	MIP: +19% (NS) Pm: +100%
Rogers et al,[73] 1992	Inpatient + outpatient	27	16 weeks	2.4	MIP: +31.5% (NS) HD: +11% 12 MW: +27.8%

*Note: All results indicate significant positive changes unless indicted (i.e., NS).
MIP = Maximum inspiratory mouth pressure; Pdi max = maximum transdiaphragmatic pressure; HD = handgrip dynamometry; SM = sternomastoid (maximum voluntary contraction); Pm = maximum sustainable mouth pressure; 12 MW = 12-minute walk distance; NS = not significant.

that weight gain achieved in the successful studies was only modest. For example, in the study by Rogers and coworkers,[73] body weight in terms of %IBW increased from a mean of 77.8% to 81.0% over the 4-month experimental period, an end point far below the lower limit of normal (i.e., 90% IBW). As no successful studies have evaluated the impact of greater than 16 weeks of nutritional supplementation, it is unclear whether progressive weight gain or normalization of a variety of nutritional parameters is possible with longer periods of nutritional supplementation.

In keeping with the modest gains in nutritional status noted in the aforementioned studies, the improvements in respiratory and peripheral muscle strength were also modest. In addition, the mechanisms underlying improvement in respiratory and peripheral muscle strength following short periods of nutritional repletion are not clear and may well reflect muscle water and electrolyte repletion rather than muscle protein anabolism and reconstitution.[72] Dyspnea and sense of well-being were assessed in only two studies[22,73] and improved in only one.[22] Of importance, the positive benefits noted with nutritional supplementation tended to wane rapidly when nutritional supplementation was discontinued (Fig. 13–6).[22] Thus, long-term supplementation appears to be necessary.

An interesting observation in some of the studies was that improvements in body weight were most marked in hospitalized patients. For example, Rogers and coworkers[73] reported a mean increment in body weight of 1.7 kg during the first month of the in-hospital intervention and a subsequent increment of only 0.7 kg (i.e., approximately 29% of the total weight increment) during the next 3 months as outpatients. Providing adequate nutritional supplementation in the outpatient arena is often difficult because outpatients often tend to reduce their food intake because of a number of side effects associated with the use of enteral formulas (such as bloating and fullness). In the studies of Lewis and colleagues[57] and Efthimiou and colleagues,[22] 70% of outpatients reduced their food intake while receiving supplemental formulas.

The provision of large quantities of carbohydrate may theoretically be a problem for patients with severe COPD in whom ventilatory reserve is limited. This is because they may not be able to augment alveolar ventilation sufficiently to cope with the resulting excess CO_2 production. The respiratory quotient (RQ) of carbohydrate is 1.0, whereas it is 8.0 with diversion to lipogenesis.[14,15,88] In the nutritional repletion studies cited previously, however, it appears that the patients were able to tolerate high carbohydrate supplements without either inducing or aggravating hypercapnia. Avoiding the provision of excess total calories may be more important than manipulating the percentage of carbohydrate versus fat (RQ=0.7) in the supplements.[93]

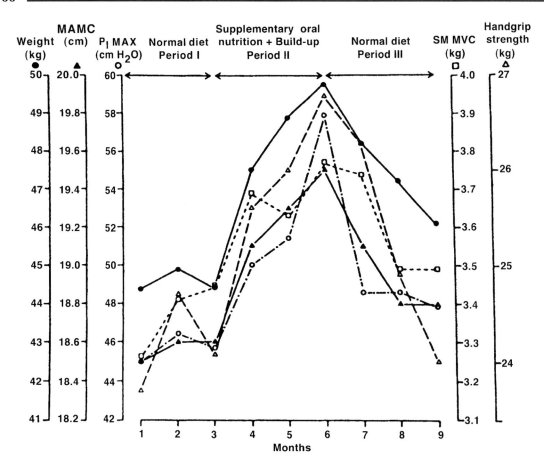

FIGURE 13–6. Graph of mean monthly values in supplemented group for midarm weight, muscle circumference (MAMC), maximal inspiratory mouth pressure (Pi_{max}), sternomastoid maximal voluntary contraction (SM MVC), and handgrip strength during the 9-month study period, showing the increase in these parameters during months 4 to 6, while receiving nutritional supplements. (From Efthimiou J, Fleming J, Gomes C, Spiro SG: The effect of supplementary oral nutrition in poorly nourished patients with chronic obstructive pulmonary disease. Am Rev Respir Dis 137:1075–1082, 1988.)

Lastly, it would appear that nutritional supplementation programs, whether in the inpatient or outpatient arena, are both time and labor intensive and costly.

BODY COMPOSITION

Studies have placed appropriate emphasis on the analysis of body composition, in terms of both better defining the nutritional status of patients and the functional sequelae of depleted states and better determining the impact of nutritional repletion. Schols and associates[83] evaluated fat free mass (using bioelectrical impedance) in 225 stable patients with COPD. Fat free mass is a useful estimate of body cell mass in the absence of fluid shifts. The patients were divided into four groups, based on body weight

(<90% IBW = reduced) and fat free mass (Table 13–4). It should be noted that 11% of the patients had reduced fat free mass, despite normal body weight, whereas a further 9% had reduced body weight with preservation of fat free mass. Patients with reduced fat free mass had greater physiologic impairment, in terms of reduced exercise capacity and reduced inspiratory mouth pressures (Fig. 13–7). The patients with reduced fat free mass also had reduced creatinine height indices, a biochemical marker of muscle mass.

A study evaluated changes in body composition induced by an aggressive nutritional support regimen in patients with severe COPD and weight loss.[18] The intervention group was randomized to receive nocturnal enteral support via a percutaneous gastrostomy tube for a period of 4 months, and the remainder received oral nutritional support. Significant weight gain

TABLE 13–4
Body Composition in Stable Patients with Chronic Obstructive Pulmonary Disease

	Body Weight (%IBW)	Fat-Free Mass	n(%)
Group 1	↓	↓	66 (26)
Group 2	↓	N	23 (9)
Group 3	N	↓	24 (11)
Group 4	N	N	138 (54)

↓ = Reduced; N = normal; n = number.
Adapted from Schols AMWJ, Soeters PB, Dingmeans AMC, et al: Prevalence and characteristics of nutritional depletion in patients with stable COPD eligible for pulmonary rehabilitation. Am Rev Respir Dis 147:1151–1156, 1993.

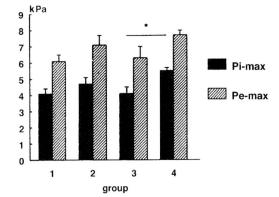

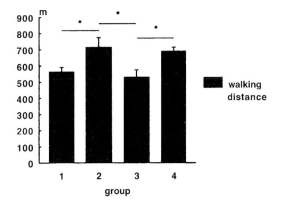

FIGURE 13–7. Bar graphs depicting maximal inspiratory (Pi_{max}) and expiratory (Pe_{max}) mouth pressures and walking distance in four groups of patients with COPD (see Table 4 for definition of groups). (From Schols AMWJ, Soeters PB, Dingmeans AMC, et al: Prevalence and characteristics of nutritional depletion in patients with stable COPD eligible for pulmonary rehabilitation. Am Rev Respir Dis 147:1151–1156, 1993.)

in the intervention group was accompanied by an increase in parameters reflecting expansion of the fat compartment, whereas no significant expansion of lean tissue mass was observed.[18] The intensive nutritional support produced "fatter" patients, which is unlikely to have an impact on important physiologic and clinical outcomes. Thus, other support measures are required that aim at expanding lean tissue mass. This provides the rationale for the evaluation of growth factors in this regard.

GROWTH FACTORS

Growth Hormone

The growth-promoting actions of growth hormone are mediated indirectly in large part through the action of polypeptide growth factors (somatomedins) produced in the liver and other extrahepatic tissues.[78] Insulinlike growth factor I (IGF-I) and IGF-II are the principal somatomedins; however, IGF-I is the more effective anabolic agent. IGF-I is bound in the plasma to binding proteins, which may modulate the effects of the circulating growth factor. It has been appreciated, however, that IGF-I can be synthesized in almost all tissues, so that an autocrine or paracrine action locally may also mediate the growth-promoting actions of growth hormone.[17] In malnourished states, circulating levels of IGF-I are reduced.[8]

Animal Studies

Lanz and coworkers[51] evaluated the effects of refeeding compared with refeeding plus growth hormone on diaphragm muscle fiber morph-

ometry in rats subjected to prolonged undernutrition. Nutritional deprivation resulted in significant atrophy of all type II (fast) fibers. Following either 5 or 9 weeks of refeeding, fiber cross-sectional areas of a proportion of the fibers were still significantly less than in free-eating controls. By contrast, in animals who received growth hormone in addition to refeeding, all fiber cross-sectional areas were similar to control values. Following acute nutritional deprivation, attenuation of body and diaphragm muscle weight was noted in mice and rats receiving IGF-I plus or minus growth hormone.[58,66]

Human Studies on COPD

Rudman[75] evaluated the hypothesis that reduced levels of IGF-I that occur with aging are responsible for a reduction in lean body mass and expansion of the fat compartment. Rudman administered growth hormone to men over 60 years of age for a period of 6 months and reported significant increases in lean body mass and vertebral bone density and a decrease in the adipose tissue mass. Growth hormone administration to malnourished elderly men over a 3-week period in addition to diet also resulted in significant weight gain, positive nitrogen balance, and improved midarm muscle circumference, whereas control patients lost weight.[44] As might be expected, a significant positive correlation was noted between weight gain and IGF-I levels.

Only preliminary results are available regarding the administration of growth hormone to malnourished patients with COPD.[69,92] These studies are limited by the small numbers of patients studied, lack of controls (patients acted as their own controls during short periods in which growth hormone was not administered), and short duration of growth hormone administration. The studies, however, did report improved nitrogen balance,[69,92] improved body weight, and improved maximum mouth pressures.[92] A dose response was noted for nitrogen balance in the study of Suchner and colleagues.[92] Growth hormone, IGF-I, or both would appear to have great therapeutic potential and a clear rationale for use in this cohort of patients, but large controlled trials are required to clarify these issues further.

Anabolic Steroids

In humans, there is much controversy regarding the effects of testosterone or synthetic derivatives with potent anabolic activity on muscle mass and strength.[37] Differences in the types of steroids used, duration of treatment, dose, route of administration, dietary protein intake, level of training, exercise, and study design may underlie some of the reasons for the varying outcomes reported. Elashoff and associates[23] performed a meta-analysis on the effects of anabolic steroids on muscle strength and concluded that a positive impact was present in trained athletes but not in untrained subjects.

In malnourished patients with COPD, anabolic steroids could theoretically improve lean body mass. In addition, low serum levels of testosterone have been reported in patients with COPD, possibly related to hypoxia-induced pituitary suppression.[15] Schols and coworkers[81] evaluated the effects of nutritional support with

and without anabolic steroids (nandrolone decanoate administered intramuscularly every 14 days over an 8-week period) in stable underweight patients with COPD (n = 233). Nutritionally depleted patients receiving nandrolone and nutritional supplementation demonstrated significant increases in fat free mass as well as in maximum inspiratory mouth pressures. No adverse side effects of note were observed (personal communication). In addition, daily administration of stanozolol to undernourished patients with COPD for 6 months was reported to be without any adverse side effects.[42]

FUTURE RESEARCH

A number of important questions remain regarding the nutritional rehabilitation of nutritionally depleted patients with COPD. These are:

1. Whether nutritional supplementation influences morbidity or mortality.
2. When to implement nutritional programs.
3. Optimal route and means of supplementation in *inpatient* and *outpatient* settings.
4. The impact of nutritional supplementation on body composition.
5. The importance of reductions in weight during exacerbations and optimal management in this setting.
6. Interactive effects of combining nutritional supplementation and various growth factors. What growth factors would be best? Evaluation during stable and decompensated phases of the condition.
7. Cost-effectiveness of nutritional interventions.

Acknowledgments

The author wishes to thank Darlene M. Ford for invaluable assistance in the preparation of this manuscript.

References

1. Arora NS, Rochester DF: COPD and human diaphragm muscle dimensions. Chest 91:719–724, 1987.
2. Arora NS, Rochester DF: Effect of body weight and muscularity on human diaphragm muscle mass, thickness, and area. J Appl Physiol 52:64–70, 1982.
3. Arora NS, Rochester DF: Effect on chronic airflow limitation (CAL) on sternocleidomastoid muscle thickness. Chest 85:58S–59S, 1984.
4. Arora NS, Rochester DF: Respiratory muscle strength

and maximal voluntary ventilation in undernourished patients. Am Rev Respir Dis 126:5–8, 1982.

5. Aubier M, Murciano D, Lecocguic Y, et al: Effect of hypophosphatemia on diaphragmatic contractility in patients with acute respiratory failure. N Engl J Med 313: 420–442, 1985.

6. Aubier M, Viires N, Piquet J, et al: Effects of hypocalcemia on diaphragmatic strength generation. J Appl Physiol 58:2054–2061, 1985.

7. Bates D: The fate of the chronic bronchitic (Amberson Lecture). Am Rev Respir Dis 108:1043–1065, 1973.

8. Bier DM: Growth hormone and insulin-like growth factor I: Nutritional pathophysiology and therapeutic potential. Acta Paediatr Scand 374 (suppl):119–128.

9. Bilbrey GL, Herbin L, Carter NW, et al: Skeletal muscle resting membrane potential in potassium deficiency. J Clin Invest 52:3011–3018, 1973.

10. Bradley TD, Chartrand A, Fitting JW, et al: The relation of inspiratory effort sensation to fatiguing patterns of the diaphragm. Am Rev Respir Dis 134:1119–1124, 1986.

11. Braun SR, Keim NL, Dixon RM, et al: The prevalence and determinants of nutritional changes in chronic obstructive pulmonary disease. Chest 87:558–563, 1984.

12. Brennan MF: Uncomplicated starvation versus cancer cachexia. Cancer 37:2359–2364, 1977.

13. Brown SE, Caschari RG, Light RW: Arterial oxygen desaturation during meals in patients with severe chronic obstructive pulmonary disease. South Med J 76:194–198, 1983.

14. Covelli HD, Waylon BJ, Olsen MS, Beekman JF: Respiratory failure precipitated by high carbohydrate loads. Ann Intern Med 95:579–581, 1981.

15. Dark DS, Pingleton SK, Kerby GR: Hypercapnia during weaning. A complication of nutritional support. Chest 88:141–143, 1985.

16. d'Asemple P, Watson WS, Beastall GH, et al: Diet, absorption and hormone studies in relation to body weight in obstructive airways disease. Thorax 34:783–788, 1979.

17. Daughaday WH, Rotwein P: Insulin-like growth factors I and II. Peptide, messenger ribonucleic acid and gene structures, serum and tissue concentration. Endocrine Rev 10:68–91, 1989.

18. Donahoe M, Mancino, J, Costantino J, et al: The effect of an aggressive nutritional support regimen on body composition in patients with severe COPD and weight loss. Am J Respir Crit Care Med 149:313A, 1994.

19. Donahoe M, Rogers RM, Wilson DO, Pennock B: Oxygen consumption of the respiratory muscles in normal and malnourished patients with chronic obstructive pulmonary disease. Am Rev Respir Dis 140:385–391, 1989.

20. Donahoe M, Rogers RM, Openbrier DR, Wilson DO: Caloric requirements for nutritional repletion of malnourished COPD. Am Rev Respir Dis 139:333A, 1989.

21. Driver AG, McAlevy MTR, Smit JL: Nutritional assessment of patients with chronic obstructive pulmonary disease and acute respiratory failure. Chest 82:568–571, 1982.

22. Efthimiou J, Fleming J, Gomes C, Spiro SG: The effect of supplementary oral nutrition in poorly nourished patients with chronic obstructive pulmonary disease. Am Rev Respir Dis 137:1075–1082, 1988.

23. Elashoff JD, Jacknow AD, Shain SG, Braunstein GD: Effects of anabolic-androgenic steroids on muscle strength. Ann Intern Med 115:387–393, 1991.

24. Farkas GA, Roussos C: Diaphragm in emphysematous hamsters: Sarcomere adaptability. J Appl Physiol 54: 1635–1640, 1983.

25. Fiaccadori E, Coffrini E, Ronda N, et al: Hypophosphatemia in the course of chronic obstructive pulmonary disease. Prevalence, mechanisms, and relationships with skeletal muscle phosphorus content. Chest 97: 857–868, 1990.

26. Fiaccadori E, Del Canale S, Coffrini E, et al: Muscle and serum magnesium in pulmonary intensive care unit patients. Crit Care Med 16:751, 1988.

27. Fitting JW, Frascarolo P, Jéquier E, Leuenberger P: Energy expenditure and rib cage-abdominal motion in chronic obstructive pulmonary disease. Eur Respir J 2: 840–845, 1989.

28. Fitting JW: Nutritional support in chronic obstructive lung disease. Thorax 47:141–143, 1992.

29. Fraser IM, Russell DM, Whittaker S, et al: Skeletal and diaphragmatic muscle function in malnourished chronic obstructive lung disease. Am Rev Respir Dis 129:269A, 1984.

30. Fuenzalida CE, Petty TL, Jones ML, et al: The immune response to short-term nutritional intervention in advanced chronic obstructive pulmonary disease. Am Rev Respir Dis 142:49–56, 1990.

31. Fuge KW, Crews EL, Pattengale PK, et al: Effects of protein deficiency on certain adaptive responses to exercise. Am J Physiol 215:660–663, 1968.

32. Goldspink G, Scutt A, Loughna PT, et al: Gene expression in skeletal muscle in response to stretch and force generation. Am J Physiol 262:R356–363, 1992.

33. Goldstein S, Askanazi J, Weissman C, et al: Energy expenditure in patients with chronic obstructive pulmonary disease. Chest 91:222–224, 1987.

34. Goldstein SA, Thomashow BM, Kvetan V, et al: Nitrogen and energy relationships in malnourished patients with emphysema. Am Rev Respir Dis 138:636–644, 1988.

35. Gravelyn TR, Brophy N, Siegert C, Peters-Golden M: Hypophosphatemia-associated respiratory muscle weakness in a general inpatient population. Am J Med 84: 870–876, 1988.

36. Green JH, Muers MF: The thermic effect of food in underweight patients with emphysematous chronic obstructive pulmonary disease. Eur Respir J 4:813–819, 1991.

37. Hickson RC, Kurowski TG: Anabolic steroids and training. Clin Sports Med 5:461–469, 1986.

38. Hoch D, Murray D, Blalock J, et al: Nutritional status as an index of morbidity in chronic airflow limitation. Chest 85(suppl):66–67, 1984.

39. Hugli O, Frascaraolo P, Shutz Y, et al: Diet-induced thermogenesis in chronic obstructive pulmonary disease. Am Rev Respir Dis 148:1479–1483, 1993.

40. Hunter AMB, Carey MA, Larsh HW: The nutritional status of patients with chronic obstructive pulmonary disease. Am Rev Respir Dis 124:376–381, 1981.

41. Jardim J, Farkas G, Prefaut C, et al: The failing inspiratory muscles under normoxic and hypoxic conditions. Am Rev Respir Dis 124:274–279, 1981.

42. Jardim J, Martins I, Verreschi I, et al: The use of 12 mg of stanozolol by COPD patients for six months does not bring any adverse effect. Am J Respir Crit Care Med 149:139A, 1994.

43. Juan G, Caverley P, Talamo C, et al: The effect of carbon dioxide on diaphragmatic function in human beings. N Engl J Med 310:874–879, 1984.

44. Kaiser FE, Silver AJ, Morley JE: The effect of recombinant human growth hormone on malnourished older individuals. J Am Geriatr Soc 39:235–240, 1991.

45. Karpatkins S, Samuels A: Effect of insulin and muscle contraction on protein synthesis in frog sartorius. Arch Biochem Biophys 121:695–702, 1967.

46. Kelsen SG, Ference M, Kappor S: The effect of prolonged undernutrition on structure and function of the diaphragm. J Appl Physiol 58:1354–1359, 1985.

47. Keys A, Brozek J, Henschel A: The biology of human starvation. The University of Minnesota Press, 1950.
48. Knowles JB, Fairbarn MS, Wiggs BJ, et al: Dietary supplementation and respiratory muscle performance in patients with COPD. Chest 93:977–983, 1988.
49. Laaban J-P, Kouchakji B, Dore M-F, et al: Nutritional status of patients with chronic obstructive pulmonary disease and acute respiratory failure. Chest 103:1362–1368, 1993.
50. Laaban JP, Grateau G, Psychoyos I, et al: Hypophosphatemia induced by mechanical ventilation in COPD patients. Am Rev Respir Dis 137:61A, 1988.
51. Lanz JK Jr, Donahoe M, Rogers RM, Ontell M: Effects of growth hormone on diaphragmatic recovery from malnutrition. J Appl Physiol 7:801–805, 1992.
52. Layman DK, Merdian-Bender M, Hegarty PVJ, Swan PB: Changes in aerobic and anaerobic metabolism in rat cardiac and skeletal muscles after total or partial dietary restrictions. J Nutr 111:994–1000, 1981.
53. Levison H, Cherniack RM: Ventilatory cost of exercise in chronic obstructive pulmonary disease. J Appl Physiol 25:21–27, 1968.
54. Lewis M, Monn S, Sieck G: Interactive effects of emphysema and malnutrition on diaphragm structure and function. J Appl Physiol 77:947–955, 1994.
55. Lewis M, Monn SA, Zhan WZ, Sieck GC: Interactive effects of emphysema and malnutrition on diaphragm contractility and fatigue properties. Am Rev Respir Dis 143:163A, 1991.
56. Lewis M, Zhan W, Sieck G: Adaptations of the diaphragm in emphysema. J Appl Physiol 72:934–943, 1992.
57. Lewis MI, Belman MJ, Door-Uyemura L: Nutritional supplementation in ambulatory patients with chronic obstructive pulmonary disease. Am Rev Respir Dis 135:1062–1068, 1987.
58. Lewis MI, LoRusso TJ, Fournier M: The influence of growth hormone (GH) and insulin-like growth factor-1 (IGF-I) on diaphragm performance in acutely malnourished adolescent rats. Am J Respir Crit Care Med 149:272A, 1994.
59. Lewis MI, Sieck GC, Fournier M, Belman MJ: The effect of nutritional deprivation on diaphragm contractility and muscle fiber size. J Appl Physiol 60:596–603, 1986.
60. Light RW, Merrill EJ, Despars JA, et al: Prevalence of depression and anxiety in patients with COPD. Chest 87:35–38, 1985.
61. Lopes J, Russell DM, Whitwell J, et al: Skeletal muscle function in malnutrition. Am J Clin Nutr 36:602–610, 1982.
62. Malloy DW, Dhingra S, Solven FS: Hypomagnesemia and respiratory muscle power. Am Rev Respir Dis 129:497–498, 1984.
63. McRussel DR, Atwood HL, Whittaker JS, et al: The effect of fasting and hypocaloric diets on the functional and metabolic characteristics of rat gastrocnemius muscle. Clin Sci 67:185–194, 1984.
64. Moriguchi S, Sone S, Kishino Y: Changes of alveolar macrophages in protein-deficient rats. J Nutr 113:40–46, 1983.
65. Niederman MS, Merril WW, Ferranti RD, et al: Nutritional status and bacterial binding in the lower respiratory tract in patients with chronic tracheostomy. Ann Intern Med 100:795–800, 1984.
66. O'Sullivan U, Gluckman PD, Breier BH, et al: Insulin-like growth factor-1 (IGF-I) in mice reduces weight loss during starvation. Endocrinology 125:2793–2794, 1989.
67. Oppenbrier DR, Irwin MN, Dauber JH, et al: Factors affecting nutritional status and the impact of nutritional support in patients with emphysema. Chest 85(suppl):67–90, 1984.
68. Otte KE, Ahlbur P, D'Amore F, Stellfeld M: Nutritional repletion in malnourished patients with emphysema. J Paren Ent Nutr 13:152–156, 1987.
69. Pape G, Friedman M, Underwood LE, Clemmons DR: The effect of growth hormone on weight gain and pulmonary function in patients with chronic obstructive lung disease. Chest 99:1495–1500, 1991.
70. Parson D, Riedy M, Moore RL, Gollnick PD: Acute fasting and fiber number in rat soleus muscle. J Appl Physiol 53:1234–1238, 1982.
71. Rochester DF, Braun NMT: Determinants of maximal inspiratory pressure in chronic obstructive pulmonary disease. Am Rev Respir Dis 132:42–47, 1985.
72. Rochester DF: Body weight and respiratory muscle function in chronic obstructive pulmonary disease. Am Rev Respir Dis 134:646–648, 1985.
73. Rogers RM, Donahoe M, Costantino J: Physiologic effects of oral supplemental feeding in malnourished patients with chronic obstructive pulmonary disease. Am Rev Respir Dis 146:1511–1517, 1992.
74. Roussos C, Macklem PT: Diaphragmatic fatigue in man. J Appl Physiol 43:189–197, 1977.
75. Rudman D: Growth hormone, body composition and aging. J Am Geriatr Soc 33:800–807, 1985.
76. Russell DM, Leiter LA, Whitwell J, et al: Skeletal muscle function during hypocaloric diets and fasting: A comparison with standard nutritional assessment parameters. Am J Clin Nutr 37:133–138, 1983.
77. Russell DM, Prendergast PJ, Darby PL, et al: A comparison between muscle function and body composition in anorexia nervosa. The effect of refeeding. Am J Clin Nutr 38:229–237, 1983.
78. Sara VR, Hall K: Insulin-like growth factors and their binding proteins. Am J Physiol 70:591–613, 1990.
79. Schols A, Mostert R, Soeters P, et al: Inventory of nutritional status in patients with COPD. Chest 96:247–249, 1989.
80. Schols AMWJ, Mostert R, Soeters PB, et al: Nutritional state and exercise performance in patients with chronic obstructive lung disease. Thorax 44:937–941, 1989.
81. Schols AMWJ, Soeters PB, Mostert R, et al: The effects of nutritional support and anabolic steroids on body composition and physiological function in patients with COPD; a placebo controlled randomized trial. Am J Respir Crit Care Med 149:313A, 1994.
82. Schols AMWJ, Soeters PB, Mostert R, et al: Energy balance in chronic obstructive pulmonary disease. Am Rev Respir Dis 143:1248–1252, 1991.
83. Schols AMWJ, Soeters PB, Dingmans AMC, et al: Prevalence and characteristics of nutritional depletion in patients with stable COPD eligible for pulmonary rehabilitation. Am Rev Respir Dis 147:1151–1156, 1993.
84. Sharp JT: The respiratory muscles in chronic obstructive pulmonary disease. Am Rev Respir Dis 136:1089–1091, 1986.
85. Sieck GC, Fournier M, Zhan W: Estimated recruitment of diaphragm motor units [abstract]. FASEB J 4:A951, 1990.
86. Sieck GC, Fournier M: Diaphragm motor units recruitment during ventilatory and nonventilatory behaviors. J Appl Physiol 66:2539–2545, 1989.
87. Sieck GC, Lewis MI, Blanco CE: Effects of undernutrition on diaphragm fiber size, SDH activity and fatigue resistance. J Appl Physiol 66:2196–2205, 1989.
88. Silberman H, Silberman AW: Parenteral nutrition, biochemistry and respiratory gas exchange. J Paren Ent Nutr 10:151–154, 1986.

89. Similowski T, Yan S, Gauthier AP, et al: Contractile properties of the human diaphragm during chronic hyperinflation. N Engl J Med 325:917–923, 1991.

90. Stauffer JL, Carbone JE, Bendoski MT: Effects of diet supplementation on anthropometric and laboratory nutritional parameters in malnourished ambulatory patients with severe chronic obstructive pulmonary disease. Am Rev Respir Dis 133:284A, 1986.

91. Stiehm EF: Humoral immunity in malnutrition. Fed Proc 39:3093–3097, 1980.

92. Suchner U, Rothkopf M, Stanislaus G, et al: Growth hormone and pulmonary disease: Metabolic effects in patients receiving parental nutrition. Arch Intern Med 150:1225–1230, 1990.

93. Talpers SS, Romberger DJ, Bunce SB, Pingleton SK: Nutritionally associated increased carbon dioxide production: Excess total calories vs high proportion of carbohydrate calories. Chest 102:551–555, 1992.

94. Vandenbergh E, Van de Woestijne KP, Gyselen A: Weight changes in the terminal stages of chronic obstructive pulmonary disease. Am Rev Respir Dis 95:556–566, 1967.

95. Whittaker JS, Ryan CF, Buckley PA, Road JR: The effects of refeeding on peripheral and respiratory muscle function in malnourished chronic obstrucive pulmonary disease patients. Am Rev Respir Dis 142:283–288, 1990.

96. Wilson DO, Donahoe M, Rogers RM, Pennock BE: Metabolic rate and weight loss in chronic obstructive lung disease. J Paren Eur Nutr 14:7–11, 1990.

97. Wilson DO, Rogers RM, Sanders MH, et al: Nutritional intervention in malnourished patients with emphysema. Am Rev Respir Dis 134:672–677, 1986.

98. Wilson DO, Rogers RM, Wright EC, Anthonisen NR: Body weight in chronic obstructive pulmonary disease: The National Institutes of Health intermittent positive pressure breathing trial. Am Rev Respir Dis 139:1435–1438, 1989.

99. Younes M: Load responses, dyspnea, and respiratory failure. Chest 97:595–685, 1990.

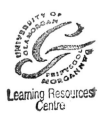

Outcomes of Pulmonary Rehabilitation

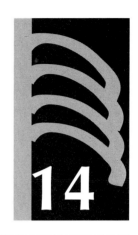

Barry J. Make, MD
Karen Glenn, RRT

Chronic obstructive pulmonary diseases (COPD) such as emphysema and chronic bronchitis represent the largest population of patients with chronic respiratory disease. Because of the frequency of these disorders, individuals with COPD have traditionally been the most common beneficiaries of pulmonary rehabilitation. Pulmonary rehabilitation, however, can also be applied to enhance the lives of individuals with intrinsic pulmonary diseases such as interstitial fibrosis and other lung disorders such as cystic fibrosis. In addition, individuals with restrictive respiratory disease such as that from advanced neuromuscular or chest wall disorders may also benefit from pulmonary rehabilitation. Because pulmonary rehabilitation is most frequently applied to patients with COPD and there is a substantial amount of medical literature on the outcomes in these patients, this chapter focuses only on the outcomes achieved by patients with COPD. COPD rehabilitation can be used as a model for pulmonary rehabilitation efforts in general, and the outcomes in COPD can be generalized to other patient populations. More specifically, this chapter (1) characterizes potential outcomes of pulmonary rehabilitation, (2) reviews models relating the various clinical dimensions of patients with COPD, and (3) presents examples of outcomes of COPD pulmonary rehabilitation programs.

POTENTIAL OUTCOMES OF PULMONARY REHABILITATION

The potential outcomes of pulmonary rehabilitation are listed in Table 14–1. A detailed consideration of these outcomes may be useful as a guide to the development and ongoing evaluation of pulmonary rehabilitation to health care professionals, patients, and third-party payers.

Medical issues are addressed by the first four possible outcomes listed in Table 14–1. In traditional medical models, avoiding mortality is the most important outcome of medical care. In COPD, supplemental oxygen is an approved therapeutic modality that is reimbursed by all third-party payers including Medicare because of the strength of the medical evidence that this therapy improves survival.[43,64,67] Avoiding mortality, however, may not be the most important outcome for the individual who suffers from the effects of COPD on a daily basis. Patients with chronic diseases frequently indicate that quality of life is much more important than longevity or the quantity of life.

Medical morbidity in patients with respiratory disease includes complications of the primary respiratory process as well as hospitalizations for acute exacerbations and the need for emergency or urgent medical care related to the

TABLE 14–1
Potential Outcomes of Pulmonary Rehabilitation

On Medical Factors

Mortality
Morbidity
Respiratory symptoms
Physiologic indices

On "Nonmedical" Factors

Functional capacity
Neuropsychological function
Health-related behaviors
Health-related quality of life
   Physical health
   Mental/emotional health
   Social health
   Role functioning
   Perception of general well-being
Ability to work
Caregiver burden
Use of assistive technology
Costs

respiratory disorder. Patients with COPD may develop pulmonary hypertension with subsequent cor pulmonale (right-sided heart failure from chronic hypoxemia and hypercapnia). Acute respiratory tract infections frequently complicate COPD and require emergency room visits.

Respiratory symptoms are prominent complaints in patients with respiratory disorders. The primary symptoms of respiratory disease include shortness of breath (dyspnea), cough, and sputum production, all of which can be disabling for patients with intrinsic lung disease but are generally minimal or nonexistent for individuals with neuromuscular disorders. Secondary symptoms related to the effects of respiratory disease, such as headaches caused by hypoxemia and fatigue, must also be considered.

Physiologic indices in individuals with respiratory disorders include standard pulmonary function tests such as forced vital capacity (FVC) and forced expired volume in 1 second (FEV_1). Both are easily obtained by simple spirometry.[42] The FEV_1 is an easy to measure index of airflow limitation that is widely used as a measure of the severity of airflow obstruction and, thus, of the physiologic severity of disease. Moreover, FEV_1 correlates with prognosis.[75] As FEV_1 declines, mortality increases; patients with a FEV_1 of less than 30% of predicted normal have a 3-year survival of 60%.[3]

Although the FEV_1 is the most common indicator of disease severity, airflow limitation is also reflected by hyperinflation. Hyperinflation is indicated by increased total lung capacity and residual volume. Other physiologic indices of pulmonary function include inspiratory and expiratory respiratory muscle strength, gas exchange, and exercise capacity. Respiratory muscle strength can be assessed most easily by measurement of maximum inspiratory and expiratory pressures measured at the mouth,[27] but more severe respiratory muscle weakness is also reflected by reductions in maximum voluntary ventilation and FVC. Gas exchange measurements include that of the partial pressure of oxygen (PaO_2) and of carbon dioxide ($PaCO_2$) in the arterial blood. Undoubtedly, one of the more important physiologic indices is the direct measurement of exercise capacity by performing a cardiopulmonary exercise tolerance test in a controlled laboratory setting. Indices that may be assessed during an exercise test include workload, oxygen consumption, heart rate, minute ventilation, arterial lactate, and arterial blood gases.[93]

The remainder of the possible outcomes of pulmonary rehabilitation listed in Table 14–1 address "nonmedical" issues that have historically been relegated as less important in the traditional medical model of patient care. These issues are of paramount importance to patients, however, and are frequently identified as the goals of rehabilitation programs. Functional capacity refers to the ability to perform tasks that are required during the course of patients' daily lives. Because walking is an important daily activity, functional capacity is commonly measured in patients with pulmonary disease as the distance walked in 6 or 12 minutes.[62] Neuropsychological function is an important and often overlooked outcome parameter. Patients with COPD are often hypoxemic and demonstrate associated reductions in neuropsychological function.[30] Health-related behaviors are important for patients with pulmonary disease. Cigarette smoking is the major cause of COPD, and smoking cessation efforts are often incorporated into rehabilitation programs. Other behavioral outcomes that foster continued health and that should, thus, be assessed during and following pulmonary rehabilitation include adherence to medication, oxygen, and exercise prescriptions.

Physical, mental, emotional, and social functioning and perception of well-being are often considered together as *health-related quality of life*. Ware[90] has argued that each of these quality-of-life factors is conceptually distinct and can be separately measured. The patients' perceptions of their own functioning can be objectively measured. Physical health is the ability to perform everyday physical activities, including self-care and mobility. Mental and emotional health evaluations include assessment of any feelings of anxiety, nervousness, and depression; control of behaviors, feelings, and thoughts; and cognitive functions such as memory, orientation, and alertness. Social health assessment includes measures of activities and interactions with others in the home and community. Role functioning refers to the performance of usual role activities, such as employment, school, and housework. A global perception of general well-being can also be assessed.

The ability to work may be important for younger individuals in the productive years of their lives, but it is not as critical for elderly, retired patients. In children, the ability to attend school and participate in the full range of school activities is considered. Decrease in lost time from work or school owing to illness can be an important outcome.

Caregiver burden refers to the effects of the patient's illness on family, friends, and others who assist in the patient's care. This includes financial issues and time lost from work for family members as well as psychological stressors on family members caring for chronically ill patients. Patients with limited function may benefit from the use of assistive technology, such as wheelchairs and vans. Ultimately, costs are always a concern. There are the direct costs of medical care, including hospitalization, emergency medical care, prescription medications, nursing and personal attendant care, and assistive equipment and supplies, and indirect costs from lost wages and the psychosocial impact on patients and families.

Careful review of the 12 potentially diverse outcomes listed in Table 14–1 indicates that pulmonary rehabilitation programs need to be multidimensional and multidisciplinary to consider all of the aspects of the daily lives of patients with respiratory disorders. The broad range of outcomes also suggests that pulmonary rehabilitation programs need to determine which outcomes are most important and continually monitor their results to ensure that beneficial effects are achieved.

Medical professionals often place mortality as the most important outcome of disease management. It appears that third-party payers have traditionally shared this view because they reimburse long-term oxygen therapy for patients with COPD based on its demonstrated ability to improve survival rather than on its ability to reduce breathlessness. Highly skilled and trained pulmonary physicians usually also emphasize the importance of objective measures of pulmonary physiology, but pulmonary function tests do not change in response to pulmonary rehabilitation. Patients who are symptomatic from chronic debilitating illnesses during much of their daily activities, however, often value other potential outcomes over survival.[56] Patients commonly express the sentiment that they would rather die than continue to exist in a restricted fashion with disabling dyspnea.

The most important possible outcome to most patients with COPD is dyspnea reduction. In the development of the Chronic Respiratory Disease Questionnaire, Guyatt and colleagues[35] noted dyspnea in daily activities as the most important symptom reported by patients, followed by fatigue; decreased mastery (feelings of being unable to control their illness, behavior, and fate); and the emotional difficulties of frustration, depression, embarrassment, and anxiety. The authors' investigations of 40 patients with COPD also indicated dyspnea reduction as the most important outcome to patients. In addition, patients indicated that other important outcomes were understanding of the disease process, increasing walking distance, improving emotional outlook, controlling their lives better, and improving ability to stairclimb. Thus, patients stress the importance of quality of life–related issues. Recognition of these issues guides the goals and content of pulmonary rehabilitation and the monitoring of its outcomes.

MODELS RELATING OUTCOMES

It may be useful to examine the relationships between potential pulmonary rehabilitation outcomes. These potential outcomes can also be considered as clinical domains or dimensions that define a population of patients with chronic respiratory disease. When viewed in this manner, these elements can be modeled to provide information on the relationship between the various pathophysiologic and psychosocial domains of an individual with an underlying respiratory disorder. In addition, relationships between these domains can suggest relationships between outcomes, aid in determining which outcomes are of greatest importance, and assist in developing goals for rehabilitation efforts.

In general, the impact of a disorder of any organ system can be considered in terms of its pathophysiology that leads to symptoms and is reflected in clinical consequences for the individual. More specifically for COPD patients, airflow limitation, disordered lung mechanics, respiratory muscle dysfunction, and altered gas exchange impair ventilation, reduce exercise capacity, and lead to dyspnea, the predominant respiratory symptom in patients with COPD. This relationship between the altered pulmonary physiology seen in COPD, limited exercise capacity, and reduced functional capacity in such patients is graphically represented in Figure 14–1. Alteration of lung mechanics with increased airway resistance and decreased elastic recoil in COPD is associated with increased work of breathing. Airflow limitation leads to increased lung volumes and hyperinflation. This places the diaphragm and respiratory muscles at a mechanical disadvantage and promotes respiratory muscle fatigue. In addition, hypoxemia and increased dead space increase the ventilatory requirement, thereby further limiting exercise capacity and aggravating dyspnea.

Shortness of breath is closely linked to psychological function and activity (Fig.14–2). Activity of any kind requires an increase in minute ventilation and, in the setting of a limited ventilatory reserve, provokes dyspnea. Because dyspnea is a frightening symptom, patients learn to avoid physical activities. This learned inactivity leads to muscle weakness and cardiac deconditioning, and the effects of deconditioning provoke further dyspnea with activity. In addition, emotions such as anxiety and anger can lead to an increased minute ventilation and provoke dyspnea. To prevent dyspnea, patients with COPD learn to avoid emotions, a situation that has been described as an "emotional straitjacket."[23] Lastly, dyspnea itself may produce fear and anxiety and lead to depression. These symptoms are commonly reported by COPD patients. As Figure 14–2 suggests, patients may become trapped in a vicious circle of shortness of breath, reduced levels of activity, and altered emotions.[54] Support for this model is available from other studies.[19,49,65] The symptom with the greatest influence on functional capacity (i.e., activity) has been shown to be dyspnea.[49] A similar model incorporating the mechanisms leading to a low level of fitness in COPD has been published by Cox and associates.[19]

Dyspnea is not the only factor that is associated with a reduction in physical activity. Psychological factors can also affect physical performance.[20] The authors examined physiologic and psychological factors affecting physical performance in 27 COPD patients before pulmonary rehabilitation.[7] These patients had severe airflow limitation as indicated by an average FEV_1 of 34% of predicted normal. The physiologic severity of the respiratory disease that was re-

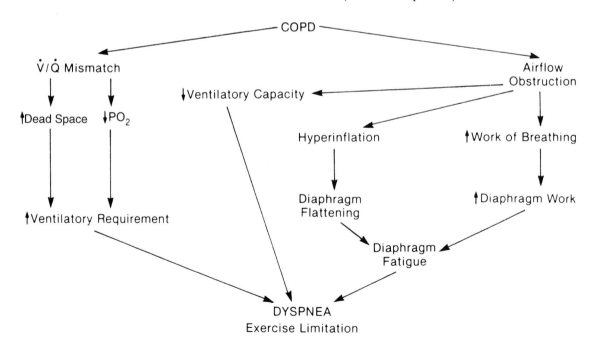

FIGURE 14–1. Physiologic mechanisms leading to dyspnea and limited exercise capacity in chronic obstructive pulmonary disease. (Modified from Belman MJ, Wasserman K: Exercise training and testing in patients with chronic obstructive pulmonary disease. Basics Respir Dis 2:1, 1981.)

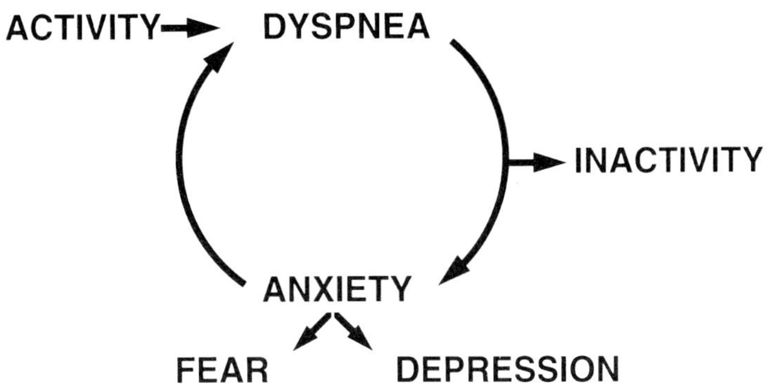

ACTIVITY➡ DYSPNEA

➡ INACTIVITY

ANXIETY

FEAR   DEPRESSION

FIGURE 14–2. The vicious circle of dyspnea. The relationships between dyspnea, activity, and psychological factors in COPD. (From Make B: COPD: Management and rehabilitation. Am Fam Phys 43:1315–1324, 1991.)

flected by the degree of reduction in FEV_1 predicted the walk distance but accounted for only 11% of its variability. The addition of other physiologic measures did not improve the ability to predict walk distance. Depressive symptoms, estimated by the Inventory to Diagnose Depression, were more closely associated with functional capacity and accounted for 16% of the variability in the 6-minute walk. The combination of FEV_1 and depressive symptoms predicted 27% of walk variability, and the addition of mental health and physical activity scales from the SF-36 Health Survey accounted of 56% of the variability in the walk distance. The highest degree of variability in the walk test (68%) was accounted for by the interactions of depression, mental health, physical activity, and physiologic severity.[7] Thus, physiologic factors alone were poor predictors of physical performance, and psychological factors strongly affected physical performance and functional capacity. This study suggests that interactions between the many domains that characterize an individual must be considered, assessed, managed, and monitored. In addition, psychological status affects patient-reported respiratory symptoms. In a group of 600 subjects without respiratory disease, more psychiatric symptoms (as measured by higher scores on the Psychiatric Symptom Index) were associated with greater degrees of respiratory symptoms.[20]

Two other models interrelating clinical domains of COPD patients have been described. McSweeny and coworkers[63] evaluated quality of life in individuals with severe COPD enrolled in an oxygen therapy trial. These authors noted impaired quality of life in most but not all patients. This suggested that disease severity was not the most important factor affecting how well patients cope with illness. They suggested a heuristic model relating clinical features that includes quality of life, neuropsychological func-

tion, physiologic measures, age, and social position for COPD patients (Fig. 14–3). Moody and associates[65] described the path analysis shown in Figure 14–4 based on evaluation of functional status, quality of life, symptoms, and disease severity (estimated by FEV_1) in 45 patients with COPD. Mastery was shown to be the most important factor related to dyspnea; low mastery was associated with increased dyspnea. Disease severity was not shown to correlate directly with dyspnea but did correlate indirectly with dyspnea through mastery. In addition, dyspnea was the most important feature affecting quality of life and functional capacity.

TOOLS TO ASSESS QUALITY-OF-LIFE OUTCOMES

Purpose of Measurement

Before selecting a measurement tool, the intent of the measurement must be well defined to maximize the ability of the instrument to assess adequately the desired outcome.[31,34,43] Based on the purposes for which they are used, measurement tools can be classified into three categories: discriminative, predictive, and evaluative. A discriminative measurement tool is designed to reflect differences within a population at a single point in time. For example, the percent predicted FEV_1 can be used to differentiate between physiologically mild, moderate, and severe COPD. A predictive measurement instrument is used when a comparative gold standard measurement exists. For example, once a baseline correlation is established, the oxygen saturation measured by pulse oximetry is predictive of arterial oxygen saturation measured by arterial blood gases. Evaluative tools are designed to detect a difference over time in a group, such as in response to an intervention or treatment.

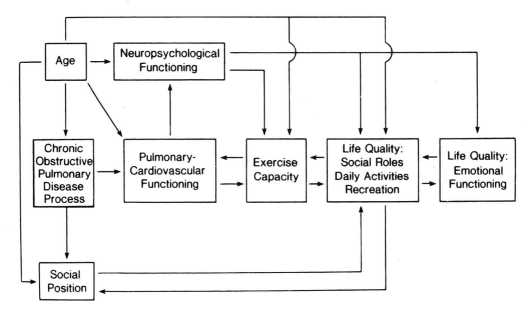

FIGURE 14–3. Heuristic model describing the relationships of various features of chronic obstructive pulmonary disease. (From McSweeney AJ, Grant I, Heaton RK, et al: Life quality of patients with chronic obstructive pulmonary disease. Arch Intern Med 142:473–478, 1982.)

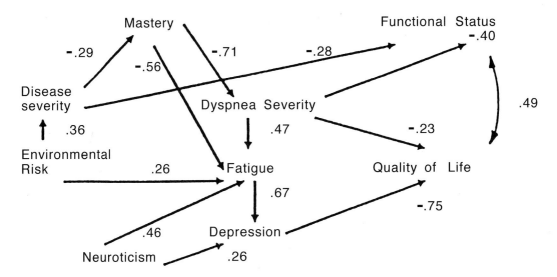

FIGURE 14–4. Path analysis relating functional status, symptoms, and quality of life in chronic obstructive pulmonary disease. (From Moody L, McCormick KM, Williams A: Disease and symptom severity, functional status, and quality of life in chronic bronchitis and emphysema. J Behav Med 13:297–306, 1990.)

The measurement of outcomes that result from pulmonary rehabilitation requires use of evaluative tools.

It should be emphasized that a particular measure may be useful for more than one purpose depending on the nature of the investigation. For example, the FEV_1 is a widely used measure of the physiologic degree of airflow limitation. As noted previously, the FEV_1 has been widely used as a discriminative tool to classify patients by the degree of their airflow limitation. The FEV_1 has also been shown to correlate with survival and, thus, may be used as a predictive tool. In patients with asthma, airflow limitation may improve as the result of treatment with bronchodilators and anti-inflammatory agents; thus, the FEV_1 may be used in this disease as an evaluative tool to assess response to therapy.

All sound evaluative measurement tools must meet three fundamental psychometric criteria: reliability, validity, and sensitivity. Although these properties are sometimes discussed in general terms, they cannot be globally confirmed. Rather, the proposed application of the measurement tool as well as the population to be studied must be taken into consideration when assessing reliability, validity, and responsiveness of a particular measurement instrument.

Reliability

The reliability of an instrument refers to the accuracy of the measurement and its stability over time.[31] Procedures to assess reliability quantify the amount of variance in the data that can be attributed to actual differences as opposed to the amount of variance due to random chance or errors. Using a ruler as an example of a reliable measurement tool for length, repeated measurements of the same piece of paper with the same ruler would yield the same results; in addition, there would be a 1:1 relationship between the measurement obtained with the ruler and the actual length of the piece of paper. Reliability coefficients are proportions and are often expressed by statistical measures, such as the Pearson correlation coefficient, paired T-test, intraclass correlation coefficient, or linear regression. One way to assess the reliability of a questionnaire is by administering the same instrument twice to a population that is thought to be stable and not subject to an intervention and then comparing the results of the two tests. This process is called test-retest reproducibility. Another form of reliability is interobserver reliability. This assesses differences in results obtained by different observers administering the same tool to the same subject.

The definition of adequate reliability varies depending on the characteristic being measured and the population being studied. Lower reliability coefficients are acceptable when comparisons are being made across groups, but much higher coefficients are generally required when comparisons are made between subjects or with repeated measurements in the same group of subjects. Ware[91] has suggested the significance of coefficients in the range of 0.50 to 0.70 for the former and greater than 0.90 for the latter.

Validity

Rather than being a precise numeric conclusion, demonstration of the validity of a quality-of-life instrument is a process of accumulating sufficient evidence to document that the tool actually measures the desired attribute.[46,48] The four frequently encountered types of validity (criterion, construct, concurrent, and face validity) assess the level of confidence that can be placed in the results generated by the tool. Criterion validity compares measurements made with the instrument under consideration to another measure considered to be a gold standard.[43] Because there is no universally agreed on gold standard measure of quality of life, criterion validity cannot be demonstrated for qualty-of-life measurement instruments. In the case of quality of life, construct validity is frequently used; investigators base the tool on expert knowledge and experience of the disease and derive the tool from such evidence combined with theories and postulations. In this case, both the instrument and the underlying theories must be assessed for accuracy. As new tools are created to measure quality of life, concurrent validity is often used to document that the scales on the new instrument correlate with similar scales on existing instruments that have been previously determined to be valid. Face validity is the general opinion that the questions appear to measure the elements under discussion. It is sometimes used for quality-of-life instruments. A joint committee of the American Psychological Association, American Education Research Association, and National Council on Measurement in Education, however, has suggested that face validity is not an appropriate or reliable basis for determining validity.[1]

Sensitivity

Pulmonary rehabilitation programs are interested in program outcomes. When measurements are repeated after an intervention using evaluative tools, the ability of an instrument to reflect a clinically relevant difference (sensitivity or responsiveness) is important.

Structure of Quality-of-Life Tools

Unfortunately, not all quality-of-life tools used for rehabilitation outcome evaluation have been evaluated for their reliability, validity, and sensitivity. Moreover, the development process for measurement instruments often does not carefully consider the proposed use of the tool nor the population to be studied. In some cases, the tool is inadequate to serve the needs of the population being studied. For example, a tool to measure the daily activities of a healthy population that includes questions about the frequency of recreational activities such as golf or going with friends to movie theaters may not be appropriate for severely disabled patients. It is strongly recommended that future studies employ tools that meet the criteria outlined here.

Quality-of-life instruments are generally structured as either general health tools or disease-specific/symptom-specific tools. Debate over the merits and drawbacks of these two structures continues.[50,70] General health or generic tools are intended to profile comprehensively the areas believed to be affected by any disease or treatment and include aspects of physical and emotional functioning and general well-being.[26] Because such instruments are designed for the public at large, they can be used across cultures, genders, populations, and diseases and, thus, allow comparison across these strata. General health profiles have the advantage of measuring the global impact of a disease state or a treatment regimen. In a drug trial of a new time-released theophylline medication, for example, patients may experience benefits beyond the expected decrease in dyspnea; they may be able to walk further and increase participation in daily activities.

General Quality-of-Life Tools

SF-36 Health Survey (SF-36)

This instrument contains 36 written questions. The questions can be answered independently by the patient in 5 to 10 minutes, and versions of the questionnaire are available in many different languages.[92] When the scoring algorithm is applied, eight subscale scores are generated: physical functioning, social functioning, role-physical, role-emotional, bodily pain, general health, vitality, and mental health. Each subscale score ranges from zero to 100, with 100 representing the most desirable score. Two summary scores (physical and mental) have been described.[89]

Sickness Impact Profile (SIP)

This tool is designed to measure the negative impact of sickness on behaviors and activities.[6] It

is composed of 136 questions that are grouped into 12 subscales and further summarized into two broad domain scores and an overall summary score. The broad domain of general physical activities includes the subscales ambulation, mobility, and body care and movement. The subscales of social interaction, communication, alertness behavior, and emotional behavior are summarized into a psychosocial domain score. The remaining subscales include sleep and rest, eating, work, home management, and recreation and pastimes. Although this questionnaire is long, it has been widely used and can be either inteviewer-administered or completed independently by the patient.

Quality of Well-Being Scale (QWB)

This rather complex tool requires significant training for interviewer administration.[45] A response coding procedure must be applied before the questionnaire can be scored. The detailed administration procedure requires the interviewer to keep an elaborate record of the subject's verbal and bodily responses to all questions posed. The QWB can be used to profile a single day or a span of several days. The interviewer probes health, symptoms, and performance. Information is recorded to characterize each day rather than merely to provide a summary response for the time period in question. Resulting subscales include the dimensions of mobility, physical activity, and social activity. Final scoring yields a QWB score for each day probed as well as summary calculations for the average QWB over the time period, a point-in-time well-being score, and a calculation of well-years.

Disease-Specific/Symptom-Specific Tools for Respiratory Disease

Although general health surveys can provide useful general information, there is little potential for their having adequate sensitivity for severely impacted populations with specific symptom complexes such as COPD. One dimension of health in which this issue can arise is physical functioning. For example, a physical functioning scale with questions about running, walking long distances, lawn mowing, or doing other strenuous activities may lack the sensitivity to differentiate among COPD patients with extremely limited functioning. In fact, a scale can inhibit detection of differences over time or between individuals or therapies if it contains a significant proportion of items to which most COPD patients would typically respond in a similar manner, either with or without any of the traditional therapeutic interventions.

Some of the disease-specific tools allow patients to identify individually impacted areas or activities and allow changes in these patient-selected activities to be followed over time with treatment. Although this individualization enhances the sensitivity to detect change for any individual, comparisons are not necessarily effective across disease groups or populations.

Chronic Respiratory Disease Questionnaire (CRDQ)

The most widely used tool to evaluate patients with respiratory disease is the CRDQ. This was designed as an evaluative rather than discriminative tool to measure the impact of chronic airflow limitation on an affected individual's quality of life. Because different individuals with chronic lung disease often identify different key physical tasks that have been affected by their lung disease, Guyatt and associates[33,35] developed this questionnaire to measure the changes each individual perceives in the performance of their key activities. For this reason, the interviewer prompts each subject to identify the five activities most affected by dyspnea on the initial administration of the CRDQ, and these same activities are queried on each subsequent questionnaire administration. This questionnaire includes 15 questions measuring the domains of dyspnea, fatigue (physical functioning), emotional functioning (encompassing anxiety and depression), and the sense of control over respiratory disease (mastery). After the initial interviewer administration, the patient may complete the questionnaire independently.

Baseline Dyspnea Index (BDI)

There are many tools to assess dyspnea.[52] The BDI is a newer widely used tool that includes three questions to grade the impact of dyspnea on the subject's activities; the questions assess functional impairment, magnitude of the task, and magnitude of effort.[53] Each question is administered by an interviewer and rated on a five-point scale that includes specific criteria for each point on the scale. An overall score results from the sum of the scores of the three questions. Follow-up evaluations are also performed by an interviewer and use the Transition Dysp-

nea Index (TDI). This tool includes three questions that examine the changes in the individual's breathlessness. A seven-point scale (-3 to $+3$) includes specific criteria to describe both positive and negative changes related to shortness of breath.

Borg Scale for Dyspnea

One widely used scale to measure dyspnea is the CR-10 scale (Borg scale) developed and later modified by Borg.[8,9] This is a 0 to 10 scale with precise descriptions attached to specific numbers at points on the scale to rate perceived effort or dyspnea (Table 14–2), usually during exercise or physical activity.[51] The scale is visually presented to the subject who reports the number that corresponds to his/her rating of dyspnea. If unable to verbalize the choice, the subject can point to the number and the technician can repeat the number to the subject to confirm it. Silverman and associates [81] demonstrated that the Borg scale reproducibly measured dyspnea during exercise for 6 patients with COPD. The average coefficient of variation for dyspnea at maximal exercise was 3%. This was similar to physiologic values for maximal oxygen consumption, minute ventilation, and heart rate obtained during three exercise tests performed to assess within-day and between-day variability.

Visual Analog Scale for Dyspnea

Another widely used dyspnea assessment method is the visual analog scale.[2,28] This scale consists of a vertical or horizontal line of a predetermined length (usually 100mm) with a descriptive phrase of opposite extremes anchored

Table 14–2
Borg Category Scale for Measurement of Dyspnea

0	Nothing at all
0.5	Very, very slight (just noticeable)
1	Very slight
2	Slight
3	Moderate
4	Somewhat severe
5	Severe
6	
7	Very severe
8	
9	Very, very severe (almost maximal)
10	Maximal

at each end of the line. The scale can be displayed on a screen or paper, and the subject rates his or her level of dyspnea by choosing a point on the line. This point is then measured from one end point and the distance is recorded. More advanced adaptations of this scale can include a dial or a slide marker the subject uses to select a point on the line. A similar measure, the oxygen-cost diagram, is anchored with tasks that cause dyspnea.[52,60]

Walk Test

Questionnaires often query for patients' perceptions of their functional capacity. This can also be directly measured, most commonly by a 6- or12-minute walk test. This assesses the ability of patients to perform a functional activity required for daily living (walking) but may not correlate with physiologic exercise capacity measured in a laboratory setting. McGavin and colleagues[62] described the 12-minute walking test to assess the exercise tolerance of patients with COPD. These authors found that the distance walked in 12 minutes correlated with maximum oxygen consumption and minute ventilation measured by bicycle ergometry but did not correlate with the FEV_1. Guyatt and coworkers,[32] however, showed that although walk distance improved with rehabilitation, there was no significant change in a cycle ergometer exercise test.

The walk test is performed according to a rigid protocol defining the number of walks and methodology to be used by the tester, both of which may affect the results. For example, it has been shown that when measured daily for 3 days, the distance walked increased on day 3. Because encouragement by the tester can increase the distance walked,[33] test administration should be standardized.

OUTCOMES OF PULMONARY REHABILITATION

Improvements in many of the domains listed in Table 14–1 have been demonstrated for COPD patients following rehabilitation. Although it is not always clear which component of pulmonary rehabilitation is most responsible for any specific outcome,[55] most of the results noted subsequently have been demonstrated in response to comprehensive multidisciplinary programs.

Mortality

Although oxygen therapy improves survival in selected patients with COPD, conclusive evidence that pulmonary rehabilitation decreases mortality is lacking. Mortality is closely related to the degree of airflow limitation as measured by the FEV_1 but is also related to age and possibly exercise tolerance and perceived physical disability.[3] Several investigators, however, have suggested that pulmonary rehabilitation may improve survival.[5,10,36,37,71,80,85]

Haas and Cardon[36] reported the mortality of 252 patients treated with pulmonary rehabilitation compared to 50 COPD patients who received only symptomatic treatment. Mortality was less in the rehabilitation patients (78% 5-year survival when considering only deaths caused by respiratory failure and 70% survival considering death from all causes) compared to control patients (58% 5-year survival considering deaths caused by respiratory failure and 42% survival considering deaths from all causes). Petty[71] also reported improved survival in patients who completed pulmonary rehabilitation compared to matched control subjects treated with standard care in the same community. Sahn and coworkers[80] compared survival in 182 patients following pulmonary rehabilitation to a historical group of patients from a Veterans Administration study in another city. Survival was 67% at 2.5 years in the rehabilitation patients compared to 50% in the earlier VA study. In these 182 rehabilitation patients with a mean FEV_1 of 0.94 L, survival was 41% at 5 years and 17% at 10 years.

Data from 75 patients reported by Hodgkin and colleagues[37] demonstrated a 63% 10-year survival, higher than most similar studies because of a higher mean FEV_1 of 1.55 L. The survival in this study, however, was higher than other reports of patients who did not have pulmonary rehabilitation but who had similar degrees of airflow limitation. In an uncontrolled study, mortality was evaluated in patients seen over an 11-year period from 1976 through 1987 in a single medical center.[85] Survival was higher in 212 patients completing rehabilitation (66% survival at 10 years) compared to 921 patients not completing the program (60% survival) and 100 randomly selected patients with COPD (53% survival). Burns and associates[10] reported a 32% survival over 10 years following pulmonary rehabilitation, which was considered better than the survival reported in historical studies of patients treated without rehabilitation.

Although these reports suggest improved survival, a definitive statement about the effects of pulmonary rehabilitation on longevity cannot be definitively made. The investigations evaluating survival lacked a concurrent control population that did not receive pulmonary rehabilitation. In addition, the available studies included patients with differing severity of underlying pulmonary disease as measured by the FEV_1 and reported widely divergent survival rates, thus making comparisons between studies difficult.

Morbidity

Several studies conducted over several decades have demonstrated a reduction in hospital days in COPD patients following pulmonary rehabilitation.[15,41,77,85] A study in the late 1960s suggested that the frequency of hospital admissions for patients with COPD could be reduced by an intensive home program.[15] Patients with frequent hospital admissions or moderately severe hypoxia and hypercapnia were enrolled in a home care program using the services of a nurse and other ancillary health care personnel when necessary. The goal of this program was to overcome functional limitations and prevent exacerbations of respiratory disease. The program focused on secretion elimination, proper use of bronchodilators, and diaphragmatic and physical activity training.

In the late 1970s, Hudson and coworkers[41] demonstrated a reduction in hospital days for 44 patients following pulmonary rehabilitation. Patients spent an average of 12 days in the hospital in the year before rehabilitation and only 3 days in the year following rehabilitation (Table 14–3). The reduction in hospital days persisted for 4 years.

More recently, a Loma Linda group demonstrated a reduction in hospital days for 80 pa-

tients from 17.4 days in the year before rehabilitation to 7.8 days in the year following rehabilitation (including a decreased hospitalization rate) to 2.7 hospital days in the third year. A decreased rate of days hospitalized persisted for 8 years after rehabilitation.[77] In Sneider et al's[85] study, patients completing rehabilitation had a reduction of 1.8 hospital days per year compared with the year before rehabilitation. The reduction in hospitalizations is even more impressive because patients only interviewed for rehabilitation had an increase in hospital days of 3.2 per year, and patients completing only an educational component had an increase in hospital days of 2.14 per year.

Respiratory Symptoms

The major respiratory symptom of interest to patients is breathlessness. Some patients cough considerably and have large amounts of sputum. Dyspnea decreases as a result of pulmonary rehabilitation, both when measured by the Baseline Dyspnea Index[29] or the CRDQ.[29,34,78,94] Breathing retraining including via pursed lips and diaphragmatic breathing[25] and exercise training decrease dyspnea.[5,17,59,83] Sputum can be more easily mobilized by using chest physical therapy modalities,[25] and medical therapy can decrease cough and sputum, particularly when associated with an infectious cause.

Functional Capacity

Pulmonary rehabilitation improves objectively assessed functional capacity as well as patient-perceived functional status. An earlier study by Moser and colleagues[66] classified patients into five functional levels based on activities that were restricted owing to dyspnea. An ac-

Table 14–3
Pulmonary Rehabilitation Reduces Hospitalizations

Year	Total Hospital Days	Mean Hospital Days per Patient
Year before rehabilitation	529	12
First year after rehabilitation	145	3
Second year	270	6
Third year	278	6
Fourth year	207	5

Data of 44 patients from Hudson LD, Tyler ML, Petty TL: Hospitalization needs during an outpatient rehabilitation program for severe chronic airway obstruction. Chest 70:606–610, 1976.

tivity of daily living index was also developed from questions about the amount of dyspnea associated with 20 normal activities. Sixteen of 29 patients improved one or more functional classes, and an additional 11 patients achieved clinically significant improvements in the index.

The walk test can be used to assess functional capacity. Vale and associates[88] showed an increase in the walk distance by 24.5% following rehabilitation, and walk distance also improved after inpatient rehabilitation.[29] Similarly, the authors have found a 21% increase in the 6-minute walk distance in 24 patients with severe COPD and an FEV_1 of 30.3% of predicted.[58] Other studies have demonstrated similar results.[38,61,78,83]

Pulmonary Physiologic Function

Although airflow limitation can be improved by bronchodilators and corticosteroids in some patients with COPD, pulmonary rehabilitation does not have an impact on pulmonary function tests, and it does not change arterial blood gases.[66,69,74] Although rehabilitation does not change the underlying respiratory disease, it does result in increased exercise capacity.

Exercise Capacity

It has been repeatedly demonstrated over the last two decades that pulmonary rehabilitation, including aerobic exercise training of the lower extremities, improves exercise tolerance as measured in the laboratory on a bicycle or treadmill.[12,13,16,66,69,74,76] Several investigators have demonstrated improved performance during steady-state exercise.[13,66] For example, Moser and colleagues[66] reported declines in oxygen consumption, heart rate, respiratory rate, and minute ventilation at the same exercise level following rehabilitation. Other investigators have noted improvement in peak exercise capacity.[11,25,39,57,59,87] For example, Toshima and coworkers[87] noted an increase in exercise endurance time, and Sneider and coworkers[85] noted an increase in treadmill walk distance. Mall and Medeiros[59] showed an increased anaerobic threshold and increased workload but similar oxygen consumption following rehabilitation in 197 patients with COPD. The authors have demonstrated a 9.2% increase in maximum oxygen consumption and a 30.3% increase in maximum workload measured on a bicycle ergometer after rehabilitation.[57] These effects were

achieved in 26 patients with FEV_1 of 43% of predicted normal without an increased maximum heart rate indicating a physiologic training effect.

A randomized, controlled study also demonstrated benefits in exercise capacity.[17] Comparing COPD patients who received exercise training to patients who did not receive training, Cockcroft and associates[17] demonstrated a 23% increase in 12-minute walk distance from 523 meters before training to 643 meters 2 months after training was initiated. Treated patients also had improvements in general well-being, dyspnea, cough and sputum production. Rehabilitation patients had sustained improvement in walk distance, but control patients improved over time and had better exercise capacity at 8 months than treated patients. Sinclair and Ingram[83] also conducted a controlled, randomized evaluation of exercise in 33 patients with COPD. Walk distance gradually improved by 25% over the course of the study.

Punzal and colleagues[76] have demonstrated that patients with COPD can train at higher intensities than previously suspected. Patients were able to train on a treadmill and walk at 84% or greater of their baseline maximum exercise workload. In addition, Casaburi and coworkers[13] have suggested that higher-intensity training is more beneficial than training conducted at a lower intensity and results in a physiologic training effect. Other potential mechanisms for improved exercise capacity following rehabilitation, such as increased motivation, increased efficiency of exercise, and desensitization to dyspnea, have also been suggested.

Most of the studies demonstrating improved quality of life have employed lower extremity aerobic training. Other forms of exercise, including strength training, respiratory muscle training, and upper extremity training, have also been employed but to a lesser extent. Strength training of the upper and lower extremities has been shown to decrease dyspnea and to improve mastery and bicycle exercise endurance time in COPD. A meta-analysis of respiratory muscle training identified 17 randomized trials.[84] Although there was little evidence of clinically important beneficial effects of respiratory muscle training, it appears that endurance and function may be improved when resistance training is performed with controlled flow breathing patterns.

The capacity for arm exercise in patients with COPD is limited by the development of dyspnea and dysynchronous use of the diaphragm and accessory muscles of ventilation.[14] Even simple arm elevation increases ventilation in patients with COPD, and there are greater demands placed on the respiratory system during unsupported arm exercise than during supported arm exercise. Training of the upper extremities in COPD reduces the increased metabolic demand and ventilation associated with arm elevation.[18] Although upper extremity training increases endurance for arm exercise, no apparent effects were demonstrated on activities of daily living in one study.[79] Moreover, upper extremity training did not improve performance in other tests not related to the training, such as steady-state treadmill exercise. A reduction in perceived dyspnea during upper extremity performance was noted. Further studies on upper extremity exercise training, however, are required before firm conclusions can be drawn.

Quality of Life

Most studies that have evaluated quality of life have demonstrated improvements following comprehensive pulmonary rehabilitation programs.[4,5,31,33,58,66] Not all studies have used standard quality-of-life tools, however. One of the earliest studies of the effects of pulmonary re-habilitation used physician and nurse interviews to determine improvement.[73] Improvement was equated with significant increases in daily home activities, a demonstrable increase in measured walk tolerance, and less dyspnea. Of 111 patients who could be evaluated 6 months following rehabilitation, 91 were considered improved, 15 unchanged, and 5 worse.

Guyatt and colleagues[33] demonstrated significant improvement in the CRDQ indices of dyspnea, fatigue, emotional function, and mastery 2 weeks after the completion of rehabilitation in 28 patients with COPD. There was no change in the CRDQ in untreated COPD patients. Interestingly, in this study, there was no change in dyspnea as assessed by the oxygen cost diagram or in the Rand physical and emotional function questionnaires. These same investigators have evaluated the long-term quality-of-life outcomes in COPD over a period of 6 months following rehabilitation (Fig. 14–5).[32] Of 31 patients enrolled in rehabilitation, 28 completed the program, and 5 patients later dropped out of the follow-up study owing to death or illness. Twenty-four of the initial 31 patients (77%) achieved a benefit from rehabilitation. Physical function, emotional function, and 6-minute walk distance were improved when remeasured

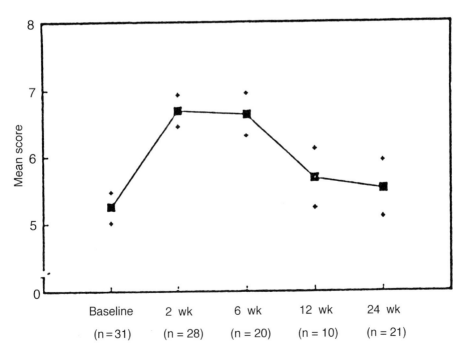

FIGURE 14–5. Scores (mean ± standard error) for physical function of the Chronic Respiratory Disease Questionnaire before and after rehabilitation in COPD. Similar results were demonstrated in emotional function and 6-minute walk distance. (From Guyatt GH, Berman LB, Townsend M: Long-term outcome after respiratory rehabilitation. Can Med Assoc J 137:1089–1095, 1987.)

at 2 weeks and 6 weeks after rehabilitation. Only 11 of these 24 patients, however, still demonstrated benefits at 6 months. This report is difficult to interpret because of the number of patients who dropped out of the study over the period of follow-up.

Vale and coworkers[88] evaluated quality of life (CRDQ) and functional capacity (12-minute walk test) in 51 of 71 patients immediately following rehabilitation and at unspecified time points several months later. These investigators found that (1) quality of life and walk distance improved immediately postrehabilitation, (2) these parameters decreased with long-term follow-up, but (3) quality of life and walk distance remained higher during long-term follow-up than before rehabilitation. Patients with the lowest baseline walk distance declined the most during long-term follow-up. Participation in a structured maintenance program in the investigators' facility did not prevent the decline in quality of life and walk distance. Vale and coworkers[88] also demonstrated improvement in quality of life using the CRDQ but a lack of effect from a maintenance exercise program (Fig. 14–6). There was no correlation between improvement in the walk distance and change in quality-of-life scores.[78] Further studies are required to evaluate the long-term benefits of rehabilitation comparing the effects of a maintenance program to a control population.

Trials of inpatient and home rehabilitation also showed improvements in quality of life measured by the CRDQ.[29,94] In a randomized trial of 2 months of inpatient rehabilitation followed by 4 months of outpatients care, there were statistical improvements in mastery, emotional function, and dyspnea as well as improvement in

walk distance.[29] The improvements in mastery and dyspnea in these patients with severe COPD (FEV$_1$ of 34.8% predicted) were at levels believed to be clinically significant. Improvements were also seen in dyspnea, emotion, and mastery indices of the CRDQ in a study of home rehabilitation.[94] In this investigation, 28 patients exercised at home with supervision by monthly home nursing visits and improved in comparison to a control group not receiving training.

The Quality of Well-Being Scale has also been used to demonstrate improved quality of life following pulmonary rehabilitation.[4] COPD patients were randomized into one of five groups (behavior modification, cognitive-behavior modification, cognitive modification, attention control, and no-treatment control) in an effort to assist them to follow a regular walking program, which was the major outcome variable. Behavior modification was used to assist patients in incorporating walking into their daily routine by specifying a specific time for walking and including self-rewards. Cognitive modification included teaching patients to replace negative thoughts, feelings, and behaviors with more positive ones. Investigators spent equivalent amounts of time with the attention-control group but did not employ other strategies to enhance patients' walking efforts. Patients in the treated groups spent significantly more time in walking, and patients in the combined cognitive-behavior therapy group had the greatest adherence to walking. Compliance with walking and increases in exercise capacity correlated with improvements in quality of life. In another study, the same group of investigators compared the effects of a rehabilitation program including exercise to an education-only

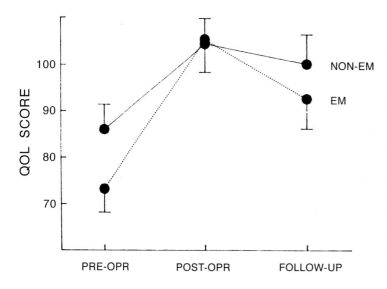

FIGURE 14–6. Quality-of-life scores measured by the Chronic Respiratory Disease Questionnaire before (pre opr), immediately after (post opr), and several months after (follow-up) pulmonary rehabilitation in COPD patients. Results are shown for patients enrolled in an exercise maintenance program (EM) and patients not participating in exercise maintenance (non-EM). Similar results were found in 12-minute walk distance. (From Vale F, Reardon JZ, ZuWallack RL: The long-term benefits of outpatient pulmonary rehabilitation on exercise endurance and quality of life. Chest 103:42–45, 1993.)

program in 129 patients with COPD.[87] Although patients in the rehabilitation group improved their exercise endurance and self-efficacy for walking, there was no improvement in quality of life.

The authors measured quality-of-life indicators using the SF-36 Health Survey and found improvements in health change, physical function, mental health, emotional role, social role, and energy/fatigue and an increase in 6-minute walk distance (Table 14–4).[58] General health and physical role were unchanged following rehabilitation in these 21 consecutive patients following the authors' 3-week outpatient rehabilitation program.

Depression also improves after rehabilitation. In 45 patients with COPD, the authors used the Inventory to Diagnose Depression (IDD) as a measure of depressive symptoms. Higher scores on the inventory indicate more depressive symptoms, and scores of greater than 21 are associated with clinical depression. Following pulmonary rehabilitation, there was a significant reduction in depressive symptoms with mean score falling from 17.0 to 9.4. In addition, 9 of the 10 patients classified as clinically depressed by this tool (IDD scores>21) had reductions in their scores indicating an improvement following rehabilitation.

Many of the studies of the results of pulmonary rehabilitation have not used a randomized, controlled design. In a randomized, controlled study, however, Toshima and coworkers[87] demonstrated that pulmonary rehabilitation for COPD improves quality of life as assessed by the Quality of Well-Being Scale. A total of 119 patients were randomized to a comprehensive 8-week rehabilitation program or an education control group. There were no significant changes in quality of life, a finding at odds with other nonrandomized studies of pulmonary rehabilitation. Improvements were demonstrated in the rehabilitation group in treadmill endurance time that persisted for at least 6 months. Self-efficacy for walking tended to increase in the rehabilitation group, but the changes were not significant.

Several studies have attempted to evaluate factors that may predict a beneficial outcome and to compare the functional and quality-of-life outcomes achieved by rehabilitation.[32,36,78] Age and sex do not appear to be predictors of outcome. The ability of baseline functional capacity and airflow limitation to predict outcome are questionable. Guyatt and coworkers[32] found that patients with less airflow limitation (higher FEV_1) were more likely to show improvement with rehabilitation, but few details were provided to support this conclusion. Haas and Cardon[36] indicated that their clinical experience suggests that rehabilitation should be started earlier in the course of COPD to achieve greater cumulative benefits. Other investigators, however, have demonstrated a greater degree of improvement in walk distance (as measured by percent increase) in patients with the lowest baseline walk distance. Whether these benefits in more functionally limited patients represent the effect of reversing more severe deconditioning or the degree of airflow limitation before rehabilitation was not evaluated. Reardon and associates[78] found that rehabilitation improved 12-minute walk distance and quality of life as measured by the CRDQ in 44 COPD patients enrolled in a 6-week outpatient program. There was no significant relationship between the change in walk distance and change in quality-of-life scores.

It appears that comprehensive programs that include exercise training are necessary to

Table 14–4
Pulmonary Rehabilitation Improves Quality of Life as Measured by the SF-36 Health Survey

Scale	Before	After	P
Physical function	29.1 ± 4.5	41.4 ± 4.5	0.004
Social function	54.5 ± 5.9	67.7 ± 5.1	0.02
Physical role	18.4 ± 6.6	30.3 ± 6.8	0.12
Emotional role	54.4 ± 10.6	77.2 ± 7.2	0.04
Mental health	69.5 ± 3.7	77.0 ± 3.2	0.03
Energy fatigue	40.7 ± 4.0	55.0 ± 3.3	0.0003
Pain	79.9 ± 4.6	88.4 ± 3.3	0.04
General health	43.0 ± 4.6	42.3 ± 4.7	0.9
Health change	31.0 ± 5.2	56.0 ± 6.2	0.0001

Data from Make B, Glenn K, Ikle D, et al: Pulmonary rehabilitation improves the quality of life of patients with chronic obstructive lung disease. Am Rev Respir Dis 145:A767, 1992.

achieve improved quality of life. Education alone does not provide significant quality-of-life benefits. In a controlled community-based study of 538 patients, Howland and coworkers[40] provided education to patients with COPD in one community and did not provide education to patients in another community. Using the Sickness Impact Profile as a quality-of-life tool, the authors found no improvement in physical function, mental health, or social function as a result of education. The education group did show improved health locus of control, that is, patients believed they were more in control of their own health.

Costs

Pulmonary rehabilitation can decrease the costs of medical care for patients with COPD. Reduced hospital days contributes to most of the cost reductions following pulmonary rehabilitation. The cost savings associated with reduced hospitalizations following pulmonary rehabilitation range from $1243 to $3817 per patient per year. Radovich and colleagues[77] noted that total costs for hospitalizations over a 5-year period for 53 survivors from an initial group of COPD patients receiving rehabilitation was $329,500 or $6216 per patient over 5 years. This amount was less than the cost of hospitalizations for the 1 year before the program ($349,600). Another investigation noted a decrease in hospital costs owing to a reduction in hospital days from 8.7 per patient to 0.6 per patient.[95] Savings were $217,610 over 1 year in these 57 rehabilitated patients or $3817 per patient over one year. A 5-year study noted a reduction in costs of $458,112 in 50 patients or $9162 per patient over 5 years.[85]

Toevs and associates[86] evaluated the cost-effectiveness of rehabilitation in patients with COPD by using the Quality of Well-Being scale to measure years of quality life (well-years) as an outcome measure. Costs of the rehabilitation program and the savings achieved by fewer hospital days were considered in the analysis; savings related to reduced hospital costs in the 56 patients equated to a reduction of only $14,000 in expenses because the rehabilitation program cost $123,000. The reduction in hospital days in this study was less than that reported by other investigators. These investigators considered the costs including both those of the rehabilitation program and those associated with hospitalization and the effectiveness of rehabilitation measured by well-years. The cost per additional year of well-being was $24,256, considered cost-effective by current standards when compared with other therapeutic modalities.

Ability to Work

It is unclear whether pulmonary rehabilitation can assist patients in returning to gainful employment. It is important to emphasize that this is not generally a goal because patients with more advanced COPD are generally older and retired as a result of a combination of age and respiratory symptoms. Pulmonary rehabilitation is generally considered more effective in maintaining employment in younger patients with less advanced disease and, thus, should be started earlier in the course of COPD. Some investigators have noted a poor compliance with vocational rehabilitation.[22]

Haas and Cardon[36] followed 252 patients receiving rehabilitation and demonstrated that 19% were able to return to work and an additional 6% were trained but never placed in a job. Only 3% of a control group not receiving rehabilitation were able to return to work.

In another study of 147 patients, 60 were working on entry to rehabilitation.[47] The same group of investigators noted that vocational rehabilitation success was related to intelligence test scores.[21] They speculated that patients with higher IQ levels might have decreased energy requirements in their jobs owing to decreased physical demands of employment, thus, allowing better vocational outcomes.

In another study of 182 consecutive COPD patients, only 57 were working at least part-time on entry to the rehabilitation program.[72] Patients who were working at entry to rehabilitation had similar pulmonary physiologic parameters but were younger and had better exercise capacity. Although only three patients who were unable to work before rehabilitation were able to return to work following rehabilitation, the authors believed that rehabilitation was helpful in allowing patients to maintain employment and adjust their work.

Other Outcomes

Little information is available concerning caregiver burden and use of assistive technology outcomes in COPD. Haas and Cardon[36] reported improved self-care ability and decreased need for nursing home care over 5 years of follow-up in patients enrolled in rehabilitation compared with patients not receiving rehabilitation. Nineteen percent of rehabilitated patients were able to care for themselves compared with only 5% of controls; 17% of controls but only 8% of rehabilitated patients were placed in nursing homes. Decreased need for skilled facility care reduces the costs of medical care for COPD patients.

SUMMARY

Although pulmonary rehabilitation can improve physiologic measures of exercise capacity, functional capacity, and health-related quality of life, additional controlled, randomized studies are needed to prove these benefits beyond any doubt. In addition, many other questions remain unanswered. Further investigations are needed to assess the relationships between these 12 domains. Further characterizations of patients with COPD may indicate distinctive patient profiles that may be useful in determining which components of pulmonary rehabilitation should be applied to individual patients with COPD. Further investigations also need to analyze which components of pulmonary rehabilitation are associated with the desired outcomes.

The variety, diversity, and number of potential outcomes of pulmonary rehabilitation (see Table 14–1) suggest that not all outcomes are of equal importance for all COPD patients. It is also difficult to measure so many disease outcomes. Based on the nature and needs of the client populations being served, pulmonary rehabilitation program directors should determine which outcomes will be the focus for their rehabilitative efforts. Periodic assessment of the outcomes achieved by rehabilitation can be used to modify the program to improve outcomes and thus enhance patient care. Outcomes can also be used to explain the need for rehabilitation to patients, health care professionals, and third-party payers.

References

1. American Psychological Association. Standards for Educational and Psychological Tests. Washington, D.C., American Psychological Association, 1974.
2. Aitken RCB: Measurement of feelings using visual analogue scales. Proc R Soc Med 62:989–993, 1969.
3. Anthonisen NR, Wright EC, Hodgkin JE: Prognosis in chronic obstructive pulmonary disease. Am Rev Respir Dis 133:14–22, 1986.
4. Atkins CJ, Kaplan RM, Timms RM, et al: Behavioral exercise programs in the management of chronic obstructive pulmonary disease. J Consult Clin Psychol 52:591–603, 1984.
5. Bebout DE, Hodgkin JE, Zorn EG, et al: Clinical and physiological outcomes of a university-hospital pulmonary rehabilitation program. Respir Care 28:1468–1473, 1983.
6. Bergner M, Bobbitt RA, Carter W, et al: The Sickness Impact Profile: Development and final revision of health status measure. Med Care 19:787–805, 1981.
7. Bethel R, Make B, Glenn K, et al: Psychological factors affect physical performance in COPD. Am Rev Respir Dis 145:A767, 1992.
8. Borg G: Perceived exertion as an indicator of somatic stress. Scand J Rehab Med 2:92–98, 1970.
9. Borg G: Psychological bases of perceived exertion. Med Sci Sports Exerc 14:377–381, 1982.
10. Burns MR, Sherman B, Madison R, et al: Pulmonary rehabilitation outcome. J Respir Care Pract 2:25–30, 1989.
11. Carter R, Nicotra B, Clark L, et al: Exercise conditioning in the rehabilitation of patients with chronic obstructive pulmonary disease. Arch Phys Med Rehabil 69:118–122, 1988.
12. Casaburi R: Exercise training in chronic obstructive lung disease. In Casaburi R, Petty TL (eds): Principles and Practice of Pulmonary Rehabilitation. Philadelphia, WB Saunders, 1993, pp. 204–224.
13. Casaburi R, Patessio A, Ioli F, et al: Reductions in exercise lactic acidosis and ventilation as a result of exercise training in patients with obstructive lung disease. Am Rev Respir Dis 143:9–18, 1991.
14. Celli B, Rassulo J, Make BJ: Dysynchronous breathing is associated with arm but not leg exercise in chronic obstructive pulmonary disease. N Engl J Med 314:1485–1490, 1986.
15. Cherniack RM, Handford RG, Svanhill E: Home care of chronic respiratory disease. JAMA 208:821–824, 1969.
16. Chester EH, Belman MJ, Bahler RC, et al: Multidisciplinary treatment of chronic pulmonary insufficiency. Chest 72:695–702, 1977.
17. Cockcroft AE, Sanders MJ, Berry G: Randomized controlled trial of rehabilitation in chronic respiratory disability. Thorax 36:200–203, 1981.
18. Couser JI, Martinez FJ, Celli BR: Pulmonary rehabilitation that includes arm exercise reduces metabolic and ventilatory requirements for simple arm elevation. Chest 103:37–41, 1993.
19. Cox NJM, van Herwaarden CLA, Folgering H, et al: Exercise and training in patients with chronic obstructive lung disease. Sports Med 6:180–192, 1988.
20. Dales RE, Spitzer WO, Schechter MT, et al: The influence of psychological status on respiratory symptom reporting. Am Rev Respir Dis 139:1459–1463, 1989.
21. Daughton DM, Fix AJ, Kass I, et al: Physiological-intellectual components of rehabilitation success in patients with chronic obstructive pulmonary disease (COPD). J Chron Dis 32:405–409, 1979.
22. Dudley DL: The Psychophysiology of Respiration in Health and Disease. New York, Appleton-Century-Crofts, 1969, pp. 313–315.
23. Dudley DL, Wermuth C, Hague W: Psychological aspects of care in the chronic obstructive pulmonary disease patient. Heart Lung 2:289–303, 1973.
24. Eakin EG, Sassi-Dambron D, Kaplan RM, et al: Clinical trial of rehabilitation in chronic obstructive pulmonary disease: Compliance as a mediator of change in exercise endurance. J Cardiopulm Rehabil 12:105–110, 1992.
25. Faling LJ: Controlled breathing techniques and chest physical therapy in chronic obstructive pulmonary disease and allied conditions. In Casaburi R, Petty TL (eds): Principles and Practice of Pulmonary Rehabilitation. Philadelphia, WB Saunders, 1993, pp. 167–182.
26. Fanshel F, Bush JW: A health status index and its appli-

cation to health services outcomes. Oper Res 18:1021–1066, 1970.

27. Ferguson G: Respiratory muscle function in chronic obstructive pulmonary disease. Semin Respir Med 14:430–445, 1993.

28. Gift AG: Validation of a vertical visual analogue scale as a measure of clinical dyspnea. Rehab Nurs 14:323–325, 1989.

29. Goldstein RS, Gort EH, Stubbing D, et al: Randomised controlled trial of respiratory rehabilitation. Lancet 344:1394–1397, 1994.

30. Grant I, Prigatano G, Heaton R, et al: Progressive neuropsychologic impairment and hypoxemia. Arch Gen Psychiatry 44:999–1006, 1987.

31. Guyatt G, Walter S, Norman G: Measuring change over time: Assessing the usefulness of evaluative instruments. J Chron Dis 40:171–178, 1987.

32. Guyatt GH, Berman LB, Townsend M: Long-term outcome after respiratory rehabilitation. Can Med Assoc J 137:1089–1095, 1987.

33. Guyatt GH, Berman LB, Townsend M, et al: A measure of quality of life for clinical trials in chronic lung disease. Thorax 42:773–778, 1987.

34. Guyatt GH, Jaeschke R: Measurements in clinical trials: Choosing the appropriate approach. In Spilker B (ed): Quality of Life Assessments in Clinical Trials. New York, Raven Press, 1990, pp. 37–46.

35. Guyatt GH, Townsend M, Berman LB, et al: Quality of life in patients with chronic airflow limitation. Br J Dis Chest 81:45–54, 1987.

36. Haas A, Cardon H: Rehabilitation in chronic obstructive pulmonary disease: A 5-year study of 252 patients. Med Clin North Am 53:593–606, 1969.

37. Hodgkin JE, Branscomb BV, Anholm JD, et al: Benefits, limitations and the future of pulmonary rehabilitation. In Hodgkin JE, Zorn EG, Connors GL (eds): Pulmonary Rehabilitation: Guidelines to Success. Boston, Butterworth, 1984, pp 403–414.

38. Holden DA, Stelmach KD, Curtis PS, et al: The impact of a rehabilitation program on functional status of patients with chronic lung disease. Respir Care 35:332–341, 1990.

39. Holle RHO, Williams DV, Vandree JC, et al: Increased muscle efficiency and sustained benefits in an outpatient community hospital-based pulmonary rehabilitation program. Chest 94:1161–1168, 1988.

40. Howland J, Nelson EC, Barlow PB, et al: Chronic obstructive airway disease: Impact of health education. Chest 90:233–238, 1986.

41. Hudson LD, Tyler ML, Petty TL: Hospitalization needs during an outpatient rehabilitation program for severe chronic airway obstruction. Chest 70:606–610, 1976.

42. Irvin CG, Corbridge T: Physiologic evaluation of patients for pulmonary rehabilitation. Semin Respir Med 14:417–429, 1993.

43. Jaeschke R, Guyatt GH: How to develop and validate a new quality of life instrument. In Spilker B (ed): Quality of Life Assessments in Clinical Trials. New York, Raven Press, 1990, pp. 47–57.

44. Kaplan RM, Atkins CJ, Timms R: Validity of a quality of well-being scale as an outcome measure in chronic obstructive pulmonary disease. J Chron Dis 37:85–95, 1984.

45. Kaplan RM, Bush JW: Health related quality of life measurement for evaluation research and policy analysis. Health Psychol 1:61–80, 1982.

46. Kaplan RM, Bush JW, Berry C: Health status: Types of validity and the indices of well-being. Health Ser Res 11:478–507, 1976.

47. Kass I, Dyksterhuis JE, Rubin H, et al: Correlation of psychophysiologic variables with vocational rehabilitation outcome in patients with chronic obstructive pulmonary disease. Chest 67:433–440, 1975.

48. Kirshner B, Guyatt GH: A mehtodologic framework for assessing health indices. J Chron Dis 38:27–36, 1985.

49. Lee RN, Graydon E, Ross E: Effects of psychological well-being, physical status, and social support on oxygen-dependent COPD patients' level of functioning. Res Nurs Health 14:323–328, 1991.

50. Lohr KN: Advances in health status assessment: An overview. Med Care 27(suppl):S1–S11, 1989.

51. Mahler DA: The measurement of dyspnea during exercise in patients with lung disease. Chest 101:242S–247S, 1992.

52. Mahler DA, Harver A: Clinical measurement of dyspnea. In Mahler DA (ed): Dyspnea. Mount Kisco, NY, Futura, 1990, pp. 75–126.

53. Mahler DA, Weinberg DH, Wells CK, et al: The measurement of dyspnea: Contents, interobserver agreement, and physiologic correlates of two clinical indices. Chest 85:751–758, 1984.

54. Make BJ: COPD: Management and rehabilitation. Am Fam Phys 43:1315–1324, 1991.

55. Make BJ: Pulmonary rehabilitation: Myth or reality. Clin Chest Med 7:519–540, 1986.

56. Make BJ: Pulmonary rehabilitation: What are the outcomes? [edit]. Respir Care 35:329–331, 1990.

57. Make B, Buchholz J: Exercise training in COPD patients improves cardiac function. Am Rev Respir Dis 143:A80, 1991.

58. Make B, Glenn K, Iklé D, et al: Pulmonary rehabilitation improves the quality of life of patients with chronic obstructive pulmonary disease (COPD). Am Rev Respir Dis 145:A767, 1992.

59. Mall RW, Medeiros M: Objective evaluation of results of a pulmonary rehabilitation program in a community hospital. Chest 94:1156–1160, 1988.

60. McGavin CR, Artvinli M, Naoe H, et al: Dyspnea, disability, and distance walked: Comparison of estimates of exercise performance in respiratory disease. BMJ 2:241–243, 1978.

61. McGavin CR, Gupta SP, Lloyd EL, et al: Physical rehabilitation for the chronic bronchitic: Results of a controlled trial of exercises in the home. Thorax 32:307–311, 1977.

62. McGavin CR, Gupta SP, McHardy GJR: Twelve-minute walking test for assessing disability in chronic bronchitis. BMJ 1:822–823, 1976.

63. McSweeney J, Grant I, Heaton RK, et al: Life quality of patients with chronic obstructive pulmonary disease. Ann Intern Med 142:473–478, 1982.

64. Medical Research Council Working Party: Long-term domiciliary oxygen therapy in chronic hypoxic cor pulmanale complicating chronic bronchitis and emphysema. Lancet 1:681–686, 1981.

65. Moody L, McCormick K, Williams A: Disease and symptom severity, functional status, and quality of life in chronic bronchitis and emphysema (CBE). J Behav Med 13:297–306, 1990.

66. Moser KM, Bokinsky GC, Savage RT, et al: Results of a comprehensive rehabilitation program. Arch Intern Med 140:1596–1601, 1980.

67. Nocturnal Oxygen Therapy Trial Group: Continuous or nocturnal oxygen therapy in hypoxemic chronic obstructive lung disease: A clinical trial. Ann Intern Med 93:391–398, 1980.

68. Mungall IPF, Hainsworth R: Assessment of respiratory function in patients with chronic obstructive airways disease. Thorax 37:254–258, 1979.

69. Olopade CO, Beck KC, Viggiano RW, et al: Exercise lim-

itation and pulmonary rehabilitation in chronic obstructive pulmonary disease. Mayo Clin Proc 67:144–157, 1992.

70. Patrick DL, Deyo RA: Generic and disease specific measures in assessing health status and quality of life. Med Care 27(suppl):S217–232, 1989.

71. Petty TL: Pulmonary rehabilitation. Am Rev Respir Dis 122 (suppl): 159, 1979.

72. Petty TL, MacIlroy ER, Swigert MA, et al: Chronic airway obstruction, respiratory insufficiency, and gainful employment. Arch Environ Health 21:71–78, 1970.

73. Petty TL, Nett LM, Finigan MM, et al: A comprehensive care program for chronic airway obstruction: Methods and preliminary evaluation of symptomatic and functional improvement. Ann Intern Med 70:1109–1120, 1969.

74. Pineda B, Haas F, Axen K: Treadmill exercise training in chronic obstructive pulmonary disease. Arch Phys Med Rehabil 67:155–158, 1986.

75. Postma DS, Koeter GH, Wijkstra PJ: Course and prognosis in patients with chronic airflow obstruction: Possible implications for therapy. *In* Casaburi R, Petty TL (eds): Principles and Practice of Pulmonary Rehabilitation. Philadelphia, WB Saunders, 1993, pp 138–150.

76. Punzal PA, Ries AL, Kaplan RM, et al: Maximum intensity exercise training in patients with chronic obstructive pulmonary disease. Chest 100:618–623, 1991.

77. Radovich JL, Hodgkin JE, Burton GG, et al: Cost effectiveness of pulmonary rehabilitation programs. *In* Hodgkin JE, Connors GL, Bell CW (eds): Pulmonary Rehabilitation: Guidelines to Success, 2nd ed. Philadelphia, JB Lippincott, 1993, pp 548–561.

78. Reardon J, Patel K, ZuWallack RL: Improvement in quality of life is unrelated to improvement in exercise endurance after outpatient pulmonary rehabilitation. J Cardiopulm Rehabil 13:51–54, 1993.

79. Ries AL, Ellis B, Hawkins RW: Upper extremity training in chronic obstructive pulmonary disease. Chest 93:688–692, 1988.

80. Sahn SA, Nett Lm, Petty TL: Ten-year follow-up of a comprehensive rehabilitation program for severe COPD. Chest 77:311–314, 1980.

81. Silverman M, Barry J, Hellerstein H, et al: Variability of the perceived sense of effort in breathing during exercise in patients with chronic obstructive pulmonary disease. Am Rev Respir Dis 137:206–209, 1988.

82. Simpson K, Killian K, McCartney N, et al: Randomised controlled trial of weightlifting exercise in patients with chronic airflow limitation. Thorax 47:70–75, 1992.

83. Sinclair DJM, Ingram CG: Controlled trial of supervised exercise training in chronic bronchitis. BMJ :519–521, 1980.

84. Smith K, Cook D, Guyatt GH, et al: Respiratory muscle training in chronic airflow limitation: A meta-analysis. Am Rev Respir Dis 145:533–539, 1992.

85. Sneider R, O'Malley JA, Kahn M: Trends in pulmonary rehabilitation at Eisenhower Medical Center: An 11-years' experience (1976–1987). J Cardiopulm Rehabil 11:453–461, 1988.

86. Toevs CD, Kaplan RM, Atkins CJ: The costs and effects of behavioral programs in chronic obstructive pulmonary disease. Med Care 22:1088–1100, 1984.

87. Toshima MT, Kaplan RM, Ries AL: Experimental evaluation of rehabilitation in chronic obstructive pulmonary disease: Short-term effects on exercise endurance and health status. Health Psychol 9:237–252, 1990.

88. Vale F, Reardon JZ, ZuWallack RL: The long-term benefits of outpatient pulmonary rehabilitation on exercise endurance and quality of life. Chest 103:42–45, 1993.

89. Ware JE Jr: SF-36 Physical and Mental Health Summary Scales: A user's Manual. Boston, The Health Institute, 1994.

90. Ware J Jr: Standards for validating health measures: Definition and content. J Chron Dis 40:473–480, 1987.

91. Ware JE Jr: Methodological considerations in selection of health status assessment procedures. *In* Wenger NK, Mattson ME, Furberg CD, et al (eds): Assessment of Quality of Life in Clinical Trials in Cardiovascular Therapies. New York, LiJacq, 1984. pp 87–111.

92. Ware JE Jr, Sherbourne CD: The MOS 36-Item Short-Form Health Survey (SF-36). Med Care 30:473–482, 1992.

93. Wasserman K, Hansen JE, Sue DY, et al: Principles of Exercise Testing and Interpretation. Philadelphia, Lea & Febiger, 1987.

94. Wijkstra PJ, van Altena R, Otten V, et al: Quality of life in patients with chronic obstructive pulmonary disease improves after rehabilitation at home. Eur Respir J 7:269–273, 1994.

95. Wright RW, Larsen DF, Moni RG, et al: Benefits of a community-hospital pulmonary rehabilitation program. Respir Care 28:1474, 1983.

Rehabilitation Considerations for the Lung Transplant Patient

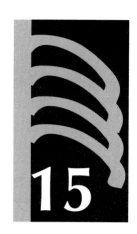

Brendan P. Madden, MD, MSC, FRCPI
Margaret E. Hodson, MD, MSc, FRCP

Lung transplantation is a realistic therapeutic option for selected patients with end-stage respiratory failure due to a variety of pulmonary vascular and parenchymal diseases. The aim of lung transplantation is to improve patient survival and quality of life. Encouraging intermediate-term results have been reported.[16,18] The major problems facing any lung transplant center are shortage of suitable donor organs and the late postoperative complication of obliterative bronchiolitis. The demand for lung transplantation will always exceed availability of donor organs, and thus, patients should only be referred for transplant assessment if, despite optimal conventional medical treatment, they have severe pulmonary disability and their conditions fail to improve.

Patients are accepted onto the transplant waiting list when severe and deteriorating chronic respiratory failure and poor quality of life are documented despite the best available medical treatment. In practice, the forced expiratory volume in one second (FEV_1) is usually <30% of the predicted value. There should also be no psychosocial instability that may interfere with the patient's ability to cope with the operation, strict postoperative follow-up, or compliance with treatment.

With increasing experience, the absolute contraindications to lung transplantation are becoming fewer[20] and include:

1. Active aspergillus or mycobacterial infection;
2. Infection with human immunodeficiency virus or hepatitis B;
3. Noncompliance with treatment;
4. Pre-existing malignant disease;
5. Prednisolone therapy >10 mg/day; and
6. Other end-organ failure unless it is also amenable to transplantation.

Although not absolute contraindications, preoperative ventilatory assistance, previous thoracic surgery (e.g. abrasion pleurodesis or pleurectomy), chemical pleurodesis, and severe liver disease necessitating combined heart-lung-liver transplantation are associated with increased early, but not late, mortality.

Many pulmonary rehabilitation techniques were initially applied to patients with severe impairment and disability from chronic obstructive pulmonary disease. The techniques and approaches to pulmonary rehabilitation are applicable to other chronic respiratory conditions, such as those associated with pulmonary fibrosis, thoracic deformities, and cystic fibrosis (CF).[26] Initially, pulmonary rehabilitation was only considered in the postoperative care of lung transplantation.[33] However, rehabilitation techniques are becoming increasingly important in pretransplantation care with important benefits to patients despite progression of the underlying lung disease.[5]

PRETRANSPLANTATION ASSESSMENT

Pretransplantation assessment involves a hospital admission for approximately 1 week that enables the patient to become familiar with the surgical center, get to know the staff, and meet some patients who have already had transplantation. A full history and physical examination (including height, weight, and chest measurements) are performed, and an assessment of the patient's quality of life and psychosocial suitability is undertaken. Measurements are made of forced vital capacity (FVC), FEV_1, and blood gas analyses at rest and on exertion. When accepted onto the transplant waiting list, patients typically have an FEV_1 of about 30% of predicted normal and oxyhemoglobin saturation (SaO_2) at rest of 80% to 90%. Furthermore, desaturation is usual with exercise. Chest radiography and computed tomography (CT) scan of the thorax are performed to assess any pleural thickening or adhesions. A detailed dental, ear, nose, and throat examination is mandatory because patients with diseases such as CF may also have chronically infected sinuses (or teeth), which may become potential sources of postoperative infection.[15] A clinical evaluation of cardiac function is performed together with electrocardiography, two-dimensional echocardiography, and 24-hour Holter monitoring.

Blood is taken for routine hematologic and biochemical investigations and grouping. When possible, abnormalities in hepatic and renal function are corrected. Cytomegalovirus, Epstein-Barr virus, Australia antigen, toxoplasma, human immunodeficiency virus, and herpes simplex serology are checked. Microbiologic examination of the sputum is undertaken for bacterial pathogens, acid-fast bacilli, and fungi.

PATIENT PREPARATION FOR TRANSPLANTATION

Following acceptance onto a transplant waiting list, patients and their families face an indeterminable wait. At this point, it is essential that patients be contactable at all times. However, it is important for patients' morale that they not be confined to their homes. A portable telephone or beeper can provide freedom within the limitations of their illness.

During the waiting period it is essential that patients receive as much support and information as possible and be fully informed of events that may follow if suitable donor organs are found. It should be stressed that due to the shortage of donor organs, being accepted onto a waiting list does not guarantee that the patient will be transplanted. Patients should also be informed of the risks of transplantation and of what to expect in the postoperative period. It should be made clear that following transplantation, life-long immunosuppressive therapy is required together with careful postoperative supervision. Furthermore, it is also important to point out that obliterative bronchiolitis may complicate successful transplantation. Despite these warnings, however, most patients realize that transplantation is the only option that offers them the possibility of prolonging survival and quality of life, and thus, even when fully informed, most patients wish to undergo transplantation.

Pulmonary Rehabilitation Goals

The aim of pulmonary rehabilitation is to maximize the functional and emotional capacity of the patient both before and after lung transplantation. This aim is usually achieved through an individually tailored, multidisciplinary program that includes elements of exercise training, education, and informed advice. Preoperative endurance training can help to prepare patients for early postoperative mobilization and may facilitate the patient's recovery to maximum possible function. Despite adverse gas exchange or pulmonary mechanics, exercise training prior to lung transplantation has been associated with increased submaximal exercise tolerance and work capacity. Furthermore, it has permitted performance of a higher workload at the same, or lower, heart rate and minute ventilation.[5,33,35] The role of ventilatory muscle training in the routine management of patients with chronic respiratory conditions remains unclear. It is hoped that research in this area will identify an appropriate population for training, the best training methods, and the role of training in the context of other rehabilitation modalities.[9] Rehabilitation aims to improve endurance by decreasing deconditioning and increasing confidence.

Rehabilitation Team and Resources

The pulmonary rehabilitation team forms an integral component of the transplantation service. Members include:

1. Transplant surgeons,
2. Pulmonologists,

3. Physiotherapists,
4. Dieticians,
5. Occupational therapists,
6. Social workers,
7. Psychologists,
8. Technicians,
9. Nurses,
10. Coordinators.

Ideally, all should be involved in the initial assessment of the candidate for transplantation.

In our units, the Rehabilitation Department is located adjacent to the transplant wards and transplant outpatient service. It is equipped with treadmills, ergometers, exercise bicycles, weight machines, and graded free weights. There are facilities for cardiac rhythm monitoring, pulse oximetry, and end-tidal carbon dioxide measurement. It includes two fully equipped resuscitation trolleys in the room which are checked on a regular basis. Staff are trained in the techniques of advanced life support by qualified instructors.

Rehabilitation Assessment

The selection and assessment of patients prior to entry into a rehabilitation program are important when judging the success of that program and the progress of any individual patient. Since conventional pulmonary function measurements do not correlate well with disability, some form of performance measure is necessary. Examples include submaximum treadmill, stair climbing, and shuttle walk tests.[32] During these tests, SaO_2 is monitored by pulse oximetry and oxygen therapy is given to maintain blood arterial SaO_2 over 90%. Patients with Eisenmenger's syndrome or primary pulmonary hypertension may respond adversely to exercise testing. Testing is, therefore, always planned on an individual basis and is supervised by a physician.

Other aspects of assessment include a reassessment of symptomatology, tobacco use, previous experience with pulmonary rehabilitation, musculoskeletal assessment, present exercise habits (if any), nutritional and quality of life assessment,[13] and employment. All patients receive a detailed psychosocial assessment, including a review of any personal care needs and other support needs.

Pretransplantation Rehabilitation Interventions

Depending on the individual clinical situation, rehabilitation programs may be inpatient, outpatient, or home-based. *Education* is very important. Patients are taught about the nature of their underlying lung disease and the rehabilitative aspects of their care. They are instructed in the optimal use of medication-delivery methods, nebulizers, and oxygen therapy. It is important that patients seek and receive prompt treatment for any exacerbations of their underlying lung disease.

Transplant *support groups* provide an important forum for patients and families throughout the waiting period.[22] These groups are often organized by a nurse specialist, social worker, or transplant coordinator and meet every 2 to 4 weeks. The groups help identify problems, such as anger or frustration, and permit the patient to work through these in a group discussion. It is most helpful for a medical member of the transplant team to attend these meetings in order to keep the group up-to-date with recent developments in the field of organ transplantation, provide encouragement, and answer questions that may arise. The improved quality of life for the successfully transplanted patient can be clearly illustrated by lung transplant recipients attending the meetings. Successfully transplanted patients share common experiences with the group and give encouragement to those on the waiting list. In this setting, patients can also learn about, and be encouraged to pursue, their maximum entitlements such as for assistance with transport or home modifications.

Physiotherapy intervention includes not only training in techniques of airway secretion management and active cycle of breathing exercises, but also the development and institution of an individualized strengthening and flexibility program. Facilitation of airway secretion elimination is particularly important for patients with suppurative lung disease, such as those with CF who are on transplant waiting lists.[19]

Malnutrition is treated aggressively. This may necessitate nasogastric or gastrostomy feedings if patients fail to gain weight adequately by maximizing their dietary caloric intake.

Exercise training for patients who are unfit or disabled does not necessarily have to be strenuous. Indeed, improvements in performance can be identified in this group with relatively low-intensity exercise training. In the United States, it is not unusual to find patients participating in exercise programs with an FEV_1 <1 liter.[28] It is most important that each patient have an individually prescribed exercise program, even if this is in a group setting. Strengthening exercises may also be incorporated into the training regimen. Oxygen therapy is used during the exercise sessions to maintain $SaO_2 > 90\%$. Inspiratory muscle training may also be added.

As a result of these efforts, many patients have improvements in quality of life, as exemplified by reduced symptoms, enhanced performance of daily activities, increased functional exercise capacity, improved quality-of-life scores, reduction in hospital stays, and return to work. It is not uncommon in our experience to note improvement in static lung function, maximum exercise capacity, arterial blood gases, rate of decline in FEV_1, or some combination of these. These findings are consistent with experience elsewhere.[6,11,13]

Throughout the waiting period, patient care is largely at the referring center, with visits to the transplant center at regular intervals. Close cooperation between centers is essential, particularly if the patient's condition deteriorates. In selected patients, nasal intermittent positive pressure ventilation (NIPPV) has been used successfully as a bridge to lung transplantation.[12] This form of treatment has a number of important advantages. Firstly, patients can be managed in familiar surroundings on the ward or at home without the necessity for hospitalization for ventilatory assistance. Secondly, because it is easily possible to adjust flow rates and inspiratory and expiratory times with instruction, the patient can adjust the support delivered by the ventilator and thus feels, to some degree, in control of the situation. Thirdly, avoidance of conventional endotracheal intubation minimizes the risk of infection or toxemia, especially in patients with CF.

SURGICAL OPTIONS

The major criteria for donor and recipient matching are ABO blood group, size of the thoracic cage, and cytomegalovirus status. Lung transplant procedures recommended for different types of pulmonary vascular and parenchymal lung diseases have recently been reviewed.[20] Surgical options include:

1. Heart-lung transplantation (HLT),
2. Double lung transplantation (DLT),
3. Bilateral single-lung transplantation (BSLT),
4. Single-lung transplantation (SLT), and
5. Lobar transplantation.

HLT involves right atrial, aortic, and tracheal anastomoses. The procedure is associated with a low incidence of tracheal dehiscence and a low incidence of accelerated coronary atherosclero-

sis. It is particularly suitable for patients with CF and other suppurative lung diseases and Eisenmenger's syndrome. However, with increasing numbers of centers worldwide performing cardiac transplantation, the number of heart-lung blocs available for HLT is declining, and the indications for this procedure are changing.

DLT involves fashioning tracheal, pulmonary arterial, and pulmonary venous (to left atrium) anastomoses. Initially the results of en bloc DLT were associated with poor results, largely because of tracheal anastomotic dehiscence.[24,25] However, the combination of improved surgical technique, shorter periods of organ ischemia, and early extubation following transplantation has contributed to the low dehiscence rates now observed after both DLT and BSLT. In addition to pulmonary arterial and venous anastomoses, bi-bronchial anastomoses are performed in BSLT. This procedure offers the advantage that airway healing is less impaired because the bronchus gathers some of its blood supply from the neighboring hilum.[4] Furthermore, the procedure frequently can be performed without the need for cardiopulmonary bypass. Early results of BSLT are encouraging,[23] and reports of intermediate-term results are awaited. HLT, DLT, and BSLT are indicated for a variety of pulmonary vascular and parenchymal conditions, which include Eisenmenger's syndrome, primary pulmonary hypertension, CF, bronchiectasis, and emphysema.

SLT is the transplant procedure of choice for patients with restrictive lung diseases, such as idiopathic pulmonary fibrosis. It has been applied successfully to patients with emphysema and primary pulmonary hypertension. Although early experience with lobar transplantation, both in vivo and cadaveric, is encouraging, further experience with this procedure is necessary.

INTENSIVE CARE MANAGEMENT

Immunosuppression

Patients are routinely immunosuppressed with cyclosporine and azathioprine after lung transplantation. Episodes of acute allograft rejection are treated with intravenous methylprednisolone, which occasionally may be supplemented with anti-thymocyte globulin.[19]

Cyclosporine whole blood levels of 500 ng/ml (monoclonal antibody assay) are maintained during the first postoperative month, and thereafter at 250–350 ng/ml, renal function permitting. Azathioprine is prescribed at up to

2 mg/kg/day. It is discontinued in the presence of leukopenia (white blood cell count < 4 × 10^9/l in peripheral blood) or thrombocytopenia. Episodes of acute rejection are diagnosed by a combination of clinical presentation, radiologic appearance, changes in pulmonary function, and histopathologic appearance of transbronchial lung biopsy specimens obtained during fiberoptic bronchoscopy.

Mechanical Ventilation

Patients routinely receive mechanical ventilatory assistance with the goal of maintaining blood arterial SaO_2 > 90% and mixed venous $SaO_2 \sim$ 70%. Weaning is commenced as soon as the patient's condition is stable. Early extubation is the goal. Patients who receive SLT for emphysema may develop hyperexpansion of the remaining native lung, leading to mediastinal shift and compression of the allograft (Fig. 15–1). In such circumstances, a cuffed double-lumen tube is inserted for endobronchial ventilation. Often, a lower respiratory rate and tidal volume are used for the native lung than for the transplanted lung. Jet ventilation may be useful for the latter. Patients who fail to respond to this treatment may receive either native lobectomy or pneumonectomy with a second SLT.

Fluid Balance and Inotropic Support

Because newly transplanted lungs are sensitive to the effects of overhydration, fluid balance, inotropic support, and diuretic therapy are carefully adjusted to maintain the lowest mean pulmonary capillary wedge pressure that achieves satisfactory tissue perfusion and renal function.

Infection Prophylaxis

Reverse barrier nursing is not routinely used in the intensive care unit. Broad-spectrum antibiotics are prescribed while central lines and chest drains are in situ. Patients who receive lung transplantation for CF receive intravenous antipseudomonal antibotics for the first 10 postoperative days. The choice of antibiotics is determined by the immediate preoperative sputum culture and sensitivity results and by body fluid specimens and wound swabs that are sent on a daily basis for microbiologic examination. Whenever possible, aminoglycosides are avoided to reduce possible synergism with cyclosporine in promoting nephrotoxicity. All patients with CF having positive sputum cultures are treated with antibiotics for the first 2 postoperative months, but thereafter, patients only receive antibiotics if there is clinical evidence of lower respiratory tract infection. Nebulized colistin sulfate is given via a facemask at a dose of 1 MU twice daily for the first 3 postoperative months, and thereafter, 1 MU daily. This may be important in reducing the incidence of postoperative lower respiratory tract infection in CF lung transplant recipients.[19] All lung transplant recipients receive life-long prophylaxis against *Pneumocystis carinii* by taking either oral co-

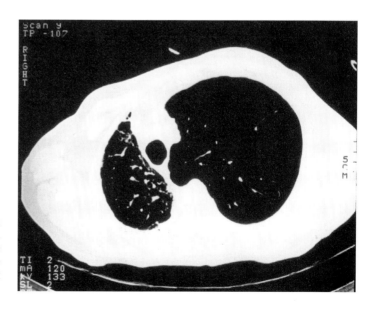

FIGURE 15–1. Thoracic CT scan of a patient with emphysema who had a right single-lung transplantation. Note the compression of the allograft by the hyperinflated native lung. This patient subsequently had a left SLT.

trimoxazole (trimethoprim-sulfamethoxazole) every third day or nebulized pentamidine isethionate biweekly.

Nutrition

It is critical to treat malnutrition vigorously. Although most pulmonary patients tolerate oral feedings soon after surgery when bowel sounds have returned, nasogastric, gastrostomy, or jejunostomy feedings are required for some patients with an elemental diet supplemented with medium-chain triglycerides and carbohydrates.[22] Patients with gastric atony secondary to vagal nerve injury who cannot tolerate nasogastric feeding receive total parenteral nutrition.

Physiotherapy

Reconditioning exercises and chest physiotherapy commence soon after surgery. In the early postoperative period, clearance of airway secretions is hampered by various factors which include endotracheal intubation, pain and discomfort, the effects of analgesia, decreased mobility,[2] loss of cough reflex, and impairment of mucociliary clearance.[33] While the patient is intubated, sterile suctioning with saline lavage is performed with the patient in each postural drainage position and as required. Immediately after extubation, deep breathing and coughing are frequently impaired and chest physiotherapy is particularly important. The intensity of chest physical therapy is indicated by the patient's clinical condition. The techniques include:

1. Breathing control,
2. Positioning (e.g., following SLT, the patient should be nursed in a lateral decubitus position with the allograft uppermost to reduce allograft edema),
3. Active cycle of breathing techniques,
4. Manual therapy,
5. Respiratory muscle exercise, and
6. Adjuncts of intermittent positive pressure breathing, periodic continuous positive airway pressure, and transcutaneous neural stimulation.[1]

The physiotherapy programs advance slowly during the first postoperative week. It is not uncommon for patients to develop oxyhemoglobin desaturation and become hemodynamically unstable during airway suctioning, chest percus-

sion, exercise, or repositioning. It is important that patients have optimal pain control and sleep well at night to enable them to participate as fully as possible with their daytime physiotherapy program.

EARLY POSTOPERATIVE MANAGEMENT FOLLOWING DISCHARGE FROM THE INTENSIVE CARE UNIT

Inotropic support is discontinued as soon as the patient's clinical condition permits, and chest drains are removed in accordance with usual surgical protocols. It is important that all medical personnel be aware of medical problems that commonly occur following lung transplantation (Table 15–1) in addition to problems particular to CF lung transplant recipients (Table 15–2).[22] Prompt diagnosis and instigation of appropriate treatment for these problems are essential.

Physiotherapy continues throughout the hospitalization and includes one or more of the previously mentioned modalities. The patient is encouraged to walk using a specially designed walking frame with wheels that can accommodate an oxygen tank and chest drain bottles if necessary. When chest drains have been removed, stair exercises commence. Oxygen therapy may be required for the first 3 or 4 days to

TABLE 15–1
Medical Problems that May Be Encountered Following Lung Transplantation

Acute allograft rejection
Opportunistic infection
Grand mal seizures
Complications of immunosuppression
Multisystem organ failure
Lymphoproliferative disorders
Obliterative bronchiolitis

TABLE 15–2
Specific Problems that May Occur in Cystic Fibrosis Lung Transplant Recipients

Malnutrition
Persisting infection in upper respiratory tract
Malabsorption of cyclosporine
Meconium ileus equivalent
Liver disease
Salt loss
Diabetes mellitus

maintain blood arterial $SaO_2 > 90\%$. If the postoperative recovery is uncomplicated, oxygen therapy is not usually required after the fifth postoperative day. Thereafter, the patient's rehabilitation is continued in the rehabilitation unit, where the program is further individualized with specifically tailored exercises on the treadmill and exercise bicycle and with free weights. During this stage, the goal of exercise training is to increase function, endurance, and confidence and to decrease deconditioning. It has been our experience that progress following lung transplantation correlates with the patient's physical condition at the time of surgery. Therefore, postoperative recovery rates are variable.

Indication for Bronchoscopy

Bronchoscopy is routinely performed perioperatively and thereafter between the 5th and 7th postoperative day. During this procedure, the anastomosis is inspected, and trap sputum and bronchoalveolar lavage fluid specimens are sent for culture, antibiotic sensitivities, and opportunistic pathogen screening. Transbronchial biopsies are taken for histopathologic examination and culture. Thereafter, bronchoscopies are only performed for one or more of the following indications:

1. Cough,
2. Dyspnea,
3. Reduction in lung function parameters, exercise capacity, or arterial SaO_2,
4. Fever of unknown origin, or
5. Abnormality noted on a chest radiograph.

Episodes of infection are diagnosed by a combination of clinical, serologic, and radiologic investigations (Fig. 15–2), together with the microbiologic and histopathologic results of specimens obtained during bronchoscopy. Patients are treated with appropriate antimicrobial agents.

Ischemia or infection can lead to granulation tissue formation in the region of the large airway anastomoses. It can be treated bronchoscopically with cryotherapy or laser fulguration and endobronchial stenting. It is important that such problems be recognized and treated early to minimize pooling of secretions in the denervated allograft that has impaired mucociliary clearance,[31] because this may lead to episodes of lower respiratory tract infection and bronchiectasis.

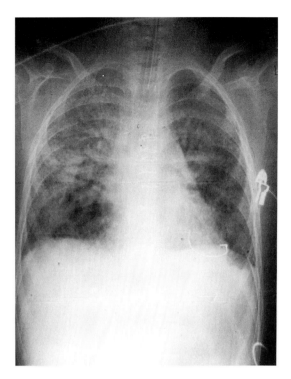

FIGURE 15–2. Chest radiograph of a patient with cytomegalovirus pneumonitis.

Psychological Support

During the early postoperative period, patients are regularly evaluated by the transplantation psychologist. It is common for patients to experience a variety of emotions, including guilt that somebody had to die to give them a chance to live. They may have difficulty in coping with the fact that an organ from somebody who has died is now keeping them alive. Patients commonly want to know about the donor and the donor family. Some of our female patients have difficulty in coping with the fact that they received male donor organs.

Partnerships may find it difficult to adjust to the role change that occurs as the patient gets progressively stronger and returns to normal quality of life. During this period, the partner on whom the patient was dependent may feel isolated, alone, and no longer needed. It is, thus, most important that support be given, not only to the patient but also to the patient's partner and family. This is also the case in the field of pediatric transplantation, where parental difficulties and sibling rivalries may emerge. The sibling rivalries can manifest in a variety of ways, which include jealousy, hiding the patient's immunosuppressive therapy, or asking the parents

"If I had a transplant, would you also love me?" The role of the pediatric transplant psychologist is to help families to readjust after transplantation.

If a patient has HLT for diseases such as CF or primary pulmonary hypertension, the native heart (with a hypertrophied or "primed" right ventricle) can be used for cardiac transplantation in patients who have moderate, reversible elevation in pulmonary vascular resistance. This practice is known as domino cardiac transplantation. Important psychological advantages have been noted following domino cardiac transplantation.[34] The cardiac recipient usually adjusts well in the knowledge that somebody did not have to die to give him or her the chance to live. Similarly, the HLT recipient is content to know that they have helped another patient.

LONG-TERM CARE AND REHABILITATION

Following discharge from the hospital and rehabilitation unit, there is close collaboration and communication between the transplant patient and referring units. Patients are given a portable spirometer (Fig. 15–3) at discharge and advised to measure FEV_1 and FVC on a daily basis. They are instructed to contact the transplant unit if they experience a >15% reduction in lung function on two consecutive daily measurements, develop a reduction in exercise capacity, or pyrexia in excess of 37.5°C. Outpatient visits to the transplant unit are initially on a weekly basis, but thereafter the frequency of appointments decreases and eventually most patients visit the center every 6 months for reevaluation. Routine hematologic and biochemical investigations are performed in a local hospital, which include determining cyclosporine levels and performing monthly lung function testing. The results are faxed to the transplant center, and any changes in immunosuppression are made as appropriate.

Each patient has an annual exercise test on the treadmill or bicycle ergometer supervised by a member of the rehabilitation team. Arterial blood gases are taken immediately before and following the exercise testing, and monitoring of heart rate and rhythm and arterial SaO_2 continues throughout the exercise test. Cardiac catheterization, right and left side, is performed on all HLT recipients at the end of the first and fourth postoperative years to monitor for the development of accelerated coronary atherosclerosis, although this complication is rare in our experience. Endomyocardial biopsies are routinely taken during the procedure. Recipients of DLT, BSLT, and SLT have cardiac catheterization studies performed at the end of the first year to measure hemodynamics and inspect the vascular anastomoses. All lung transplant recipients have annual technetium-99m-labeled diethylenetriamine penta-acetic acid (DTPA) and ultrafast CT scans. In addition, routine clinical examination is performed, as are routine hematologic and biochemical investigations, lung function tests, chest radiographs, and electrocardiographs.

Continued patient well-being depends on well-coordinated multidisciplinary postoperative care. Patients are educated about possible postoperative complications and advised to contact the unit if there are any problems. The importance of returning to as normal a lifestyle as

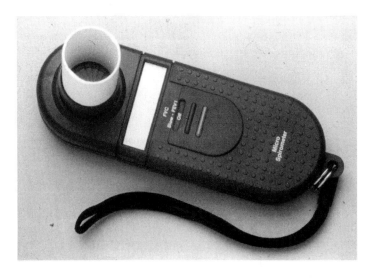

FIGURE 15–3. A home spirometer.

possible is stressed. Each patient receives information leaflets on discharge, giving advice on issues such as immunosuppression, diet, exercise, sexual activity, foreign travel, support groups, and possible postoperative problems. With a regular exercise program, general deconditioning is often relatively quickly reversed in these patients.

Survival Results

One- and 2-year survivals of 61% and 51%, respectively, were reported in a series of 303 pediatric and adult patients who underwent HLT for a variety of pulmonary vascular (57%) and parenchymal (43%) lung diseases.[18] No statistically significant difference in survival was noted between those patients who underwent HLT for pulmonary vascular disease when compared to those who had HLT for parenchymal lung disease.[18] The International Society for Heart and Lung Transplantation reported a similar 1-year survival of 59% for HLT.[14] The largest number of HLTs for CF patients was reported in two surveys in the United Kingdom.[16,29] In both series, 1-year survival was approximately 70% and intermediate (5.5 year) survival was also encouraging.[18] A North American Group reported a 43% 1-year survival in 33 HLT recipients with CF. Sepsis was the major cause of death.[7] More recently, centers are favoring the techniques of BSLT for CF and are reporting survival rates similar to that of the UK experience with HLT.[23,27] One-year survival as high as 62% for DLT and 69% for SLT, performed for a variety of pulmonary vascular and parenchymal diseases, has been reported.[14]

Lung Function

In general, lung function improves rapidly after transplantation and attains 70% of predicted normal values or higher by the third postoperative month. Studies have shown that the improvement in lung function is maintained to the third postoperative year.[16]

Quality of Life

There is no doubt that the quality of life improves significantly for the successfully transplanted patient. Many patients have returned to school, work, or higher education after surgery. Some have gone on overseas holidays. Some have married; and three of our female patients have delivered healthy children. Using the Nottingham Health Profile, HLT recipients have been shown to enjoy improved levels of social and emotional well-being.[3]

Obliterative Bronchiolitis

Obliterative bronchiolitis is the most serious late complication following lung transplantation, with a cumulative probability of occurrence of 40% by the third postoperative year.[18] The incidence is higher in children under age 10 years. The diagnosis is made clinically in patients with progressive airflow obstriction, often in the presence of infection. Cough, reduced exercise capacity, and deterioration in lung function are typical presenting features. The chest radiograph is usually normal, although it may reveal hyperinflated lung fields. The diagnosis may be supported by a ^{99m}Tc DPTA lung scan, ultrafast CT scan, and transbronchial lung biopsies.

The etiology of obliterative bronchiolitis remains unclear. An association with acute episodes of viral infection has been suggested.[10] Further evidence suggests that obliterative bronchiolitis may represent a final common pathway to pulmonary injury from a variety of etiologies, which include acute and chronic allograft rejection and viral and bacterial infection.[21,30] It is essential, therefore, that early diagnosis of acute rejection and pulmonary infection be made, and early intervention be undertaken to reduce the incidence of this complication. Once the diagnosis is made, immunosuppression is augmented with oral prednisolone, 1 mg/kg/day for a period of up to 1 month, and thereafter, the dose is reduced over a period of time to a maintenance dose of 0.2 mg/kg/day, in addition to cyclosporine and azathioprine. Unfortunately, only a minority of patients regain lost lung function on this regimen. The majority either stabilize at lower levels of lung function or deteriorate progressively to end-stage respiratory failure. Those patients who fail to respond to steroid therapy and their families need support and counseling during this period. It can be very difficult to readjust to recidive illness once a formerly chronically unwell patient has had his or her quality of life transformed by successful lung transplantation. It is also of paramount importance to be honest with patients during this time about their future. At present, the only remaining treatment option for patients with end-stage respiratory failure secondary to obliterative bronchiolitis is retransplantation.[7,17,18] However, many centers do not retransplant patients with obliterative bronchiolitis because of limited donor organ availability and the poor results associated with retransplantation. One-year survival of 30% following retransplantation for obliterative bronchiolitis has been reported.[14]

References

1. Bray CE: Transcutaneous neural stimulation. In Webber BA, Pryor JA (eds): Physiotherapy for Respiratory and Cardiac Problems. Edinburgh, Churchill Livingstone, 1993, p 343.
2. Breslow MJ, Mill CF, Rogers M: Perioperative management. St. Louis, CV Mosby, 1990.
3. Caine N, Sharples LD, Smyth R, et al: Survival and quality of life of cystic fibrosis patients before and after heart-lung transplantation. Transplant Proc 23:1203–1204, 1991.
4. Cooper J: Current status of lung transplantation. Transplant Proc 23:2107–2114, 1991.
5. Craven JL, Bright J, Dear CL: Psychiatric, psychological and rehabilitative aspects of lung transplantation. Clin Chest Med 11:247–257, 1990.
6. Curtis JR, Deyo RA, Hudson LD: Health-related quality of life among patients with chronic obstructive pulmonary disease. Thorax 49:162–170, 1994.
7. Frist WH, Fox PW, Campbell SB, et al: Cystic fibrosis treated with heart-lung transplantation: North American results. Transplant Proc 23:1205–1206, 1991.
8. Glanville AR, Baldwin JC, Burke CM, et al: Obliterative bronchiolitis after heart-lung transplantation: Apparent arrest by augmented immunosuppression. Ann Intern Med 107:300–304, 1987.
9. Goldstein RS: Ventilatory muscle training. Thorax 48:1025–1033, 1993.
10. Griffith BP, Paradis IL, Zeevi A, et al: Immunologically mediated disease of the airways after pulmonary transplantation. Ann Surg 208:371–378, 1988.
11. Guyatt GH, Berman LB, Townsend M: Long term outcome after pulmonary rehabilitation. Can Med Assoc J 137:1089–1095, 1987.
12. Hodson ME, Madden BP, Steven MH, et al: Non-invasive mechanical ventilation for cystic fibrosis patients: A bridge to transplantation. Eur Respir J 4:524–527, 1991.
13. Jones P, Quirk FH, Baeystock CM, Littlejohns P: A self-completed measure of health status for chronic airflow limitation: The St. George's Respiratory Questionnaire. Am Rev Respir Dis 145:1321–1372, 1992.
14. Kaye M: The Registry of the International Society of Heart and Lung Transplantation: Ninth Official Report. J Heart Lung Transplant 11:599–606, 1992.
15. Lewiston N, King, V, Umetsu D, et al: Cystic fibrosis patients who have undergone heart-lung transplantation benefit from maxillary sinus antrostomy and repeated sinus lavage. Transplant Proc 23:1207–1208, 1991.
16. Madden BP, Hodson ME, Tsang V, et al: Intermediate-term results of heart-lung transplantation for cystic fibrosis. Lancet 339:1583–1587, 1992.
17. Madden B, Khaghani A, Yacoub M: Successful retransplantation of the heart and lungs in an adult with cystic fibrosis. J R Soc Med 84:561, 1991.
18. Madden B, Radley-Smith R, Hodson ME, et al: Medium term results of heart and lung transplantation. J Heart Lung Transplant 11:S241–S243, 1992.
19. Madden B, Kamalvand K, Chan CM, et al: The medical management of patients with cystic fibrosis following heart-lung transplantation. Eur Resp J 6:965–970, 1993.
20. Madden B, Geddes DM: Which patients should receive lung transplants? Monaldi Arch Chest Dis 48:346–352, 1993.
21. Madden BP, Siddiqi AJ, Pomerance A, Burke M: Possible ethological factors in obliterative bronchiolitis following lung transplantation. Pediatr Pulmonol (Suppl 9):273, 1993.
22. Madden B: Lung transplantation for cystic fibrosis. In Hodson ME, Geddes DM (eds): Cystic Fibrosis. London, Chapman and Hall, 1994, p 329.
23. Pasque M, Cooper JD, Kaiser LR, et al: Improved technique for bilateral lung transplantation: Rationale and initial clinical experience. Ann Thorac Surg 49:785–791, 1990.
24. Patterson GA: Double lung transplantation. Pediatr Pulmonol 4:456–457, 1989.
25. Patterson GA, Todd TR, Cooper JD, et al: Airway complications after double lung transplantation. J Thorac Cardiovasc Surg 99:14–21, 1990.
26. Petty TL: Pulmonary rehabilitation in perspective: Historical roots, present status and future projections. Thorax 48:855–862, 1993.
27. Ramirez JC, Patterson GA, Winton TL, et al: Bilateral lung transplantation for cystic fibrosis. J Thorac Cardiovasc Surg 13:287–294, 1992.
28. Ries AL: Position paper of the American Association of Cardiovascular and Pulmonary Rehabilitation: Scientific basis of pulmonary rehabilitation. J Cardiopulm Rehabil 10:418–441, 1990.
29. Scott J, Higenbottam T, Hutter, J, et al: Heart-lung transplantation for cystic fibrosis. Lancet ii:192–194, 1988.
30. Scott JP, Sharples L, Mullis P, et al: Further studies on the natural history of obliterative bronchiolitis following heart-lung transplantation. Transplant Proc 23:1201–1202, 1991.
31. Shankar S, Fulsham L, Read R, et al: Mucociliary function after lung transplantation. Transplant Proc 23:1222–1223, 1991.
32. Singh SJ, Morgan MDL, Scott SC, et al: The development of the shuttle walking test of disability in patients with chronic airways obstruction. Thorax 47:1019–1024, 1992.
33. Toronto Lung Transplant Group: Experience with single lung transplantation for pulmonary fibrosis. JAMA 259:2258–2262, 1988.
34. Wallis S: Domino cardiac transplantation. Paediatr Nurs 5:24–26, 1993.
35. Williams TJ, Grossman RF, Maurer JR: Long term functional follow-up of lung transplant recipients. Clin Chest Med 11:347–358, 1990.

Sexuality and Individuals with Respiratory Impairment

16

Marca L. Sipski, MD

Sexuality is an important part of life from the time we are born until the time we die. Unfortunately the importance of sexuality is often overlooked by clinicians, who place their emphasis on medical and not psychosocial concerns. For those individuals who suffer from pulmonary dysfunction, their sexual function may be impaired because of fear related to lack of knowledge, psychological, or organic factors. Left alone, patients may be reluctant to voice concerns related to their sexuality. Therefore, it is important for the clinician who works with pulmonary patients to accept that sexuality is an integral part of living a full life and to encourage patients to address their concerns. One model by which this may be done is through the PLISSIT (permission/limited information/ specific suggestions/intensive therapy) model of Annon.[2] In this manner, the patients are given permission to discuss their sexuality with any one of their health care providers. Next, they are provided limited information by the practitioner when concerns come up—to the extent the practitioner is able. Specific suggestions are the next level of care that is appropriate. This may include giving information on modifying sexual positions or timing of sexual activity. Finally, intensive therapy is reserved for those instances in which individual or couples counseling is necessary regarding psychological issues or aggressive medical or surgical management.[2]

IMPACT OF PULMONARY DISEASE ON LIFE IN GENERAL AND SEXUAL FUNCTION

Lung disease affects the whole life of an individual. Consequently, declining pulmonary function leads to diminished ability to perform all activities. Individuals who suffer from chronic obstructive pulmonary disease (COPD) commonly feel a loss of control over their lives.[7] Marital and family roles may be reversed when the disabled individual must give up his or her source of employment. This can result in relationship stressors and anxiety in addition to a loss of self-esteem in the person with pulmonary disease. The added assistance that the disabled individual may need from his or her significant other may also create anger and frustration in both parties. These psychological issues, including loss of self-esteem, anger, fear, depression, and feeling a loss of self-control, can cause a diminution in desire for sexual activity. Moreover, they can cause psychogenic problems with sexual response and orgasm.

Physical changes associated with lung disease are numerous. The most predominant symptom is dyspnea, and it occurs with increasing frequency and intensity as the respiratory impairment worsens. Chronic fatigue is also commonly present, and as pulmonary reserves decrease an individual may find his or her mobility extremely limited. Prescribed medications can also cause physical problems. Equipment that the individual with pulmonary disease may need to use, such as oxygen or medication delivery equipment or a portable ventilator, can be cumbersome. Each of these physical changes, in turn, can contribute to decreased interest and ability to participate in sexual activity.

Pulmonary disease has many causes. Patients may suffer from chronic bronchitis, asthma, emphysema, or carcinoma of the lung. They may also suffer from pulmonary disease as a result of cystic fibrosis (CF), muscular dystrophy, or spinal cord injury. Depending on the cause of the person's lung disease, there may be concomitant medical issues that must be treated, such as paralysis, spasticity, infections, or decubiti. In addition, the elderly individual with chronic lung disease frequently suffers from other nonrelated medical conditions, such as diabetes mellitus, peripheral vascular disease, or systemic hypertension. The impact of these other conditions must also be taken into account when one considers the sexual function of any individual with pulmonary disease.

Although diminished respiratory capacity can cause a person to have less energy for and during sexual activity, it should not prohibit sexual activity. The physiologic demands of activity are described in Mets—the amount of oxygen consumed per kilogram of body weight per minute. Penis-vagina sexual intercourse uses the equivalent amount of energy as walking 3 miles per hour: 3 to 4 Mets. Different positions and different types of activities require more or less energy use. Therefore the individual with pulmonary disease should approach sexual activity with an aim at minimizing energy expenditure while maximizing pleasure. Although pulmonary disease itself generally does not cause physical changes in genital sexual responsiveness, concomitant medical problems or medications can do so and need to be addressed.

EFFECT OF AGING
ON SEXUAL RESPONSE

Many patients with pulmonary disease are elderly. Therefore, it is important to know how aging affects sexual response. Aging results in a number of predictable changes in sexual response that can lead to psychological distress if the individual is not aware of them. Older men have been found to need a longer time and

more direct penile stimulation to achieve an erection. Erections are also less firm, and detumescence occurs more readily and rapidly. Although it is easier for older men to delay ejaculation, the force of semen expulsion and the number of muscular contractions during ejaculation is decreased. Moreover, older men generally exhibit an increase in their refractory period such that they may need several days between orgasms.[13]

Women who are postmenopausal experience thinning of the vaginal mucosa and loss of elasticity related to the loss of estrogen. Hormonal replacement can be useful to restore normal vaginal function. Masters and Johnson[13] studied sexual response and aging. They found that aging women required prolonged stimulation to produce vaginal lubrication and that the amount of lubrication was decreased. With orgasm, the women's sensation was the same; however, fewer and weaker pelvic muscle contractions occurred. Although changes in sexual response occur in both sexes with aging, under normal circumstances they should not interfere with sexual activity. Unfortunately, when individuals lack knowledge of the age-related changes (e.g., taking a longer time to have an erection), they may become distressed. This psychological distress can then lead to further problems (e.g., psychogenic impotence). The vicious cycle that ensues may be resolved only by educating the individual.

PATTERNS OF SEXUAL DYSFUNCTION
AFTER PULMONARY DISEASE

Sexual dysfunction associated with pulmonary disease can be divided into four categories: (1) inhibited sexual desire, (2) inhibited sexual arousal, (3) inhibited orgasm, and (4) other problems.[6] To understand fully the impact of pulmonary disease on an individual's sexual functioning, one must understand how the disease has affected the individual, the concomitant medical problems, and psychological issues. Then the sexual dysfunction can be evaluated and categorized.

Inhibited sexual desire can occur with pulmonary disease as with any other chronic medical illness. The individual with pulmonary disease must spend a lot of energy to perform activities of daily living. He or she may also be fatigued, dyspneic, and hypoxic. This may result in diminished libido. Decreased sexual desire can also occur owing to fear of dyspnea during sexual activity or that medical harm may occur. With chronic illness, men and women may also experience an altering of their body shapes and find themselves unattractive and undesirable. These feelings can also lead to a decrease in sexual desire. Common medications, such as theophylline, sympathomimetic bronchodilators, and corticosteroids, can cause secondary effects that interfere with the individual's interest in sex.[19] Theophylline, for example, can cause nausea, restlessness, headache, and irritability leading to diminished libido. In contrast, corticosteroids can cause truncal obesity, fluid retention, easy bruising, and moon facies. These physical changes can lead to decreased self-esteem and resultant lack of interest in sexual activity.

Inhibited sexual arousal refers to the inability of an individual to achieve erection or lubrication successfully during sexual activity. Various studies have examined the frequency of impotence with pulmonary disease. One report noted that 6 of 20 men with COPD suffered from erectile dysfunction,[8] whereas another found that 6 of 23 men with COPD who completed a rehabilitation program reported complete impotence for 1 year.[1] In a larger study of 90 men with COPD, Kass and associates[10] noted that 17 men admitted to problems attaining an erection. Impotence in the man with COPD may be due to a number of factors. Depression about chronic illness, loss of self-esteem, fear of hypoxia, and relationship conflicts can all contribute to psychogenic impotence. Lack of knowledge regarding the effects of aging on erectile function can also contribute to psychogenic impotence. Concomitant medical conditions, such as diabetic neuropathy or spinal cord injury, can lead to physical causes of impotence. Medications such as some antihypertensives can also cause erectile dysfunction. Moreover, it has been suggested that COPD may result in male impotence in the absence of other known causes.[8]

Female sexual function has been studied less than male sexual function. As such, little information is available on the effect of pulmonary disease on lubrication. It follows, however, that similar problems apparently occur in women with pulmonary disease. Psychological issues, such as depression and loss of self-esteem, may lead to inability to be aroused. Medications can also cause an absence of lubrication. Finally, an overwhelming concern over dyspnea can cause a woman to be unable to achieve lubrication.

Inhibited orgasm occurs less frequently than impairment of the excitement phase of sexual response; however, it can still occur for a number of reasons.[16] Concomitant neurologic disease may result in decreased ability to achieve orgasm. Moreover, some medications impair the ability to achieve orgasm. For instance, in men, phenothiazines can interfere with both emission and the sensory experience of orgasm.[17] Women often experience orgasmic dysfunction when taking antidepressant drugs. As with the other types of sexual dysfunction, psychological issues can also contribute to the inability to achieve orgasm.

Other problems of sexual functioning that can occur in the individual with pulmonary disease include premature ejaculation, priapism, dyspareunia, and vaginismus. As with the other categories, these problems may have, at least in part, a psychological cause or be due to concomitant medical problems.

SPECIFIC DISORDERS AND THEIR IMPACT ON SEXUALITY

CF is a genetically determined chronic illness. Although previously these patients died at a young age, they are now living longer and can be expected to lead active sexual lives. One study evaluated married CF patients to investigate their sexual functioning.[12] Twenty percent of patients 19 years of age and older were found to be married. All 30 of these married patients were interviewed, as were 21 of their spouses. Nineteen of the 30 patients were female and 11 were male. Seventeen couples, including 11 women and 7 men with CF, were found to have good sexual relationships. Thirteen couples, including 12 women and 5 men with CF, were noted to have minor to serious sexual problems. These problems included infrequent orgasm in one woman who was not considered to have impaired pulmonary function. One man complained of psychogenic impotence during a period when he was considering divorce. Nine patients complained of significantly decreased sexual desire. Sixteen patients complained that sexual intercourse often provoked coughing, and nine patients complained of occasional difficulties during intercourse owing to the weight of their partner on their chests. Severity of disease was evaluated in this study and found not to correlate with the presence or absence of sexual difficulties.

Asthma is a disorder characterized by reversible obstructive airway disease. The airways of asthmatics react to a variety of stimuli with edema and bronchoconstriction. Asthma can occur at any time in life.[20] It is often associated with allergies, and acute episodes can be precipitated by emotional or physical overactivity. Sexual activity can be a source of emotional excitement and thus can precipitate an asthmatic episode. This is even more likely if it is a first sexual encounter or if the individual is concerned about performing well. If an acute episode does occur, the individual may react by avoiding future sexual encounters. It is important, therefore, for these individuals to receive sex education and counseling.[27] This way early parental prohibitions, fears, or misconceptions can be addressed, eliminating, it is hoped, some of the individual's anxiety and diminishing the possibility of provoking an acute episode. Bronchodilator medication can also be useful when taken before sexual activity.[18]

Patients with neuromuscular disease are considered elsewhere in this text.

TREATMENT OF IMPOTENCE

In the past 10 years, the treatment of impotence has greatly improved. The silicone penile prosthesis, first used in 1968,[11] began a new era of medical treatment for erectile dysfunction. These devices all require a surgical procedure and are placed in the cavernous bodies of the penis. They are available in three basic types: malleable, inflatable, and self-contained inflatable. The malleable prosthesis has the advantage of having a low complication rate of from 5% to 10%; however, it has the disadvantage of causing permanent penile rigidity. Inflatable prostheses have the advantage of allowing the penis to be in both semiflaccid and erect states; unfortunately, their complication rates at 5% to 15% tend to be higher than with the malleable devices. The traditional inflatable prosthesis has cylinders placed in the cavernous bodies that are connected by tubing to a reservoir and pump contained in the scrotum. With this prosthesis, to stimulate an erection, the man squeezes the pump between his fingers, forcing the saline solution into the cylinders. The newest inflatable prosthesis has two cylinders with deep and middle chambers. The penis is semiflaccid when fluid is in the deep chamber. Fluid is pumped into a middle chamber to produce an erection.[17]

None of the penile prostheses recreates a normal erection. They cannot improve sensation, desire, or other aspects of a man's sexual response cycle. Although complication rates in the nonneurologically impaired are low, complication rates as high as 33% have been noted in individuals with spinal cord injury.[5] The destructive aspect of prosthesis insertion, in addition to the potential for complications, should make this a last choice effort in treatment of impotence. In addition, it is important that those individuals who are considering prosthesis surgery be provided with the opportunity for psychological consultation to understand contributing psychogenic factors involved in impotence.

Another alternative for treating impotence is the vacuum pump. These devices are available from many manufacturers. A large cylinder connected to a pump that produces a vacuum is placed over the flaccid penis. After 4 to 6 minutes in the vacuum, an erection is stimulated. It is most beneficial if the man is sitting or standing during the pumping.[14] The erection is then maintained by placement of a band or constricting ring of some sort at the base of the penis. When used as directed, these erections are relatively safe; however, they can cause ecchymoses or petechiae. Users should also be cautioned not to fall asleep with the ring on and should limit their use to 30 minutes because after this time risk of penile ischemia and resulting complications increases. It should be noted that with the vacuum, there is engorgement of both corporeal and extracorporeal tissues; therefore the erection that occurs has greater girth than normal. The penis may also appear cyanotic with dilation of superficial veins, and pivoting can occur at the base.

Other treatments available for erectile dysfunction include the use of rings at the base of the penis without the pump for those men who are able to obtain but not sustain an erection. The same precautions should be used with the rings alone as with the pump. Most recently, surface applications of various vasoactive drugs have also been advocated to treat impotence. These have included nitroglycerin[15] and minoxidil.[4] Yohimbine, a presynaptic alpha$_2$-adrenergic blocker with action on blood vessels similar to reserpine, is also commonly used as an oral agent for treatment of impotence. Double-blind studies have shown, however, that although it was effective for psychogenic impotence, it was not better than placebo in patients with organic impotence.[3]

RECOMMENDATIONS FOR HELPING PATIENTS MAINTAIN SEXUAL ACTIVITY DESPITE PULMONARY DISEASE

For the health care professional to assist patients in maintaining sexual activity despite pulmonary disease, it is important for the professional to be comfortable with the topic and to express a nonjudgmental attitude toward the patient's sexual desires.[9] Without this, communication is stifled, and the patient should be referred to another health care professional who is more able to discuss the subject.

It is better for the physician, than for the patient, to bring up the topic of the effect of the patient's illness on sexual function. In this way, even though patients may choose not to discuss the subject at the time, they have permission to do so in the future. It is also appropriate to address sexual issues with the patient's spouse or significant other. Of course, the physician should have a basic understanding of sexual physiology as well as of the impact of pulmonary disease on sexuality.

Patients should be apprised of the metabolic requirements of sexual activity. They should be told that increases in respiratory and heart rates are normal with sexual activity. The impact of pulmonary disease and any other illness they may have on sexual functioning should be discussed. Medications should be reviewed, and discussion with the patient of potential side effects on sexual functioning may be appropriate. Patients and their partners should consider varying positions to limit energy expenditure during sexual activity (see later), and suggestions can be made to time sexual activity during the day when the affected individual's energy level is optimal. Sexual activity should not occur after a full meal owing to the limitations in respiratory capacity caused by abdominal compression. Performance of bronchial hygiene or chest physical therapy before sexual activity may be helpful for some individuals.

Suggestions can also be given to the patient and partner to try mutual masturbation as a way to relieve sexual tension with low energy expenditure or to use various sexual aids such as a vibrator. Use of a waterbed may facilitate movement during sexual activity, and supplemental oxygen may also be helpful.

In addition to providing general information, the clinician should also give patients with pulmonary disease opportunities to address their concerns regarding sexuality and sexual function. One way to discuss the psychological issues concerning the individual, such as low self-esteem or depression, is to ask how he or she feels about sexual activity then to discuss the specific concerns and fears. If the patient is married or has a significant other, the significant other should also be invited to voice feelings and concerns. An open, assertive approach allows the patient to explore sexuality, and when a sexual problem occurs, he or she feels comfortable addressing the issue and seeking help.

POSITIONING FOR SEXUAL ACTIVITIES WITH RESPIRATORY DISEASE

Practical suggestions can help the individual with pulmonary disease save energy during sexual activity. Proper ventilation and a cool comfortable room are important to allow the individual to be comfortable. Certain sexual positions are also less taxing than others and may be recommended. For couples in which one individual is afflicted by respiratory disease, it is important to avoid applying pressure on the affected individual's chest. Sidelying with the woman turned away or with both individuals facing each other is also a good position that may be useful when either the man or woman suffers from pulmonary dysfunction. Having the man seated with the woman on top with her back toward him is another position with low energy requirement that is good for either men or women who need to use oxygen (Figs. 16–1 through 16–3). Couples can also sit in bed with their legs straddled and face each other, or the woman can kneel or lean on a table or dresser while the man enters her from behind (Figs. 16–4 through 16–6).

Certainly, there are other options for sexual activity aside from genital intercourse. Oral sex can be even more enjoyable than intercourse for the man or woman and can easily be performed on the affected man or woman who is lying down with the head up on pillows or is seated (Figs. 16–7 and 16–8). Comfortable positioning can also be found for individuals with pulmonary disease to perform oral sex on their partners; however, care must be taken so that they are able to breathe properly. Other activities, such as masturbation, or the use of assistive devices, such as vibrators, can also help diminish the energy requirements for sexual activity while maximizing the pleasure involved.

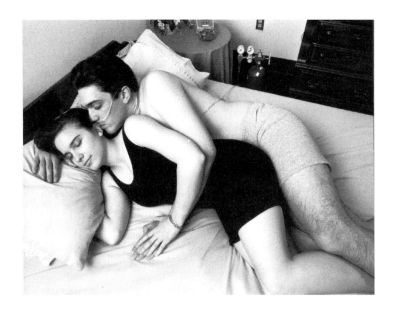

FIGURE 16–1. Sidelying intercourse position for impaired man.

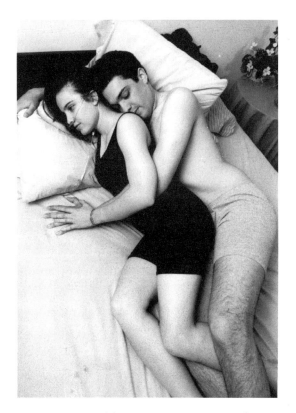

FIGURE 16–2. Sidelying intercourse position for impaired woman.

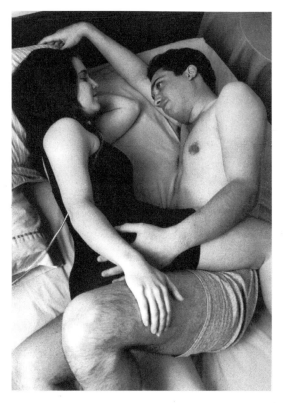

FIGURE 16–3. Face-to-face sidelying intercourse position.

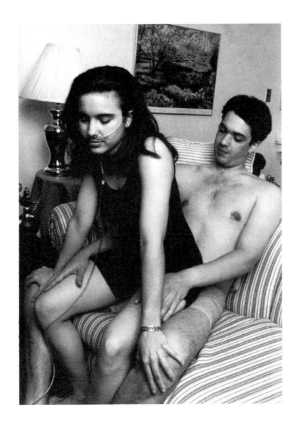

FIGURE 16–4. Seated intercourse position for impaired woman.

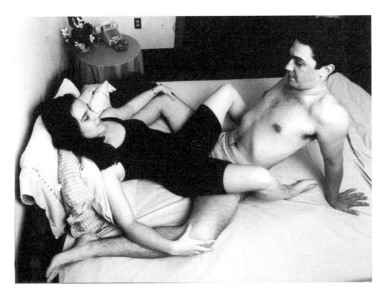

FIGURE 16–5. Restful intercourse position with couples face to face.

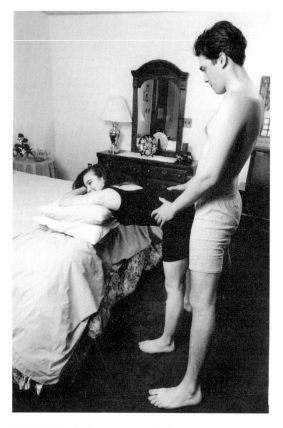

FIGURE 16–6. Rear entry restful intercourse position for impaired woman.

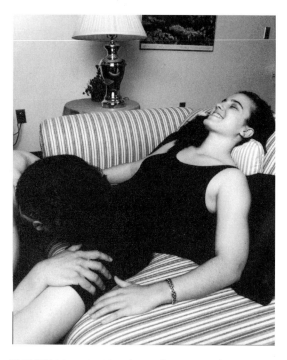

FIGURE 16–7. Position for performing oral sex on impaired woman.

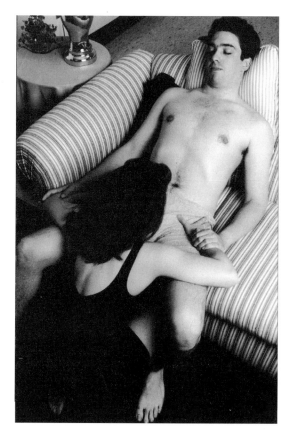

FIGURE 16–8. Position for performing oral sex on impaired man.

Acknowledgment

Grateful acknowledgment is made to Susan M. Gilbert and Ruth Abujudeh for their support in the preparation of this manuscript.

References

1. Agle DP, Baum GL: Psychological aspects of chronic obstructive pulmonary disease. Med Clin North Am 61: 749–758, 1977.
2. Annon JS: The Behavioral Treatment of Sexual Problems. Honolulu, Enabling Systems, 1976.
3. Basile G, Goldstein I: Medical treatment of neurogenic impotence. Sexuality Disability 12:81–94, 1994.
4. Cavallini G: Minoxidil versus nitroglycerin: A prospective double-blind controlled trial in transcutaneous erection facilitation for organic impotence. J Urol 146:50–53, 1991.
5. Collins K, Hackler R: Complications of penile prostheses in the spinal cord injury population. J Urol 240:984–985, 1988.
6. Constain JS, Haas SS, Salazer-Schicchi J: Sexual aspects of the pulmonary-impaired person. In Haas F, Axen K (eds): Pulmonary Therapy and Rehabilitation: Principles and Practice, ed 2. Baltimore, Williams & Wilkins, 1991, pp 315–326.
7. Dudley DL, Sitzman J, Rugg M: Psychiatric aspects of patients with chronic obstructive pulmonary disease. Adv Psychosom Med 14:64–77, 1985.
8. Fletcher EC, Martin RJ: Sexual dysfunction and erectile impotence in chronic obstructive pulmonary disease. Chest 81:413–421, 1982.
9. Francoeur RT: Sexual components in respiratory care. Respir Manage 18(2):35–39, 1988.
10. Kass I, Updegraff K, Muffly RB: Sex in chronic obstructive pulmonary disease. Med Aspects Hum Sex 6:33–42, 1972.
11. Lash H: Silicone implant for impotence. J Urol 100:709, 1968.
12. Levine SB, Stern RC: Sexual function in cystic fibrosis. Chest 81:422–428, 1982.
13. Masters WH, Johnson VE: Human Sexual Response. Boston, Little, Brown, 1966.
14. Nadig PW: Vacuum constriction devices in patients with neurogenic impotence. Sexuality Disability 12:99–106, 1994.
15. Owen JA, Saunders F, Harris C, et al: Topical nitroglycerin: A potential treatment for impotence. J Urol 141:546–658, 1989.
16. Schover LR: Sexual problems in chronic illness. In Leiblum SR, Rosen RC (eds): Principles and Practice of Sex Therapy. New York, Guilford Press, 1989, p 326.
17. Schover LR, Jensen SB: Sexuality and Chronic Illness: A Comprehensive Approach. New York, Guilford Press, 1988.
18. Sipski ML: Spinal cord injury: What is the effect on sexual response? J Am Paraplegia Soc 14:40–43, 1991.
19. Thompson WL: Sexual problems in chronic respiratory disease. Sexual Dysfunction 79:41–52, 1986.
20. Thompson WL, Thompson TL: Psychiatric aspects of asthma in adults. Adv Psychosom Med 14:33–47, 1985.

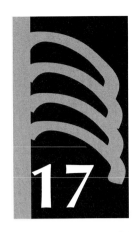

Disability Evaluation

Horacio D. Pineda, MD

Respiratory disease affects the physical, psychological, social, and vocational aspects of a person's life. Not infrequently, physicians are asked to evaluate how diseases in general and respiratory diseases in particular affect total body function. Among disability evaluators, the question is often how much functional loss has resulted from a disease process. This considers the problem from a negative viewpoint. Rehabilitation specialists are trained to view the problem from a more positive perspective. They are usually more interested in how much functional potential remains to be developed.

Evaluation of degree of functional loss or potential, however, is difficult. This is because of the multitude of systems being used in disability and capacity evaluation. No single universally acceptable method exists. Evaluation techniques for determining impairment or disability caused by respiratory disease have been suggested by the American Thoracic Society (ATS), the American Medical Association (AMA), and the Social Security System (SSS), among others. Although some of their criteria overlap, it is unclear which system is most accurate.

The impact of respiratory disease on function correlates with the severity, permanency, and rate of progression of the disease. As with other diseases, lung disease may be mild, moderate, or severe. Although in most instances respiratory disease is relentlessly progressive (as with emphysema), in some cases respiratory status can improve (high-level Guillain Barré Syndrome). Some diseases such as chronic obstructive pulmonary disease (COPD) leave permanent sequelae, whereas others affect the patient only temporarily. Therefore, one must consider whether the actual disease course is stable or progressive for any particular patient. After pneumonectomy, an individual finds breathing and general function significantly altered. Provided that remaining lung is healthy, however, the patient's condition should remain fairly stable. For most diseases, however, including COPD and sarcoidosis, slow steady progression is the rule. Consequently, progressively increasing disability and decreasing functional capacity occur.

The role of oxygen consumption, nutrition, work of breathing, dyspnea, and deconditioning cannot be overstated. Mammals depend primarily on aerobic metabolism to function. Simply stated, mammals need oxygen to satisfy the energy requirements of various bodily functions. Unfortunately, lung disease adversely affects oxygen consumption ($\dot{V}O_2$). The raw materials for this energy come from food and are therefore dependent on the individual's nutritional status. Too little food intake, as often occurs in severe COPD, leads to weakness and cachexia, but too much food may lead to obesity. This, in turn, can contribute to respiratory volume restriction and increased work of breathing.

Physical deconditioning occurs frequently as lung disease progresses. Dyspnea may be an important factor in the development of deconditioning. Dyspnea results from physical exertion, and it occurs at lower levels of energy expenditure, the more severe the respiratory disease process. To avoid dyspnea, most patients refrain from exercising. With time, this leads to physical and cardiovascular deconditioning, reducing exercise capacity beyond levels that can be explained by the primary disease pathology. Being deconditioned, patients discover that they experience dyspnea at ever lower levels of physical exertion, which leads to less exercise and more deconditioning. Unchecked, this cycle of dyspnea and deconditioning may totally disable the patient. Finally, the cost of breathing at rest has been found by most investigators to be 0.5 to 1 mL/L of ventilation.[4] The more severe the lung disease, however, the higher the energy cost of breathing, leaving much less energy for other activities.

The terms *normal, impairment, disability,* and *handicap* deserve reconsideration. The term *normal* has been defined as "the state of being healthy, efficient, free of obvious physical defects, free of symptoms, and having ability to withstand physical effort or strain, and the capacity to work."[7] *Impairment* is the loss of, loss of use of, or derangement of any body part, system, or function, which may be permanent or temporary and mild, moderate, or severe.[1] Impairment refers to a purely medical condition. The much broader term *disability* indicates "the total effects of impairment on a person's life."[2] It is also defined as the inability to engage in substantial gainful activity by reason of any medically determinable physical or mental impairment that has lasted or can be expected to last for a continuous period of not less than 12 months.[10] It considers factors such as age, sex, socioeconomic status, education, and occupation that can result in an individual's inability to meet certain physical, social, vocational, and economic responsibilities. Handicap occurs when an individual's work, mobility, and interpersonal and social roles are impeded because of a negative interplay of disability and environment. By changing the environment with wheelchair-accessible homes, transportation, and workplaces, wheelchair-bound patients' handicaps can be minimized.

EVALUATION OF IMPAIRMENT AND DISABILITY

Evaluating a patient with respiratory disease is a difficult and complex process. It entails making an accurate diagnosis of the condition and assessing its severity and permanence. The physician must understand the pathophysiology of the disease as well as its natural course. It also includes evaluating the treatment and its effects. In some cases, the treatment can result in more disability. To aid the clinician, a complete history and physical examination are vital. Laboratory tests and procedures such as radiologic studies (chest radiographs and computed tomography), bronchoscopy, cytology, pulmonary function testing, blood gas analyses, and exercise testing are important.

Respiratory disease can affect the airways, the lung parenchyma, the respiratory muscles, and the vascular and neurologic connections. Airway diseases such as emphysema, chronic bronchitis, asthma, and bronchiectasis all cause an increase in airway resistance. They, however, have individual differences in terms of symptoms, clinical course, treatment, prognosis, and ultimately outcome. Bronchitis and bronchiectasis manifest profuse tracheobronchial secretions. Bronchitis also predisposes to early hypoventilation and perfusion abnormalities that result in cyanosis and plethora. Emphysema patients have progressive, irreversible destruction of alveoli and terminal airways with expiratory airway obstruction leading to air trapping. In contrast to patients with bronchitis, they are not cyanotic until late in the disease. Asthmatics suffer from periodic bronchospastic episodes or attacks sometimes triggered by allergies, infections, or other noxious agents, which result in acute respiratory distress and wheezing. Patients generally respond well to bronchodilation and steroid medications and can sometimes enjoy relatively symptom-free periods between attacks. Asthma, bronchitis, and emphysema can coexist in a patient. These conditions are generally progressive and can ultimately lead to respiratory failure and cor pulmonale.

Restrictive diseases result in reduced lung volumes. Reduced lung volumes may result from parenchymal diseases, such as sarcoidosis, asbestosis, infections, or neoplastic diseases; musculoskeletal deformities, such as kyphoscoliosis or pectus excavatum; or neuromuscular diseases, such as muscular dystrophy, poliomyelitis, or Guillain-Barré syndrome. Musculoskeletal and neuromuscular restrictive diseases frequently involve more than the respiratory system and thus cause much greater disability. Clinical presentations and prognoses differ as well. A C-5 complete quadriplegic, for example, may have adequate inspiratory function but complete paralysis of expiratory muscles making coughing ineffective. A muscular dystrophy patient presents with progressive weakness of inspiratory, expiratory, and skeletal muscles. A severe kyphoscoliotic patient may present with compression of one hemithorax and a relative overexpansion of the opposite side. This results in uneven distribution of ventilation. At times, the condition itself presents no obvious disability, but the resulting treatment can. A patient with an asymptomatic malignant lung tumor may function normally but after surgical pneumonectomy may be at least partially disabled. As in other illnesses, restrictive diseases may be progressive (sarcoid) or static (polio, spinal cord injury), gradual in development (muscular dystrophy, sarcoid) or sudden (pneumonectomy), permanent or temporary.

Impairment from respiratory disease, a purely medical condition, adversely affects the patient's physical functioning in general and respiratory functioning in particular. Disability from respiratory disease results from the effects of respiratory impairment on the patient's life as a whole. Proper evaluation of the effects of disease include assessment of physical, psychological, social, vocational, and economic implications.

PULMONARY FUNCTION TESTING

Pulmonary function testing (PFT) evaluates the functional status of the different components of respiration. Airway integrity, lung volumes, lung and chest wall mechanics, the alveolar membrane, ventilation, and blood gas parameters are measured. The patient's results are compared with values from the *normal* population of the same age, sex, height, and weight. The effects of respiratory disease on lung function can, therefore, be quantitated. Based on the results, it can be determined that the disease process has primarily impaired airway integrity (obstructive lung disease), static lung volumes (restrictive lung disease), or both. Severity is estimated by calculating the percentage of difference between the patient's values and those of the normal population.

PFT parameters are widely used to evaluate impairment and disability in patients with pulmonary disease. Spirometry measures static and dynamic lung volumes and ventilation parameters. The total lung capacity (TLC) and its subdivisions can be mapped out and changes qualitatively and quantitatively compared to normal predicted values. These tests are especially important in the diagnosis of restrictive disease. Airflow parameters, whether measured using timed forced vital capacity (FVC) or a flow vol-ume loop, can be used to assess changes in airway resistance during inspiration and expiration. These tests are especially important in diagnosing obstructive lung diseases and can differentiate whether the obstruction is intrathoracic or extrathoracic, variable, or fixed.

Diffusion capacity to carbon monoxide (DLCO) is particularly important in assessing gas transfer in restrictive parenchymal disease. It is also important when the severity of the patients' disease seems to be more than what spirometry values indicate.

Finally, blood gas analysis is used to assess the sum total effect of the different pulmonary subfunctions in terms of oxygenation and ventilation.

Measurement of maximum oxygen consumption ($\dot{V}O_2$max) is important for estimating the individual's capacity for physical work. This can be accurately and noninvasively measured during exercise testing with a metabolic analyzer (clinical exercise testing). Aerobic metabolism is the primary means by which energy is derived from food. The higher the patient's $\dot{V}O_2$max, the higher the capacity to do physical work. Not surprisingly, *fitness* can be determined by the value of the $\dot{V}O_2$max. The energy cost of different activities is assessed by how much oxygen is consumed during their performance (Table 17–1).[9] If a patient's $\dot{V}O_2$max is known, one can use the energy cost table to determine which activities the patient can or cannot do. Activities for which the oxygen cost is less than the $\dot{V}O_2$max are theoretically tolerable.

One metabolic equivalent (Met) is 3.5 mL/kg/minute of oxygen consumed or the amount of basal oxygen consumption at rest. Oxygen consumption can easily be assessed in Mets, that is, in multiples of basal metabolic rate. The European Society for Clinical Respiratory Physiology recommended that respiratory disability assessments be based on maximal oxygen uptake. One hundred percent disability was defined as an "inability to achieve during exercise a rate of energy expenditure in excess of twice that used at rest, that is, more than 2 Mets."[3]

The American Medical Association uses $\dot{V}O_2$max and the PFT parameters FVC, forced expiratory volume in 1 second (FEV_1), FEV_1/FVC ratio, and extent of dyspnea to evaluate and classify impairment from respiratory disease (Table 17–2).[1] By contrast, the American Thoracic Society uses the same three PFT parameters and DLCO (Table 17–3).[6] Impairment is rated as none, mild, moderate, or severe. Mildly impaired individuals usually do not have diminished ability to perform most jobs. Moderate im-

TABLE 17–1
Energy Cost of Some Occupational
and Recreational Activities

Activity	Cal/Min	METS	Activity	Cal/Min	METS
Rest, supine	1.0	1.0	Hand sewing	1.4	1.0
Sitting	1.2	1.0	Sweeping floor	1.7	1.5
Standing, relaxed	1.4	1.0	Machine sewing	1.8	1.5
Eating	1.4	1.0	Polishing furniture	2.4	2.0
Conversation	1.4	1.0	Peeling potatoes	2.9	2.5
Dressing, undressing	2.3	2.0	Scrubbing, standing	2.9	2.5
Washing hands, face	2.5	2.0	Washing clothes	3.0	2.5
Bedside commode	3.6	3.0	Kneeding dough	3.3	2.5
Walking, 2.5 mph	3.6	3.0	Scrubbing floors	3.6	3.0
Showering	4.2	3.5	Cleaning windows	3.7	3.0
Using bedpan	4.7	4.0	Making beds	3.9	3.0
Walking downstairs	5.2	4.5	Ironing, standing	4.2	3.5
Walking, 3.5 mph	5.6	5.5	Mopping	4.2	3.5
Propulsion, wheelchair	2.4	2.0	Wringing by hand	4.4	3.5
Ambulation, braces	8.0	6.5	Hanging	4.5	3.5
and crutches			Beating carpets	4.9	4.0
Watch repairing	1.6	1.5	Painting, sitting	2.0	1.5
Armature winding	2.2	2.0	Playing piano	2.5	2.0
Radio assembly	2.7	2.5	Driving car	2.8	2.0
Sewing at machine	2.9	2.5	Canoeing, 2.5 mph	3.0	2.5
Bricklaying	4.0	3.5	Horseback riding,	3.0	2.5
Plastering	4.1	3.5	slow		
Tractor ploughing	4.2	3.5	Volleyball	3.0	2.5
Horse ploughing	5.9	5.0	Bowling	4.4	3.5
Wheeling barrow 115	5.0	4.0	Cycling, 5.5 mph	4.5	3.5
lbs, 2.5 mph			Golfing	5.0	4.0
Carpentry	6.8	5.5	Swimming, 20 yd/	5.0	4.0
Mowing lawn by hand	7.7	6.5	min		
Felling tree	8.0	6.5	Dancing	5.5	4.5
Shoveling	8.5	7.0	Gardening	5.6	4.5
Ascending stairs 17 lb	9.0	7.5	Tennis	7.1	6.0
load, 27 ft/min			Trotting horse	8.0	6.5
Planing	9.1	7.5	Spading	8.6	7.0
Tending furnace	10.2	8.5	Skiing	9.9	8.5
Ascending stairs 22 lb	16.2	13.5	Squash	10.2	8.5
load, 54 ft/min			Cycling, 13 mph	11.0	9.0

From Rusk HA (ed): *Rehabilitation Medicine.* St. Louis, CV Mosby, 1977.

pairment indicates diminished ability to meet the physical requirements of many jobs, and severe impairment indicates inability to meet the physical demands of most jobs. The Social Security System uses spirometry (FEV_1, FVC), blood gas analysis, DLCO, and exercise testing in evaluating impairment (Table 17–4).[10]

If significant impairment is noted from the results of spirometry, arterial blood gas analysis can help determine whether an impairment meets or is equivalent in severity to a disability listing (Table 17–5).[10] Whenever the blood gases are chronically impaired, DLCO and steady-state blood gases sampled while the pa-

tient is exercising at a workload of about 12 mL O_2/kg/minute or 5 Mets may also be useful. DLCO determination is necessary whenever existing evidence, including spirometry, is inadequate to establish the level of functional impairment. DLCO values less than 10.5 mL/minute (single breath method) or less than 40% of normal predicted values establish chronic impairment of gas exchange from any cause.

ESTIMATING FUNCTIONAL CAPACITY

The physician interested in the rehabilitation of patients with lung disease must be interested

TABLE 17–2
Classes of Respiratory Impairment

	Class 1 0% No Impairment	Class 2 10%–25% Mild Impairment	Class 3 30%–45% Moderate Impairment	Class 4* 50%–100% Severe Impairment
Dyspnea	The subject may or may not have dyspnea. If dyspnea is present, it is for nonrespiratory reasons or it is consistent with circumstances of activity	Dyspnea with fast walking on level ground or when walking up a hill; patient can keep pace with persons of same age and body build on level ground but not on hills or stairs	Dyspnea while walking on level ground with person of the same age or walking up one flight of stairs. Patient can walk a mile at own pace without dyspnea but cannot keep pace on level ground with others of same age and body build	Dyspnea after walking more than 100 M at own pace on level ground. Patient sometimes is dyspneic with less exertion or even at rest
	or	or	or	or
Tests of ventilatory function[†]				
FVC FEV_1 FEV_1/FVC ratio (as percent)	Above the lower limit of normal for the predicted value as defined by the 95% confidence interval	Below the 95% confidence interval but greater than 60% predicted for FVC, FEV_1 and FEV_1/FVC ratio	Less than 60% predicted but greater than 50% predicted for FVC, 40% predicted for FEV_1, 40% actual value for FEV_1/FVC ratio	Less than 50% predicted for FVC, 40% predicted for FEV_1, 40% actual value for FEV_1/FVC ratio, 40% predicted for DCO
	or	or	or	or
$\dot{V}O_2$max	Greater than 25 mL/(kg·min)	Between 20–25 mL/(kg·min)	Between 15–20 mL/(kg·min)	Less than 15 mL/(kg·min)

*An asthmatic patient who, despite optimum medical therapy, has had attacks of severe bronchospasm requiring emergency room or hospital care on the average of 6 times per year is considered to be severely impaired.
[†]FVC=Forced vital capacity; FEV_1=forced expiratory volume in 1 second. At least one of the three tests should be abnormal to the degree described for classes 2, 3, and 4.
From American Medical Association: Guides to the Evaluation of Permanent Impairment, 2nd ed. Chicago, American Medical Association, 1984.

TABLE 17–3
American Thoracic Society Rating of Impairment*

Impairment	FVC	FEV_1	FEV_1/FVC	DLCO
Normal	≥80%	≥80%	≥75%	≥80%
Mild	60%–79%	60%–79%	60%–74%	60%–79%
Moderate	51%–59%	41%–59%	41%–59%	41%–59%
Severe	50% or <	40% or <	40% or <	40% or <

*All values represent percent of predicted.
Data from American Thoracic Society: Evaluation of impairment/disability secondary to respiratory disorders. Am Rev Respir Dis 133:1205–1209, 1986.

in knowing not only the extent of functional loss, but also, more importantly, how much function remains. A patient's remaining functional capacity determines whether he or she can be a productive member of society. In addition to knowing a patient's capacity, the medical community and society as a whole must collaborate in developing it. The criteria used to determine disability play a role in functional capacity determinations. Remaining pulmonary or ventilatory function can be estimated from the patient's PFTs and arterial blood gases. In addi-

TABLE 17–4
Social Security System Respiratory Impairment Classification

COPD

Height without shoes (cm)	Height without shoes (in.)	FEV$_1$ equal to or less than (L, BTPS)
154 or less	60 or less	1.05
155–160	61–63	1.15
161–165	64–65	1.25
166–170	66–67	1.35
171–175	68–69	1.45
176–180	70–71	1.55
181 or more	72 or more	1.65

Chronic Restrictive Pulmonary Syndrome

Height without shoes (cm)	Height without shoes (in.)	FVC equal to or less than (L, BTPS)
154 or less	60 or less	1.25
155–160	61–63	1.35
161–165	64–65	1.45
166–170	66–67	1.55
171–175	68–69	1.65
176–180	70–71	1.75
181 or more	72 or more	1.85

tion, a clinical exercise test is crucial because it allows estimation of how much actual physical work can be done and at what metabolic cost. Disability parameters focus on the time-honored pulmonary function subtests: FEV$_1$, FVC, FEV$_1$/FVC, maximum voluntary ventilation (MVV), and DL$_{CO}$. Other subtests that may indicate early, presymptomatic disease are no less important, particularly from the point of view of prevention. Maximum midexpiratory flow rates (MMEF or FEV 25 to 75), closing volume, and volume of isoflow can sometimes show abnormalities even before FEV$_1$, FVC, MVV, or blood gases show significant changes. Knowing these early changes is important for instigating primary prevention even before clinical disease is apparent.

Pulmonary function and resting blood gas values, however, do not permit accurate estimation of remaining functional capacity. A study of severely impaired COPD patients showed poor correlation between PFT parameters and exercise capacity. Even the best statistical correlation, that of FEV$_1$, was shown to account for only 56% and 60% of the observed variation in $\dot{V}O_2$ and external work.[8]

When evaluating exercise capacity, therefore, the energy requirement of certain activi-

ties (household task, job requirements, sports activities) and the patient's biologic capacity to do physical work must be estimated. One yardstick that can be used is the patient's $\dot{V}O_2$max. Because most biologic activities use aerobic metabolism, not surprisingly, $\dot{V}O_2$max had been used by many as a tool to estimate exercise capacity. Assmussen and Orbach, for example, proposed grading work capacity based on different percentages of aerobic capacity:

10% of aerobic capacity = light work.
10% to 30% of aerobic capacity = moderate work.
30% to 50% of aerobic capacity = hard work.
50% or more of aerobic capacity = exceedingly hard work.

Oxygen consumption is a reflection of how efficiently the heart and lungs function as a unit. It is expressed by the product of the arteriovenous oxygen difference and the cardiac output. The better the patient's lung and heart function, the more oxygen can be delivered to meet metabolic demands. During exercise, the interrelationship of the lungs, cardiovascular system, and skeletal muscles is closely interwoven for proper coupling of cellular and pulmonary res-

TABLE 17–5
Respiratory Impairment Defined by
Arterial Blood Gas Sampling
(Social Security System)

A*†

Arterial Paco$_2$ (mm Hg)	Arterial Pao$_2$ equal to or less than (mm Hg)
30 or below	65
31	64
32	63
33	62
34	61
35	60
36	59
37	58
38	57
39	56
40 or above	55

B‡

30 or below	60
31	59
32	58
33	57
34	56
35	55
36	54
37	53
38	52
39	51
40	52

C§

30 or below	55
31	54
32	53
33	52
34	51
35	50
36	49
37	48
38	47
39	46
40 or above	45

*Disability indicated by arterial blood gas values measured while at rest (breathing room air, awake, and sitting or standing), with the patient clinically stable, on at least two occasions, 3 or more weeks apart within a 6-month period.
†Applicable at test sites 3000 feet above sea level.
‡Same as A but applicable at test sites 3000 through 6000 feet above sea level.
§ Same as A but applicable at test sites 6000 feet above sea level.

piration. Failure in any of these three systems can seriously compromise gas transfer and consequently adversely affect exercise capacity.

Training, likewise, plays a role in exercise tolerance. The better trained the individual is at a certain activity, the better and more efficient his or her performance. During work evaluation, therefore, the exercise testing modality must, as much as possible, approximate the main tasks that the patient needs to perform. It is inappropriate, for example, to use an arm crank ergometer rather than a treadmill to assess a patient's capability for long distance running. By doing so, the testing does not reflect the task the patient was trained for and does not provide accurate results.

Efficiency is another important factor in assessing functional capacity. Efficiency is generally defined as:

$$E = output/input \times 100$$

During exercise, output represents external work usually expressed in calories, and input is the oxygen consumption (converted to calories) needed to do the work. An efficient, well-trained patient can do more physical work with a minimum cost in oxygen consumption. Without considering efficiency, one might mistakenly believe that if the energy cost of walking 2.5 mph equals 3 Mets (according to published tables), a patient with a $\dot{V}O_2$max of at least 3 Mets can always perform this activity. The truth is that these tables are usually derived from young, healthy populations of individuals without the complicating medical conditions so common in elderly patients with pulmonary disease, such as arthritis or coronary artery disease. Patients with such concomitant conditions cannot be expected to walk as efficiently as the *normals* and may actually require a higher oxygen consumption than otherwise expected.

Task-specific exercise testing is important for evaluating functional capacity. Figure 17–1 represents an idealized exercise testing technique.[5] The patient is given an exercise modality that closely resembles the activity he or she wishes to accomplish. To assess cardiovascular parameters during exercise, blood pressure and electrocardiographic monitoring are done. Respiratory monitoring is accomplished using a metabolic analyzer with a spirometer and flow volume loop set up interfaced in between. Chest wall excursions and respiratory rate are measured using accelerometers or strain gauge monitors attached to the chest. Using this technique, simultaneous measurement of ventilation, chest wall motion, airflow (to detect

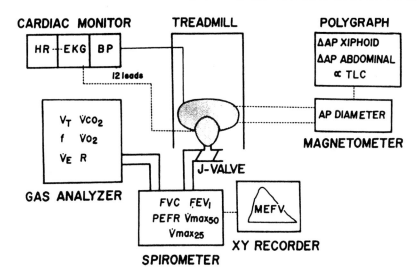

FIGURE 17–1 Idealized exercise testing setup in which, at any given exercise lead, pulmonary, cardiac, and chest wall parameters can be simultaneously monitored. *HR*=Heart rate; *EKG*=electrocardiogram; *BP*=blood pressure; V_T=tidal volume; $\dot{V}_E$=minute ventilation; *f*=frequency of breathing; *R*=respiratory exchange ratio; $\dot{V}CO_2$=CO$_2$ production; $\dot{V}O_2$=O$_2$ consumption; *FVC*=forced vital capacity; *PEFR*=peak expiratory flow rate; *FEV$_1$*=forced expiratory volume after 1 second; $\dot{V}MAX_{50}$=maximum expiratory flow at 50% forced vital capacity; $\dot{V}MAX_{25}$=maximum expiratory flow at 25% forced vital capacity; *MEFV*=maximum expiratory flow volume curve; *AP*=change in AP diameter.

exercise-induced bronchospasm), and aerobic parameters ($\dot{V}O_2$, $\dot{V}CO_2$, anaerobic threshold, respiratory quotient) can be accomplished at any time during rest, exercise, and recovery. Knowledge of the cardiac and respiratory limits of the patient in relation to external work allows a safe, objective means of prescribing or advising physical exercise to respiratory patients.

DISABILITY PREVENTION

The World Health Organization expert committee on disability prevention and rehabilitation describes three levels of prevention. The first level is aimed at reducing the occurrence of impairment. The second level is aimed at limiting or reversing disability caused by impairment. The third level is aimed at preventing the transition of disability into handicap. To accomplish these requires the combined efforts of the medical community, industry, government, and the country as a whole. It is unfortunate that the present system of medical reimbursement is aimed at secondary prevention. This implies that the patient must first get sick before receiving appropriate help. Primary prevention or preventing occurrence of or probability of developing respiratory disease before it happens may be the better approach. More effort should be paid at stopping smoking, giving immunizations, providing a safe work environment, and

giving better education. These practical methods should be as universally accessible as are curative and rehabilitative services.

References

1. American Medical Association: American Medical Association Guides to the Evaluation of Permanent Impairment, 2nd ed. Chicago, American Medical Association, 1984, pp 85–101.
2. American Thoracic Society: Evaluation of impairment/disability secondary to respiratory disorders. Am Rev Respir Dis 133:1205–1209, 1986.
3. Coles JE, Chinn DJ, Reed JW, et al: Experience of standardised method for assessing respiratory disability. Eur Respir J 7:875–880, 1994.
4. Fenn W, Rahn H: Respiration. In Handbook of Physiology. Baltimore, Waverly Press, 1964, p 463.
5. Goodgold J: Rehabilitation Medicine. St. Louis, CV Mosby, 1988, p 378.
6. Haas F, Axen F: Pulmonary Therapy and Rehabilitation: Principles and Practice, 2nd ed. Baltimore, Williams * Wilkins, 1991, p 111.
7. Kessler HH: Disability Determination and Evaluation. Baltimore, Williams & Wilkins, 1979, p 8.
8. Pineda H, Haas F, Axen K, et al: Accuracy of pulmonary function testing in predicting exercise tolerance in chronic obstructive pulmonary disease. Chest 86:564–567, 1984.
9. Rusk HA: Rehabilitation Medicine, 4th ed. St. Louis, CV Mosby, 1977, pp 552, 557.
10. U.S. Department of Health and Human Services: Disability Evaluation Under Social Security. SSA, Publication No. 05-10089. Washington, D.C., U.S. Government Printing Office, 1986, pp. 28–34; and Program Operations Manual System, Part 04, Chapter 340, 1994.

Vocational Rehabilitation for Persons with Pulmonary Disease

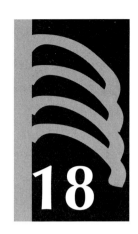

Theresa Keegan, MA, CRC

In 1942, *rehabilitation* was described as the restoration of the individual to the fullest medical, mental, emotional, social, and *vocational* potential of which he or she is capable.[6] The aim of rehabilitation programs is to return the client to maximum potential functioning. Most pulmonary rehabilitation programs described in the medical literature, however, do not have a vocational component. In fact, it appears that little has been attempted or accomplished in this area, and the need for the vocational rehabilitation of persons with disabilities continues to be underestimated. Nevertheless, returning to gainful employment is important for optimizing the patient's sense of well-being, psychosocial functioning, and quality of life. This chapter explores the underlying principles and structure of a vocational rehabilitation program and applications to persons with pulmonary disorders.

VOCATIONAL REHABILITATION AND CAREER GUIDANCE

The generally accepted goal of vocational rehabilitation is to assist the person with disability to return to work and to be self-sufficient.[14] This process began in 1909 with Parsons, the primary architect of vocational guidance in the United States. Parsons's most enduring contribution was the three-step outline of the vocational guidance process that he referred to as *true reasoning*. This involved establishing a clear understanding of the individual's aptitudes, abilities, interests, resources, limitations, and other qualities; a knowledge of the requirements and conditions for a successful return to gainful employment and the advantages and disadvantages, potential compensation opportunities, and prospects in different lines of work; and true reasoning of the relations of these two groups of facts.[1] When considering this, it becomes evident that a comprehensive vocational rehabilitation program must encompass a holistic and individualized course of action if optimal results are to be achieved.

Why do people work? If you were to take a poll, many might answer "because I have to." In the rehabilitation setting, however, when respiratory disease renders someone unable to work, that person loses much more than just a job. He or she may be faced with an identity crisis—because people often define "who they are" by "what they do," and when that role is taken away, even temporarily, it can lead to anxiety, depression, loss of self-esteem, agitation, anger, and feelings of helplessness that can magnify the patient's respiratory symptoms.

Work is a multifaceted human enterprise, done for intrinsic, social, and extrinsic rewards. A number of variables can influence a disabled individual's vocational potential and choice. For someone growing up with disability, low expectations and restricted opportunities impair social development to the point that "the work personality simply remains undeveloped."[15]

Later onset of disability can also have an impact on vocational development. Kunce[10] reported that "difficulties involved in rehabilitation vary directly with the interference that the given disability has upon the individual's lifestyle." Specifically, he found that individuals experiencing physical disabilities, who valued physical activity highly, encountered more problems in restructuring their lifestyles than those who did not.[10]

Environmental and cultural factors also play a large role in what vocation a person chooses. Temperature, pollutants, odors, and other factors can determine the environment in which one can perform. Likewise, in some ethnic groups, it is not "acceptable" for a man to work in a traditionally female occupation even though the environment of that employment might be cleaner and advantageous with regards to his medical condition.

Work setting factors should also be addressed when attempting to choose a career. Structural features include locale, proximity of work site to the client's home, transportation, length of the work day, and the essential functions of the job.[15]

The amount of interpersonal support needed can affect whether or not someone is ready for competitive employment or work adjustment training. The latter is appropriate if the person needs considerable support and is therefore not job-ready. Another consideration is the social implications of a particular work site. The client must conform to certain rules of appearance, conduct, and manner appropriate to that particular setting.[16]

In working with a person with chronic obstructive pulmonary disease (COPD), the greatest benefits can be achieved by early referral to vocational rehabilitation services. Unfortunately, service delivery schedules in rehabilitation programs usually place vocational services at the bottom of the list (Table 18–1) and list them as additional (not essential) services.[6] Perhaps this should not be surprising given the fact that so few published studies consider vocational outcomes in COPD rehabilitation programs.[12] Those that do, however, demonstrate positive results. Haas and Cardon compared a rehabilitation group of 252 COPD patients with a group that did not receive rehabilitation. At 5 years after rehabilitation, twice as many patients in the rehabilitation group were able to return to their former jobs; another 13% in the rehabilitation group (and 0% in the unrehabilitated group) were employed in other jobs.[4a] Whereas vocational benefits may be difficult to achieve in the presence of severely disabling conditions, even severely disabled ventilator users can maintain gainful employment despite their reliance on computers and voice synthesizers to

TABLE 18–1
Rehabilitation Program Services

Essential Services

Initial medical evaluation and care plan
Patient education, evaluation, and program coordination
Respiratory therapy techniques
Physical therapy techniques
Daily performance evaluation
Social service evaluation
Nutritional evaluation

Additional Services

Psychological evaluation
Psychiatric evaluation
Vocational evaluation

function and communicate. Clearly a referral for vocational evaluation is appropriate regardless of the extent of physical disability.

Consultation from a vocational/career guidance counselor is appropriate when the patient is medically stable and ready to participate. Generally, a vocational referral encompasses the following order of services:

1. *Vocational intake.* The client is interviewed by the counselor to gather background information, including a work and educational history, environmental and social circumstances, and goals and interests. This information is considered along with the client's abilities and physical limitations to plan for individualized testing and planning strategies.
2. *Vocational evaluation.* Appropriate tests are selected for each client based on the goals established during the intake interview. Evaluations are then administered to assess aptitudes, interests, work-samples, personality profiles, and other measures to determine potential. The results establish realistic employment or educational goals and the skills that the client can use in a potential school or work setting.
3. *Vocational/guidance counseling.* This is provided on an ongoing basis from the time the counselor first meets the patient and may continue even after work placement. Counseling provides ongoing support, helps the person realize potential, and assists with the formulation and achievement of vocational goals. Often, during this phase, the counselor develops a rapport with the client that results in mutual trust and respect.

4. *Job development training and placement.* Once a realistic job, skill, or educational goal is determined, the counselor contacts and visits employers to facilitate the client's return to work or to develop new jobs for the client if returning to the former job is not feasible. Additional job sources may include business directories, family and friends, job banks, placement advisory boards, and government agencies. If the person requires occupational retraining or wants to attend college, the counselor refers him or her to the Division of Vocational Rehabilitation (DVR) (to be discussed) and explores financial resources.

5. *Labor market survey.* The counselor often performs a labor market survey to determine a client's potential for employment before sending the client on interviews. The counselor contacts local companies (based on the client's geographic location) and presents the person's skills, education, abilities, and work history to the prospective employers. The counselor is then able to determine whether or not there are appropriate jobs available in the local labor market for someone with the client's background.

6. *Job-site analysis.* In the event that a client can return to his or her employer or if a new job placement has been achieved, the counselor visits the employer (or school when appropriate) and assesses whether the environment and work conditions are in accordance with the Americans with Disabilities Act. The counselor also offers consultation for job modifications to insure that the client's surroundings are comfortable, safe, and accessible.

The importance of ongoing vocational rehabilitation counseling must be emphasized. Someone going through a rehabilitation program is almost always referred to as a "patient." Although this may be true in a medical sense, such individuals tend to lose their identities as spouses, students, parents, or workers. Most decisions are made for them during rehabilitation, including what they eat, where they go and when, what their goals are, and the proposed length and extent of their rehabilitation programs. This facilitates dependence and indecisiveness, and individuals lose control over many, if not all, aspects of their lives. The same person is then referred for vocational rehabilitation and instructed to be motivated, decisive, goal-oriented, independent, and responsible for his or her livelihood. I often say to clients, "Reality begins here." It is no small wonder that these individuals become overwhelmed by the thought of career planning and returning to a job when they have been conditioned to be passive. This phenomenon can often lead to client dissatisfaction because they expect the vocational counselor to "do everything for them."[2,4,12,13,19]

Consumer satisfaction, however, is a central component of quality management. According to Johansson and McArthur,[9] "quality is first and foremost a perception in the consumer's eyes," and according to Hutchens,[8] "in searching for a usable and quantifiable basis for an organization's quality strategy, the focus changes from internal to external—to the customer."

The focus of any quality vocational rehabilitation program is the client. His or her opinions, beliefs, and personality traits are considered—using the results of testing as a guide in the overall evaluation. For example, why try to convince someone with an aptitude to become an engineer to obtain training in this field if he or she wants to be a security guard? It may be true that the individual is working below his or her aptitude, but if that is the career the client chooses, a good vocational counselor does not try to convince the client otherwise—as long as the client is made aware of his or her abilities and potential.

The flip side is also true. If someone wants to become an engineer but demonstrates a low aptitude in that area, it is the counselor's responsibility to point that out to the individual and to make it clear that he or she would be taking on an uphill battle. It is not, however, the counselor's responsibility to discourage someone from striving to achieve his or her desired goals. It has been proven that some people overcome their limitations despite overwhelming odds:

> While you flex your muscles in front of your morning mirror and congratulate yourself on your nimble brain, consider this: The light over your mirror was perfected by a deaf man. While your morning radio plays, remember the hunchback who helped invent it. If you listen to contemporary music, you may hear an artist who is blind. If you prefer classical, you may enjoy a symphony written by a composer who couldn't hear. The President who set an unbeatable American political record could hardly walk. A woman born unable to see, speak, or hear stands as a great achiever in American history. The handicapped can enrich our lives. Let's enrich theirs.

Others may not be able to overcome limitations. Either way, the person must discover that for himself or herself.

To ensure that the client is getting the best quality of service to achieve the greatest poten-

---

KESSLER INSTITUTE FOR REHABILITATION, INC.
CAREER GUIDANCE AND PLACEMENT SERVICES
CLIENT SATISFACTION PHONE SURVEY

Hello, I am calling from the Career Guidance and Placement Service office at Kessler Institute (formerly Vocational Services).

May I speak with _____.
Name

I am following up with some clients to find out how our department can better provide services and help our clients return to work.
Have you ever received vocational rehabilitation services from our department?

Yes   or   No

Would you be willing to help us by answering some questions about your experience with us?

Questions

1. Are you currently attending school?
2. If so, which school?
3. What is your major?
4. When are you graduating?
5. If not in school, are you interested in attending?

Yes   or   No

6. Were you treated with respect and courtesy by our staff?
7. Did your counselor promptly schedule appointments?
8. Do you feel your counselor took time to listen to your needs?
9. Were your questions answered and valuable information provided?
10. Did you feel involved in making decisions about and planning your future.
11. Did the counselor help you get or keep a job?
12. Are you working now?
13. If so, is it the same job you had prior to your injury?
14. How would you rate your experience with our department?

Very Good	Satisfactory	Fair	Poor
1	2	3	4

15. What are 1 or 2 things that caused you satisfaction or dissatisfaction?

AT THIS POINT THANK THE INDIVIDUAL FOR RESPONDING AND GIVE THEM THE KESSLER TOLL-FREE NUMBER AND MY NAME AND EXTENSION IN CASE THEY HAVE ANY QUESTIONS ABOUT SERVICE OR NEED ANYTHING ELSE FROM OUR DEPARTMENT.

THERESA KEEGAN 1 (800) 248-3221
Extension 305

FIGURE 18–1. One-month postdischarge phone survey for client satisfaction.

---

tial, a vocational rehabilitation program should survey client satisfaction. Two surveys developed by our facility are shown in Figures 18–1 and 18–2. They represent the 1-month postdischarge phone survey and follow-up mail-in surveys that are performed at 6-month and 1-year intervals.

First, the purpose of these questionnaires is to improve the quality of services extended to the clients by considering and possibly implementing any suggestions they might have. Second, it is interesting to note whether the re-sponses on the phone surveys correlate with the follow-up mailings.

STATE VOCATIONAL REHABILITATION AGENCIES

The DVR was established pursuant to the Rehabilitation Act of 1973. Every state has established a network of DVR offices that facilitate the employment of individuals with disabilities. In New Jersey, DVR is administratively a division of the New Jersey Department of Labor. DVR is

KESSLER INSTITUTE FOR REHABILITATION, INC.

In order to assist me in improving the Career Guidance & Placement Services for future patients, I would appreciate it if you would complete the following questions about your present rehabilitation status.

CURRENT WORK STATUS

1. Are you still receiving outpatient therapy?   Yes   or   No
2. Are you attending college?   Yes   or   No
   Name of college: _____
   Major (if declared): _____
   Date you expect to complete your degree: _____
3. Are you receiving vocational training?   Yes   or   No
   Name of school: _____
   Type of training _____
4. Are you employed? _____   Yes   or   No
   Name of employer: _____
   Type of employment: _____
   Part-time? _____ Full-time? _____
5. Are you retired?   Yes   or   No

FURTHER INFORMATION

6. Please indicate the TOPICS OF PROGRAMS you would be interested in attending if offered (check all that apply).
   _____ Employment opportunities for the disabled
   _____ Part-time employment
   _____ Social security inservice
   _____ Information—the division of vocational rehabilitation
   _____ Other suggested topics: _____
7. Are you interested in discussing vocational planning at this time?
8. Would you like active assistance in the following (check off desired answers):
   _____ Job-seeking skills
   _____ Resume writing
   _____ How to choose a career
   _____ Training and academic opportunities
   _____ Job interviewing
   _____ Filling out employment applications
   _____ Assistance in finding employment
   _____ Other: _____
9. _____ Transportation (circle desired answers):
   a. Do you have a current N.J. drivers' license?   Yes   or   No
   b. Do you have a car?   Yes   or   No
   c. Do you have a van?   Yes   or   No
   d. Do you need driver training?   Yes   or   No
   e. Are you ready for driver training?   Yes   or   No
10. Have you even been referred to DVR?   Yes   or   No
    If so, do you know who your DVR counselor is?   Yes   or   No

Please contact me if you have any questions concerning your vocational plans.

Thank you,

Theresa Keegan, M.A., C.R.C., Director of Career Guidance and Placement Services Department/West

FIGURE 18–2. Mail-in survey.

an eligibility program, not an entitlement, for persons with disabilities. To be eligible, one must have a physical or mental disability that results in a substantial handicap to employment and a reasonable expectation that vocational rehabilitation services may facilitate employability.

Often, DVR counselors' roles become that of financial facilitators because they rely heavily on the clients' vocational counselors' evaluations and recommendations. When the DVR counselor agrees with the vocational experts, he or she can authorize payment for the provisions noted in Table 18–2.

There may be no cost to the client for any of these services. Expenses for medical services, training, books, supplies, tools, and equipment, however, as authorized by the agency, are subsidized based on each individual's ability to pay. The DVR's financial criteria are less restrictive than those of many other agencies.[7] The DVR counselor is required to exhaust other possible third-party payer options before authorizing subsidies. For example, persons seeking training are required to apply for PELL and other educational grants. The PELL grant, for example, is a federally funded grant that is based on financial need and can be applied for by individuals accepted to college.

PATIENT APPLICATIONS

Every vocational rehabilitation program has to be individualized for specific patient needs if it is to meet the standards of the profession and be effective. Several guidelines assist the physician, social worker, and rehabilitation counselor in determining the likelihood for the successful vocational rehabilitation of COPD clients.[3]

1. If the patient's forced expiratory volume in 1 second (FEV_1) is less than 50% of the forced vital capacity (FVC), the likelihood for

TABLE 18–2
Division of Vocational Rehabilitation Supported Services

Rehabilitation evaluation
Vocational guidance and counseling
Medical appliances and prosthetic device(s)
Training—at colleges, trade, on the job, or in workshops
Occupational equipment and tools
Job placement and follow-up
Postemployment services

achieving work placement is poor. The greater the FEV_1/FVC over 50%, the better the likelihood for return to gainful employment.
2. Individuals whose pulmonary perfusion scans demonstrate impaired perfusion in less than 50% of the total lung area can be good candidates to return to work. Less involvement correlates with better work potential.
3. The presence of moderate to marked right-sided heart failure (cor pulmonale) is a contraindication to inclusion in a vocational rehabilitation program.

Potential candidates for vocational rehabilitation should be referred to vocational counselors as early as possible. The probability for success is greatest with early intervention when the client is first confronted with the need to change lifestyle.

Several factors must be considered when placing the person with COPD in an employment or educational setting, including whether

- The client has the capacity to meet the oxygen requirement needs of the job.[6]
- The client has an effective cough technique and has learned patterned breathing.[5]
- The environment is appropriately controlled —properly ventilated; free of dust, fumes, and odors; and free of temperature extremes.
- Stress and job-related pressures have been minimized.

An on-the-job work evaluation is helpful to restore the client's confidence in his or her capability for future employment. When an on-the-job evaluation is coupled closely with optimal medical treatment, it can be an effective way of initiating career renewal. If the person is returning to his or her job, it may be feasible to alter the work responsibilities without fundamentally changing the client's vocation. If it is obvious that one cannot return to one's usual employment, even with modifications, retraining is necessary. This undertaking depends on patient acceptance of a retraining program and whether the ultimate results will be worth the effort. Clearly, this is a highly individualized consideration that is almost impossible to answer for the hundreds of thousands of people who are disabled by COPD. Nevertheless, even if it is apparent that gainful employment is not feasible, emphasis should be placed on achieving maximal self-reliance and minimizing dependence on the family and community.[11]

Quality of life and the individual's self-concept and sense of dignity are of utmost importance. To optimize these, we must make every effort to help clients return to the mainstream and achieve life fulfillment. Properly devised and applied physical and vocational rehabilitation techniques can help accomplish this, but society must invest the necessary resources.

References

1. Cramer SH: Introduction. In Herr EL, Cramer SH (eds): Through the Life Span. Boston, Little, Brown, 1984, p 3.
2. Downes SC, McFarland FS, Alston PP: Survey of the NRCA membership regarding the basis for evaluating counselor performance. J Appl Rehabil Counsel 5:196–200, 1974.
3. Dyksterhuis JE: Vocational rehabilitation of chronic pulmonary disease patients. Rehabil Lit 33:136–138, 1972.
4. Emener W, Placido D: Client feedback a valuable source of counselor development. J Appl Rehabil Counsel 13:18–23, 1982.
4a. Haas A, Cardon H: Rehabilitation in chronic obstructive pulmonary disease: a 5-year study of 252 male patients. Med Clin North Am 53:593–607, 1969.
5. Hall LK: The structuring of pulmonary rehabilitation services: a new concept. J Cardiopulm Rehabil 13:251–254, 1993.
6. Hodgkin JE: Pulmonary rehabilitation. Clin Chest Med 11:447–460, 1990.
7. Hoens HE: Disability Law: A Legal Primer, 2nd ed., Washington, DC, Vocational Rehabilitation. General Accounting Office, 1992, p 23.
8. Hutchens D: Quality is everybody's business. Management Decisions 23–36, 1986.
9. Johansson H, McArthur D: Rediscovering the fundamentals of quality. Management Review 77:34–37, 1988.
10. Kunce J: Vocational interest, disability and rehabilitation. Rehab Counsel Bull 12:204–210, 1969.
11. Lertzman MM, Cherniack RM: Rehabilitation of patients with chronic obstructive pulmonary disease. Am Rev Respir Dis 114:1145–1165, 1978.
12. Lorenz JR: Setting performance objectives and evaluating individual performance in rehabilitation. Rehabil Administ 3:5–8, 1979.
13. Moriarity JB: Issues in the evaluating of vocational rehabilitation. Professional Psychology 8:641–649, 1977.
14. Mund S: Vocational rehabilitation, employment, self-employment: Vocational rehabilitation process. In Goldenson RM (ed): Disability and Rehabilitation Handbook. New York, McGraw-Hill, 1978, pp 67–71.
15. Neff WS: Work and Human Behavior. New York, Atherton, 1968, pp. 213–234.
16. Neff WS: The world of work. In Herr E (ed): Vocational Guidance and Career Development. Boston, Houghton Mifflin, 1974, pp. 156–179.
17. Petty TL: Chronic Obstructive Pulmonary Disease, 2nd ed. New York, Marcel Dekker, 1985, p 512.
18. Ries AL: Pulmonary rehabilitation. Respir Manag 17:39, 1987.
19. Roessler RT: Vocational counseling consideration for the disabled. In Stanford RE, Roessler RT (eds): Foundations of the Vocational Rehabilitation Process, vol. 2. Baltimore, University Park Press, 1978, p 113.
20. Vernon M, Bussey P, Day DA: The "closure system" and accountability in vocational rehabilitation. J Rehabil 45:45–47, 1979.
21. Wett LM, Petty TL: Effective treatment for emphysema and chronic bronchitis. J Rehabil 33:5, 1967.

Chest Physical Therapy: Mucus Mobilizing Techniques

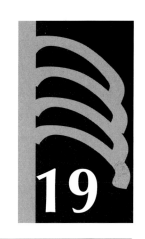

19

Cees P. van der Schans, PT, PhD
Thomas W. van der Mark, PhD
Bruce K. Rubin, MD
Dirkje S. Postma, PhD, MD
Gerard H. Koëter, PhD, MD

AIRWAY SECRETIONS AND TRANSPORT FROM THE LOWER RESPIRATORY TRACT

Healthy Subjects

In adults, at least 10,000 L of air per day expose airway membranes to toxic gases, dust, and microorganisms, some of which are deposited in the lower airways. Effective defense mechanisms are, therefore, required to clear the airways of foreign matter and to keep the lungs sterile. One of the most important lung defense mechanisms is the production of bronchial secretions and the continuous transport of the debris carried by these secretions from the peripheral to the central airways and the oropharynx. Bronchial secretion is a heterogeneous fluid that consists mainly of water (about 95%), dialysable constituents (mainly electrolytes, amino acids, and sugars) and macromolecules.[13,76,78,99,100,142,166] Fundamentally the bronchial secretions, or mucus, are a colloidal suspension of various macromolecular glycoproteins.[78,100]

Mucus is produced throughout the bronchial tree by serous cells, goblet or mucus cells, Clara cells, and type II alveolar cells.[75,76,99,100] The amount of mucus produced at any level in the bronchial tree depends on the number of mucus-producing cells at that level, and the number of these cells is related to the total airway surface. Airway surface decreases from the peripheral to the central airways. The amount of mucus produced in the peripheral airways is, therefore, higher than in the central airways. In normal situations, without pulmonary disease, the total amount of mucus that reaches the trachea is about 10 to 100 mL/day.[76,174]

Transport of material is governed by external mechanical action; that is, forces are needed to transport airway secretions. These forces are counteracted by frictional and inertial forces. In fluid mechanics, the most important frictional forces are internal and determined by the rheologic properties of the fluid. Surface interfacial and adhesive forces between mucus and epithelium, however, may predominate in the airways. Rheology is the science of how a material deforms or stores energy as a result of an applied stress. One of the most important rheologic properties of mucus is viscosity. Viscosity is the resistance to flow and represents the capacity of a material to absorb energy while it moves. In an "ideal" or newtonian fluid, viscosity is a constant for any specific fluid. Mucus, however, is not a newtonian fluid. Thus, viscosity is not a constant but is dependent on the shear rate, the velocity at which the shear stress is applied. Elasticity is the capacity to store energy used to move or deform material. The shear modulus is a measure of the stress needed to induce alterations in the shape of the material. When the shear modulus is high, at comparable forces, less energy is stored in deformation. Consequently, mucus with a high shear modulus may be more easily transported.[83] The ratio between viscosity and elasticity appears to be an important determinant of the transport rate. This ratio is called tangent d, or the loss tangent, and is inversely related to mucus recoil.

Bronchial secretions in the airways can be considered as being separated into two layers: (1) the periciliary sol layer and (2) the gel layer, overlying the periciliary layer (Fig. 19–1). Although the rheology of the sol layer has never been studied, it has a low concentration of glycoproteins and presumably a low viscosity. It is, therefore, always liquid and has no elastic properties. The gel layer consists mainly of mucus. The concentration of cross-linked glycoproteins in this layer is high, making it a nonnewtonian viscoelastic gel. It is likely that only the gel layer is transported. The sol layer, however, is also essential for mucus transport[98] because it provides a low resistance medium for ciliary beating to move debris up the airway.

The transporting surface at any level in the bronchial tree is determined by the cross-sectional diameter of the airways and by the number of airways at any level. Airway diameter decreases but the number of airways increases exponentially from the central to the peripheral airways.[196] As a result, the transporting surface of the airways decreases from the peripheral to the central airways. In the peripheral airways, the transporting surface is somewhat reduced at bifurcations.[66] Owing to the small transporting surface in the central airways, mucus could potentially accumulate. In healthy subjects, accumulation is prevented by the fact that the transport rate of mucus is higher in the central airways than in the peripheral airways[7,95] and possibly by a reduction of the amount of mucus lingering in the central airways owing to reabsorption of its watery constituents.[81,177] In healthy subjects, mucus transport is decreased during sleep.[123] The reasons for this are as yet unknown.[18] In addition, especially during non-REM sleep, the diminished sleep tidal volumes may decrease airway pressure–dependent transport from the peripheral airways.

The most important transport mechanism of mucus in the bronchial tree is mucociliary transport. This takes place by coordinated activity of cilia that cover the bronchial surface of the airways.[178] Ciliated cells are found in the airways from the trachea to terminal bronchioles. Each cell contains about 200 cilia,[116,164,189] which end in little claws.[74] The cilia beat in the direction of the oropharynx with a frequency of about 8 to

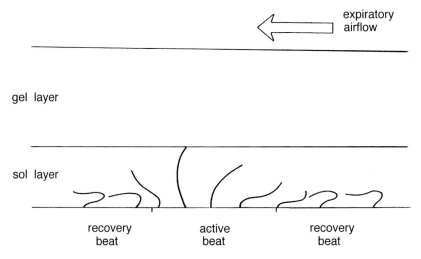

FIGURE 19–1. Respiratory secretions in the airways are separated into two layers: a sol layer and a gel layer. Respiratory cilia have an effective beat in the direction of the trachea (to the left) and a recovery beat in the direction of the bronchiole (to the right). (Modified after Sleigh MA: The nature and action of respiratory tract cilia. In Brain JD, Proctor DF, Reid LM [eds]: Respiratory Defense Mechanisms. New York, Marcel Dekker, 1977, p 247.)

15 Hz. The claws of the cilia reach the mucus gel layer and push this layer toward the oropharynx (see Fig. 19–1). The recovery beat in the direction of the bronchioles takes place only in the periciliary sol layer.[67] Mucus transport by ciliary beating is influenced by the viscoelastic and surface properties of the mucus.[148] Theoretic models suggest that a decrease in the ratio of viscosity to elasticity (loss modulus or tangent d) can lead to an increase in mucociliary transport.[87]

The decrease of the total airway surface and the decreased number of ciliated cells per unit airway surface from the peripheral to the central airways result in a lower mucus transport capacity by ciliary beat in the central airways.[74] This is partly compensated by a higher beat frequency of the cilia in the central airways.[154]

Patients with Airways Diseases

Stasis of secretions in the lower airways and chronic expectoration of mucus are physically and socially disabling symptoms of underlying pulmonary pathology. Stasis of mucus in the airways may contribute to bronchial obstruction in patients with chronic bronchitis and in patients experiencing an acute asthmatic episode. Mucus retention can cause pathologic changes in the lungs[115] and is thought to contribute to the progression of airway disease.[114] Hypersecretion of mucus also appears to be associated with increased mortality,[92,170] and it is thought to contribute to the development of respiratory tract infections. Basically, two mechanisms are responsible for the retention of mucus: hypersecretion and impaired clearance.

Hypersecretion

In healthy individuals, the amount of mucus in the bronchial tree is small. In pathologic conditions, such as bronchitis, however, the production of mucus increases considerably,[71] and the development of sputum arises from a mixture of mucus, inflammatory cells, cellular debris, and sometimes bacteria. Hypersecretion can be caused by inhalation of smoke, by inhalation of antigens triggering inflammation, and by other airway irritants or mechanical stimulation of the upper airways.[130,143] Irritation of the airways also causes changes in the molecular constituents of bronchial secretions. Initially the increased volume of secretions is caused by increased secretion per secretory cell; later on, increases are also due to an increased number of secretory cells.[140,150]

Impaired Mucus Clearance

Mucus transport is often decreased in patients with pulmonary diseases such as asthma,[16] chronic obstructive pulmonary disease (COPD),[23,54,71,158] and cystic fibrosis (CF).[89,204,205] The causes of reduced mucus transport vary depending on the disease processes.

Asthma

Asthma is characterized by sudden episodes of dyspnea and bronchospasm, which can usually be almost completely reversed with therapy.[3] Hypersecretion, which is usually present during these episodes, is a result of mediator release after antigen exposure. Even with resolution of dyspnea and pulmonary dysfunction, there is ongoing airway inflammation and hyperplasia of the mucus glands and cells. Bronchodilation probably has no effect on bronchial mucus transport in these patients.[73] In patients with asthma, a ciliary inhibiting *factor* has been postulated to be present during exacerbations,[43,190] which reduces ciliary activity, disorganizes ciliary beating, and thereby reduces the efficacy of ciliary activity.[198] This *factor* may actually be the result of abnormal physical properties of mucus rather than an intrinsic ciliary inhibitor. Mucociliary transport is markedly reduced in association with unfavorable increases in viscosity and loss tangent—to the lowest levels observed in any clinical situation—in patients with fatal asthma.[137] Mucus hypersecretion and changes in the rheologic or surface properties of mucus may also cause a reduction of ciliary activity.[1,135,139,147] Mucociliary transport, therefore, can be severely reduced in these patients, with a further reduction observed during sleep.[125] After an exacerbation, when the patients are symptom free, mucus transport can recover[53] and become comparable to that of healthy subjects[16,110,113] or remain reduced,[124,125] despite favorable changes in mucus viscoelasticity.

Chronic Obstructive Pulmonary Disease

In patients with COPD, there is persistent dyspnea and airway obstruction with some day-to-day variability and incomplete reversibility with therapy.[31] Although mucociliary transport may be normal in patients with emphysema associated with alpha$_1$-antitrypsin deficiency,[114] in other forms of pulmonary emphysema and COPD it is usually reduced. Mucus transport may also be decreased by smoking-induced ciliary paralysis[43,72,152] and by bacterial infections.[42,199,200] In contrast to patients with asthma, mucociliary transport does not fully recover, and it may progressively decrease owing to a loss of ciliated epithelium by recurrent infections.[200] Hypersecretion, which is usually present in these patients, may also reduce mucociliary transport.

Cystic Fibrosis

Patients with CF initially have normal functioning cilia and an efficient cough.[89] During the course of the disease, however, mucus transport may decrease. The bronchial mucus transport rate in CF patients appears to correlate with the degree of pulmonary function impairment.[138] An inverse correlation between residual volume, expressed as a percentage of total lung capacity, and bronchial mucus clearance rate has been described.[138] Because the coefficient of correlation was low (-0.39), however, only about 16% of the variance in pulmonary function can be explained by differences in the mucus clearance rate. Although bronchial mucus is considered to be a bigger problem in CF than in COPD, the rheologic characteristics of CF sputum are comparable to those of sputum from chronic bronchitis patients.[84,149] Sputum hydration has been postulated to be decreased, but experimental evidence does not support this contention.[149,172] It is more likely that poor mucus clearance in CF airways results from abnormal mucus adhesiveness and tenacity.[151] The small peripheral airways can be completely obstructed by secretions. Recurrent respiratory tract infections in combination with hypersecretion can further reduce mucociliary transport by the mechanisms described previously.

CONTROL OF MUCUS HYPERSECRETION AND CHEST PHYSICAL THERAPY

There are two therapeutic approaches to treat stasis of secretions in the lower airways: medical inhibition of secretion production and facilitation of mucus clearance from the airways.[191] Chest physical therapy (CPT) can be defined as the use of physical measures or techniques, usually applied externally to the chest wall, to facilitate airway secretion elimination and thereby improve respiratory symptoms and prevent complications.[33]

Assessment of the patient should include information concerning:

1. The balance between mucus production and mucus transport and expectoration. Mucus expectoration itself is not an indication for intervention. The indication for intervention is retention of mucus in the airways. Information concerning retention of mucus can be obtained from auscultation and percussion.
2. Ease of expectoration. The patient should be asked if it takes a long time or a lot of effort to expectorate mucus. The patient's technique is evaluated. Difficulties in expectoration are an indication for CPT.
3. The impact of mucus retention on pulmonary function and gas exchange. Patients with severe airway obstruction have more difficulties expectorating mucus.
4. Possible contraindications with regards to specific interventions. CPT interventions can be hazardous for certain patients, especially those who are critically ill. Therefore, these patients should be closely observed before, during, and after intervention.

CPT can include the use of special breathing techniques, chest percussion or vibration, and postural drainage, all with or without directed coughing. Sometimes this combination of techniques is also called postural drainage.[22] The authors prefer to reserve this term for the facilitation of airway drainage by assuming the gravity-assisted positions that are discussed later in this chapter. Other methods to augment mucus clearance include the use of special devices, such as positive expiratory pressure (PEP) masks, flutter valves, or high frequency chest wall or airway oscillation devices.[62]

In animal studies, it was found that percussion combined with postural drainage increased tracheal mucus transport velocity.[28] Likewise, CPT has been found to improve mucus transport in the airways of patients with COPD.[14] When compared to coughing, the results are conflicting, however. Some authors found an improvement in mucus transport using CPT and directed coughing by comparison with coughing alone in patients with COPD[15] and in others with copious sputum production.[168] Others did not observe mucus transport improvement by using CPT in CF patients.[146] Differences in application and treatment duration as well as differences in disease pathology may account for the different outcomes.

Likewise, some studies demonstrated improvement in pulmonary function parameters, gas exchange, or both in COPD[34,46] and CF patients receiving CPT.[39,46,171,197] Other studies failed to confirm beneficial effects of CPT in COPD[24,103,107,111,117] and CF patients.[80,210] In some CF studies, CPT and coughing appeared to have similar effects on pulmonary function.[10,38] In general, improvements in mucus transport and mucus expectoration were not found to be associated with improvements in pulmonary function.

In acute COPD patients[24] and in patients with acute pulmonary disease,[59] undesirable side effects, such as increased bronchial airway obstruction and oxyhemoglobin desaturation, have been associated with CPT. In patients in critical condition with severe hypoxia or bronchial hyperreactivity, care must be taken when applying CPT, and the patient should be closely monitored.[175] The elderly and patients with cardiac disorders appear to have an increased risk of arrhythmias during CPT.[59]

CPT does not appear to benefit patients during recovery from acute exacerbations of COPD[4,117] or pneumonia.[21,55] These conditions are characterized by interstitial pathology, which cannot be influenced by physical interventions in the airways. When impaired mucus transport and hypersecretion are present, however, CPT appears to be useful. Inhalation of nebulized saline, water, or terbutaline can further improve the effects of CPT on mucus transport.[36,169] This improvement may be due to increased ciliary beat frequency, to increased hydration of bronchial secretions, or to bronchodilation leading to a higher and thus more effective airflow. Systemic hydration, however, has been shown to impair mucociliary transport during allergic mucociliary dysfunction.[104] Although CPT can probably be effective in increasing mucus transport, its effects on pulmonary function are unclear.

Forced Expirations and Coughing

Cough is the primary defense mechanism against foreign bodies in the lower airways. It is also an important compensating mechanism when production and clearance of secretions are out of balance. During cough, high peak intrapulmonary pressures are reached when the glottis is closed, and with opening of the glottis, high expiratory flows are generated. When using a forced expiration technique known as *huffing*, forced expiratory flows are created through an open glottis, and the intrapulmonary pressures are much lower than when coughing.[93] Coughing and huffing may be performed from different lung volumes. Forced expirations combined with breath control (diaphragmatic breathing) exercises are known as the forced expiration technique (FET). FET combined with thoracic expansion exercises is known as the active cycle of breathing (ACB).[195]

Forced expirations and coughing derive from the fact that airflow through a tube lined with viscous liquid can transport the liquid. This is called two-phase gas-liquid flow.[32,97] Mucus transport by two-phase gas-liquid flow can arise in airways that are closed by mucus as well as in open airways thickly lined with mucus. Mucus transport in a closed airway can be achieved only during forced expirations because it requires a high pressure. Mucus transport in an open airway may be achieved both by forced expirations and to some degree by tidal breathing.[82,155,192] Mucus is, however, especially well mobilized by linear expiratory airflow velocities of 1 to 2.5 m/sec (annular flow) or flow velocities greater than 2.5 m/sec (misty flow).[32] High airflow velocities are reached when airflow is high and airway diameter is small. In healthy individuals, the total airway diameter depends on the airway level and on dynamic compression.

Because the total airway diameter decreases from the peripheral to the central airways, airflow velocity increases centrally (Fig. 19–2). Forced expirations and coughing are, therefore, mainly effective in the central airways.[159]

During a forced expiration or cough, dynamic compression of the airways occurs. The alveolar pressure, which is the sum of the elastic recoil pressure and the pleural pressure, is the driving pressure to produce expiratory flow. During the coughing maneuver, the pressure in the bronchi decreases from the peripheral airways to the mouth owing to frictional pressure loss and convective acceleration pressure loss.[127] There exists a point within the airways where the intrabronchial pressure equals the pleural pressure. This point is called the equal pressure point (EPP) (Fig. 19–3). Upstream, in the direction of the alveoli, bronchial pressure is higher than pleural pressure, and no compression takes place. Downstream, in the direction of the mouth, the surrounding pleural pressure is higher than the bronchial pressure, and compression of the airways can take place depending on the stiffness of the airway wall.[108] In the event of severe obstruction to airflow, the frictional pressure loss in the bronchi is higher and results in a shift of the EPP in the direction of the alveoli. A lower elastic recoil pressure as

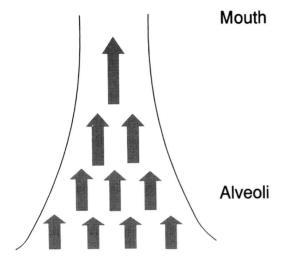

Mouth

Alveoli

FIGURE 19–2. The total airway diameter decreases from the peripheral to the central airways, and consequently airflows increase from the peripheral to the central airways.

seen in pulmonary emphysema, forced expiration from a lower lung volume, and higher pleural pressures owing to higher expiratory forces all lead to an upstream shift of the EPP. Less obstruction to airflow, higher elastic recoil pressure, and lower pleural pressures lead to a shift of the EPP downstream, in the direction of the mouth. The degree of compression is related to the compliance of the airway wall. The more compliant the peripheral airways by comparison to the central airways, the greater is the degree of compression when the EPP is located more upstream. Dynamic compression contributes to the development of local high airflow ve-

locities in these airways. In experimental animal models, it has been shown that cough-induced mucus transport is much greater when airways are constricted (Fig. 19–4).[2,183] This supports the hypothesis that dynamic compression of the airways can be used to assist mucus clearance during CPT and maneuvers which attempt to maintain maximal airway patency may reduce cough effectiveness.

When the force of the expiratory muscles is severely reduced, as in tetraplegic patients, the dynamic compression of the airways is less pronounced, which may thereby limit the effectiveness of coughing.[6] However, in a considerable number of these patients, sufficient airway compression may occur owing to contraction of the clavicular part of the pectoralis major muscle.[44] When airway compression is too great, airways collapse, as often occurs for patients with severe pulmonary emphysema, and cough-induced mucus transport is reduced.[181] In certain pathologic states, smooth muscle contraction, inflammatory processes and edema, and dynamic compression reduce the diameter of the peripheral airways. This limits peripheral airflow and thereby airflow velocity in the more central airways, and it may result in airway collapse.

Another aspect of forced expirations and coughing is that during a forced expiration a high expiratory flow is generated within approximately 0.1 seconds; thereby, a high shear rate is created. Mucus viscosity varies inversely with shear rate. This phenomenon is called pseudoplastic flow or shear thinning. Viscosity of mucus in the same sample may vary by a factor of up to 500 depending on the applied shear.

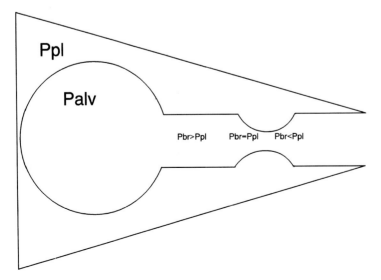

Ppl

Palv

Pbr>Ppl Pbr=Ppl Pbr<Ppl

FIGURE 19–3. During a forced expiration, there is a point in the airways where bronchial pressure (Pbr) equals pleural pressure (Ppl). This point is called the equal pressure point (EPP). Downstream from the EPP, compression of the airways can take place and lead to high linear airflow velocities.

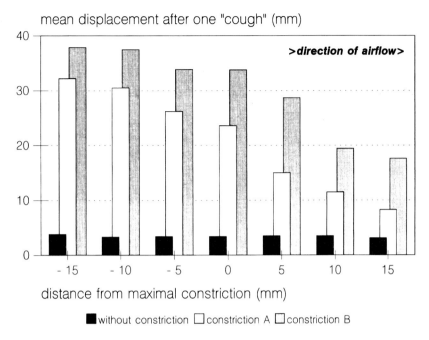

FIGURE 19–4. Cough-induced transport of a mucus simulant gel (MSG), with viscoelastic properties similar to human sputum, was measured in an artificial trachea. A constriction with a length of 73 mm and a maximal diameter of 7.5 mm (*constriction A*) and a constriction with a length of 87 mm and a maximal diameter of 10 mm (*constriction B*) were used. MSG samples of 40 μL were spread linearly over the width of the trachea under the point of maximal constriction and 5, 10, and 15 mm both upstream and downstream from the maximal constriction point. Measurements without the constriction were made at the same positions. Displacement of the MSG was measured after a single simulated cough. The application of the constrictive elements significantly increased mucus displacement (ANOVA $P<0.001$). The position of the MSG relative to the point of maximal airway constriction significantly influenced cough displacement with constriction A (ANOVA $P<0.001$) and constriction B (ANOVA $P<0.001$). The displacement was higher in the upstream positions than in the downstream positions. Without constriction, the displacement was unrelated to the position of the MSG (ANOVA $P>0.2$). (From van der Schans CP, Ramirez OE, Postma DS, et al: Effect of airway constriction on the cough transportability of mucus. Am J Respir Crit Care Med 149:A1023, 1994.)

This decrease in mucus viscosity can be explained by a temporary realignment of macromolecular glycoproteins[100] as a result of the applied force. Repeated forced expiratory flows, therefore, may improve mucociliary and cough-induced transport by temporarily reducing mucus viscosity. This hypothesis is supported by the work of Zahm and colleagues.[209] These authors found in an experimental model that transport of a mucus gel simulant in an artificial trachea was higher when the interval between the coughs was reduced. Bennett and coworkers[17] found that in healthy subjects both forced expirations and forced inspirations increased mucus transport. The explanation for this surprising phenomenon is not entirely clear but can be explained at least in part by the reduction in mucus viscosity owing to the additional shear effects of the forced inspirations.

Mucus transport by expiratory airflow also depends on the properties of the mucus layer. The critical airflow to transport mucus decreases with increasing thickness of the mucus layer.[82] Thus, patients with more hypersecretion probably need less effort to expectorate their mucus by coughing than patients with less pronounced hypersecretion.

Results of Clinical Trials

Forced expirations and coughing are probably the most effective aspects of CPT for improving mucus transport.[38,133,146,184,194] They are even effective in patients who do not expectorate any mucus.[63] It is probably for this reason that Lannefors and Wollmer[94] found no difference in mucus transport in a study of CF patients when comparing forced expirations plus postural drainage, forced expirations plus PEP mask use, and forced expirations plus physical exercise. Forced expirations have been shown to be as effective as coughing for patients with COPD or bronchiectasis even though patient effort is less when performing forced expirations.[64] In a long-term study of CF patients, however, it was shown that the annual decrease in the forced expiratory flow of the middle one-half of the expiratory volume (FEF$_{25-75\%}$) was less in a group that received CPT, including postural drainage, percussion, and FET, by comparison with a group that applied self-administered FET. No statistically significant differences between the two groups were found in decline in forced vital capacity (FVC), forced expiratory volume in 1 second (FEV$_1$), or number of hospitalizations.[141] The reasons for the difference between the groups is not clear, although both treatment efficacy and differences in patients' compliance may be responsible.

It has been suggested by Zach and coworkers[208] that in patients with CF the use of bronchodilators may decrease the stability of the airway wall and, thus, reduce the effectiveness of forced expirations and coughing because of airway collapse. This suggestion, however, was not confirmed in a study by Desmond and associates.[40] Bennett and coworkers[18] showed that mucus clearance by cough in patients with stable COPD was diminished after inhalation of ipratropium bromide. According to these authors, this was possibly the result of alteration of airway compression characteristics or possibly due to changes in the rheologic properties of the mucus. From the present data, it can be concluded that bronchodilation does not a priori increase the effectiveness of forced expirations and coughing. The effects of bronchodilators on the effectiveness of forced expirations and coughing need to be investigated in future studies to determine which if any patients may benefit.

Practice

Forced expirations or coughing are considered the first choice of physical therapeutic intervention. Each patient learns to perform the techniques most effective for himself or herself. The first factor to determine is whether to use dynamic airway compression or to decrease it.

In patients with severe airflow obstruction or with reduced elastic recoil of lung tissue, compression of the airways can result in complete

airway collapse, which can reduce forced expiration or cough effectiveness and can cause a sudden cessation of airflow during these activities. Collapse of airways, however, arises inhomogeneously and may, therefore, be difficult to assess without pulmonary function testing. In the generation of a maximum expiratory flow volume (MEFV) curve, airway collapse is reflected by a typical sharp bend convex to the volume axis at a volume shortly after the peak expiratory flow (PEF) has been reached (Fig. 19–5). When there are signs of airway collapse, forced

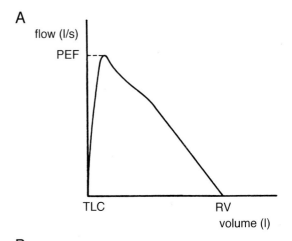

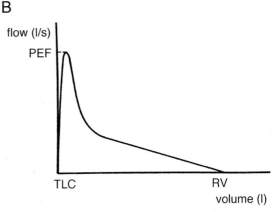

FIGURE 19–5. *A,* Relationship between expiratory airflow and lung volume during a forced expiration in a healthy subject. A maximal forced expiration is performed after a maximal inspiration. Peak expiratory flow (PEF) is reached at high lung volume. Thereafter, the flow decreases. *B,* Relationship between expiratory airflow and lung volume during a forced expiration in a patient with pulmonary emphysema. The PEF is mildly reduced, but after the PEF is reached the airflow is suddenly severely curtailed owing to airway collapse.

expiration should be started from a lung volume nearer the total lung capacity (TLC) and with submaximal or less expiratory force. In this way, the compression takes place predominantly in the large central airways and collapse may be partly prevented.

In patients with less severe airflow obstruction and normal or increased elastic recoil of lung tissue, forced expiration and coughing can be performed with higher force and can also be initiated at lower lung volumes. By doing so, the site of dynamic airway compression is shifted toward the small peripheral airways. The force and lung volume should be chosen in a way that mucus mobilization can be heard or felt by the patient. Using forced expirations instead of coughing, lung volume and expiration force may more easily be varied than by coughing. Patients with tracheostoma can also be taught more effective coughing by capping the tracheostomy tube or, preferably, by having the tube removed and a button placed if necessary. This clears the airway of the obstructing tube. These patients can then learn to use forced expirations to expectorate their mucus effectively.

If the experimental data of Zahm and colleagues[209] are clinically relevant, it is important that repetitive forced expirations be performed with short intervals and that high expiratory flows be reached quickly for a high shear rate. This can occur more easily by coughing than by forced expiration with an open glottis. In case of severe respiratory muscle weakness, inspiration can be supported by glossopharyngeal breathing,[195] and expiration can be assisted by manual compression of the thorax and abdomen or by mechanical exsufflation.[8,9,12]

Exercise

Many patients with chronic hypersecretion and impaired mucus transport improve their expectoration by general physical exercise, such as running or bicycling.

Mechanism

The increased expiratory flow rates, minute volumes, and sympathetic activity during exercise increase ciliary beat, decrease mucus viscosity, and increase mucus transport.[201] Assuming that the expiratory flows are the most important factor, the exercise must have sufficient intensity and duration to increase ventilatory demand.

Results of Clinical Trials

Exercise may improve bronchial mucus transport both in healthy subjects[201] and in patients with COPD[119] or CF.[207] The addition of exercise to CPT has been shown to result in a significant increase in the amount of expectorated mucus.[11] It has been suggested by some authors that exercise may be a substitute for CPT,[25,206] a supposition not supported by the results of some studies on CF patients.[19,157] It has also been shown that exercise may improve pulmonary function in CF patients,[207] possibly by improving mucus transport or by the bronchodilating effect of exercise itself.[101] Exercise reconditioning is considered elsewhere in this text.

Postural Drainage

Gravitational forces can enhance mucus transport when bronchi are vertically positioned. Postural drainage is probably most effective when there are relatively large quantities of mucus with low adhesiveness in the airways. Nine postural positions have been described for draining the large bronchi.[195]

Results of Clinical Trials

In an animal model, Chopra and associates[28] found an increase in tracheal mucus transport velocity during postural drainage. Other studies found improved mucus transport in patients with CF,[187,203] but in a study of patients with chronic bronchitis, no improvement was seen.[119]

Practice

Localization of airway mucus is essential. The object is to position vertically the secretion-encumbered bronchus for sufficient duration, generally about 20 minutes, to drain it. The time required probably depends on the amount of mucus, its viscoelasticity, and its adhesiveness. If the patient can tolerate it, he or she sleeps in a postural drainage position. Positioning of the patient in this manner, however, may affect his or her ventilation, perfusion, and oxyhemoglobin saturation.[26,41,52,102,145] One study of patients with COPD, however, showed that lung volumes were conserved and oxyhemoglobin desaturation and dyspnea did not occur in postural drainage positions.[105] Thus the effect of postural drainage positioning on oxygenation remains unclear, and close monitoring is recommended. Positioning can also place the patient at risk for skin and cardiac complications, cerebral flood flow or intracranial pressure changes, and gastroesophageal reflux. Nevertheless, postural drainage may be a good alternative when forced expirations and exercise are not possible or are inadequate. Disadvantages are that it is relatively time-consuming, and it may necessitate use of a specially modified bed or table on which the patient may become dependent.

Percussion, Vibration, High Frequency Oscillation

Manual percussion and vibration techniques are probably the best-known and most debated techniques of CPT.[51] Several mechanisms are thought to be responsible for their apparent beneficial effects on mucus transport. They may decrease mucus viscosity and act to induce small coughs or resonance with ciliary action.[61]

Results of Clinical Trials

In healthy subjects, high frequency oscillation increases mucus transport.[53] Chest vibration at 41 Hz and an amplitude of 2 mm, however, had no effect on mucus transport in patients with COPD.[126] Percussion also had no effect on mucus transport in a mixed group of patients with hypersecretion[167] and only a small effect on mucus transport in patients with COPD (Fig. 19–6).[182] Effects on mucus transport seemed to be frequency dependent.[85,136,143,153] In animal models, a frequency of 13 Hz was most effective in improving tracheal mucus transport[85,153] and bronchial mucus transport.[27] In one animal model, a frequency of 25 to 35 Hz appeared to be most effective.[136] Differences in animals used in these models might be responsible for the different results. In a study of CF patients, the intrathoracic pressures induced by vibration also appeared to be frequency dependent with the highest pressures reached at frequencies of about 15 Hz.[47] In most studies, a frequency of 10 to 15 Hz, which is outside the range of possible manual techniques but lower than most commercial vibrators, seems to have had the best effect on mucus transport. Oscillation or vibration has also been shown to be more effective when expiratory flows are greater than inspiratory flows.[27,49,86,88] The experiments of

Chang and associates[27] also indicated that intervention is more effective on thicker mucus layers.

Most studies on COPD and CF patients, however, have failed to demonstrate benefit from percussion or vibration on mucus transport (see Fig. 19–6).[132,168,182,186] One study found an improvement in the rate of expectoration of mucus, expressed as grams per minute, when percussion or vibration was added to CPT for patients with chronic bronchitis.[50] Another study suggested that the combination of percussion and postural drainage may be more effective for patients with COPD in terms of volume of expectorated mucus than coughing alone.[106] In a study of CF patients recovering from an acute pulmonary exacerbation, no difference was found in pulmonary function and amount of expectorated mucus between conventional CPT and high frequency chest wall compression.[5] Warwick and Hansen[193] found long-term increases in FVC and FEV_1 for CF patients when treated with high frequency chest wall compression as compared to when receiving conventional CPT alone. The improved pulmonary function was thought to be related to improved mucus clearance.

Beneficial effects of vibration may also be the result of mechanisms not related to mucus transport. Piquet and coworkers[131] found an improvement in gas exchange during high frequency oscillation, probably owing to changes in breathing pattern. Sibuya and colleagues[163] found that chest wall vibration decreased dyspnea, and Holody and Goldberg[70] found an increase in oxygenation in acutely ill patients with atelectasis or pneumonia.

Side effects of percussion and vibration include increasing obstruction to airflow for patients with COPD.[24] In an animal model, the application of vibration and percussion was associated with the development of atelectasis.[211]

From these studies, it can be concluded that there is not enough evidence to justify the routine use of percussion, vibration, or oscillation techniques. The experimental results of high frequency oscillation are promising, but more clinical studies are needed to investigate its effects on mucus transport and to indicate the circumstances in which it may be effective. Further studies are also needed into the side effects of these interventions.

Practice

Manual percussion is performed with cupped hands on the ventral, lateral, and dorsal side of

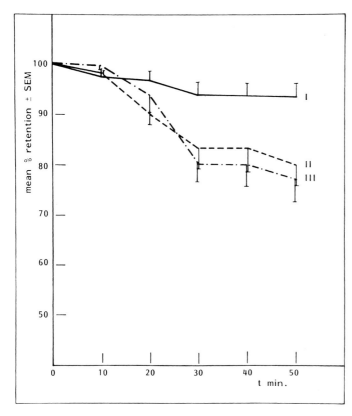

FIGURE 19–6. Clearance of a radioactive tracer deposited on airway mucus, from the peripheral lung regions, expressed as percentages of the starting value (mean and standard error of the mean [SEM]), in patients with COPD during three different protocols. During protocol 1, chest percussion was performed between 20 and 30 minutes. It resulted in a small but statistically significant increase in mucus clearance. During protocol 2, the patients were lying in a 20-degree head-down position and percussion, breathing exercises, and coughing were performed for 10 to 30 minutes. This resulted in a significantly greater clearance as compared with protocol 1. Protocol 3 was the same as protocol 2 but without percussion. No significant differences were found between protocols 2 and 3. (From van der Schans CP, Pilas DA, Postma DS: Effect of manual percussion on tracheobronchial clearance in patients with chronic airflow obstruction and excessive tracheobronchial secretion. Thorax 41: 448–452, 1986.)

the thorax of the patient with a frequency of approximately 3 to 6 Hz. Mechanical vibration is performed at frequencies up to 40 Hz. Percussion and vibration are applied during both expiration and inspiration or only during expiration. Oscillations can be applied at the mouth or on the thorax using special devices. In individual patients in which forced expirations, exercise, and postural drainage are ineffective, it may be useful to apply these techniques for a limited time. Their application should be closely monitored and should be continued only when there are convincing signs of clinical improvement.

Positive Expiratory Pressure Breathing

Application of PEP breathing is based on the hypothesis that mucus in peripheral small airways is more effectively mobilized by coughing or forced expirations if alveolar pressure and volume behind mucus plugs are increased. PEP is usually applied by breathing through a face mask or mouth piece with an inspiratory tube containing a one-way valve and an expiratory tube containing a variable expiratory resistance. It results in PEP throughout expiration. Expiratory pressures of 10 to 20 cm H_2O are generally used. PEP increases the pressure gradient between open and closed alveoli, thus tending to maintain alveoli patency, and increases functional residual capacity, which reduces the resistance in collateral and small airways.[109,128]

Results of Clinical Trials

The results of studies on the effect of PEP breathing are conflicting. One study in patients with CF suggests that the addition of PEP increases mucus expectoration more than conventional CPT or coughing,[45] but other studies failed to confirm this for patients with CF[69,112,176,179,180] or COPD.[120,185] Some authors have shown that physiotherapy that includes PEP breathing improves pulmonary function in patients with CF[45,56,173] and arterial blood gas values in patients with various disorders,[65] but other studies were unable to confirm these results.[69,79,176,179] PEP breathing is one of the few CPT interventions for which long-term effects have been investigated.[29,30] The results of two studies are, however, conflicting. Christensen and coworkers[29] found over a 12-month treatment period a decrease in exacerbation frequency and antibiotics utilization. Christensen and associates,[30] however, found no effect of PEP on exacerbation frequency and antibiotics use over a 6-month treatment period.

A variation of PEP breathing has been developed by Oberwaldner and coworkers.[118] In this high pressure PEP technique, the patient is asked to expire forcefully through a PEP mask. The purpose of this is to prevent airway compression during forced expiration. It is believed by these authors that airway compression leads to airway collapse in patients with CF making mucus transport impossible and that this is preventable.

The possible benefit of PEP and high pressure PEP on mucus transport remains to be proven. PEP may be useful when there are indications to (temporarily) increase lung volume.

Flutter Breathing

Flutter breathing is a combination of PEP and vibration or oscillation applied at the mouth. The patient expires through a small pipe. The expiratory opening of the pipe is closed by a small stainless steel ball. During expiration, the stainless steel ball is pushed upward, producing a positive expiratory pressure, and falls downward again producing an interruption of the expiratory flow. The mucus mobilizing effect is thought to be due to both a widening of the airways owing to the increased expiratory pressure and the occurrence of airflow oscillations owing to the oscillating ball.[160]

Results of Clinical Trials

The results of clinical trials have been conflicting. Konstan and associates[90] found a significantly greater amount of expectorated sputum in CF patients during flutter breathing by comparison with during voluntary coughing or CPT, but there was no improvement in pulmonary function or patient well-being demonstrated after the use of this modality. Pryor and colleagues,[134] however, found that the ACB technique resulted in a significantly greater amount of expectorated mucus than flutter breathing in a study of CF patients but also failed to demonstrate changes in lung function or oxygenation. Use of the flutter device is demanding, and it cannot be easily used by patients with severe disease. Carefully controlled studies need to be conducted before this technique can be recommended.

Autogenic Drainage

Autogenic drainage is based on the hypothesis that a mucus mobilizing *milking* or squeezing effect occurs in the peripheral airways when the patient breathes with low expiratory flows at lung volumes between the functional residual capacity and residual volume. After this so-called mobilizing phase, a *collection phase* follows during which mucus is thought to be transported to the larger airways by increasing tidal volumes. The last phase of this technique is the *expectoration phase* during which mucus is expectorated by low volume forced expirations.[161] There are no studies on the effect of this intervention on mucus transport or mucus expectoration.

Nasotracheal Suctioning

Nasotracheal suctioning is the last resort when other methods have failed to improve mucus transport. To perform this, a catheter is passed through the vocal cords into the trachea or a main stem bronchus and mucus is suctioned. It is easier to enter the right main stem bronchus than the left main stem bronchus for anatomic reasons.[58] The procedure may induce coughing, which may mobilize mucus from more peripheral airways. During the procedure, saline may be instilled through the suction catheter into the trachea to liquefy the mucus. The instillations reach the trachea only because of the cough reflex and probably have no liquefying or diluting effect on mucus in the main stem bronchi.[60] The practice of introducing saline into an endotracheal tube and driving it into the airway by positive pressure *bagging* is to be condemned because this may cause mucus to be loosened and driven deeper into the airway, occluding airways beyond the reach of suction catheters. The direct bronchoscopic aspiration of secretions may be preferable to endotracheal or nasotracheal suctioning because the bronchoscope permits visual inspection of the airway and direction of the suction pressure.

Results of Clinical Trials

Nasotracheal suctioning can lead to damage of the bronchial epithelium[68,77,156] without apparently significantly diminishing mucociliary transport[91] and to hypersecretion of mucus.[130] The procedure may also cause severe hemodynamic complications,[20,57,162,165,188] arterial oxyhemoglobin desaturation,[129,144] bronchospasm, and bacteremia[96] as well as tracheal puncture, suction catheter granuloma formation with airway obstruction, and inadvertent esophageal intubation with blind introduction of the catheter.

Practice

Nasotracheal suctioning is extremely unpleasant and often poorly tolerated. Thus, in view of its risks and complications, it should be used only when it is absolutely necessary, that is, when there is a risk of acute ventilatory insufficiency owing to accumulation of mucus in the airways and the patient cannot expectorate the mucus sufficiently. A sterile disposable catheter is brought into the trachea through the nose or mouth. Hypoxic patients should receive supplemental oxygen before starting the procedure. Suctioning is done in intervals of a few seconds with negative pressures between 8 and 20 kPa depending on the viscoelasticity of the mucus.[195] In case of large airways instability, the negative pressure may lead to tracheobronchial collapse, and suction pressures are decreased. A few milliliters of saline can be instilled through the catheter into the trachea. The patient is monitored closely for complications. After removing the catheter, ventilation is checked in both lungs by auscultation.

Mechanical Insufflation-Exsufflation

Mechanical insufflation-exsufflation involves the use of an airflow generator to provide about 10 L/sec of expiratory flow directly to the airways. It can be applied via an oral-nasal interface, via a mouth piece, or directly via an endotracheal or tracheostomy tube. Its application for both patients with obstructive and with restrictive pulmonary syndromes is discussed elsewhere in this text.

CONCLUSION

Patterson and coworkers[122] found in a 10-year study of CF patients that good patient compliance with daily CPT was associated with a slower rate of loss of FEV_1. Patient compliance with mucus mobilizing interventions is generally poor, however.[37,48,121] Independence in administering therapy improves compliance. Methods to facilitate independence and the development of other strategies need to be explored to improve patient compliance with treatment.

CPT, including forced expirations and directed coughing, is a treatment of choice to enhance mucus transport. Exercise and postural drainage may be alternatives or be complementary techniques. When inadequate, other methods, including the use of mechanical devices, may be tried to mobilize secretions. Further studies are needed to investigate in more detail which patients may benefit most from the use of these techniques and their side effects.

References

1. Adler KB, Wooten M, Dulfano MJ: Mammalian respiratory mucociliary clearance. Arch Environ Health 27:364–369, 1973.
2. Agarwal M, King M, Rubin BK, Shukla JB: Mucus transport in a miniaturized simulated cough machine: Effect of constriction and serous layer simulant. Biorheology 26:977–988, 1989.
3. American Thoracic Society Committee on Diagnostic Standards: Definition and classification of chronic bronchitis, asthma, and pulmonary emphysema. Am Rev Respir Dis 85:762–769, 1962.
4. Anthonisen P, Riis P, Søgaard-Andersen T: The value of lung physiotherapy in the treatment of acute exacerbations in chronic bronchitis. Acta Med Scand 175:715–719, 1964.
5. Arens R, Gozal D, Omlin KJ, et al: Comparison of high frequency chest compression and conventional chest physiotherapy in hospitalized patients with cystic fibrosis. Am J Respir Crit Care Med 150:1154–1157, 1994.
6. Arora NS, Gal TJ: Cough dynamics during progressive expiratory muscle weakness in healthy curarized subjects. J Appl Physiol 51:494–498, 1981.
7. Asmundsson T, Kilburn KH: Mucociliary clearance rates at various levels in dogs lungs. Am Rev Respir Dis 102:388–397, 1970.
8. Bach JR: Mechanical insufflation-exsufflation. Comparison of peak expiratory flows with manually assisted and unassisted coughing techniques. Chest 104:1553–1562, 1993.
9. Bach JR, Smith WH, Michaels J, et al: Airway secretion clearance by mechanical exsufflation for post-poliomyelitis ventilator assisted individuals. Arch Phys Med Rehabil 74:170–177, 1993.
10. Bain J, Bishop J, Olinsky A: Evaluation of directed coughing in cystic fibrosis. Br J Dis Chest 82:138–148, 1988.
11. Baldwin DR, Hill AL, Peckham DG, Knox AJ: Effect of addition of exercise to chest physiotherapy on sputum expectoration and lung function in adults with cystic fibrosis. Respir Med 88:49–53, 1994.
12. Barach AL, Beck GJ: Exsufflation with negative pressure. Arch Intern Med 93:825–841, 1954.
13. Barton AD, Lourenço RV: Bronchial secretions and mucociliary clearance. Biochemical characteristics. Arch Intern Med 131:140–144, 1973.
14. Bateman JRM, Newman SP, Daunt KM, et al: Regional lung clearance of excessive bronchial secretions during chest physiotherapy in patients with stable chronic airways obstruction. Lancet 1:294–297, 1979.
15. Bateman JRM, Newman SP, Daunt KM, et al: Is cough as effective as chest physiotherapy in the removal of exces-

sive tracheobronchial secretions? Thorax 36:683–687, 1981.

16. Bateman JRM, Pavia D, Sheahan NF, et al: Impaired tracheobronchial clearance in patients with mild asthma. Thorax 38:463–467, 1983.

17. Bennett WD, Foster WM, Chapman WF: Cough-enhanced mucus clearance in the normal lung. J Appl Physiol 69:1670–1675, 1990.

18. Bennett WD, Chapman WF, Mascarella JM: The acute effect of ipratropium bromide bronchodilator therapy on cough clearance in COPD. Chest 103:488–495, 1993.

19. Bilton D, Dodd M, Abbot JV, Webb AK: The benefits of exercise combined with physiotherapy in the treatment of adults with cystic fibrosis. Respir Med 86:507–511, 1992.

20. Boutros AR: Arterial blood oxygenation during and after endotracheal suctioning in the apneic patient. Anaesthesiology 32:114–118, 1970.

21. Britton S, Bejstedt M, Vedin L: Chest physiotherapy in primary pneumonia. BMJ 290:1703–1704, 1985.

22. Bronchial Hygiene Guidelines Committee: AARC Clinical practice guidelines. Postural drainage therapy. Respir Care 36:1418–1426, 1991.

23. Camner P, Mossberg B, Philipson K: Tracheobronchial clearance and chronic obstructive lung disease. Scand J Respir Dis 54:272–281, 1973.

24. Campbell AH, O'Connell JM, Wilson F: The effect of chest physiotherapy upon the FEV1 in chronic bronchitis. Med J Aust 1:33–35, 1975.

25. Cerny F: Relative effects of bronchial drainage and exercise for in-hospital care of patients with cystic fibrosis. Phys Ther 69:633–639, 1989.

26. Chang SC, Chang HI, Shiao GM, Perng RP: Effect of body position on gas exchange in patients with unilateral central airway lesions. Down with the good lung. Chest 103:787–791, 1993.

27. Chang HK, Weber ME, King M: Mucus transport by high frequency nonsymetrical airflow. J Appl Physiol 65:1203–1209, 1988.

28. Chopra SK, Taplin GV, Simmons DH, et al: Effects of hydration and physical therapy on tracheal transport velocity. Am Rev Respir Dis 115:1009–1014, 1977.

29. Christensen EF, Nedergaard T, Dahl R. Long-term treatment of chronic bronchitis with positive expiratory pressure mask and chest physiotherapy. Chest 97:645–650, 1990.

30. Christensen HR, Simonsen K, Lange P, et al: PEEP-mask in patients with severe obstructive pulmonary disease: A negative report. Eur J Respir Dis 3:267–272, 1990.

31. Ciba Guest Symposium Report: Terminology, definitions and classification of chronic pulmonary emphysema and related conditions. Thorax 14:286–299, 1959.

32. Clarke SW, Jones JG, Oliver DR: Resistance to two-phase gas-liquid flow in airways. J Appl Physiol 9:359–372, 1970.

33. Clarke SW: Management of mucus hypersecretion. Eur J Respir Dis 71(suppl 153):136–144, 1987.

34. Cochrane GM, Webber BA, Clarke SW: Effects of sputum on pulmonary function. BMJ 2:1181–1183, 1977.

35. Connors AF, Hammon WE, Martin RJ, Rogers RM: Chest physical therapy. The immediate effect on oxygenation in acutely ill patients. Chest 78:559–564, 1980.

36. Conway JH, Fleming JS, Perring S, Holgate SD: Humidification as an adjunct to chest physiotherapy in aiding tracheo-bronchial clearance in patients with bronchiectasis. Respir Med 86:110–116, 1992.

37. Currie DC, Munro C, Gaskell D, Cole PJ: Practice, problems and compliance with postural drainage: A survey of chronic sputum producers. Br J Dis Chest 80:249–253, 1986.

38. de Boeck C, Zinman R: Cough versus chest physiotherapy. A comparison of the acute effects on pulmonary function in patients with cystic fibrosis. Am Rev Respir Dis 129:182–184, 1984.

39. Desmond KJ, Schwenk WF, Thomas E, et al: Immediate and long-term effects of chest physiotherapy in patients with cystic fibrosis. J Pediatr 103:538–542, 1983.

40. Desmond KJ, Demizio DL, Allen PD, et al: Effect of salbutamol on gas compression in cystic fibrosis and asthma. Am J Respir Crit Care Med 149:673–677, 1994.

41. Dhainaut JF, Bons J, Bricard C, Monsallier JF: Improved oxygenation in patients with extensive unilateral pneumonia using the lateral decubitus position. Thorax 35:792–793, 1980.

42. Dormehl I, Ras G, Taylor G, Hugo N: Effect of pseudomonas aeruginosa-derived pyocyanin and 1-hydroxyphenazine on pulmonary mucociliary clearance monitored scintigraphically in the baboon model. Nucl Med Biol 18:455–459, 1991.

43. Dulfano MJ, Luk CK: Sputum and ciliary inhibition in asthma. Thorax 37:646–651, 1982.

44. Estenne M, van Muylem A, Gorini M, et al: Evidence of dynamic airway compression during cough in tetraplegic patients. Am J Respir Crit Care Med 150:1081–1085, 1994.

45. Falk M, Kelstrup M, Andersen JB, et al: Improving the ketchup bottle method with positive expiratory pressure, PEP. A controlled study in patients with cystic fibrosis. Eur J Respir Dis 65:57–66, 1984.

46. Feldman J, Traver GA, Taussig LM: Maximal expiratory flows after postural drainage. Am Rev Respir Dis 119:239–245, 1979.

47. Flower KA, Eden RI, Lomax L, et al: New mechanical aid to physiotherapy in cystic fibrosis. BMJ 2:630–631, 1979.

48. Fong SL, Dales RE, Tierney MG: Compliance among adults with cystic fibrosis. Drug Intell Clin Pharm 24:689–692, 1990.

49. Freitag L, Long WM, Kim CS, Wanner A: Removal of excessive bronchial secretions by asymmetric high-frequency oscillations. J Appl Physiol 67:614–619, 1989.

50. Gallon A: Evaluation of chest percussion in the treatment of patients with copious sputum production. Respir Med 85:45–51, 1991.

51. Gallon A: The use of percussion. Physiotherapy 78:85–89, 1992.

52. Gillespie DJ, Rehder K: Body position and ventilation-perfusion relationships in unilateral pulmonary disease. Chest 92:75–79, 1987.

53. George RJD, Johnson MA, Pavia D, et al: Increase in mucociliary clearance in normal man induced by oral high frequency oscillation. Thorax 40:433–437, 1985.

54. Goodman RM, Yergin BM, Landa JF, et al: Relationship of smoking history and pulmonary function tests to tracheal mucous velocity in nonsmokers, young smokers, ex-smokers, and patients with chronic bronchitis. Am Rev Respir Dis 117:205–214, 1978.

55. Graham WGB, Bradley DA: Efficacy of chest physiotherapy and intermittent positive pressure breathing in the resolution of pneumonia. N Engl J Med 199:624–627, 1978.

56. Groth S, Stafanger G, Dirksen H, et al: Positive expiratory pressure (PEP mask) physiotherapy improves ventilation and reduces volume of trapped gas in cystic fibrosis. Bull Eur Physiopathol Respir 21:339–343, 1985.

57. Gunderson LP, Stone KS, Hamlin RL: Endotracheal suctioning-induced heart rate alterations. Nurs Res 40:139–143, 1991.

58. Haberman PB, Green JP, Archibald C, et al: Determinants of successful selective tracheobronchial suctioning. N Engl J Med 289:1060–1063, 1973.

59. Hammon WE, Connors AF, McCaffree DR: Cardiac arrhythmias during postural drainage and chest percussion of critically ill patients. Chest 102:1836–1841, 1992.

60. Hanley MV, Rudd T, Butler J: What happens to intratracheal saline instillations. Am Rev Respir Dis 117 (suppl):124, 1978.

61. Hansen LG, Warwick WJ, Hansen KL: Mucus transport mechanisms in relation to the effect of high frequency chest compression (HFCC) on mucus clearance. Pediatr Pulmonol 17:113–118, 1994.

62. Hardy KA: A review of airway clearance: New techniques, indications, and recommendations. Respir Care 39:440–455, 1994.

63. Hasani A, Pavia D, Agnew JE, Clarke SW: The effect of unproductive coughing/FET on regional mucus movement in the human lungs. Respir Med 85:23–26, 1991.

64. Hasani A, Pavia D, Agnew JE, Clarke SW: Regional lung clearance during cough and forced expiration technique (FET): Effects of flow and viscoelasticity. Thorax 49:557–561, 1994.

65. Herala M, Gislason T: Chest physiotherapy. Evaluation by transcutaneous blood gas monitoring. Chest 93:800–802, 1988.

66. Hilding AC: Ciliary streaming in the lower respiratory tract. Am J Physiol 191:404–410, 1957.

67. Hilding AC: Phagocytosis, mucous flow, and ciliary action. Arch Environ Health 6:67–79, 1963.

68. Hilding AC: Experimental bronchoscopy in calves: Injury and repair of tracheobronchial epithelium after passage of bronchoscope. Am Rev Respir Dis 98:646–652, 1968.

69. Hofmeyer JL, Webber BA, Hodson ME: Evaluation of positive expiratory pressure as an adjunct to chest physiotherapy in the treatment of cystic fibrosis. Thorax 41:951–954, 1986.

70. Holody B, Goldberg HS: The effect of mechanical vibration physiotherapy on arterial oxygenation in acutely ill patients with atelectasis or pneumonia. Am Rev Respir Dis 124:372–375, 1981.

71. Iravani J, van As A: Mucus transport in the tracheobronchial tree of normal and bronchitic rats. J Pathol 116:81–93, 1972.

72. Iravani J, Melville GN: Long term effect of cigarette smoke on mucociliary function in animals Respiration 31:358–366, 1974.

73. Isawa T, Teshima T, Hirano T, et al: Effect of bronchodilation on the deposition and clearance of radioaerosol in bronchial asthma in remission. J Nucl Med 28:1901–1906, 1987.

74. Jeffery PK, Reid L: New observations of rat airway epithelium: A quantitative and electron microscopic study. J Anat 120:295–320, 1975.

75. Jeffery PK: The respiratory mucous membrane. In Brain JD, Proctor DF, Reid LM (eds): Respiratory Defense Mechanisms. New York, Marcel Dekker, 1977, p 193.

76. Jeffery PK: The origins of secretions in the lower respiratory tract. Eur J Respir Dis 71(suppl 153):34–42, 1987.

77. Jung RC, Gottlieb LS: Comparison of tracheobronchial suction catheters in humans. Visualization by fiberoptic bronchoscopy. Chest 69:179–181, 1976.

78. Kaliner M, Marom Z, Patow C, Shelhamer J: Human respiratory mucus. J Allergy Clin Immunol 73:318–323, 1984.

79. Kaminska TM, Pearson SB: A comparison of postural drainage and positive expiratory pressure in the domiciliary management of patients with chronic bronchial sepsis. Physiotherapy 74:251–254, 1988.

80. Kerrebijn KF, Veentjer R, Bonzet-van de Water E: The immediate effect of physiotherapy and aerosol treatment on pulmonary function in children with cystic fibrosis. Eur J Respir Dis 63:35–42, 1982.

81. Kilburn KH: A hypothesis for pulmonary clearance and its implications. Am Rev Respir Dis 98:449–463, 1968.

82. Kim CS, Rodriguez CR, Eldridge MA, Sackner MA: Criteria for mucus transport in the airways by two-phase gas-liquid flow mechanism. J Appl Physiol 60:901–907, 1986.

83. King M, Macklem PT: Rheological properties of microliter quantities of normal mucus. J Appl Physiol 42:797–802, 1977.

84. King M: Is cystic fibrosis mucus abnormal? Pediatr Res 15:120–122, 1981.

85. King M, Phillips DM, Gross D, et al: Enhanced tracheal mucus clearance with high frequency chest wall compression. Am Rev Respir Dis 128:511–515, 1983.

86. King M, Phillips DM, Zidulka A, Chang HK: Tracheal mucus clearance in high-frequency oscillation. Am Rev Respir Dis 130:703–706, 1984.

87. King M, Rubin BK: Rheology of airway mucus. Relationship with clearance function. In Takishima T, Shimura S (eds): Airway Secretion. Physiological Bases for the Control of Mucus Hypersecretion. New York, Marcel Dekker, 1994, p 283.

88. King M, Zidulka A, Phillips DM, et al: Tracheal mucus clearance in high-frequency oscillation: Effect of peak flow rate bias. Eur Respir J 3:6–13, 1990.

89. Kollberg H, Mossberg B, Afzelius BA, et al: Cystic fibrosis compared with the immotile-cilia syndrome. A study of mucociliary clearance, ciliary ultrastructure, clinical picture and ventilatory function. Scand J Respir Dis 59:297–306, 1978.

90. Konstan MW, Stern RC, Doershuk CF: Efficacy of the flutter device for airway mucus clearance in patients with cystic fibrosis. J Pediatr 124:689–693, 1994.

91. Landa JF, Epstein S, Sackner MA: Effects of bronchoscopy on mucociliary transport. Chest 3:452–453, 1980.

92. Lange P, Nyboe J, Appleyard M, et al: Relation of ventilatory impairment and of chronic mucus hypersecretion to mortality from obstructive lung disease and from all causes. Thorax 45:579–585, 1990.

93. Langlands J: The dynamics of cough in health and in chronic bronchitis. Thorax 22:88–96, 1967.

94. Lannefors L, Wollmer P: Mucus clearance with three chest physiotherapy regimes in cystic fibrosis: A comparison between postural drainage, PEP and physical exercise. Eur Respir J 5:748–753, 1992.

95. Lee PS, Gerrity TR, Hass FJ, Lourenço RV: A model for tracheobronchial clearance of inhaled particles in man and comparison with data. IEEE Transactions on Biomedical Engineering 26:624–630, 1979.

96. LeFrock JL, Klainer AS, Wu WH, Turndor FH: Transient bacteremia associated with nasotracheal suctioning. JAMA 236:1610–1611, 1976.

97. Leith DE: Cough. Phys Ther 48:439–447, 1968.

98. Litt M: Mucus rheology relevance to mucociliary clearance. Arch Intern Med 126:417–423, 1970.

99. Lopez-Vidriero MT, Das I: Airway secretion: Source, biochemical and rheological properties. In Brain JD, Proctor DF, Reid LM (eds): Respiratory Defense Mechanisms. New York, Marcel Dekker, 1977, p 288.

100. Lopez-Vidriero MT: Airway mucus production and composition. Chest 80:799–804, 1981.

101. Mahler DA: Exercise-induced asthma. Med Sci Sports Exerc 25:554–561, 1993.

102. Mahler DA, Snyder PE, Virgulto JA, Loke J: Positional dyspnea and oxygen desaturation related to carcinoma of the lung: Up with the good lung. Chest 83:826–827, 1983.

103. March H: Appraisal of postural drainage for chronic obstructive pulmonary disease. Arch Phys Med Rehabil 52:528–530, 1971.

104. Marchette LC, Marchette BE, Abraham WM, Wanner A: The effect of systemic hydration on normal and impaired mucociliary function. Pediatr Pulmonol 1:107–111, 1985.

105. Marini JJ, Tyler ML, Hudson LD, et al: Influence of head-dependent positions on lung volume and oxygen saturation in chronic air-flow obstruction. Am Rev Respir Dis 129:101–105, 1984.

106. May DM, Munt PW: Physiologic effects of chest percussion and postural drainage in patients with stable chronic bronchitis. Chest 75:29–31, 1979.

107. Mazzocco MC, Owens GR, Kirilloff LH, Rogers RM: Chest percussion and postural drainage in patients with bronchiectasis. Chest 88:360–363, 1985.

108. Mead J, Turner JM, Macklem PT, Little JB: Significance of the relationship between lung recoil and maximum expiratory flow. J Appl Physiol 22:95–108, 1967.

109. Menkes HA, Traystman RJ: State of the art. Collateral ventilation. Am Rev Respir Dis 116:287–309, 1977.

110. Messina MS, O'Riordian TG, Smaldone GC: Changes in mucociliary clearance during acute exacerbations of asthma. Am Rev Respir Dis 143:993–997, 1991.

111. Mohsenifar Z, Rosenberg N, Goldberg HS, Koerner SK: Mechanical vibration and conventional chest physiotherapy in outpatients with stable chronic obstructive lung disease. Chest 87:483–485, 1985.

112. Mortensen J, Falk M, Groth S, Jensen C: The effects of postural drainage and positive expiratory pressure physiotherapy on tracheobronchial clearance in cystic fibrosis. Chest 100:1350–1357, 1991.

113. Mossberg B, Strandberg K, Philipson K, Camner P: Tracheobronchial clearance in bronchial asthma: Response to beta-adrenoceptor stimulation: Scand J Respir Dis 57:119–128, 1976.

114. Mossberg B, Camner P, Afzelius BA: The immotile-cilia syndrome compared to other obstructive lung diseases: a clue to their pathogenesis. Eur J Respir Dis 64(suppl 127):129–136, 1983.

115. Mullen JBM, Wright JL, Wiggs BR, et al: Structure of central airways in current smokers and ex smokers with and without mucus hypersecretion: Relation to lung function. Thorax 42:843–848, 1987.

116. Newhouse M, Sanchis J, Bienenstock J: Lung defense mechanisms. N Engl J Med 195:990–998, 1976.

117. Newton DAG, Stephenson A: Effect of physiotherapy on pulmonary function. Lancet 228–230, 1978.

118. Oberwaldner B, Evans JC, Zach MS: Forced expirations against a variable resistance: A new chest physiotherapy method in cystic fibrosis. Pediatr Pulmonol 2:358–367, 1986.

119. Oldenburg FA, Dolovich MB, Montgomery JM, Newhouse MT: Effects of postural drainage, exercise and cough on mucus clearance in chronic bronchitis. Am Rev Respir Dis 120:730–745, 1979.

120. Olséni L, Midgren B, Hörnblad Y, Wollmer P: Chest physiotherapy in chronic obstructive pulmonary disease: Forced expiratory technique combined with either postural drainage or positive expiratory pressure breathing. Respir Med 88:435–440, 1994.

121. Passero MA, Remor B, Salamon J: Patient-reported compliance with cystic fibrosis. Clin Pediatr 20:264–268, 1981.

122. Patterson JM, Budd J, Goetz D, Warwick WJ: Family correlates of a 10-year pulmonary health trend in cystic fibrosis. Pediatrics 91:383–389, 1993.

123. Pavia D, Agnew JE, Clarke SW: Physiological, pathological and drug-induced alterations in tracheobron-chial mucociliary clearance. In Isles AF, Wichert von P (eds): Sustained-Release Theophylline and Nocturnal Asthma. Amsterdam, Excerpta Medica, 1985, p 44.

124. Pavia D, Bateman JRM, Sheahan NF, et al: Tracheo-bronchial mucociliary clearance in asthma: Impairment during remission. Thorax 40:171–175, 1985.

125. Pavia D, Lopez-Vidriero MT, Clarke SW: Mediators and mucociliary clearance in asthma. Bull Eur Physio-pathol Respir 23(suppl 10):89s-94s, 1987.

126. Pavia D, Thomson ML, Phillipakos D: A preliminary study of the effect of a vibrating pad on bronchial clearance. Am Rev Respir Dis 113:92–96, 1976.

127. Pedersen OF, Nielsen TM: The critical transmural pressure of the airway. Acta Physiol Scand 97:426–446, 1976.

128. Peters RM: Pulmonary physiologic studies of the perioperative period. Chest 76:576–584, 1979.

129. Petersen GM, Pierson DJ, Hunter PM: Arterial oxygen saturation during nasotracheal suctioning. Chest 76:283–287, 1979.

130. Phipps RJ, Richardson PS: The effects of irritation at various levels of the airway upon tracheal mucus secretion in the cat. J Physiol 261:561–581, 1976.

131. Piquet J, Brochard L, Isabey D, et al: High frequency chest wall oscillation in patients with chronic air-flow obstruction. Am Rev Respir Dis 136:1355–1359, 1987.

132. Pryor JA, Parker RA, Webber BA: A comparison of mechanical and manual percussion as adjuncts to postural drainage in the treatment of cystic fibrosis in adolescents and adults. Physiotherapy 6:140–141, 1981.

133. Pryor JA, Webber BA, Hodson ME, Batten JC: Evaluation of the forced expiration technique as an adjunct to postural drainage in treatment of cystic fibrosis. BMJ 2:417–418, 1979.

134. Pryor JA, Webber BA, Hodson ME, Warner JO: The Flutter VRP1 as an adjunct to chest physiotherapy in cystic fibrosis. Respir Med 88:677–681, 1994.

135. Pucchelle E, Polu JM, Zahm JM, Sadoul P: Role of the rheological properties of bronchial secretion in the mucociliary transport at the bronchial surface. Eur J Respir Dis 61(suppl 111):29–34, 1980.

136. Radford R, Barutt J, Billingsley JG, et al: A rational basis for percussion augmented mucociliary clearance. Respir Care 27:556–563, 1982.

137. Ramirez O, Rubin BK, Green F, et al: The properties of respiratory mucus from patients with stable asthma and fatal asthma. Chest 100:47S, 1991.

138. Regnis JA, Robinson M, Bailey DL, et al: Mucociliary clearance in patients with cystic fibrosis and in normal subjects. Am J Respir Crit Care Med 150:66–71, 1994.

139. Reid L: An experimental study of hypersecretion of mucus in the bronchial tree. Br J Exp Pathol 44:437–445, 1963.

140. Reid LM, O'Sullivan DD, Bhaskar KR: Pathophysiology of bronchial hypersecretion. Eur J Respir Dis 71(suppl 153):19–25, 1987.

141. Reisman JJ, Rivington-Law B, Corey M, et al: Role of conventional physiotherapy in cystic fibrosis. J Pediatr 113:632–636, 1988.

142. Richardson PS: The physical and chemical properties of airway mucus and their relation to airway function. Eur J Respir Dis 61(suppl 111):13–15, 1980.

143. Richardson PS, Peatfield AC: The control of airway secretion. Eur J Respir Dis 71(suppl 153):43–51, 1987.

144. Rindfleisch SH, Tyler ML: Duration of suctioning: An important variable. Respir Care 28:457–459, 1983.

145. Ross J, Dean E, Abboud RT: The effect of postural drainage positioning on ventilation homogeneity in healthy subjects. Phys Ther 72:794–799, 1992.

146. Rossman CM, Waldes R, Sampson D, Newhouse MT:

Effect of chest physiotherapy on the removal of mucus in patients with cystic fibrosis. Am Rev Respir Dis 126: 131–135, 1982.

147. Rubin BK: Immotile cilia syndrome (primary ciliary dyskinesia) and airways inflammation. Clin Chest Med 9:657–668, 1988.

148. Rubin BK, Ramirez O, King M: Mucus-depleted frog palate as a model for the study of mucociliary clearance. J Appl Physiol 69:424–429, 1990.

149. Rubin BK, Ramirez O, Zayas JG, King M: Is cystic fibrosis sputum abnormal? Chest 98:81S, 1990.

150. Rubin BK, Ramirez O, Zayas JG, et al: Respiratory mucus from asymptomatic smokers is better hydrated and more easily cleared by mucociliary action. Am Rev Respir Dis 145:545–547, 1992.

151. Rubin BK: A superficial view of mucus and the cystic fibrosis defect. Pediatr Pulmonol 13:4–5, 1993.

152. Rubin BK, King M: The physiologic effects of smoking in COPD. Eur J Respir Dis 4:S19, 1993.

153. Rubin EM, Scantlen GE, Chapman GA, et al: Effect of chest wall oscillation on mucus clearance: Comparison of two vibrators. Pediatr Pulmonol 6:123–127, 1989.

154. Rutland J, Griffin WM, Cole PJ: Human ciliary beat frequency in epithelium from intrathoracic and extrathoracic airways. Am Rev Respir Dis 125:100–105, 1982.

155. Sackner MA, Kim CS: Phasic flow mechanisms of mucus clearance. Eur J Respir Dis 71(suppl 153):159–164, 1987.

156. Sackner MA, Landa JF, Greeneltch N, Robinson MJ: Pathogenesis and prevention of tracheobronchial damage with suction procedures. Chest 64:284–290, 1973.

157. Salh W, Bilton D, Dodd M, Webb AK: Effect of exercise and physiotherapy in aiding sputum expectoration in adults with cystic fibrosis. Thorax 44:1006–1008, 1989.

158. Santa Cruz R, Landa J, Hirsch J, Sackner MA: Tracheal mucous velocity in normal man and patients with obstructive lung disease: Effects of terbutaline. Am Rev Respir Dis 109:458–463, 1974.

159. Scherer PW: Mucus transport by cough. Chest 80:830–833, 1981.

160. Schibler A, Casaulta C, Kraemer R: Rational of oscillatory breathing in patients with cystic fibrosis. Pediatr Pulmonol 8:301S, 1992.

161. Schöni MH: Autogenic drainage: A modern approach to physiotherapy in cystic fibrosis. J R Soc Med 82 (suppl 16):32–37, 1989.

162. Shim C, Fine Fernandez R, Williams MH: Cardiac arrhythmias resulting from tracheal suctioning. Ann Intern Med 71:1149–1153, 1969.

163. Sibuya M, Yamada M, Kanamaru A, et al: Effect of chest wall vibration on dyspnea in patients with chronic respiratory disease. Am J Respir Crit Care Med 149:1235–1240, 1994.

164. Sleigh MA: The nature and action of respiratory tract cilia. In Brain JD, Proctor DF, Reid LM (eds): Respiratory Defense Mechanisms. New York, Marcel Dekker, 1977, p 247.

165. Stone KS, Preuser BA, Groch KF, et al: The effect of lung hyperinflation and endotracheal suctioning on cardiopulmonary hemodynamics. Nurs Res 40:76–80, 1991.

166. Sturgess J, Palfrey AJ, Reid L: Rheological properties of sputum. Rheol Acta 10:36–43, 1971.

167. Sutton PP, Lopez-Vidriero MT, Pavia D, et al: Assessment of percussion, vibratory-shaking and breathing exercises in chest physiotherapy. Eur J Respir Dis 66:147–152, 1985.

168. Sutton PP, Parker RA, Webber BA, et al: Assessment of the forced expiration technique, postural drainage and directed coughing in chest physiotherapy. Eur J Respir Dis 64:62–68, 1983.

169. Sutton PP, Gemell HG, Innes N, et al: Use of nebulized saline and nebulized terbutaline as an adjunct to chest physiotherapy. Thorax 43:57–60, 1988.

170. Takishima T, Shimura S: Airway hypersecretion in bronchial asthma and chronic obstructive pulmonary disease. In Takishima T, Shimura S (eds): Airway Secretion. Physiological Bases for the Control of Mucus Hypersecretion. New York, Marcel Dekker, 1994, p 527.

171. Tecklin JS, Holsclaw DS: Evaluation of bronchial drainage in patients with cystic fibrosis. Phys Ther 55:1081–1084, 1975.

172. Tomkiewicz RP, App EM, Boucher RC, et al: Amiloride inhalation therapy in cystic fibrosis: Its influence on ion content, hydration and rheology of sputum. Am Rev Respir Dis 148:1002–1007, 1993.

173. Tonnesen P, Stovring S: Positive expiratory pressure (PEP) as lung physiotherapy in cystic fibrosis: A pilot study. Eur J Respir Dis 65:419–422, 1984.

174. Toremalm NG: The daily amount of tracheobronchial secretions in man. Acta OtoLaryngol 53(suppl 185):43–53, 1960.

175. Tyler ML: Complications of positioning and chest physiotherapy. Respir Care 27:458–466, 1982.

176. Tyrrell JC, Hiller EJ, Martin J: Short reports. Face mask physiotherapy in cystic fibrosis. Arch Dis Child 61:598–611, 1986.

177. van As A: Pulmonary airway clearance mechanisms: A reappraisal. Am Rev Respir Dis 115:721–726, 1977.

178. van As A: Pulmonary airway defense mechanisms: An appreciation of integrated mucociliary activity. Eur J Respir Dis 61(suppl 111):21–24, 1980.

179. van Asperen PP, Jackson L, Hennessy P, Brown J: Comparison of positive expiratory pressure (PEP) mask with postural drainage in patients with cystic fibrosis. Aust Paediatr J 23:283–284, 1987.

180. van der Schans CP, van der Mark ThW, de Vries G, et al: Effect of positive expiratory pressure breathing in patients with cystic fibrosis. Thorax 46:252–256, 1991.

181. van der Schans CP, Piers DA, Beekhuis H, et al: Effect of forced expirations on mucus clearance in patients with chronic airflow obstruction: Effect of lung recoil pressure. Thorax 45:623–627, 1990.

182. van der Schans CP, Piers DA, Postma DS: Effect of manual percussion on tracheobronchial clearance in patients with chronic airflow obstruction and excessive tracheobronchial secretion. Thorax 41:448–452, 1986.

183. van der Schans CP, Ramirez OE, Postma DS, et al: Effect of airway constriction on the cough transportability of mucus. Am J Respir Crit Care Med 149:A1023, 1994.

184. van Hengstum M, Festen J, Beurskens C, et al: Conventional physiotherapy and forced expiration maneuvers have similar effects on tracheobronchial clearance. Eur J Respir Dis 1:758–761, 1988.

185. van Hengstum M, Festen J, Beurskens C, et al: The effect of positive expiratory pressure versus forced expiration technique on tracheobronchial clearance in chronic bronchitis. Scand J Gastrenterol 23(suppl 143):114–118, 1988.

186. van Hengstum M, Festen J, Beurskens C, et al: No effect of oral high frequency oscillation combined with forced expiration maneuvers on tracheobronchial clearance in chronic bronchitis. Eur Respir J 3:14–18, 1990.

187. Verboon JML, Bakker W, Sterk PJ: The value of the forced expiration technique with and without postural

drainage in adults with cystic fibrosis. Eur J Respir Dis 69:169–174, 1986.

188. Walsh JM, Vandenwarf C, Hoscheit D, Fahey PJ: Unsuspected hemodynamic alterations during endotracheal suctioning. Chest 95:162–165, 1989.

189. Wanner A: Clinical Aspects of mucociliary transport. Am Rev Respir Dis 115:73–125, 1977.

190. Wanner A: The role of mucociliary dysfunction in bronchial asthma. Am J Med 67:477–485, 1979.

191. Wanner A: Possible control of airway hypersecretion. In Takishima T, Shimura S (eds): Airway Secretion. Physiological Bases for the Control of Mucus Hypersecretion. New York, Marcel Dekker, 1994, p 629.

192. Warwick WJ: Mechanisms of mucous transport. Eur J Respir Dis 64(suppl 127):162–167, 1983.

193. Warwick WJ, Hansen LG: The long-term effect of high-frequency chest compression therapy on pulmonary complications of cystic fibrosis. Pediatr Pulmonol 11:265–271, 1991.

194. Webber BA, Hofmeyer JL, Morgan MD, Hodson ME: Effects of postural drainage: Incorporating forced expiration technique on pulmonary function in cystic fibrosis. Br J Dis Chest 80:353–359, 1986.

195. Webber BA, Pryor JA: Physiotherapy skills: Techniques and adjuncts. In Webber BA, Pryor JA (eds): Physiotherapy for Respiratory and Cardiac Problems. London, Churchill Livingstone, 1993, p 113.

196. Weibel ER: Morphometry of the Human Lung. Berlin, Springer-Verlag, 1963.

197. Weller PH, Bush E, Preece MA, Matthew DJ: Short-term effects of chest physiotherapy on pulmonary function in children with cystic fibrosis. Respiration 40:53–56, 1980.

198. Wilson R, Roberts D, Cole P: Effect of bacterial products on human ciliary function in vitro. Thorax 40:125–131, 1985.

199. Wilson R, Sykes DA, Currie D, Cole PJ: Beat frequency of cilia from sites of purulent infection. Thorax 41:453–458, 1986.

200. Wilson R: Secondary ciliary dysfunction. Clin Sci 75:113–120, 1988.

201. Wolff RK, Dolovich MB, Obminski G, Newhouse MT: Effects of exercise and eucapnic hyperventilation on bronchial clearance in man. J Appl Physiol 43:46–50, 1977.

202. Wollmer P, Ursing K, Midgren B, Eriksson L: Inefficiency of chest percussion in the physical therapy of chronic bronchitis. Eur J Respir Dis 66:233–239, 1985.

203. Wong JW, Keens TG, Wannamaker EM, et al: Effects of gravity on tracheal mucus transport rates in normal subjects and in patients with cystic fibrosis. Pediatrics 60:146–152, 1977.

204. Wood P, Wanner A, Hirsch J, Farrel P: Tracheal mucociliary transport in patients with cystic fibrosis and its stimulation by terbutaline. Am Rev Respir Dis 111:733–738, 1975.

205. Yeates D, Sturgess J, Kahn S, et al: Mucociliary transport in the trachea of patients with cystic fibrosis. Arch Dis Child 51:28–33, 1976.

206. Zach MS, Oberwaldner B, Häusler F: Cystic fibrosis: Physical exercise versus chest physiotherapy Arch Dis Child 57:587–589, 1982.

207. Zach MS, Purrer B, Oberwaldner B: Effect of swimming on forced expiration and sputum clearance in cystic fibrosis. Lancet 2:1201–1203, 1982.

208. Zach MS, Oberwaldner B, Forche G, Polgar G: Bronchodilators increase airway stability in cystic fibrosis. Am Rev Respir Dis 131:537–543, 1985.

209. Zahm JM, King M, Duvivier C, et al: Role of simulated repetitive coughing in mucus clearance. Eur Respir J 4:311–315, 1991.

210. Zapletal A, Stefanova J, Horak J, et al: Chest physiotherapy and airway obstruction in patients with cystic fibrosis—a negative report. Eur J Respir Dis 64:426–433, 1983.

211. Zidulka A, Chrome JF, Wight DW, et al: Clapping or percussion causes atelectasis in dogs and influences gas exchange. J Appl Physiol 66:2833–2838, 1989.

Management of Acute Exacerbations of Chronic Obstructive Pulmonary Disease

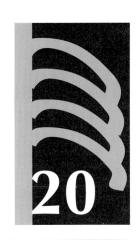

William D. Marino, MD

NATURE OF OBSTRUCTION IN CHRONIC OBSTRUCTIVE PULMONARY DISEASE

Chronic obstructive pulmonary disease (COPD) is a disease characterized by the presence of the mucosal changes of bronchitis and the parenchymal changes of emphysema. Its fundamental physiology is that of airway dysfunction leading to impaired mass exchange of gas. There are four basic mechanisms that contribute to this airway dysfunction.

First, there is, in some individuals with COPD, a measurable degree of reversible bronchospasm. This reflects mucosal inflammation causing airway hyperactivity owing either to chronic bronchitis or to allergic airway inflammation as is seen in asthma.[10] A second factor contributing to airway obstruction in COPD in patients with a significant bronchitic component is accumulation and inspissation of secretions.[63] A third component, also related to the bronchitic component of the disease, is airway compromise caused by thickening of the bronchial mucosa, although this seems less important than other factors.[49,57]

The final, and probably the most important, disease-specific factor causing airways obstruction in COPD is loss of the elastic recoil force of the lungs owing to emphysematous change.[57] Normal tidal expiration requires a substantial component of elastic recoil of the lungs themselves (Fig. 20–1).[53,66] Figure 20–1A shows the origin of expiratory pressure during tidal expiration in the normal lung. Alveolar pressure (Palv) is generated entirely by elastic recoil pressure (Pel). In Figure 20–1B, forced expiration raises intrapleural pressure (Ppl) and, thus, alveolar pressure. The increased pleural pressure, however, also causes some compression of the airway downstream from the equal pressure point (EPP). In Figure 21–1C, showing an asthmatic lung during forced expiration, a normal elastic force with an elevated pleural pressure still produces an alveolar pressure equal to that in the normal lung, but the low airway pressure distal to the site of obstruction causes a considerable exaggeration of the dynamic compression of the airway that is seen during forced expiration in the normal lung. Finally, in Figure 20–1D, the emphysematous lung, elastic force is much reduced. To achieve the same Palv present in A and B, the component of Palv provided by pleural pressure is much greater. This, however, means that a much greater compressive force is exerted on the airways, again moving the equal pressure point upstream and causing exaggerated dynamic airway compression. In addition, in the emphysematous lung, it seems that the airways are more prone to collapse, at least in part because of loss of supporting parenchymal tissue and loss of connective tissue in the airway walls themselves.[19,26,52]

Evaluating these phenomena in another way, we can consider the compliance curves of the normal and emphysematous lungs (Fig. 20–2). It is clear that at normal tidal lung volumes

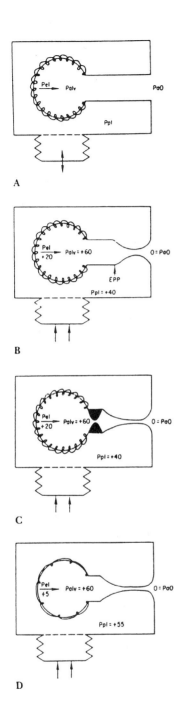

A

B

C

D

FIGURE 20–1. Model of forced expiratory airflow. See text for explanation. *A* and *B,* Normal relationships. *C,* Effects of intrinsic airways obstruction on forced expired airflow. *D,* Effects of decreased lung elastic recoil, as might occur with emphysema. Pel = Elastic recoil pressure; Palv = alveolar pressure; PaO = airway-opening pressure; Ppl = intrapleural pressure; EPP = equal-pressure point. (From Baum G, Wolinski E: Textbook of Pulmonary Diseases, 5th ed. Boston, Little, Brown, 1994.)

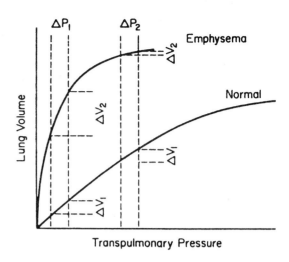

FIGURE 20–2. Pressure-volume relationships in normal and emphysematous lungs. At small lung volumes, the emphysematous lung is more compliant than the normal lung, but the reverse is true at large lung volumes. delta P = Change in pressure; delta V = change in volume. (From Baum G, Wolinski E: Textbook of Pulmonary Diseases, 5th ed. Boston, Little, Brown, 1994.)

(delta P_1), there is a much larger volume excursion for a given delta P in the emphysematous than in the normal lung. The implication of this is that for any given volume change, a much smaller elastic recoil force is generated. Consequently, the person with emphysema, to breathe at a normal or near-normal functional residual capacity (FRC), would need to employ active muscle effort in exhalation, with its attendant problems as noted in Fig. 20–1*D*. Instead, however, the emphysematous patient maintains an artificially elevated end-expiratory volume in part by using constant inspiratory muscle activity[50,58] to recruit greater elastic recoil by operating toward the top of the compliance curve (Fig. 20–2, delta P_2). There is another beneficial consequence of hyperinflation. As noted previously, the airways of the emphysematous lung are predisposed to collapse. Breathing at a higher setpoint within the total lung capacity (TLC) maintains a higher total lung volume. This permits not only higher parenchymal volumes, but also higher airway volumes, thus helping prevent airway collapse.

Clearly, in such a system, if tidal ventilation is conducted at a lung volume that permits expiratory airway patency, the lungs are relatively clear to auscultation. If the end-expiratory volume falls into that region of lung volumes in which the airways can collapse and forced expiration may become necessary because of inadequate elastic recoil force, wheezing occurs even in the absence of bronchospasm, secretions, or mucosal hypertrophy. Similarly, if, in a limited respiratory system, a sudden demand is made that requires a substantial proportion of the total respiratory capacity, forced expiration is employed, again producing the expiratory wheezing found in *COPD in exacerbation.*

Of major importance here is the need to maintain an elevated end-expiratory volume, distinct from the actual FRC, at least in part by constant activity of inspiratory muscles.[58,67] This importance stems from the fact that if these muscles develop weakness, particularly from fatigue or malnutrition, one of the consequences of this weakness is a decrease in end-expiratory volume. The result of this decrease is impaired gas exchange and progressive obstruction (wheezing), which results in progressive muscle fatigue and further deterioration. Alternatively, if a sudden demand is made for ventilation beyond the capacity of the diseased respiratory system, again wheezing and impaired gas exchange result from active expiration, and a disproportionate amount of the increase in ventilation is required to provide for the gas exchange needs of the stressed respiratory muscles, again potentially leading to progressive deterioration. For this reason, apparently acute obstruction can develop in an emphysematous lung in the absence of any obvious inciting event such as bronchospasm. This obstruction is caused by decreased structural integrity of the lung and active expiratory effort, both of which contribute to airway collapse owing to dynamic compression. Respiratory muscle weakness, which may be due in part to the disadvantageous length tension relationship of the muscles of respiration during chronic hyperinflation, and which may be acutely exacerbated by fatigue, can cause a decrease in this compensatory hyperinflation and thus precipitate an apparently acute attack.[67]

In severe COPD, this fatigue results from four factors that can markedly increase either the total respiratory workload or the workload for each breath. The total respiratory workload is increased by any factor that increases dead space and, thus, necessitates an increase in the total ventilation required to achieve any given alveolar ventilation.[79] The second factor is the continuous activity of the inspiratory muscles during expiration as well as inspiration that is needed to maintain the artificial elevation of end-expiratory volume referred to previously. Although the chest wall muscles and diaphragm alternate their activity (*paradoxic breathing*) and thus can avoid, to some extent, progressive fatigue, still the demand for continuous inspiratory muscle contraction contributes to the fatiguing workload. These are the two features that contribute to the total work of breathing.[58,67]

The two other factors contribute to an increase in the work required for each breath. First, it must be noted (see Fig. 20–2) that when the patient with COPD breathes at a high end-expiratory volume to increase elastic recoil, he or she is distending a hyperinflated structure with primarily nondistensible collagen and little elastic (elastin) tissue. As a result, the pressure required for a given change in volume is much higher than is required to distend the normal lung at FRC.[39] The second factor increasing the work required for each breath is intrinsic positive end-expiratory pressure (PEEP), the elevated end-expiratory pressure in the parenchyma and airways caused by air trapping in the obstructed lung. PEEP results in a substantial increase in trans-pulmonary pressure at end expiration that must be overcome by inspiratory muscle activity before inspiratory flow can begin.[28]

ACUTE EXACERBATIONS OF CHRONIC OBSTRUCTIVE PULMONARY DISEASE

Intrinsic factors such as emphysematous changes and decreased elastic recoil, coupled with generally reversible intercurrent airway effects (bronchospasm, infection, bronchitic mucosa, mucous plugging), can exacerbate chronic airflow obstruction. When these events are not adequately reversed by medical therapy, they can increase the respiratory workload in a positive feedback–type loop and ultimately result in respiratory failure.

Potentially precipitating extrapulmonary factors include left ventricular failure, right ventricular failure, fluid overload of noncardiac (e.g., renal) origin, and pulmonary thromboembolism. An extrathoracic respiratory condition that can also increase respiratory workload and cause progressive respiratory muscle dysfunction is obstructive sleep apnea syndrome (OSAS). OSAS is characterized by repetitive powerful efforts by the diaphragm and other respiratory muscles, exerted during sleep against a passively collapsed hypopharynx. This fatiguing workload, in combination with hypercapnia, which is known to cause diaphragmatic dysfunction,[37] is clearly involved in the deterioration of ventilatory function observed in certain patients with COPD. It is useful to note that sedatives can cause or exacerbate OSAS in some individuals, and the decision on the part of a susceptible patient as simple as that of having a cocktail just before bedtime can potentially begin a cycle of sleep-disordered breathing leading to respiratory muscle fatigue and acute respiratory embarrassment.

Thus, there are numerous factors, both pulmonary and extrapulmonary, that can affect the delicately balanced respiratory system of the COPD patient. All factors are capable of abruptly increasing respiratory work, inducing respiratory muscle fatigue and dysfunction, and resulting in progressive deterioration in gas exchange and, at times, respiratory failure.

Patient Evaluation

The treatment of acute exacerbations of COPD follows logically from the pathophysiology of the precipitating factors. The first and most rapid step is the evaluation and management of contributing nonpulmonary processes. Left ventricular failure with pulmonary vascular congestion or pulmonary edema would be manifested by some combination of the presence of dyspnea, rales on lung auscultation, a third heart sound on cardiac auscultation, and vascular congestion or pulmonary edema on chest radiograph. Pulmonary embolism is characterized by sudden onset of dyspnea, signs of deep venous thrombosis, and sometimes fever.

Potentially reversible respiratory factors include pulmonary infection. This can increase the work of breathing and cause dyspnea by increasing sputum production, which obstructs the airways, and by causing fever that necessitates increased gas exchange. If fever, increased sputum production, an increased sputum thickness or purulence, or physical findings suggestive of consolidation or an infiltrate on chest radiograph are found, antibiotic therapy has been shown to help resolve the acute exacerbation of COPD.[77]

Another potentially reversible factor is bronchospasm. Its presence can be deduced from a history of paroxysmal episodes of dyspnea, allergy, and asthma; from a physical examination significant for inspiratory wheezing in the absence of endobronchial lesions; and by the immediate beneficial effects of an inhalation treatment with beta-agonist medication. This evaluation is important to determine whether or not there is a quantifiable benefit from bronchodilator medication.

Exacerbations of COPD can cause hypercapnic respiratory failure. Clinical signs include lethargy (or even stupor), plethora with cyanosis, and signs of cor pulmonale—either acute or chronic edema, pleural effusions, elevated jugular venous pressure, and a right ventricular third heart sound, all in the absence of a left ventricular third sound or rales.

Impending respiratory failure is suggested by a normal to mildly elevated blood carbon dioxide level in combination with a disproportionately elevated respiratory workload. Respiratory muscle fatigue is signaled by tachypnea and paradoxic abdominal motion with respiration.[16,30,71] In addition, it has been shown that at levels of ventilation greater than 55% of maximum capacity, the respiratory muscles, probably exclusive of the diaphragm, enter a state of anaerobic metabolism.[45] Recruitment of paraspinal, scalenus anterior, and sternocleidomastoid muscles or gasping strongly suggests an elevated ventilatory workload that could cause fatigue and must be addressed.[13,31,34,40,48,81]

Treatment

The COPD patient with an acute exacerbation without evidence of reversible bronchospasm is virtually always treated with a full regimen of bronchodilators, including beta-agonists, for which there is no documented efficacy. Similarly, in the author's experience, anticholinergics (inhaled atropine, glycopyrrolate, or ipratroprium bromide) appear to improve airway function in COPD, either when used alone or in combination with beta-agonists, but no convincing controlled study has yet documented a beneficial effect from the use of these medications on the outcome of acute exacerbations of COPD. The other component of bronchodilator therapy is corticosteroid medication. For asthmatics, steroids reduce hypersensitivity by relieving airway inflammation and by preserving beta-agonist responsiveness. This may be true for the inflamed airway mucosa of chronic bronchitis as well. In any case, well-constructed studies have reported substantial improvement in the clinical status of acutely ill COPD patients treated with corticosteroids.[1,72]

In view of these data, it seems reasonable to treat all patients with acute exacerbations of COPD for potentially reversible bronchospasm as noted previously. This approach should not cause undue complacency, however. The following is of primary importance.

Therapy directed at correcting a disproportion between respiratory workload and respiratory pump capacity can take two forms: that of increasing the work capacity of the muscles or employing strategies to reduce the workload imposed on the muscles.

Relatively few ways exist to increase respiratory muscle work capacity and even fewer appropriate to the setting of acute respiratory insufficiency. Thus, inspiratory muscle exercise and other aspects of pulmonary rehabilitation are discussed elsewhere in this text. The one intervention that can increase respiratory muscle capacity in the COPD patient with carbon dioxide retention is the administration of theophylline, an important therapy for all patients with COPD in exacerbation. Theophylline has been shown to increase diaphragmatic contractility in normal as well as in COPD patients with carbon dioxide retention.[3] It also causes a primary increase in respiratory drive independent of muscle function.[47] The other pharmacologic intervention that may have utility in the setting of respiratory failure with cor pulmonale is gentle diuresis of the accumulated total body water. Great care must be taken, however, to avoid bicarbonate accumulation with a resultant *contraction alkalosis,* which can be deleterious by decreasing respiratory drive. Acetazolamide, potassium chloride, and arginine monohydrochloride can be of some use in this regard. All three agents act to deplete the extracellular fluid of bicarbonate.

There are two major approaches to the reduction of respiratory muscle workload. The first, oxygen therapy, is used to maintain oxygenation while permitting a decrease in ventilation. The second, mechanical ventilation, reduces the respiratory muscle workload.

With regard to oxygen therapy, it has long been common knowledge that hypercapnic patients have reduced respiratory center activity and are dependent on hypoxic drive. Consequently, it has been thought that high oxygen concentrations are to be avoided to avoid hypoventilation leading to intubation. What has in recent years become clear, however, is that even during therapy with 100% oxygen flows, hypercapnic COPD patients can have significant elevations of respiratory drive as compared with normals. Although the respiratory drive of these hypercapnic COPD patients is lower while breathing 100% oxygen than it is on room air,[4] the decrease in minute ventilation observed with administration of 100% oxygen is not adequate to explain observed rises in $PaCO_2$. This may instead be related to changes in dead space ventilation or carbon dioxide production during oxygen administration. The significance of

these findings is, however, that oxygen administration decreases ventilation and, thus, respiratory work, with a frequently concomitant rise in $PaCO_2$ that is multifactorial and is not necessarily life-threatening. Understanding this and that maintenance of tissue oxygen delivery is ultimately the major concern,[12] it can be appreciated that one may safely allow mild increases in carbon dioxide levels to decrease the work of breathing, while maintaining tissue oxygenation by supplemental oxygen administration. It is also worth noting at this time the fact that administration of either theophylline[51] or oxygen[41,81,80] can improve pulmonary hemodynamics.

Despite all of the above-listed measures, however, deterioration progresses for some patients with severe dysfunction. Thus, a means of unloading some or all of the respiratory muscle workload must at times be employed. This means mechanical ventilatory support of some type, either full time or intermittently.

For the past 25 years, the type of support has been endotracheal intubation with volume cycled intermittent positive-pressure ventilation (IPPV) along with medical therapy, followed by weaning from mechanical ventilation by any of a number of protocols. This form of mechanical ventilation is, of course, effective at supporting ventilation and protecting the airway of patients whose consciousness may be impaired by exhaustion, hypercapnia, or hypoxemia. Endotracheal intubation is invasive, is uncomfortable in the extreme, and presents certain inherent difficulties in evaluation for independent ventilation after acute therapy has been completed. In addition, because of these factors, the decision to intubate has become somewhat of a benchmark in therapy, to be avoided if possible. Clearly, this attitude raises the possibility that some patients may be harmed because of attempts to defer intubation.

As a consequence of these problems, and in view of the fact that the clinical course of acute exacerbations of COPD is generally a relatively short one, various noninvasive alternatives of mechanical ventilation have been evaluated in the treatment of acute exacerbations of COPD.

The negative pressure body ventilator, in the form of either the cuirass or the tank ("iron lung") respirator, has been widely used since the late 1940s in the management of acute respiratory failure.[17,29,65] This form of mechanical ventilation can be effective in reducing hypercapnia, but its use is attended by difficulties including gastroesophageal reflux and the development of hyperinflation with auto-PEEP.[44] In addition, negative pressure ventilation can confine patients and render them relatively helpless. Negative pressure ventilation is also labor intensive compared to noninvasive IPPV methods.

With the development of snug-fitting full face masks and nasal interfaces for the treatment of obstructive sleep apneas with continuous positive airway pressure (CPAP) and their observed usefulness in providing IPPV to patients with neuromuscular ventilatory insufficiency,[5,21,38] the utility of IPPV applied via such interfaces has been evaluated in the acute care setting.[11,43,55] There have been several series[7,24,54,62] that have generally demonstrated a 60% to 80% success rate in improving clinical status and blood gases, while avoiding intubation in patients with acute exacerbations of COPD who were otherwise thought to require it. One series[15] reported no success with nasal IPPV in exacerbations of COPD and a substantial increase in the nursing workload associated with such therapy. No other group has reported such an increase in nursing workload. The author intensively interviewed nursing personnel at his institution. It was clear that the nursing staff does not consider nasal IPPV to influence their workload significantly in caring for patients with acute exacerbations of COPD. One cooperative study[25] reported no benefit from nasal IPPV in the acute setting. There were significant problems, however, related to patient selection and lack of controls in this study.

More recently, prospective, randomized, controlled studies[9,78] have shown substantial success in improving outcomes and avoiding intubation by nasal IPPV. Further, some reports have shown that long-term nocturnal nasal IPPV following respiratory failure associated with acute exacerbations of COPD improves functional status and reduces the frequency of subsequent hospital admissions for selected patients.[27,43]

The benefits of using nasal IPPV for acute exacerbations of COPD derive, no doubt, from multiple mechanisms. A major mechanism is probably that of resting the respiratory muscles, increasing their endurance, and, thus, permitting respiration at higher tidal volumes. A number of studies have provided electromyographic and physiologic data demonstrating respiratory muscle rest during the use of nasal IPPV.[2,6,14,59] The results of these studies have been quite similar to those found in studies on the use of negative pressure ventilation by patients with hypercapnic respiratory failure.[42,68]

A second mechanism is the improvement in bulk gas exchange achieved by nasal IPPV. It must be noted, however, that hyperinflation may occur when any method of IPPV is used by the COPD patient,[28,39] and this can increase physiologic dead space (V_D/V_T), thus offsetting the bulk gas exchange improvement achieved by mechanical ventilation. Increased total ventilation by nasal IPPV allows for improved oxygenation without the danger of the development of severe hypercapnia, which has been observed during oxygen therapy for severe COPD. Assisting ventilation can allow time for the institution of other treatments (steroids, antibiotics) that may alleviate respiratory compromise sufficiently to eliminate or delay the need for intubation. This can be a major benefit from the use of nasal IPPV during the acute exacerbation of COPD. Further, improved gas exchange can benefit diaphragmatic contractility either by decreasing the $PaCO_2$[37] or by increasing arterial oxygenation.[32,36,71] Some investigators have suggested that nocturnal nasal IPPV may exert a beneficial effect by improving the disordered nocturnal breathing of patients with respiratory failure[27] and, similar to CPAP, may splint the upper airway to prevent obstructive apneas.[73,75] Such obstruction causes impaired bulk gas exchange and increases in the inspiratory workload. In the author's experience, however, hypercapnic patients use nasal IPPV at various times during the day or night according to their need, preference, and convenience, and all appear to benefit. Indeed, CPAP alone has been applied to patients with acute respiratory failure caused by COPD in levels of 5 to 10 cm H_2O with some apparent benefit in clinical status and blood gas tensions, although this may not be related to its effects on airway patency but rather to auto-PEEP and alterations in respiratory muscle activity patterns.[20,56]

The third effect of nasal IPPV on hypercapnic respiratory failure in COPD seems to be a resetting of the constitutive drive level of the respiratory center and possibly of chemoreceptor sensitivity.[22,23,70,76] In the face of a fatiguing workload, the respiratory center may decrease its constitutive activity, thus avoiding the imposition of a fatiguing workload on the respiratory muscles. This is done at the expense of carbon dioxide retention and is sometimes referred to as central fatigue.[60,71,74] Evidence for such a progressive desensitization of the respiratory center and decreased constitutive respiratory drive associated with progressive bicarbonate retention and metabolic alkalosis, and its reversal with treatment, exists in the sleep apnea literature.[8] In studies of patients using negative pressure body ventilators[33] or IPPV techniques,[35] reduction of hypercapnia during autonomous breathing appears to be independent of changes in muscle function. Although these reports are compelling, however, it is not clear that the measurement of muscle function parameters and of constitutive respiratory drive were sufficiently accurate to confirm a change in respiratory center activity without a change in muscle function.

Thus, nasal IPPV in acute respiratory failure in COPD can stabilize the hypoventilating patient, after which its salutary effects on respiratory muscle function and respiratory drive can improve lung, airway, and ventilatory function as well.

PRACTICAL ASPECTS OF INSTITUTING NONINVASIVE INTERMITTENT POSITIVE PRESSURE VENTILATION IN ACUTE RESPIRATORY FAILURE

Advanced COPD patients with hypercapnia and some patients with hemodynamic instability are appropriate candidates for the use of noninvasive IPPV alternatives to intubation.

Choice of Ventilators

Any microprocessor ventilator capable of assist control (A/C) and pressure support ventilation (PSV) can be used to deliver nasal IPPV. Although bilevel positive airway pressure ventilators can provide adequate ventilatory support for some, the monitoring capabilities and alarms of more sophisticated volume-cycled machines make them more useful in the treatment of acute respiratory failure by facilitating individualization of ventilator adjustment and use.

A/C and PSV modes have been shown to be equally effective for the acute treatment of COPD in exacerbation.[7,9,11,24,43,54,55,62,78] Generally, however, pressure support ventilation allows for excellent patient-ventilator synchrony while unloading each inspiratory effort and is more comfortable and thus preferable.[78] In the author's experience, the only scenario in which A/C is clearly more useful than PSV is for the patient with decreased respiratory drive and lethargy in which the patient's autonomous respiratory rate is inadequate in a ventilatory mode, such as PSV, that is dependent on patient triggering.

Air leak occasioned by opening of the mouth (insufflation air leakage) during nasal IPPV and by poorly fitting nasal interfaces must be managed by trying interfaces of various designs, sometimes in combination with nasal or oral airways, until an optimal one is found.

Three general designs have been shown to be useful in the acute provision of noninvasive IPPV. The initially used interfaces were the so-called bombardier full face masks (Vital Signs, Inc., Totowa, NJ) typified by the Downs CPAP mask.[55] This type of interface is effective because it provides both mouth and nose coverage, but its use is beset by problems with pressure at the nasal bridge, air leaks in the area of the cheeks, and rather uncomfortable retention harness arrangements. In addition, this type of tightly fitting interface has a small volume and, in covering both mouth and nose, provides a certain risk of aspiration in the event of vomiting.

More recent studies have evaluated the use of nasal interfaces, both nostril prongs and nose-covering interfaces, produced by a number of companies.[9,11,43] These interfaces, initially developed to deliver CPAP, have little or no buccal leak and do not increase risk of aspiration. They are relatively comfortable and allow for free speech during use. The problem of pressure points remains, however, and there is an additional difficulty of severe insufflation air leakage when the mouth opens during sleep. This problem has been addressed by various strategies, including the use of chin straps and changes in ventilator settings.[14,27] Although these strategies may help, many patients continue to have leak-associated oxyhemoglobin desaturations. A third interface type has been evaluated for the provision of IPPV in both long-term[18] and acute[46] settings. This is a full face mask, similar in shape to a fencing mask with a soft gasket around its entire perimeter to create a seal around the perimeter of the face during IPPV. This mask obviates difficulties with discomfort, pressure points, mouth leaks, and focal perimeter leaks. Although it covers the entire face, its volume is large enough to minimize the risk of aspiration in the event of vomiting. It has been shown to be effective for the delivery of IPPV for COPD patients in acute exacerbation,[46] even for patients obtunded by hypercapnia. Its major drawback is its volume, which contributes considerably to dead space and thus makes this mask relatively impractical for use with A/C ventilation. For PSV, however, in which there is an ample continuous flow of air to clear interface-associated dead space, this mask is efficient and efficacious. It is currently in the prototype stage but may soon be available on a limited production basis (Respironics, Inc., Murrysville, PA).

Protocol

Essentially, one or more physiologic parameters were monitored in all studies of IPPV use by patients with COPD in exacerbation. The author evaluated the response to, initially, 6 to 10 hours of IPPV on respiratory rate, heart rate, and $PaCO_2$. A reduction in respiratory rate or heart rate suggests effective ventilatory support; then blood gases are measured to document improved alveolar ventilation.

After initial evaluation, all studies report the use of daily intermittent periods of IPPV. Total use varies from 8 to 20 hours and is provided in short (2 to 3 hours), long (8 to 10 hours), or short daily plus overnight treatment periods. No study has clearly addressed the issue of cessation of noninvasive IPPV assistance. This may be because the majority of patients for whom this is an appropriate acute treatment appear to benefit from it for long-term management of chronic hypercapnic respiratory failure.[43]

The author has had success in maintaining respiratory stability in patients with chronic respiratory insufficiency by providing noninvasive IPPV during admissions for acute upper gastrointestinal bleeding, often accompanied by hypotension. Patients with hypotension from sepsis, from cardiogenic shock, or associated with cardiac dysrhythmias should have airways secured and protected by endotracheal intubation. Similarly, it has been recommended by some that patients not be considered for noninvasive IPPV unless they are fully alert and cooperative. Although stuporous and lethargic patients do, indeed, frequently require intubation, it is the author's experience that many such patients can be successfully ventilated by use of full face masks. They can exhibit a rapid improvement in mental status as exhaustion and hypercapnia are relieved. COPD patients with copious quantities of mucus may require intubation, not only for mechanical ventilation, but also to facilitate airway secretion management. Likewise, upper airway obstruction, most often from bulbar muscle dysfunction or trauma, can also preclude the successful use of noninvasive IPPV. Finally, many intubated patients who were otherwise candidates for noninvasive IPPV but who have instead been intubated can be quickly extubated and "weaned" using noninvasive IPPV.

Thus, any patient with a hypercapnic exacerbation of COPD who does not demonstrate concurrent cardiac ischemia or instability, who shows no evidence of difficult to reverse hemodynamic instability, and whose mental status is, at the worst, hypercapnic lethargy is a candidate for noninvasive IPPV. This may be critical for patients with end-stage cystic fibrosis awaiting lung transplantation and for many patients who refuse intubation.[7] Endotracheal intubation precludes cystic fibrosis patients from consideration for transplantation.[64]

CONCLUSION

Thus, COPD can be exacerbated by paroxysmal disease processes (bronchospasm, infection) and by the loss of compensatory hyperinflation from respiratory muscle weakness and fatigue. Therapy involves treatment for paroxysmal disease processes, including bronchodilator medications, steroids, diuretics, theophylline, and antibiotics. This, in combination with oxygen therapy, improves about 60% of patients with a hypercapnic exacerbation.[69] The remaining patients require some form of ventilatory assistance, which can be provided by various invasive and noninvasive means. After the acute episode is resolved, decisions are made regarding the need for any form of long-term assistance.

References

1. Albert R, Martin T, Lewis S: Controlled clinical trial of methylprednisone in patients with chronic bronchitis and acute respiratory insufficiency. Ann Intern Med 92:753–758, 1980.
2. Ambrosino N, Nava S, Bertone P, et al: Physiologic evaluation of pressure support ventilation by nasal mask in patients with stable COPD. Chest 101:385–391, 1992.
3. Aubier M: Effect of theophylline on diaphragmatic muscle function. Chest 92:27S-31S, 1987.
4. Aubier M, Murciano D, Fournier M, et al: Central respiratory drive in acute respiratory failure of patients with chronic obstructive pulmonary disease. Am Rev Respir Dis 122:191–199, 1980.
5. Bach J, Alba A, Mosher R, Delaubier A: Intermittent positive pressure ventilation via nasal access in the management of respiratory insufficiency. Chest 92:168–170, 1987.
6. Belman M, SooHoo G, Kuei J, Shadmehr R: Efficacy of positive vs. negative pressure ventilation in unloading the respiratory muscles. Chest 98:850–856, 1990.
7. Benhamoud, Girault C, Faure C, et al: Nasal mask ventilation in acute respiratory failure. Experience in elderly patients. Chest 102:912–917, 1992.
8. Berthon-Jones M, Sullivan C: Time course of change of the ventilatory response to CO2 with long term CPAP therapy for obstructive sleep apnea. Am Rev Respir Dis 135:144–147, 1987.
9. Bott J, Carroll M, Conway J, et al: Randomized controlled trial of nasal ventilation in acute ventilatory failure due to chronic obstructive airways disease. Lancet 342:1555–1557, 1993.
10. Boushy SF: The use of expiratory forced flows for determining bronchodilator therapy. Chest 62:534–541, 1972.

11. Brochard L, Isabey D, Piquet J, et al: Reversal of acute exacerbations of chronic obstructive lung disease by inspiratory assistance with a face mask. N Engl J Med 323:1523–1530, 1990.

12. Campbell EJM: The management of acute respiratory failure in chronic bronchitis and emphysema. Am Rev Respir Dis 96:626–639, 1967.

13. Campbell EJM, Agostoni E, Newsome-Davis J: The Respiratory Muscles—Mechanics and Neural Control. Philadelphia, WB Saunders, 1970, pp 181–199.

14. Carrey Z, Gottfried S, Levy R: Ventilatory muscle support in respiratory failure with nasal positive pressure ventilation. Chest 97:150–158, 1990.

15. Chevrolet J, Jolliet P, Abajo B, et al: Nasal positive pressure ventilation in patients with acute respiratory failure: Difficult and time consuming procedure for nurses. Chest 100:775–782, 1991.

16. Cohen C, Zagelbaum G, Gross P, et al: Clinical manifestations of inspiratory muscle fatigue. Am J Med 73:308–316, 1982.

17. Corrado A, DePaola E, Messori A, et al: The effect of intermittent negative pressure ventilation and long term therapy for patients with COPD: A 4-year study. Chest 105:95–99, 1994.

18. Criner G, Travaline J, Brennan K, Kreimer D: Efficacy of a new full face mask for non-invasive positive pressure ventilation. Chest 106:1109, 1994.

19. Dayman H: Mechanics of airflow in health and emphysema. J Clin Invest 30:1175–1190, 1951.

20. de Lucas P, Tarancón C, Puente L, et al: Nasal continuous positive airway pressure in patients with COPD in acute respiratory failure: A study of the immediate effects. Chest 104:1694–1697, 1993.

21. Ellis E, Bye P, Bruderer J, Sullivan C: Treatment of respiratory failure during sleep in patients with neuromuscular disease: Positive pressure ventilation via nasal mask. Am Rev Respir Dis 135:148–152, 1987.

22. Ellis E, Grunstein R, Chen S, et al: Non-invasive ventilatory support during sleep improves respiratory failures in kyphoscoliosis. Chest 94:811–815, 1988.

23. Ellis E, McCauley V, Mellis C, Sullivan C: Treatment of alveolar hypoventilation in a six-year-old girl with intermittent positive pressure ventilation through a nose mask. Am Rev Respir Dis 136:188–191, 1987.

24. Fernandez R, Blanch L, Valles J, et al: Pressure support ventilation via face mask in acute respiratory failure in hypercapnic COPD patients. Intens Care Med 19:456–461, 1993.

25. Foglio C, Vitacca M, Quadri A, et al: Acute exacerbations in severe COLD patients: Treatment using positive pressure ventilation by nasal mask. Chest 101:1533–1538, 1992.

26. Fry DL, Ebert RV, Stead WW, Brown CC: Mechanics of pulmonary ventilation in normal subjects and in patients with emphysema. Am J Med 16:80–97, 1954.

27. Gay P, Patel A, Viggiano R, Hubmayer R: Nocturnal nasal ventilation for treatment of patients with hypercapnic respiratory failure. Mayo Clin Proc 66:695–703, 1991.

28. Gay PC, Rodante JR, Hubmayr RJ: The effects of positive end-expiratory pressure on isovolume flow and dynamic hyperinflation in patients receiving mechanical ventilation. Am Rev Respir Dis 139:621–626, 1989.

29. Gigliotti F, Spinelli A, Duranti R, et al: Four week negative pressure ventilation improves respiration function in severe hypercapnic COPD patients. Chest 105:87–94, 1994.

30. Gilbert R, Ashutosh K, Auchincloss J: Clinical value of observations of chest and abdominal motion in patients with pulmonary emphysema. Am Rev Respir Dis 119:155–158, 1979.

31. Goldman M, Grimby G, Mead J: Mechanical work of breathing derived from rib cage and abdominal V-P partitioning. J Appl Physiol 41:752–763, 1976.

32. Goldstein R, DeRosie J, Avendaro M, Dulmage T: Influence of non-invasive positive pressure ventilation on inspiratory muscles. Chest 99:408–415, 1991.

33. Goldstein R, Molotiu N, Skrastins R, et al: Reversal of sleep induced hypoventilation and chronic respiratory failure by nocturnal negative pressure ventilation in patients with restrictive ventilatory impairment. Am Rev Respir Dis 135:1049–1055, 1987.

34. Grimby G, Goldman M, Mead J: Respiratory muscle activity inferred from rib cage and abdomen V-P partitioning. J Appl Physiol 41:739–751, 1976.

35. Hill N, Eveloff S, Carlisle C, Goff S: Efficacy of nocturnal nasal ventilation in patients with restrictive thoracic disease. Am Rev Respir Dis 145:365–371, 1992.

36. Jardim J, Farkas G, Prefaut C, et al: The failing inspiratory muscles under normoxic and hypoxic conditions. Am Rev Respir Dis 124:274–279, 1981.

37. Juan G, Calverly P, Talamo C, et al: Effect of carbon dioxide on diaphragmatic function in human beings. N Engl J Med 310:874–879, 1984.

38. Kerby G, Mayer L, Pingleton S: Nocturnal positive pressure ventilation via nasal mask. Am Rev Respir Dis 135:738–740, 1987.

39. Kimball W, Leith D, Robins A: Dynamic hyperinflation and ventilator dependence in chronic obstructive pulmonary disease. Am Rev Respir Dis 126:991–995, 1982.

40. Konno K, Mead J: Measurement of the separate volume changes of rib cage and abdomen during breathing. J Appl Physiol 22:407–422, 1967.

41. Lee J, Read J: Effect of oxygen breathing on distribution of pulmonary blood flow in chronic obstructive lung disease. Am Rev Respir Dis 96:1173–1180, 1967.

42. Marino W: The acute effects of negative pressure mechanical ventilation on patients with chronic respiratory insufficiency. Am Rev Respir Dis 133:A167, 1986.

43. Marino W: Intermittent volume cycled mechanical ventilation via nasal mask in patients with respiratory failure due to COPD. Chest 99:681–684, 1991.

44. Marino W: Reversal of negative pressure ventilation induced lower esophageal sphincter dysfunction with metoclopramide. Am J Gastroenterol 87:190–194, 1992.

45. Marino W: Anaerobic metabolism in the respiratory muscles: A possible link between hyperventilation and panic attacks. Chest 102:118S, 1992.

46. Marino W: The efficacy and comfort of mask positive pressure ventilation via a unique full face mask. Chest 106:159S, 1994.

47. Marino W, Canada F: Theophylline really does increase respiratory drive. Chest 98:21S, 1990.

48. Marino W, Estepan H: Transdiaphragmatic pressure and spirometry during quiet breathing and the MVV maneuver. Am Rev Respir Dis 135:A196, 1987.

49. Martin C, Katsura S, Cochran T: The relationship of chronic bronchitis to the diffuse obstructive pulmonary syndrome. Am Rev Respir Dis 102:362–369, 1970.

50. Martin J, Powell E, Shore S, et al: The role of respiratory muscles in the hyperinflation of bronchial asthma. Am Rev Respir Dis 121:441–447, 1980.

51. Matthay R: favorable cardiovascular effects of theophylline in COPD. Chest 92:22S-26S, 1987.

52. Mead J, Lindgren I, Gaensler EA: The mechanical properties of the lungs in emphysema. J Clin Invest 34:1005–1016, 1955.

53. Mead J, Turner J, Macklem P, Little JB: Significance of the relationship between lung recoil and maximum expiratory flow. J Appl Physiol 22:95–108, 1967.

54. Meduri G, Abu-Shala N, Fox R, et al: Non-invasive face

mask ventilation in patients with hypercapnic respiratory failure. Chest 100:445–454, 1991.

55. Meduri G, Conoscenti C, Menashe P, Nair S: Non-invasive face mask ventilation in patients with acute respiratory failure. Chest 95:865–870, 1989.

56. Miro A, Shivaram V, Mertig I: Continuous positive airway pressure in COPD patients in acute hypercapnic respiratory failure. Chest 103:266–268, 1993.

57. Mitchell R, Stanford R, Johnson J, et al: The morphologic features of the bronchi, bronchioles and alveoli in chronic airway obstruction: A clinico-pathologic study. Am Rev Respir Dis 114:137–145, 1976.

58. Muller N, Bryan AC, Zamel N: Tonic inspiratory muscle activity as a cause of hyperinflation in histamine-induced asthma. J Appl Physiol 49:869–874, 1981.

59. Nava S, Ambrosino N, Rubini F, et al: Effect of nasal pressure support ventilation and external peep on diaphragmatic activity in patients with severe stable COPD. Chest 103:143–150, 1993.

60. NHBLI Workshop: Summary, respiratory muscle fatigue—report of the respiratory muscle fatigue workshop group. Am Rev Respir Dis 142:474–480, 1990.

61. Pardaens J, Van de Woestijne KP, Clément J: A physical model of expiration. J Appl Physiol 33:479–490, 1972.

62. Pennock B, Kaplan B, Curlin B, et al: Pressure support ventilation with a simplified ventilatory support system administered with a nasal mask in patients with respiratory failure. Chest 100:1371–1376, 1991.

63. Petty TL: The national mucolytic study results of a randomized, double-blind placebo controlled study of iodinated glycerol in chronic obstructive bronchitis. Chest 97:75–83, 1990.

64. Piper A, Parker S, Torzillo P, et al: Nocturnal nasal IPPV stabilizes patients with cystic fibrosis and hypercapnic respiratory failure. Chest 102:846–850, 1992.

65. Plum F, Lukas DS: An evaluation of the cuirass respirator in acute poliomyelitis with respiratory insufficiency. Am J Med Sci 221:417–424, 1951.

66. Pride NB, Permutt S, Riley RC, Bromberger-Burnea B: Determinants of maximal expiratory flow from the lungs. J Appl Physiol 23:646–662, 1967.

67. Rochester DF, Braun NMT, Aurora NS: Respiratory muscle strength in chronic obstructive pulmonary disease. Am Rev Respir Dis 119:151–154, 1979.

68. Rochester D, Braun N, Laine S: Diaphragmatic energy expenditure in chronic respiratory failure: The effect of assisted ventilation with body ventilators. Am J Med 63:223–232, 1977.

69. Rogers R, Weiler C, Ruppenthal B: The impact of the intensive care unit on survival of patients with acute respiratory failure. Chest 621:94–97, 1972.

70. Roussos C: Function and fatigue of respiratory muscles. Chest 88:124S-132S, 1985.

71. Roussos C, Macklem P: The respiratory muscles. N Engl J Med 307:786–797, 1982.

72. Rubini F, Rampulla C, Nava S: Acute effect of corticosteroids an respiratory mechanics in mechanically ventilated patients with chronic airflow obstruction and acute respiratory failure. Am J Respir Crit Care Med 149:306–310, 1994.

73. Sanders M: Nasal CPAP Effect on patterns of sleep apnea. Chest 86:839–844, 1984.

74. Shapiro S, Ernst P, Gray-Donald K, et al: Effect of negative pressure ventilation in severe chronic obstructive pulmonary disease. Lancet 340:1425–1429, 1992.

75. Shivaram V, Cash M, Beal A: Nasal continuous positive airway pressure in decompensated hypercapnic respiratory failure as a complication of sleep apnea. Chest 104:770–774, 1993.

76. Strumpf D, Millman R, Hill N: The management of chronic hypoventilation. Chest 98:474–480, 1990.

77. Toews GB: Use of antibiotics in patients with chronic obstructive pulmonary disease. Semin Respir Med 8:165–169, 1986.

78. Vitacca M, Rubini F, Foglio K, et al: Non-invasive modalities of positive pressure ventilation improve the outcome of acute exacerbations in COLD patients. Intens Care Med 19:450–455, 1993.

79. Wagner PD, Dantzker DR, Dvede R, et al: Ventilation perfusion inequality in chronic obstructive pulmonary disease. J Clin Invest 59:203–216, 1977.

80. Weitzenbaum E, Hirth C, Roeslin N, et al: Pulmonary hemodynamic changes during acute respiratory failure in patients with chronic obstructive lung disease. Respiration 28:539–554, 1971.

81. Wilson R, Hoseth W, Dempsey M: Effects of breathing 99.6% oxygen on pulmonary vascular resistance and cardiac output in patients with pulmonary emphysema and chronic hypoxia. Ann Int Med 42:629–637, 1955.

Neuromuscular and Skeletal Disorders Leading to Global Alveolar Hypoventilation

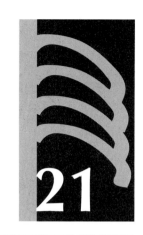

John R. Bach, MD

CANDIDATES FOR PHYSICAL MEDICINE RESPIRATORY INTERVENTIONS

Patients with respiratory impairment can be divided into those who have primarily oxygenation impairment and those with primarily impairment of alveolar ventilation. This section focuses only on the latter—that is, patients whose conditions result in the development of global alveolar hypoventilation (GAH).

GAH can result from any neuromuscular or skeletal disorder that causes respiratory muscle dysfunction. Patients who can most benefit from physical medicine as well as from general rehabilitation interventions must be able to learn and have adequate bulbar muscle function to use specific respiratory techniques and equipment.[7] These include various inspiratory and expiratory muscle aids and biofeedback approaches that can optimize pulmonary function. Patients with the diagnoses listed in Table 21–1 can retain adequate bulbar muscle and cognitive function to be candidates for the use of the physical medicine alternatives to endotracheal intubation or long-term ventilatory support via an indwelling tracheostomy tube. Some patients whose bulbar weakness precludes safe use of noninvasive inspiratory aids may still benefit from manual and mechanical cough assist methods. In addition, virtually any patient with adequate cognition and at least one reliable volitional movement, such as eye blink, can also use robotics and computers to communicate and operate sophisticated environmental control systems.

For the purpose of developing treatment strategies, disorders can be divided into those with acute, those with relapsing, and those with insidious development of ventilatory failure. The *acute courses* of certain conditions such as poliomyelitis[12,54] and traumatic high-level spinal cord injury[3,4,77] (traumatic tetraplegia) can be complicated by acute respiratory failure. Ventilatory failure may persist or recovery of ventilatory function may occur and last for decades before chronic late-onset ventilatory insufficiency develops.[8] Other individuals with certain degenerative central nervous system conditions can have *relapsing or intermittently exacerbating courses* with periods of ventilatory failure. They, too, can eventually develop chronic GAH.[1] Finally, patients with *progressive neuromuscular conditions* develop GAH insidiously.[5] Except for individuals with isolated phrenic neuropathies, some of whom go on to develop multiple sclerosis or motor neuron disease, virtually all patients with GAH also have skeletal muscle and, at times, cardiac muscle dysfunction and can also benefit from general physical medicine and rehabilitation interventions.

THE RELEVANT DIAGNOSES AND THEIR PRESENTATIONS

An in-depth discussion of the disorders of all candidates for physical medicine respiratory

TABLE 21–1
Common Neuromusculoskeletal Conditions Leading to Global Alveolar Hypoventilation
with Functional Bulbar Musculature

Myopathies
  Muscular dystrophies[6,10,14]
    Dystrophinopathies—Duchenne and Becker dystrophies
    Other muscular dystrophies—limb-girdle, Emery-Dreifuss, facioscapulohumeral, congenital, childhood,
      autosomal recessive, and myotonic dystrophy[10,14,51]
  Non-Duchenne myopathies[10,14]
    Congenital and metabolic myopathies such as acid maltase deficiency[75,124]
    Inflammatory myopathies such as polymyositis[26]
    Diseases of myoneural junction, such as myasthenia gravis,[99] mixed connective tissue disease[80]
    Myopathies of systemic disease, such as carcinomatous myopathy, cachexia/anorexia nervosa,[110]
      medication-associated myopathies
Neurologic disorders
  Spinal muscular atrophies[18]
  Motor neuron diseases[6,14]
  Poliomyelitis[10,12,14]
  Neuropathies
    Hereditary sensory motor neuropathies, including familial hypertrophic interstitial polyneuropathy
    Phrenic neuropathies—associated with cardiac hypothermia, surgical or other trauma, radiation, phrenic
      electrostimulation, familial, paraneoplastic or infectious etiology, lupus erythematosus[37]
    Guillain-Barré syndrome
  Multiple sclerosis[1,13,14]
  Disorders of supraspinal tone such as Friedreich's ataxia
  Myelopathies of rheumatoid, infectious, spondylitic, vascular, traumatic,[3,4,11] or idiopathic etiology[27,28]
  Tetraplegia associated with pancuronium bromide,[57] botulism
Sleep disordered breathing, including obesity hypoventilation,[10,14] central and congenital hypoventilation
  syndromes,[78,97] and hypoventilation associated with diabetic microangiopathy[114] or familial dysautonomia
Skeletal pathology such as kyphoscoliosis,[10,14,17] osteogenesis imperfecta, and rigid spine syndrome[47]
After lung resection[14,133]
Chronic obstructive pulmonary disease[14,79,85]

interventions is beyond the scope of this book.[49,58,107,108,134,135] A discussion of key clinical aspects of the most common pertinent diagnoses follows.

Myopathies

The term *myopathy* applies to disorders attributed to pathologic, biochemical, or electrical changes in muscle fibers or in the interstitial tissues of the skeletal musculature in the absence of nervous system dysfunction.[126] In 1891, Erb described the histopathology of *muscular dystrophy*.[50] Walton suggested that this term be reserved for cases of progressive, genetically determined, primary, degenerative myopathy in which active muscle degeneration and regeneration is observed in muscle biopsy specimens.[126] Thus, myopathies are recognized and differentiated by characteristic histopathologic findings, electromyographic (EMG) findings, and increased serum titers of muscle enzymes.

Dystrophin-Deficient Muscular Dystrophies

Duchenne muscular dystrophy (DMD), the most common severe myopathy, and Becker muscular dystrophy (BMD) are caused by a defect in the 21 region on the short arm (p) of the X-chromosome (Xp21 defect).[94] The nature and precise position of the defect or deletion impact on the quantity and quality of the encoded dystrophin and thereby on phenotypic expression.[73] DMD, in which little or no dystrophin is seen in biopsy specimens, has an incidence of 1/3000 to 3500 male births.[48,91] BMD, with reduced quantity or abnormal dystrophin, has an incidence of 1/25,000.

Children with DMD may be somewhat hypotonic from birth, but weakness is often not evaluated before 3 years of age. They have pseudohypertrophic calves and a relentless, progressive, fairly symmetrical and predictable pattern of muscle weakness, contractures, and wasting. The child may be slow in attaining the motor "milestones," but no correlation has been found between late walking and rapid progression (Fig. 21–1).[62] The average age at wheelchair dependence is 8.6 to 9.5 years (range, 6–15).[40,56,106] Children with DMD do not walk unassisted beyond 13 years of age. Most BMD patients have a much milder course with later onset, up to 25 years of age, and slower progression. The genetics, evaluation, and management principles are basically the same as for DMD.

Medical and surgical strategies for treating DMD date back to 1845.[86] Most medical treatment attempts have been unsuccessful, but, corticosteroid trials have, in some reports, been associated with mild slowing of muscle deterio-

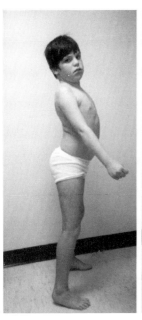
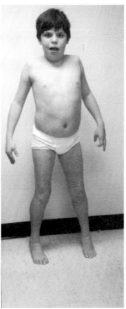

FIGURE 21–1. Seven-year-old with Duchenne muscular dystrophy. Hip extensor weakness leads to anterior pelvic tilt, hip flexor contractures, and increased lumbar lordosis to keep the weight line behind the hips. Tensor fascia lata and iliotibial band contractures lead to a wide-based gait. With increasing quadriceps weakness, the patient must stabilize the knee by keeping the weight line anterior to the knee. The stronger plantar flexors encourage toe walking and lead to equinus deformity which early on helps to stabilize the knee. Iliotibial tract tightness increases torque on the femur to flex the knee and eventually prevents adequate hyperextension of the hip and lumbar spine. With knee flexion contractures, it becomes impossible to keep the center of gravity both behind the hip and in front of the knee, and imbalance of foot evertor strength with the stronger tibialis posterior destabilizing the subtalar joint leads to falls on uneven and eventually on all surfaces.

ration.[42,45] Glucocorticoids, though, have side effects, may increase surgical and anesthetic risks, and have not been shown to significantly change serum creatine kinase concentrations[45,84,113] or prolong life.[39] A new corticosteroid, deflazacort, has fewer side effects than prednisone.[46] Efficacy studies using deflazacort are ongoing. About 8,000,000 myoblasts cloned from satellite cells derived from a rectus femoris muscle biopsy of the father were injected into the left extensor digitorum brevis muscle of a 9-year-old boy with DMD. Cyclosporine was administered for immunosuppression. The donor myoblasts survived, developed, and produced dystrophin, and dystrophin-positive fibers developed in clusters.[70] Although results have been positive for this muscle, further studies have not demonstrated benefit from the transfer of normal myoblasts. In more extensive, ongoing work, gene therapy (i.e., the introduction of genes into tissue using viral vectors or direct gene transfer) is being attempted for the dystrophin gene.

When not optimally treated, progressive spinal deformity occurs in at least 90% of DMD patients.[60] Incidence approaches 100% and severity is greatest for patients with plateau (lifetime best) vital capacities below 1500 ml.[102] Scoliosis can now be prevented or minimized (Table 2).[41]

It has been estimated that 55%[33,92] to 90%[64,101,125] of DMD patients die from the *pulmonary complications* associated with untreated GAH between 16.2 and 19 years of age and uncommonly after age 25 (Fig. 21–2).[48,101] When inadequately treated, patients with DMD develop pneumonias and episodes of respiratory failure, most often during otherwise benign upper respiratory tract infections. These episodes lead to intubation and possibly tracheostomy tube placement.[48] Despite or, at times, because

TABLE 21–2
Reasons for Scoliosis Prevention

1. To permit intermittent abdominal pressure ventilator use as an option to treat alveolar hypoventilation
2. To prevent associated cardiopulmonary compromise
3. To prevent loss of sitting balance and need for seating support systems
4. To prevent losing the possibility of assuming the sitting position
5. To prevent lumbar radiculopathies and lower limb radicular pain
6. To prevent ischial skin pressure pain and pressure ulcers.

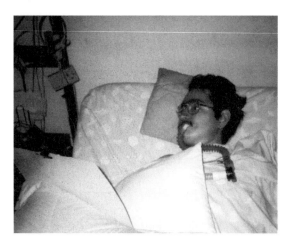

FIGURE 21–2. Twenty-six-year-old patient with Duchenne muscular dystrophy who has required 24-hour use of mouthpiece intermittent positive pressure ventilation (IPPV) since age 12. He has had no ventilator-free breathing time for the last 5 years but has had no respiratory complications or hospitalizations.

of these invasive interventions, respiratory complications remain the most common cause of death for patients with DMD and other severe neuromuscular conditions.[48]

Cardiomyopathy is also a common complication of many myopathies and especially the muscular dystrophies. The incidence of congestive heart failure was reported to be 9.4% (5/53 cases) in DMD.[52] However, evidence of myocardial damage is present in 96% of DMD patients.[120] Cor pulmonale and right ventricular failure also result from untreated GAH. Most myopathic patients who die before developing GAH or who die suddenly despite effective use of noninvasive respiratory muscle aids die from complications of cardiomyopathy.[33] Although progressive,[95,121] there is little or no correlation between the severity of cardiac involvement and skeletal or respiratory muscle involvement in DMD[118] or apparently in other myopathies. Cardiac involvement can range from virtually nonexistent in certain individuals with DMD prior to 18 years of age, to severe in female DMD carriers[89,134] as well as in Becker, Emery-Dreifuss, and limb-girdle muscular dystrophy (LGMD).[71] Indeed, an X-linked dystrophin-deficient cardiomyopathy exists with no evidence of skeletal muscle pathology.

Although for many patients with DMD, non-Duchenne muscular dystrophies, and other myopathies, the most frequent cause of death has been respiratory failure, the great majority of these patients also have varying degrees of car-

diomyopathy. As life is now being prolonged for many of these patients by the use of ventilatory assistance, attention should now be turned to the new medications and treatment approaches that are reversing dilated cardiomyopathy and congestive heart failure.[65]

Children with DMD have delayed *gastric emptying*, up to three times longer than normal.[20] Gastrointestinal motility is decreased in association with smooth muscle dystrophin deficiency.[90] Constipation can result from decreased intestinal motility and from the loss of effective Valsalva maneuver due to abdominal muscle weakness. This is a common problem for patients with neuromuscular disorders. Complaints of malaise, anxiety, epigastric pain, and effortless vomiting have been reported to be of gastrointestinal etiology. Acute episodes of gastric and intestinal distention and tenderness, vomiting, diarrhea, and tachycardia may result in dehydration, impaired diaphragm excursion, and cardiopulmonary failure.[66,105] In such patients, degeneration of the outer, longitudinal, smooth-muscle layer of the stomach has been observed at autopsy.[72] It has been noted that such episodes can follow anesthesia, complicate respiratory tract infections, and be associated with emotional factors and fatigue. Intestinal obstruction, pseudo-obstruction, malabsorption, and possibly volvulus are also more common in neuromuscular disorders and can cause or contribute to ventilatory insufficiency.[112] In the author's experience, however, retching, vomiting, and tachycardia are more commonly associated with GAH and can be reversed by the use of noninvasive inspiratory muscle aids.

Patients with DMD and others with severe neuromuscular conditions have a high incidence of dysphagia and choking associated with bulbar muscle dysfunction.[66] However, in the author's experience, bulbar muscle weakness so severe as to necessitate tracheostomy and interdiction of oral food intake occurs in less than 2% of DMD patients (1/82 > 20 years of age), even after 20 years or more of ventilatory support by noninvasive means.[16]

Other Muscular Dystrophies

Emery-Dreifuss muscular dystrophy is a disease of unknown etiology with X-linked recessive (distal long arm at Xq27–28)[122] inheritance, although autosomal dominant inheritance has been described.[88] The target protein has been identified and named emerin. Prominent flexion contractures characteristically develop at the elbows and heel cords before muscle weakness becomes prominent. The cervical spine is hyperextended and neck flexion limited. The two typical patterns of weakness are those of (1) elbow flexion and extension and peroneal muscle weakness (humeroperoneal dystrophy) and (2) elbow and pelvic muscle weakness (humeropelvic dystrophy). Most patients are able to walk until the third decade.[106] Cardiac arrhythmias, including atrial fibrillation, atrial paralysis, and atrioventricular heart block, are common and prolonged bradycardia may lead to dilated cardiomyopathy.[130] Some patients present with syncopal episodes and arrest.[55] Individuals who do not succumb to cardiac impairment often develop GAH.

The *autosomal recessive muscular dystrophies* include autosomal recessive muscular dystrophy of childhood, LGMD, and the congenital muscular dystrophies. The specific histochemical natures of these disorders have not yet been determined; however, defects at loci on chromosomes 5 and 15 have been identified for LGMD. The diagnoses are made on the basis of muscle biopsy histopathology and the identification of characteristic patterns of muscle weakness. As such, on occasion, an autosomal dominant inheritance has been described for individuals phenotypic for congenital and LGMDs. These conditions are expressed in either sex.

Onset of LGMD is between 5 and 30 years of age. Initial involvement is of the shoulder and pelvic girdle muscles, and rate of progression is highly variable. Calf hypertrophy may occur. Severe disability, muscular contractures, skeletal deformities, cardiomyopathy, and GAH are common (Fig. 21–3).

Autosomal recessive muscular dystrophy of childhood is often confused with DMD and its course may be almost as severe.[128] Muscle dystrophin content is normal, however, and there is no Xp21 defect. History of parental consanguinity may help in establishing the diagnosis. Wheelchair dependence occurs at the mean age of 18 years[100] but may occur from age 10 to 45. If untreated, scoliosis can become severe and respiratory failure may begin as early as age 20, although it more commonly appears after age 25.

Congenital muscular dystrophy without cerebral involvement usually presents as hypotonia at birth or soon thereafter.[83] Static to rapidly progressive forms have been described.[96,131,136] Except for some static, relatively mild forms such as the stick man type, these patients develop predominantly proximal muscle weakness, joint contractures, and occasionally facial muscle weakness, but other cranial musculature is generally spared. About 50% remain severely disabled and never achieve the ability to walk. Scoliosis and GAH may become early and severe problems.

Autosomal dominant forms of muscular dystrophy include, most commonly, facioscapulohumeral muscular dystrophy (FSH) and myotonic dystrophy. Autosomal recessive forms have also been described for FSH.[128] FSH can present in adult, juvenile, or infantile forms.[21] It can vary greatly in severity and in each form lead to the development of life-threatening GAH. The pattern of weakness is distinct. Facial muscles are markedly weakened, and scapular winging becomes prominent. Limb weakness usually begins in the upper arm but typically spares the biceps. Weakness in the legs may be more prominent in distal musculature. Patients may

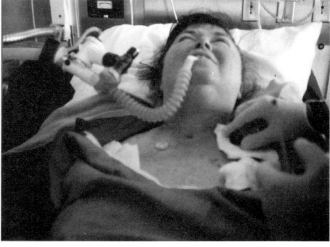

FIGURE 21–3. Woman with limb-girdle muscular dystrophy (LGMD), onset at age 5, diagnosed at age 10, wheelchair dependent at age 22, and tracheostomized for continuous ventilatory support at age 37. After 6 years of 24-hour tracheostomy IPPV, she was converted to daytime mouthpiece IPPV (*see* case 12 in Chapter 25 for details).

lose the ability to close their eyes, speech may become indistinct, and smiling and whistling are impossible.

Myotonic dystrophy is common, with an incidence of 13/100,000 (Fig. 21–4).[32] The defective gene, a triplet repeat sequence of DNA abnormally expanded many times, has been located on chromosome 19.[2] Clinical severity increases with the number of triplet repeats. An increase in the size of the expansion can occur in succeeding generations, particularly when the affected parent is the mother. With few exceptions, the most severe form, congenital myotonic dystrophy, is maternally inherited.[109] Myotonic dystrophy can present from birth until 50 years of age with some combination of myotonia, hand weakness, gait difficulties, temporal muscle atrophy, frontal baldness (in the male), and complaints of poor vision, ptosis, weight loss, impotence, and hypertrichosis. There is a predilection for neck flexor and distal limb muscle weakness. Systemic manifestations may include cataracts, gonadal atrophy, and other endocrine anomalies, cardiomyopathy, GAH, bony changes, and abnormalities of serum immunoglobulins. Mental retardation may be present and especially pronounced for congenital myotonic dystrophy patients. Dysarthria is a common problem. Creatinine kinase is usually normal. Ankle and occasionally other musculotendinous contractures may develop along with weakness and wasting of the limbs. Pulmonary involvement[23,24,53,76,103] is discussed elsewhere in this text. Cardiac involvement is also common, with 65% of patients having electrocardiographic abnormalities[38]; however, involvement is usually much less consequential than for patients with Emery-Dreifuss dystrophy.

Non-Duchenne Myopathies

The term *congenital myopathy* relates to conditions defined by specific morphologic abnormalities observed in muscle biopsy specimens. Childhood-onset congenital myopathy patients are often floppy neonates (Table 21–3). The best characterized congenital myopathies include central core disease, centronuclear myopathies, and nemaline myopathies. Although central core disease usually presents as hypotonia at birth, is usually autosomal dominant, and is generally a mild nonprogressive condition, centronuclear and nemaline myopathies can have mildly to rapidly progressive courses leading to severe disability and GAH.[37,83,104] Nemaline myopathy also has a rapidly progressive adult-onset form.[34] Spheroid body myopathy can also be rapidly progressive and lead to GAH.[80] Dilated cardiomyopathies can occur in these conditions. Most other congenital myopathies are less well characterized and have mild or nonprogressive courses (Fig. 21–5). It is possible that some severe myopathies thought to be of congenital origin are of viral etiology.[36]

Except for certain mitochondrial myopathies, *metabolic myopathies* are autosomal recessive disorders for which defects have been identified, or are suspected, in muscle metabolism. The defects can be in lipid, glycogen, or purine metabolism. For most metabolic myopathies,

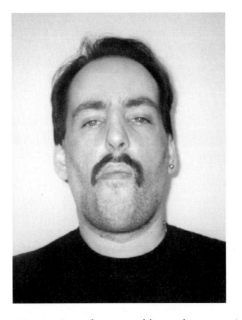

FIGURE 21–4. Forty-five-year-old man demonstrating the temporal atrophy, frontal baldness, and typical facies of myotonic dystrophy. He has the severe global alveolar hypoventilation typical of this disorder.

TABLE 21–3
Neuromuscular Diseases of Floppy Infants in Order of Incidence

Spinal muscular atrophy
Congenital myopathies
Congenital muscular dystrophies
Congenital myotonic dystrophy
Congenital myasthenic syndrome
Acid maltase deficiency (Pompe's disease)
Debranching enzyme deficiency (type 3 glycogen
   storage disease)
Branching enzyme deficiency (type 4 glycogen
   storage disease)
Carnitine deficiency
Mitochondrial myopathies
Congenital peripheral neuropathies

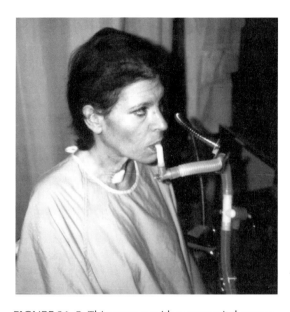

FIGURE 21–5. This woman with a congenital myopathy was able to walk until age 16 and remained stable until age 49, at which point respiratory failure led to her undergoing tracheostomy for ventilatory support. After 5 months of unsuccessful ventilator weaning attempts, she was converted to noninvasive IPPV (*see* case 16 in Chapter 25 for details).

These patients may still be able to walk and work despite GAH and intercurrent pulmonary complications (Fig. 21–6).

Mitochondrial myopathies are metabolic disorders in which abnormalities in mitochondria are suspected and can often be detected by electron microscopy. The most common indication of mitochondrial neuromuscular disease is progressive external ophthalmoplegia (PEO) and possibly ptosis.[58] Nonmuscular manifestations may include lipomas, ichthyosis, cataracts, retinitis pigmentosa, cardiac arrhythmias, cardiomyopathy, intestinal pseudo-obstruction, short stature, diabetes, goiter, primary ovarian failure, deafness, ataxia, neuropathy, seizures, and strokes. In Kearns-Sayre syndrome, a defect in mitochondrial DNA, PEO is accompanied by a myriad of other symptoms and signs,[58] including pigmentary degeneration of the retina, heart block, and depressed ventilatory drive (lack of response to hypercapnia and hypoxia) (Fig. 21–7).[19] Familial PEO syndromes, in which there is little risk of heart block, have been separated into a maternally inherited mitochondrial abnormality and an autosomal dominant disorder.[58] Maternally inherited PEO does not

patients present with fatigue, muscle cramps, and exercise intolerance and ultimately have only mild muscle weakness. The diagnoses are suspected by elevated creatinine kinase levels and myoglobinuria and are confirmed by muscle biopsy. However, progressive generalized muscular weakness resembling LGMD is characteristic of acid maltase deficiency and both branching and debranching enzyme deficiencies, which are disorders of glycolysis, and carnitine deficiency, a disorder of lipid storage. For these disorders, generalized, predominantly proximal, often painless muscle weakness and possibly severe cardiomyopathy are key findings. There is no medical treatment for acid maltase deficiency; the use of small frequent meals is recommended for individuals with debranching enzyme deficiency; and liver transplantation has been very effective in treating branching enzyme deficiency.[111] Some patients with carnitine deficiency respond well to restrictions in dietary fat and treatment with oral L-carnitine.[116] The clinical courses of these conditions, and especially acid maltase deficiency, can closely resemble that of LGMD. Acid maltase deficiency, which leads to accumulation of glycogen in lysosomes, not uncommonly presents with GAH due to respiratory muscle involvement, particularly in the adult-onset disorder.

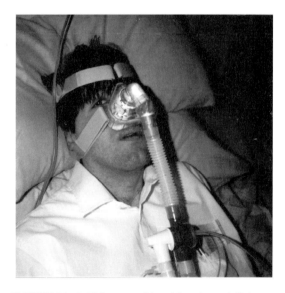

FIGURE 21–6. This man with acid maltase deficiency was a successful high school athlete. Onset of weakness was noted at age 24, diagnosis was made at age 28, and severe dyspnea and chronic global alveolar hypoventilation led to his using a rocking bed ventilator for nocturnal ventilatory assistance from 30 to 35 years of age. At this point, the rocking bed was minimally effective and he required periods of daytime ventilatory assistance. He was switched to daytime mouthpiece IPPV and nocturnal nasal IPPV, which he has used for 5 years.

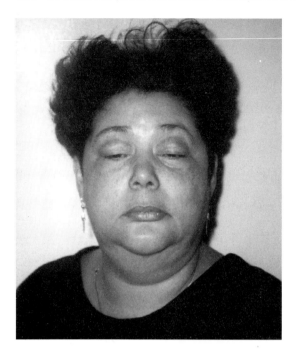

FIGURE 21–7. External ophthalmoplegia (PEO) and ptosis due to Kearns-Sayre syndrome. This patient had both depressed ventilatory drive and respiratory muscle weakness which lead to severe chronic alveolar hypoventilation and four episodes of respiratory failure before institution of respiratory muscle aids.

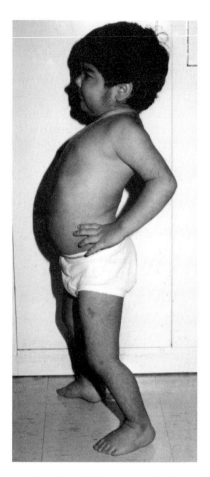

FIGURE 21–8. This child presented with rapid onset of generalized weakness at age 2. His condition appeared to stabilize with glucocorticoid therapy, and he remained stable subsequently without medications. However, he lost the ability to walk at age 7 and had a severe restrictive pulmonary syndrome. He developed chronic alveolar hypoventilation in his early teen years.

have multisystem involvement like Kearns-Sayre syndrome or autosomal dominant PEO, in which tremor, ataxia, sensorimotor peripheral neuropathy, and hearing loss may be present. Other than for some suggestion that coenzyme Q administration may be helpful, there are no medical treatments for the mitochondrial myopathies. For patients with other mitochondrial myopathy syndromes, such as mitochondrial myopathy plus myoclonic epilepsy and ragged red fibers (MERRF), and mitochondrial myopathy plus encephalopathy, lactic acidosis, and stroke-like episodes (MELAS), severe systemic involvement and intellectual deterioration preclude the use of noninvasive respiratory muscle aids.[35]

Polymyositis is an *inflammatory myopathy* that does not affect more than one member of a family. It uncommonly presents before age 20; however, childhood and infantile cases have been reported (Fig. 21–8).[123] Progression may be very rapid or insidious, with symmetric, predominantly proximal and neck muscle weakness. Dysphagia is common; pseudohypertrophy is rare; muscular atrophy is often not severe; and deep tendon reflexes are relatively spared. Creatinine kinase levels can be markedly elevated during disease activity but may otherwise be normal. There may be skin changes (dermatomyositis) or other manifestations of systemic disease. Inflammation is not always seen in the muscle biopsies of inflammatory myopathies. Such conditions may imitate progressive myopathies with limb-girdle weakness.[55] When diagnosed and treated in a timely manner with corticosteroids or other immunosuppressives, an excellent response may be achieved. These patients are susceptible to both acute[26] and late-onset ventilatory failure.

Myasthenia gravis is characterized by intermittent exacerbations of muscle weakness following repetitive muscle activation or with fatigue. There is at least partial recovery after a period of inactivity, especially with treatment. Bulbar and respiratory muscles may be markedly affected, particularly during acute exacerbations, and there is often moderate irreversible involvement of both. Despite this, bulbar muscle function is usually adequate for effective physical medicine interventions.

Prevalence of myasthenia gravis is about 1 in 10,000 with females predominating. The modal age of onset is about 20 years[115]; however, incidences are highest in young women and in middle-aged men. The onset is usually insidious but may be sudden. Diagnosis is made on the basis of the characteristic clinical picture, which often includes asymmetric ptosis and ophthalmoplegia, the presence of anti-acetylcholine receptor site antibodies, characteristic EMG findings including decremental evoked action potential amplitudes during repetitive supramaximal stimulation, and therapeutic response to anticholinesterases. These patients respond well to currently available treatments including corticosteroid therapy, anticholinesterase administration, and plasmapheresis (Fig. 21–9).

Many *systemic diseases* lead to muscle weakness, myopathic changes in muscle groups, or both. Usually, treating the primary medical disorder prevents the extent of respiratory muscle deterioration that would otherwise necessitate the use of respiratory muscle aids. On some occasions, however, conditions such as cancer, collagen disease, or endocrine disease may be complicated by one or more of the following risk factors: advanced age,[129] obesity,[30] cardiopulmonary disease, malnutrition, ongoing glucocorticoid therapy, or the use of certain chemotherapeutic agents or agents such as penicillamine and cimetidine which can produce an inflammatory myopathy. For many such patients, the risk of pulmonary complications and even overt respiratory failure can be prevented or managed strictly by noninvasive respiratory muscle aids.

Disease Affecting the Motor Neurons

Motor neurons are affected in the *spinal muscular atrophies* (SMAs), poliomyelitis, and amyotrophic lateral sclerosis (ALS). The SMAs are inherited as autosomal recessive disorders. The incidence is about 1/5,000.[32] Severity ranges from severe generalized paralysis and need for ventilatory support from birth, to relatively mild, slowly progressive conditions presenting in the second or third decade. They have been arbitrarily separated into three types based on severity. In infantile SMA type 1 (Werdnig-Hoffmann disease), onset is up to 6 months of age and the developmental milestones of rolling, sitting, and walking are not achieved. Ventilatory failure occurs by 2 to 3 years of age (Fig. 21–10). In chronic infantile SMA type 2, onset is up to age 2. In chronic proximal SMA type 3 (Kugelberg-Welander disease), onset is after 2 years of age and ventilatory insufficiency is rare before 10 years of age.[98] Eighty percent of SMA type 3 patients achieve some early developmental milestones but lose the ability to walk before adulthood.[22] Bulbar muscle weakness and inability to cooperate preclude the effective use of noninvasive respiratory muscle aids for severe type 1 patients, but most type 2 and all type 3 patients can be managed indefinitely without resort to tracheostomy. For these patients, oropharyngeal musculature is usually adequate for functional speech and the taking of at least some nu-

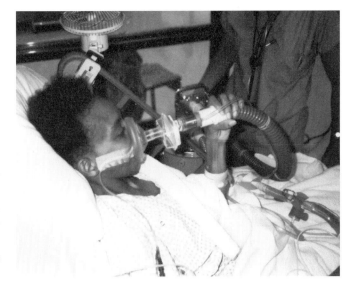

FIGURE 21–9. This patient with myasthenia gravis has relied heavily on auto-administration of mechanical insufflation-exsufflation, nocturnal nasal IPPV, and during acute exacerbations, continuous noninvasive IPPV for 3 years, during which she has been free of hospitalization despite intermittent exacerbations. Prior to this time she was hospitalized and underwent endotracheal intubation on numerous occasions during exacerbation-associated episodes of respiratory failure.

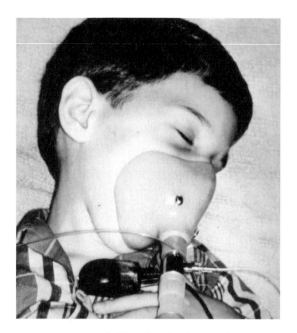

FIGURE 21–10. Child with infantile spinal muscular atrophy, onset at 3 months of age, ability to walk lost at age 4, began nocturnal ventilatory assistance at age 6 receiving IPPV via a strapless oral nasal interface, and continues to use noninvasive IPPV at age 15.

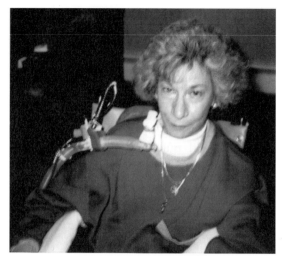

FIGURE 21–11. A woman with onset of amyotrophic lateral sclerosis at age 59, diagnosed 6 months later, developed hypophonia from alveolar hypoventilation 13 months from onset and quickly became dependent on daytime mouthpiece and nocturnal nasal IPPV with no ventilator-free breathing time.

trition by mouth, although bulbar musculature can be acutely weakened during acute respiratory tract infections.[87] Musculotendinous contractures and especially scoliosis are invariably present in type 1 and 2 patients and are a primary concern in early management.

Amyotrophic lateral sclerosis is a disease of unknown etiology of upper and lower motor neurons. Five to 10% of cases have an autosomal dominant pattern of transmission. Although the disease affects about 10% of the population of Guam, it has an incidence of about 1/1800 in the United States. ALS most often presents in middle age but can begin before age 30. The first symptoms and signs are usually muscle cramps, weakness, and fasciculations; however, fatigue, dyspnea, slurred speech, dysphagia, and hypophonia may be initial symptoms (Fig. 21–11). Flaccid paralysis and atrophy usually coexist with cramps, fasciculations, and spasticity. The rate of disease progression is highly variable. It has been estimated that 15% to 20% of all patients have greater than 5-year survival without ventilatory support.[93]

It is possible that the majority of the survivors of the midcentury *poliomyelitis* pandemic are still alive. Over 500,000 people were afflicted in the United States at that time (Fig. 21–12).[63] There have also been several hundred indigenous

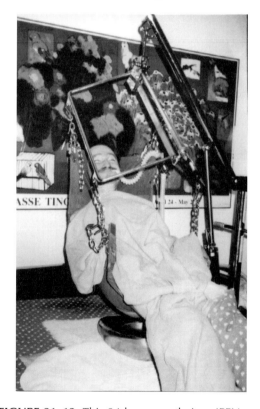

FIGURE 21–12. This 24-hour mouthpiece IPPV user with poliomyelitis has had no measurable vital capacity and no volitional extremity movement since 1952 but has never been intubated. He is using a Hoyer lift as part of his bowel program. This approach has reduced the time needed to complete his bowel movements from 3 hours to 15 to 20 minutes.

cases and many immigrants in this country with *post-polio* sequelae.[117] Late complications of poliomyelitis present as a form of motor neuron disease with a constellation of symptoms that include fatigue, dysphagia, dyspnea, and increased functional difficulties.[59] It is the result of senescent loss of remaining anterior horn cells. Post-polio survivors are developing pulmonary complications associated with GAH and, rarely, with bulbar muscle weakness. Many patients who require ventilatory assistance are able to walk.

Neuropathies

The most common hereditary peripheral neuropathy is *Charcot-Marie-Tooth disease.* It is an autosomal dominant disorder with variable penetrance and symmetric distal greater than proximal weakness and sensory involvement. EMG demonstrates severe nerve conduction slowing; however, an axonal form has been described in which conduction may be within normal limits while amplitudes are diminished. Although ankle deformities and distal extremity weakness and sensory loss are usually the only impairments, weakness can on occasion (four patients in the author's experience) progress to severe generalized tetraplegia and need for permanent ventilatory support.

Familial hypertrophic interstitial polyneuropathy (Dejerine-Sottas disease) is a rare disease of generalized weakness. It is diagnosed by peripheral nerve biopsy. Bulbar muscle involvement often precludes the optimal use of noninvasive inspiratory muscle aids because the lips are often too weak to grasp a mouthpiece, and scoliosis can prevent the effective use of an intermittent abdominal pressure ventilator. Expiratory muscle aids, however, can be very helpful to assist cough.

A multitude of conditions can cause *phrenic neuropathies* (Table 1). With bulbar and expiratory musculature sparing, these patients only require the use of inspiratory muscle aids.

Acute post-infectious polyneuropathy or the *Guillain-Barré syndrome* is an acquired inflammatory segmental demyelinating neuropathy. Two-thirds of cases present with a history of preceding viral infection, immunization, surgery, or immunologic disorder.[74] Sensory loss is usually slight and is absent in one-third of patients.[74] Ascending weakness and parasthesias begin in the hands and feet and usually progress for 1 to 2 weeks. Partial to almost complete recovery usually takes 3 to 6 months. Cerebrospinal fluid protein concentration is elevated at some time during the illness. The diagnosis is made on the basis of the history, clinical and laboratory picture, and the observation of characteristically severe nerve conduction slowing. With recovery, residual weakness ranges from mild ankle dorsiflexion weakness to, uncommonly, essentially complete paralysis necessitating permanent ventilatory support.

Multiple sclerosis is a disease of unknown etiology characterized by widespread patches of central nervous system demyelination followed by gliosis. Its incidence is 1 to 8/10,000 population.[126] Symptoms and signs most commonly include optic neuritis and nystagmus. Focal or generalized paralysis, incoordination, dysarthria, sensory abnormalities, bowel and bladder incontinence, vertigo, and mental symptoms are also common. The diagnosis is made by the characteristic appearance of high cerebrospinal fluid gamma globulin levels, occasionally elevations of mononuclear cell levels, and by the characteristic appearance of central nervous system plaques viewed during nuclear magnetic resonance imaging. Remissions and relapses are characteristic and usually occur over many years.[81,82] Acute relapses often respond well to administration of high doses of corticosteroids (Fig. 21–13). Interferon therapy is also becoming popular.

Friedreich's ataxia is an inherited, autosomal recessive (rarely autosomal dominant), progres-

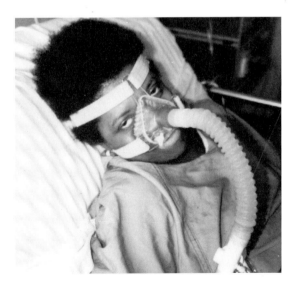

FIGURE 21–13. A 36-year-old woman, blind from optic neuritis, presented with rapid onset of tetraplegia and acute ventilatory failure (vital capacity decreased to 100 ml). She received 24-hour nasal IPPV instead of intubation (*see* case 1 in Chapter 25 for details).

sive condition with symptoms first appearing after 5 years of age. There is generalized central nervous system, and especially spinal cord, degeneration and reactive gliosis. The anterior horn cells may also be involved.[126] About 50% of patients die from cardiomyopathy.[61] GAH and severely impaired cough occur late in this disorder.

The most common cause of *myelopathy* is traumatic spinal cord injury (SCI). This most commonly results from motor vehicle accidents, diving accidents, and gunshot wounds. The incidence of acute SCI in the United States is 28 to 50/million/year.[44] The number of tetraplegics slightly exceeds that of paraplegics.[68] The prevalence of individuals with SCI in the United States has been estimated at about 200,000[69] and is increasing yearly due to the increasing longevity of this population.[68] Untimely and inadequate treatment for impaired cough are the principle reasons that pulmonary complications are the leading cause of death for at least the first 12 years after injury (Fig. 21–14).[43]

Myelitis refers to any condition that causes inflammation of the spinal cord. Myelitis usually involves both the gray and white matter and may involve any level of the spine. When limited to a few segments, it is noted as transverse myelitis. It is most often due to neurotrophic viruses and is associated with smallpox, measles, chickenpox, mononucleosis, herpes zoster, influenza, certain vaccinations, and tuberculosis.[126] An episode of apparent transverse myelitis may be a precursor to multiple sclerosis. Myelopathies also result from radiation exposure, tumors, vascular disease (especially of the anterior and posterior spinal arteries), fibrocartilaginous emboli

to the spine,[27] cervical spondylosis, spondylitis associated with connective tissue diseases, and electric shock to the spine, but most often, they are of unknown etiology (Fig. 21–15). Myelopathies can be of sudden onset or develop over a period of months or years and result in ventilatory failure. Bulbar musculature is most often spared.

Tetraplegia can occur following administration of pancuronium bromide[57] or other curarization agents that are often used to prevent patients from self-tracheal extubation. Botulism, the generalized paralysis resulting from the toxin of intestinal *Clostridium botulinum* spores, has also been treated by noninvasive ventilatory support rather than endotracheal intubation.[25] Botulism immune globulin, which neutralizes the toxin in the intestine, has been developed recently and may be effective in limiting paralysis.

Skeletal Pathology

Kyphoscoliosis invariably develops in progressive pediatric neuromuscular diseases and is frequently seen in neurofibromatosis, osteogenesis imperfecta, tuberculosis of the spine, rigid spine syndrome,[47] familial dysautonomia, and especially familial autosomal dominant idiopathic kyphoscoliosis. Patients with neuromuscular weakness develop collapsing spines because of a lack of supporting muscular structure. Spinal deformity progresses throughout life. The pathogenesis of kyphoscoliosis is less clear for patients with generally intact skeletal muscle strength. Kyphoscoliosis can cause or exacer-

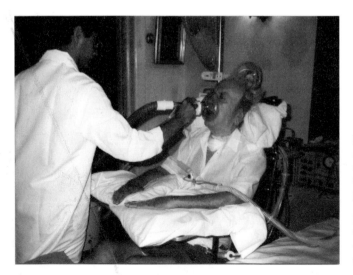

FIGURE 21–14. A 72-year-old man suffered a C2 fracture and complete C2 quadriplegia on falling from a tree. His tracheostomy tube, which was placed in the immediate post-injury period, was removed, and he relied on continuous noninvasive IPPV. Here, he is using mechanical insufflation-exsufflation to eliminate food that he aspirated while eating because of swallowing dysfunction.

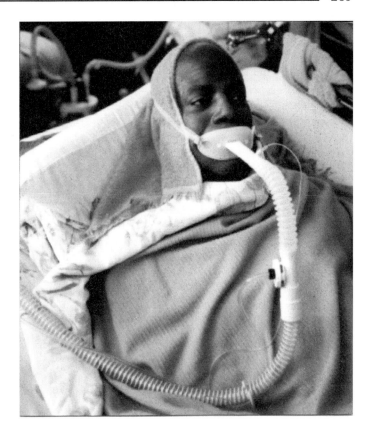

FIGURE 21–15. A man with idiopathic C2 transverse myelitis developed complete tetraplegia over a several-month period in 1967 and has relied on continuous mouthpiece IPPV since then.

bate GAH. These patients also develop ventilation perfusion mismatching and have a higher incidence of obstructive sleep apneas when the skeletal deformities involve the upper cervical region and, therefore, the hypopharynx. Kyphoscoliosis must be prevented or minimized for the reasons noted in Table 2. Perhaps the worst complication of severe kyphoscoliosis results when the lower ribs on the convex side impinge into the abdomen, physically precluding the assumption of the sitting position. These patients then lose most remaining function. Management of kyphoscoliosis is disease-specific.[15]

Individuals with *pulmonary restrictive syndromes* following lung resection or from any intrinsic lung or chest wall pathology often develop GAH. Provided that noninvasive IPPV can normalize ventilation and PaO_2 levels at airway pressures under 50 cm H_2O tracheostomy can be avoided.[14]

Chronic Obstructive Pulmonary Disease

Although not a neuromusculoskeletal disorder per se, chest wall distortions occur in patients with chronic obstructive pulmonary disease (COPD), and the resulting stretching of inspiratory musculature alters normal length-contraction relationships and lends to respiratory muscle weakness and fatigue.

For patients with severe COPD, hypercapnia results from the low tidal volumes used to avoid acute respiratory muscle fatigue. Hypercapnia is associated with increased mortality in COPD patients[29] as it is in patients with any diagnosis. There is a strong physiologic rationale to rest[31] the respiratory musculature of hypercapnic patients.[119] The use of ventilatory assistance for patients with normocapnic respiratory failure may also be beneficial by reducing oxygen consumption related to the increased work of breathing for patients with intrinsic lung disease. Unlike for certain hypercapnic COPD patients, the use of ventilatory assistance by normocapnic COPD patients has not been proved to be useful.

References

1. Aisen M, Arlt G, Foster S: Diaphragmatic paralysis without bulbar or limb paralysis in multiple sclerosis. Chest 98:499–501, 1990.
2. Aslanidis C, Jansen G, Amemiya C, et al: Cloning of the essential myotonic dystrophy region and mapping of the putative defect. Nature 355:548–551, 1992.
3. Bach JR: Alternative methods of ventilatory support for

the patient with ventilatory failure due to spinal cord injury. J Am Paraplegia Soc 14:158–174, 1991.

4. Bach JR: New approaches in the rehabilitation of the traumatic high level quadriplegic. Am J Phys Med Rehabil 70:13–20, 1991.

5. Bach JR: Pulmonary rehabilitation considerations for Duchenne muscular dystrophy: The prolongation of life by respiratory muscle aids. Crit Rev Phys Rehabil Med 3:239–269, 1992.

6. Bach JR: Amyotrophic lateral sclerosis: Communication status and survival with ventilatory support. Am J Phys Med Rehabil 72:343–349, 1993.

7. Bach JR: Comprehensive rehabilitation of the severely disabled ventilator-assisted individual. Monaldi Arch Chest Dis 48:331–345, 1993.

8. Bach JR: Inappropriate weaning and late onset ventilatory failure of individuals with traumatic quadriplegia. Paraplegia 31:430–438, 1993.

9. Bach JR: Management of post-polio respiratory sequelae. Ann N Y Acad Sci 753:96–102, 1995.

10. Bach JR, Alba AS: Management of chronic alveolar hypoventilation by nasal ventilation. Chest 97:52–57, 1990.

11. Bach JR, Alba AS: Noninvasive options for ventilatory support of the traumatic high level quadriplegic. Chest 98:613–619, 1990.

12. Bach JR, Alba AS: Pulmonary dysfunction and sleep disordered breathing as post-polio sequelae: Evaluation and management. Orthopedics 14:1329–1337, 1991.

13. Bach JR, Alba A, Mosher R, Delaubier A: Intermittent positive pressure ventilation via nasal access in the management of respiratory insufficiency. Chest 92:168–170, 1987.

14. Bach JR, Alba AS, Saporito LR: Intermittent positive pressure ventilation via the mouth as an alternative to tracheostomy for 257 ventilator users. Chest 103:174–182, 1993.

15. Bach JR, Lieberman JS: Rehabilitation of the patient with disease affecting the motor unit. In DeLisa JD (ed): Rehabilitation Medicine: Principles and Practice. Philadelphia, JB Lippincott, 1993, pp 1099–1110.

16. Bach JR, O'Brien J, Krotenberg R, Alba A: Management of end stage respiratory failure in Duchenne muscular dystrophy. Muscle Nerve 10:177–182, 1987.

17. Bach JR, Robert D, Leger P, Langevin B: Sleep fragmentation in kyphoscoliotic individuals with chronic alveolar hypoventilation treated by nasal IPPV. Chest 107:1552–1558, 1995.

18. Bach JR, Wang TG: Noninvasive long-term ventilatory support for individuals with spinal muscular atrophy and functional bulbar musculature. Arch Phys Med Rehabil 76:213–217, 1995.

19. Barohn RJ, Clanton T, Sahenk Z, Mendell JR: Recurrent respiratory insufficiency and depressed ventilatory drive complicating mitochondrial myopathies. Neurology 40:103–106, 1990.

20. Barohn RJ, Levine EJ, Olson JO, Mendell JR: Gastric hypomotility in Duchenne's muscular dystrophy. N Engl J Med 319:15–18, 1988.

21. Bailey RO, Marzulo DC, Hans MB: Infantile fascioscapulohumeral muscular dystrophy: New observations. Acta Neurol Scand 74:51–58, 1986.

22. Barois ィ, Estournet B, Duval-Beaupere G, et al: Amyotrophie spinale infantile. Rev Neurol (Paris) 145:299–304, 1989.

23. Begin R, Bureau MA, Lupien L, et al: Pathogenesis of respiratory insufficiency in myotonic dystrophy. Am Rev Respir Dis 125:312–318, 1982.

24. Begin R, Bureau MA, Lupien L, Lemieux B: Control and

25. Blackney DA: Negative pressure conquers infant botulism. Lifecare's Alert Newsletter Sep/Oct, 1994.

26. Blumbergs PC, Byrne E, Kakulas BA: Polymyositis presenting with respiratory failure. J Neurol Sci 65:221–229, 1984.

27. Bockenek W, Bach JR: Fibrocartilaginous emboli to the spinal cord: A review of the literature. J Am Paraplegia Soc 13:18–23, 1990.

28. Bockenek W, Bach JR, Alba AS, Cravioto A: Cartilagenous emboli to the spinal cord: A case study. Arch Phys Med Rehabil 71:754–757, 1990.

29. Boushy SF, Thompson HK Jr, North LB, et al: Prognosis in chronic obstructive pulmonary disease. Am Rev Respir Dis 108:1373–1383, 1973.

30. Bradley TD, Phillipson EA: Pathogenesis and pathophysiology of the obstructive sleep apnea syndrome. Med Clin North Am 69:1169–1185, 1985.

31. Braun NMT, Arora NS, Rochester DF: Respiratory muscle and pulmonary function in polymyositis and other proximal myopathies. Thorax 38:616–623, 1983.

32. Brooke MH: A Clinician's View of Neuromuscular Diseases, 2nd ed. Baltimore, Williams & Wilkins, 1986, pp 194–212, 243–331.

33. Brooke MH, Fenichel GM, Griggs RC, et al: Duchenne muscular dystrophy: Patterns of clinical progression and effects of supportive therapy. Neurology 39:475–480, 1989.

34. Brownell AKW, Gilbert JJ, Shaw DT, et al: Adult onset nemaline myopathy. Neurology 28:1306–1309, 1978.

35. Byrne E, Dennett X, Trounce I, Burdon J: Mitochondrial myoneuropathy with respiratory failure and myoclonic epilepsy. J Neurol Sci 71:273–281, 1985.

36. Carpenter S, Karpati G, Holland P: New observations in reducing body myopathy. Neurology 35:818–827, 1985.

37. Chan CK, Loke J, Virgulto JA, et al: Bilateral diaphragmatic paralysis: Clinical spectrum, prognosis, and diagnostic approach. Arch Phys Med Rehabil 69:967–979, 1988.

38. Church SC: The heart in myotonia atrophica. Arch Intern Med 119:176–181, 1967.

39. Cohen L, Morgan J, Babbs Jr R, et al: Fast walking velocity in health and Duchenne muscular dystrophy: A statistical analysis. Arch Phys Med Rehabil 65:573–578, 1984.

40. Demos J: Early diagnosis and treatment of rapidly developing Duchenne de Boulogne type myopathy Am J Phys Med 50:271_84, 1971.

41. Duport G, Gayet E, Pries P, et al: Spinal deformities and wheelchair seating in Duchenne muscular dystrophy: Twenty years of research and clinical experience. Semin Neurol 15:9–17, 1995.

42. DeSilva S, Drachman DB, Mellits D, Kunel RW: Prednisone treatment in Duchenne muscular dystrophy: Long-term benefit. Arch Neurol 44:818–822, 1987.

43. DeVivo MJ, Black KJ, Stover SL: Causes of death during the first twelve years after spinal cord injury [abstract]. J Am Paraplegia Soc 14:113, 1991.

44. DeVivo MJ, Fine PR, Maetz HM, Stover SL: Prevalence of spinal cord injury: A re-estimation employing life table techniques. Arch Neurol 37:707–708, 1980.

45. Drachman DB, Toyka RV, Myer E: Prednisone in Duchenne muscular dystrophy. Lancet 2:1409–1412, 1974.

46. Dubrovsky AL, Mesa L, Marco P, et al: Deflazacort treatment in Duchenne muscular dystrophy. Neurology 41 (suppl 1):136–141, 1991.

47. Efthimiou J, McLelland J, Round J, et al: Diaphragm paralysis causing ventilatory failure in an adult with rigid spine syndrome. Am Rev Respir Dis 136:1483–1485, 1987.

48. Emery AEH: Duchenne muscular dystrophy: Genetic aspects, carrier detection and antenatal diagnosis. Br Med Bull 36:117–122, 1980.

49. Engel AG, Franzini-Armstrong C (eds): Myology: Basic and Clinical, vol 2. New York, McGraw Hill, 1994.

50. Erb W: Dystrophia muscularis progressiva: klinische und pathologischanatomische studien. Dtsch Z Nervenheilkd 1:13–94,173–261, 1891.

51. Estenne M, Borenstein S, De Troyer A: Respiratory muscle dysfunction in myotonia congenita. Am Rev Respir Dis 130:681–684, 1984.

52. Farah MG, Evans EB, Vignos PJ: Echocardiographic evaluation of left ventricular function in Duchenne's muscular dystrophy. Am J Med 69:248–254, 1980.

53. Fernandez JM, Lara I, Gila L, et al: Disturbed hypothalamic-putuitary axis in idiopathic recurring hypersomnia syndrome. Acta Neurol Scand 82:361–363, 1990.

54. Fischer DA: Poliomyelitis: Late respiratory complications and management. Orthopedics 8:891–894, 1985.

55. Fowler WM, Nayak NN: Slowly progressive proximal weakness: Limb-girdle syndromes. Arch Phys Med Rehabil 64:527–538, 1983.

56. Gardner-Medwin D: Clinical features and classification of the muscular dystrophies. Br Med Bull 36:109–115, 1980.

57. Giostra E, Magistris MR, Pizzolato G, et al: Neuromuscular disorder in intensive care unit patients treated with pancuronium bromide: Occurrence in a cluster group of seven patients and two sporadic cases, with electrophysiologic and histologic examination. Chest 106:210–220, 1994.

58. Griggs RC, Mendell JR, Miller RG: Evaluation and Treatment of Myopathies. Philadelphia, FA Davis, 1995.

59. Halstead LS: Post-polio sequelae: Assessment and differential diagnosis for post-polio syndrome. Orthopedics 14:1209–1217, 1991.

60. Heckmatt J, Rodillo E, Dubowitz V: Management of children: Pharmacological and physical. Br Med Bull 45: 788–801, 1989.

61. Hewer RL: Study of fatal cases of Friedreich's ataxia. BMJ 3:649–652, 1968.

62. Hinge HF, Hein-Sorensen O, Reske-Nielsen E: X-linked Duchenne muscular dystrophy. Scand J Rehabil Med 21:27–31, 1989.

63. Historical Statistics of the United States: Colonial Times to 1970, Bicentennial Edition, Pt 1. Washington, DC, U.S. Department of Commerce, Bureau of the Census. 1975, pp. 8, 77.

64. Inkley SR, Oldenberg FC, Vignos PJ: Pulmonary function in Duchenne muscular dystrophy related to stage of disease. Am J Med 56:297–306, 1974.

65. Ishikawa Y, Bach JR, Sarma RJ, et al: Cardiovascular considerations in the management of neuromuscular disease. Semin Neurol 15:93–108, 1995.

66. Jaffe KM, McDonald CM, Ingman E, Haas J: Symptoms of upper gastrointestinal dysfunction in Duchenne muscular dystrophy: Case-control study. Arch Phys Med Rehabil 71:742–744, 1990.

67. Jerusalem F, Ludin H, Bischoff A, Hartmann G: Cytoplasmic body neuromyopathy presenting as respiratory failure and weight loss. J Neurol Sci 41:1–9, 1979.

68. Kennedy EJ (ed): Spinal Cord Injury: The Facts and Figures. Birmingham, AL, University of Alabama at Birmingham, 1986, p 27, 59.

69. Kraus JF: Epidemiological aspects of acute spinal cord injury: A review of incidence, prevalence, causes, and outcome. In Becker DP, Povlishock JT (eds): Central Nervous System Trauma Status Report—1985. Bethesda, MD, National Institute of Neurological and Communicative Disorders and Stroke, National Institutes of Health, 1985, p 313–322.

70. Law PK, Bertorini TE, Goodwin TG, et al: Dystrophin production induced by myoblast transfer therapy in Duchenne muscular dystrophy. Lancet 336:114–115, 1990.

71. Lazzeroni E, Favaro L, Botti G: Dilated cardiomyopathy with regional myocardial hypoperfusion in Becker's muscular dystrophy. Int J Cardiol 22:126–129, 1989.

72. Leon SH, Schuffler MD, Kettler M, Rohrmann CA: Chronic intestinal pseudoobstruction as a complication of Duchenne's muscular dystrophy. Gastroenterology 90:455–459, 1986.

73. Liechti-Gallati S, Koenig M, Kunkel LM, et al: Molecular deletion patterns in Duchenne and Becker type muscular dystrophy. Hum Genet 81:343–348, 1989.

74. Lisak RP: The immunology of neuromuscular disease. In Walton JN (ed): Disorders of Voluntary Muscle, 5th ed. London, Churchill Livingstone, 1988, pp 345–371.

75. Maayan C, Springer C, Armon Y, et al: Nemaline myopathy as a cause of sleep hypoventilation. Pediatrics 77:390–395, 1986.

76. Manni R, Zucca C, Martinetti M, et al: Hypersomnia in dystrophia myotonica: A neurophysiological and immunogenetic study. Acta Neurol Scand 84:498–502, 1991.

77. Mansel JK, Norman JR: Respiratory complications and management of spinal cord injuries. Chest 97:1446–1452, 1990.

78. Marcus CL, Livingston FR, Wood SE, Keens TG: Hypercapnic and hypoxic ventilatory responses in parents and siblings of children with congenital central hypoventilation syndrome. Am Rev Respir Dis 144:136–140, 1991.

79. Marino W: Intermittent volume cycled mechanical ventilation via nasal mask in patients with respiratory failure due to COPD. Chest 99:681–684, 1991.

80. Martyn JB, Wong MJ, Huang SHK: Pulmonary and neuromuscular complications and mixed connective tissue disease: A report and review of the literature. J Rheumatol 15:703–705, 1988

81. McAlpine D, Comston N: Some aspects of the natural history of disseminated sclerosis. Q J Med 21:135–167, 1952.

82. McIntyre HD, McIntyre AP: Prognosis of multiple sclerosis. Arch Neurol Neurosurg Psychiat 50:431–439, 1943.

83. McMenamin JB, Becker LE, Murphy EG: Congenital muscular dystrophy: A clinicopathologic report of 24 cases. J Pediatr 100:692–697, 1982.

84. Mendell JR, Moxley RC, Griggs RC, et al: Randomized, double-blind six-month trial of prednisone in Duchenne's muscular dystrophy. N Engl J Med 320:1592–1597, 1989.

85. Meduri GU, Conoscenti CC, Menashe P, Nair S: Noninvasive face mask ventilation in patients with acute respiratory failure. Chest 95:865–870, 1989.

86. Meryon E: On granular or fatty degeneration of the voluntary muscles. Med-Chir Trans 35:73–84, 1852.

87. Mier-Jedrzejowicz A, Brophy C, Green M: Respiratory muscle weakness during upper respiratory tract infections. Am Rev Respir Dis 138:5–7, 1988.

88. Miller RG, Layzer RB, Mellenthin MA, et al: Emery-Dreifuss muscular dystrophy with autosomal dominant transmission. Neurology 35:1230–1233, 1985.

89. Mingo PU, Romero JT, Barbero JLT, Jalon EI: Miocardiopatia dilatada en une mujer portadora de la enfermedad de Duchenne de Boulogne. Rev Clin Esp 181: 468, 1987.

90. Miyatake M, Miike T, Zhao J, et al: Possible systemic smooth muscle layer dysfunction due to a deficiency of dystrophin in Duchenne muscular dystrophy. J Neurol Sci 93:11–17, 1989.

91. Monckton G, Hoskin V, Warren S: Prevalence and incidence of muscular dystrophy in Alberta, Canada. Clin Genet 21:19–24, 1982.

92. Mukoyama M, Kondo K, Hizawa K, et al: Life spans of Duchenne muscular dystrophy patients in the hospital care program in Japan. J Neurol Sci 81:155–158, 1987.

93. Mulder DW, Howard FM: Patient resistance and prognosis in amyotrophic lateral sclerosis. Mayo Clin Proc 51:537–541, 1976.

94. Murray JM, Davies KE, Harper PS, et al: Linkage relationship of a cloned DNA sequence on the short arm of the X chromosome to Duchenne muscular dystrophy. Nature 300:69–71, 1982.

95. Nigro G, Comi LI, Limongelli FM, et al: Prospective study of X-linked progressive muscular dystrophy in Campania. Muscle Nerve 6:253–262, 1983.

96. O'Brien MD: An infantile muscular dystrophy: Report of a case with autopsy findings. Guy's Hosp Rep 111: 98–106, 1962.

97. Oren J, Kelly DH, Shannon DC: Long-term follow-up of children with congenital central hypoventilation syndrome. Pediatrics 80:375–380, 1987.

98. Paern JH, Wilson J: Acute Werdnig-Hoffmann disease. Arch Dis Child 48:425–430, 1973.

99. Quera-Salva MA, Guilleminault C, Chrevret S, et al: Breathing disorders during sleep in myasthenia gravis. Ann Neurol 31:86–92, 1992.

100. Rideau Y, Delaubier A, Foucault P, et al: Une forme meconnue de myopathie: II. Definition et caractéres cliniques. Semin Hôp Paris 67:1343–1349, 1991.

101. Rideau Y, Gatin G, Bach J, Gines G: Prolongation of life in Duchenne muscular dystrophy. Acta Neurol 5:118–124, 1983.

102. Rideau Y, Glorion B, Delaubier A, et al: Treatment of scoliosis in Duchenne muscular dystrophy. Muscle Nerve 7:281–286, 1984.

103. Rimmer KP, Golar SD, Lee MA, Whitelaw WA: Myotonia of the respiratory muscles in myotonic dystrophy. Am Rev Respir Dis 148:1018–1022, 1993.

104. Rimmer KP, Whitelaw WA: The respiratory muscles in multicore myopathy. Am Rev Respir Dis 148:227–231, 1993.

105. Robin GC, Falewski de Leon GH: Acute gastric dilatation in progressive muscular dystrophy. Lancet 2:171–172, 1963.

106. Rowland LP, Fetell M, Olarte M, et al: Emery-Dreifuss muscular dystrophy. Ann Neurol 5:111–117, 1979.

107. Rowland LP, Laycer RB: The X-linked muscular dystrophies. In Vinken PJ, Bruyn GW (eds): Handbook of Clinical Neurology. New York, North Holland Publishing Co., 1979, pp 349–414.

108. Rowland LP, Wood DS, Schon EA, DiMauro S (eds): Molecular Genetics in Diseases of Brain, Nerve, and Muscle. New York, Oxford University Press, 1989.

109. Rutherford MA, Heckmatt JZ, Dubowitz V: Congenital myotonic dystrophy: Respiratory function at birth determines survival. Arch Dis Child 64:191–195, 1989.

110. Ryan CF, Whittaker JS, Road JD: Ventilatory dysfunction in severe anorexia nervosa. Chest 102:1286–1288, 1992.

111. Selby R, Starzl TE, Yunis E, et al: Liver transplantation for type IV glycogen storage disease. N Engl J Med 324:39–42, 1991.

112. Siegel IM: Update on Duchenne muscular dystrophy. Compr Ther 15:45–52, 1989.

113. Siegel IM, Miller JE, Ray RD: Failure of corticosteroid in the treatment of Duchenne (pseudo-hypertrophic) muscular dystrophy: Report of a clinically matched three year double-blind study. Ill Med J 145:32–33, 1974.

114. Silverstein D, Michlin B, Sobel HJ, Lavietes MH: Right ventricular failure in a patient with diabetic neuropathy (myopathy) and central alveolar hypoventilation. Respiration 44:460–465, 1983.

115. Simpson JA: Myasthenia gravis and myasthenic syndromes. In Walton JN (ed): Disorders of Voluntary Muscle, 5th ed. London, Churchill Livingstone, 1988, pp 628–665.

116. Stanley CA, DeLeeuw S, Coates PM, et al: Chronic cardiomyopathy and weakness or acute coma in children with a defect in carnitine uptake. Ann Neurol 30:709–716, 1991.

117. Statistical Abstracts of the United States, 110th ed. Washington, DC, U.S. Department of Commerce, Bureau of the Census, 1990, p 116.

118. Stewart CA, Gilgoff I, Baydur A, et al: Gated radionuclide ventriculography in the evaluation of cardiac function in Duchenne's muscular dystrophy. Chest 94:1245–1248, 1988.

119. Stoller JK: Physiologic rationale for resting the ventilatory muscles. Respir Care 36:290–296, 1991.

120. Tamura T, Shibuya N, Hashiba K, et al: Evaluation of myocardial damage in Duchenne's muscular dystrophy with thalium-201 myocardial SPECT. Jpn Heart J 34:51–61, 1993.

121. Tanaka H, Nishi S, Katanasako H: Natural course of cardiomyopathy in Duchenne muscular dystrophy. Jpn Circ J 43:974–984, 1979.

122. Thomas NST, Williams H, Elsas LJ, et al: Localisation of the gene for Emery-Dreifuss muscular dystrophy to the distal long arm of the X chromosome. J Med Genet 23:596–598, 1986.

123. Thompson CE: Infantile myositis. Dev Med Child Neurol 24:307–313, 1982.

124. Vercken JB, Raphael JC, De Lattre J, et al: Adult maltase acid deficiency myopathy: Treatment with long-term home mechanical ventilation. Biomed Pharmacother 42:343–349, 1988.

125. Vignos PJ: Respiratory function and pulmonary infection in Duchenne muscular dystrophy. Isr J Med Sci 13:207–214, 1977.

126. Walton JN: Brain's Diseases of the Nervous System, 8th ed. Oxford, Oxford University Press, 1977, pp 548–549, 672–674, 779–786.

127. Walton JN, Gardner-Medwin D: Progressive muscular dystrophy and the myotonic disorders. In Walton J (ed): Disorders of Voluntary Muscle, 3rd ed. London, Churchill Livingstone, 1974, pp 561–613.

128. Walton JN, Gardner-Medwin D: The muscular dystrophies. In Walton J (ed): Disorders of Voluntary Muscle, 5th ed. London, Churchill Livingstone, 1988, pp 519–568.

129. Wang TG, Bach JR: Pulmonary dysfunction in residents of chronic care facilities. Taiwan J Rehabil 21:67–73, 1993.

130. Waters DD, Nutter DO, Hopkins LC, Dorney ER: Cardiac features of an unusual X-linked humeroperoneal neuromuscular disease. N Eng J Med 293:1017–1022, 1975.

131. Wharton BA: An unusual variety of muscular dystrophy. Lancet 1:603–604, 1965.
132. Wiegand V, Rahlf G, Meinck M, Kreuzer H: Kardiomyopathie bei tragerinnen des Duchenne-gens. Z Kardiol 73:188–191, 1984.
133. Yang GF, Alba A, Lee M: Respiratory rehabilitation in severe restrictive lung disease secondary to tuberculosis. Arch Phys Med Rehabil 65:556–558, 1984.
134. Younger DS (ed): Paralysis: Pt 1. Semin Neurol 13:241–315, 1991.
135. Younger DS (ed): Paralytic syndromes: Pt II. Semin Neurol 13:319–379, 1991.
136. Zellweger H, Afifi A, McCormick WF, Mergner W: Severe congenital muscular dystrophy. Am J Dis Child 114:591–602, 1967.

Pathophysiology of Paralytic-Restrictive Pulmonary Syndromes

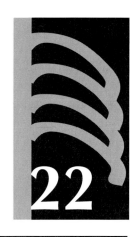

22

John R. Bach, MD

As noted in the previous chapter,[7] paralytic-restrictive disorders, or individuals with primarily impairment of alveolar ventilation, can be divided into those with sudden, permanent respiratory muscle dysfunction; those with rapidly developing or relapsing conditions; and those with insidious, late-onset ventilatory failure. Some patients, such as those with spinal cord injury or poliomyelitis, can fall into any of the three categories.

PULMONARY FUNCTION IN RESTRICTIVE PULMONARY SYNDROMES

Normally the vital capacity (VC) plateaus at 19 years of age then decreases by 1% to 1.2% per year throughout life.[6] Individuals with restrictive pulmonary syndromes, however, have a reduction in total lung volumes, VC, expiratory reserve volume, and usually functional residual capacity. Restriction can be due to a combination of respiratory muscle weakness, paralysis, and mechanical factors involving the chest wall and lungs. Mechanical problems associated with global alveolar hypoventilation (GAH) include thoracic deformities, obesity, the use of improperly fitting thoracolumbar orthoses, and sleep-associated hypopharyngeal collapse or other upper airway narrowing.[8] Acute conditions that decrease pulmonary function, such as bronchial mucus plugging, pulmonary infiltrations, pleural diseases, pneumothoraces, and other respiratory complications, can exacerbate hypercapnia or trigger acute respiratory failure.

For patients with paralytic-restrictive disorders who do not receive deep mechanically assisted insufflations, a rapid, shallow breathing pattern and inability to take occasional deep breaths can lead to microatelectasis in 1 hour.[62] The long-term inability to take deep breaths, or chronic hypoinflation, leads to chronic microatelectasis and permanent loss or, for children, underdevelopment of lung tissues as well as a decreased chest wall elasticity[30,32,34] and static pulmonary compliance.[31,32,39] Thus, decreased pulmonary compliance results initially from microatelectasis and ultimately from increased stiffness of the chest wall and lung tissues themselves.[34] Pulmonary deterioration is exacerbated by suboptimal treatment of acute respiratory tract infections that lead to repeated pneumonic processes, pulmonary scarring, and further loss of elasticity. The presence of scoliosis exacerbates the loss of compliance, which, in turn, increases the work of breathing.

Inadequacy of inspiratory muscle function can be from primary neuromuscular dysfunction, thoracic cage deformity, loss of respiratory exchange membrane and decreased pulmonary compliance, obstructive airway disease, severe sleep-disordered breathing, or some combination. The atelectasis and increased work of breathing associated with respiratory muscle dysfunction leads to GAH.[8] Hypercapnia is likely when the VC falls below 55% of predicted normal, and it is insidiously progressive.[26] This results directly from the resort to shallow breathing to avoid overloading inspiratory muscles[19] and can in itself decrease respiratory muscle strength.[73,81] The risk of pulmonary morbidity and mortality from acute respiratory failure correlates with increasing hypercapnia.[24,47] Hypoxia and hypercapnia are exacerbated when intrinsic lung disease, kyphoscoliosis, sleep-disordered breathing, or obesity complicates inspiratory muscle weakness. When not corrected by appropriate use of inspiratory muscle aids, respiratory control centers reset to accommodate hypercapnia,[8] and a compensatory metabolic alkalosis develops. The resulting elevated central nervous system bicarbonate levels contribute to depression of the ventilatory response to hypoxia and hypercapnia. This permits worsening of GAH and may decrease the effectiveness of the nocturnal use of inspiratory muscle aids once instituted.[8] Right ventricular strain and serum acid-base imbalance are reversible with the effective use of inspiratory muscle aids.[33]

Patients with paralytic-restrictive pulmonary syndromes have weakness of expiratory muscles as well as inspiratory muscles. Indeed, the former is usually more marked than the latter.[26,42] Expiratory muscle weakness decreases peak cough flows (PCF). PCF are also decreased by any inspiratory muscle weakness that decreases the inspiratory capacity below 2.5 L[52]; bulbar muscle weakness that impairs the retention of an optimal breath with a closed glottis or leads to aspiration of food or saliva; upper airway obstruction whether from tracheal stenosis, laryngeal muscle incompetence, or postintubation vocal cord adhesions or paralysis; lower airway obstruction from concomitant obstructive pulmonary disease; or any other impediment to the generation of optimal cough airflows. These patients have difficulty clearing secretions, particularly during upper respiratory tract infections, when their spontaneous or assisted PCF cannot exceed 5 L/second. They require an indwelling tracheostomy tube when PCF cannot exceed 3 L/second.[3] In this case, mucus plugging can lead to ventilation perfusion imbalance, gross atelectasis, airway collapse, pulmonary infiltrates and scarring, further loss of lung compliance, cor pulmonale, and eventually cardiopulmonary arrest. The cough reflex is also suppressed during sleep, when mucus plugs may be more likely to cause sudden hypoxia and acute respiratory failure. Many patients with myopathic disease have varying degrees of cardiomyopathy that render them susceptible to hypoxia-triggered arrhythmias and cardiac decompensation.

Smoking, the presence of an endotracheal cannula, or bronchorrhea for any other reason increases the tendency to develop chronic mucus plugging. For patients managed conventionally, that is, without physical medicine–assisted coughing and assisted ventilation methods, chronic mucus plugging often leads to repeated intubation, bronchoscopy, and possibly permanent tracheostomy. The last-mentioned also reduces PCFs, and failure of suction catheters to enter the left main stem bronchus during routine suctioning can also lead to morbidity.

The first significant blood gas abnormalities seen in individuals with restrictive pulmonary syndromes owing to Duchenne muscular dystrophy, and probably in others with neuromuscular weakness, usually occur during rapid eye movement (REM) sleep as short periods of hypercapnia and eventually hypoxemia.[69] These periods gradually extend throughout most of sleep before significant blood gas disturbances occur with the patient awake.[76,78] As noted, the ventilatory responses to hypoxia and hypercapnia are diminished during sleep,[74] and because the threshold for arousal is lower to hypoxia and higher to hypercapnia, more severe, prolonged blood gas alterations can occur without arousing the patient. Unless treated, this may result in increased risk of cardiac arrhythmia and cor pulmonale. For patients who have a $PaCO_2$ of greater than 50 mm Hg when awake, nocturnal oxyhemoglobin desaturation below 85% is common.[64] Increasing $PaCO_2$ and decreasing PaO_2 levels cross at about 60 mm Hg, a point at which it is tempting, but an error, to provide supplemental oxygen.

Nocturnal blood gas alterations ultimately extend to 24 hours a day as GAH. Wake hypercapnia tends to occur when the VC falls below 40%[27] to 55%[26] of predicted normal. Severe carbon dioxide retention itself has been demonstrated to decrease muscle strength further.[50] Normocapnic hypoxemia is also common[47] and may be due to decreased total oxygen diffusion across a diminished respiratory exchange membrane from microatelectasis and pulmonary fibrosis. Ventilatory insufficiency progresses insidiously and the risk of acute respiratory failure increases with the loss of pulmonary volumes.

Medications such as calcium channel blockers, aminoglycosides, steroids, and benzodiazepines can reduce the ventilatory response to hypercapnia and hypoxia and exacerbate GAH, especially during sleep. Beta-blockers may increase airway resistance. Malnutrition, acidosis, electrolyte disturbances, cachexia, infection, fatigue, and muscle disuse or overuse can all exacerbate ventilatory insufficiency. The risk of pulmonary complications may also be increased by oxygen administration to give the "patient a comfortable night's rest."[78] Although oxyhemoglobin saturation (SaO_2) can be improved by oxygen therapy, oxygen therapy depresses ventilatory drive, exacerbates GAH, and hastens the inevitable occurrence of respiratory arrest in these patients who do not benefit from physical medicine interventions.[8,13] Oxygen therapy has been shown to prolong hypopneas and apneas by 33% during REM sleep and 19% otherwise in Duchenne muscular dystrophy individuals with still good ventilatory function (average vital capacity 1.4 L).[77] It also suppresses the central nervous system–mediated reflex muscular activity needed to support ventilation overnight by noninvasive intermittent positive-pressure ventilation (IPPV) methods.[8,13] These complications are avoidable by application of physical medicine principles.

SUDDEN, PERMANENT RESPIRATORY MUSCLE FAILURE

Patients with sudden, permanent respiratory muscle failure, typically those with acute complete C-1 to C-3 spinal cord injury, lose VC and expiratory reserve volume suddenly as the result of interruption of the corticospinal tracts to the cell bodies of the nerves to the diaphragm and other respiratory muscles. Usually these patients are apneic from the time of injury. Those who survive receive cardiopulmonary support within a few minutes of injury and usually undergo endotracheal intubation before arriving at the hospital. They may or may not have concomitant lung damage.

RAPIDLY DEVELOPING OR RELAPSING VENTILATORY FAILURE

Rapidly developing or relapsing ventilatory failure most commonly occurs in patients with spinal cord injury lesions below the C-3 level, acute cervical myelitis and other myelopathies, Guillain-Barré syndrome, myasthenia gravis, acute poliomyelitis, and multiple sclerosis and in any patient with GAH complicated by an intercurrent respiratory tract infection with bronchorrhea. These patients can develop ventilatory failure over a period of hours or days. Once weaned from ventilator use, many of these patients require the use of respiratory muscle aids only during intercurrent respiratory tract infec-

tions. Many eventually develop insidious late-onset GAH and require ongoing ventilatory assistance.[4]

Any myelopathy at the C-5 level or above affects the corticospinal efferents to the C-3 through C-5 anterior horn cells of the phrenic nerves. Likewise, C-3 through C-5 nerve root injuries can also affect the phrenic nerves and diaphragm function. Some accessory inspiratory muscle function, that is, essentially function of the scalenes, sternocleidomastoid, and neck extensors, is retained unless spinal cord damage is complete and above C-2. Lower cervical and lumbar spine lesions spare the diaphragm but impair intercostal and abdominal muscle function. The intercostal muscles assist in both inspiratory and expiratory efforts, and the abdominal muscles are important for forced expiration or coughing. Patients with lesions of only the sacral spine have intact diaphragm and inspiratory muscle function in general, but inspiratory capacity is decreased because of inability to stabilize the pelvic floor and abdominal wall for optimal diaphragm excursion. Expiratory reserve volume and maximum generated expiratory pressures and flows are also severely reduced, resulting in impaired cough and inadequate ability to clear airway secretions. This can result in bronchial mucus plugging and atelectasis. Ventilatory failure is triggered in 74% of patients with spinal cord injury who develop atelectasis or pneumonia in the acute postinjury period.[36]

For patients with traumatic cervical spinal cord injury, 25%,[48] to in some reports as many as 79%,[63] develop ventilatory failure and require ventilatory assistance from hours to up to 7 days after injury. This is often caused by ascending spinal cord edema that extends the area of injury. Acute respiratory decompensation is conventionally managed by endotracheal intubation. When early ventilator weaning is not possible, the patients undergo tracheostomy for IPPV and transtracheal suctioning. Although only about 4% require ventilatory support following hospital discharge, more than 11% of all spinal cord injury patients have been reported to undergo tracheostomy.[21]

Despite reports to the contrary,[59,60] respiratory muscle weakness and pulmonary dysfunction are not uncommon in multiple sclerosis, especially in those with severe limb or bulbar muscle paralysis and, in particular, during acute relapses.[82] Diaphragm paralysis can also occur without concomitant bulbar or limb paralysis.[1] Respiratory muscle dysfunction develops from plaque involvement of the spinal cord and from lesions of the reticular activating system and reticulospinal tract, which can cause central hypoventilation, particularly during sleep when conscious triggering of the nerves to respiratory muscles cannot occur via the corticospinal tract. It was noted as early as 1977 that the VC and respiratory status of multiple sclerosis patients in general can vary from day to day[10] and month to month.[2] For any given patient, the difference between the lowest and highest values found on a monthly basis over a 6-month period varied from 8% to 40%, and for 10 patients, VC ranged from 8% to 99% of predicted normal.[2] Patients with moderate to severe but otherwise stable disease also have a lower ventilatory response to carbon dioxide. These phenomena have been explained by the presence of chronic respiratory muscle weakness, lack of coordination, or both.[82]

Pulmonary complications usually result from aspiration of food or secretions owing to bulbar muscle dysfunction. Despite diminished VC and volitional PCF, effective reflex coughs may be triggered in many patients with predominantly central nervous system pseudobulbar involvement. These patients may also manifest occasional reflex deep breaths (sighs) but may not be able to produce an effective cough or deep breath on command. Late-onset chronic GAH is uncommon but can develop in these patients.

Patients with myasthenia gravis often present with rapid shallow breathing, a blunted ventilatory response to hypercapnia, and GAH, despite often apparently adequate VC and inspiratory muscle strength. This occurs from some combination of impaired neuromuscular transmission,[20] respiratory center depression, and attenuated respiratory muscle endurance. Obesity, intercurrent respiratory tract infections, bulbar muscle weakness, and resort to surgical thymectomy may add to or trigger respiratory muscle compromise and ventilatory failure. Thus, the development of chronic GAH is often insidious, and early on, patients usually require the use of respiratory muscle aids only during recurrent disease exacerbations and during respiratory tract infections, both of which typically weaken bulbar and respiratory muscles.[61] At least early on, these episodes usually clear with medical treatment.

In Guillain-Barré syndrome, demyelinization affects the neural input to the respiratory and bulbar musculature. Twenty percent to 30% of patients require ventilatory support.[41] The diaphragm is often more severely affected than other respiratory musculature. This often leads to disproportionate pulmonary dysfunction with the patient supine, resulting in severe orthopnea and need for ventilatory assistance only when the patient is recumbent. Bulbar muscles are usually, but not always, too severely involved to permit the use of noninvasive respiratory aids as alternatives to endotracheal intubation early on. Permanent 24-hour need for ventilatory support from onset and late-onset GAH are uncommon but do occur.

INSIDIOUS, LATE-ONSET VENTILATORY FAILURE

Most patients with severe paralytic-restrictive pulmonary syndromes have insidiously progressive disorders, such as most of those listed in Table 21–1.[7] Chronic GAH results from progressive disease; ongoing senescent loss of residual myoneural function; and previously mentioned complicating factors such as obesity, thoracic cage and spinal deformities, loss of pulmonary compliance, concomitant sleep-disordered breathing, and possibly complicating chronic medical conditions.

For patients with pediatric-onset neuromuscular disease, the VC plateau occurs prematurely and at less than normal pulmonary volumes. For individuals with Duchenne muscular dystrophy, the VC plateaus between ages 10 and 14 years[6] at 1000 to about 2800 mL. The magnitude of the plateau VC is an indication of the severity of the disorder and of life expectancy for those who are managed conventionally.[70] With or without concomitant chest wall deformity, VC is then lost at a rate of 200 to 250 mL per year with the rate of loss tapering off below 400 mL (Fig. 22–1). In contrast to many patients with non-Duchenne myopathies or motor neuron diseases, there is usually little difference between upright and recumbent lung volumes and flow rates for individuals with Duchenne muscular dystrophy. This is an indication that the diaphragm is relatively preserved by comparison with skeletal muscle and that the chest wall does not retract significantly with diaphragm contraction.

Although onset during adolescence has been reported,[28] patients with motor neuron disease are most often afflicted after their natural VC plateau is reached.[28] Following onset of symptoms, there is often little or no clearly discernible change in VC for 2 to 4 years. Once the VC begins to decrease, however, the subsequent rate of loss is high and often 1 to 2 L are lost per year. Typically, patients able to ambulate with generalized respiratory muscle weakness and relatively intact bulbar muscle function develop

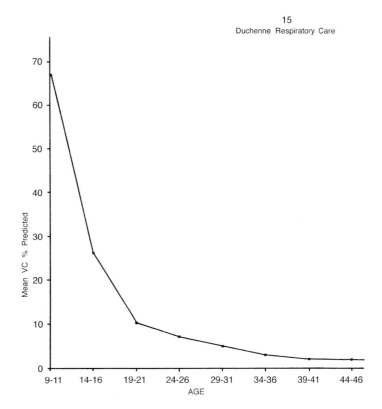

15
Duchenne Respiratory Care

FIGURE 22–1. Deterioration of vital capacity as a function of age for 29 Duchenne muscular dystrophy ventilator users. (From Bach J, Alba A, Pilkington LA, Lee M: Long-term rehabilitation in advanced stage of childhood onset, rapidly progressive muscular dystrophy. Arch Phys Med Rehabil 62:328–331, 1981.)

symptoms of GAH.[8] An early sign of impending ventilatory failure is decrease in voice volume. Patients whose respiratory muscle weakness is complicated by severe bulbar muscle involvement have difficulty managing saliva and airway secretions and present with dyspnea or acute respiratory failure caused by atelectasis or pneumonia despite having VCs that are often greater than 50% of predicted normal. Although amyotrophic lateral sclerosis survival can vary from less than a year to more than a decade with,[40] or occasionally without, ventilatory support, average survival without ventilator use is 3 to 4 years. Conventionally managed amyotrophic lateral sclerosis patients are typically hypercapnic during the last 20% of unaided survival.[80]

Patients with spinal muscular atrophy may present with ventilatory failure in the neonatal period (for severe type 1 patients), but failure is more frequently triggered after this period by a respiratory tract infection during which respiratory muscle weakness is exacerbated[61] and the airways are obstructed by mucus. Despite early spinal instrumentation and spinal fusion, most patients develop moderate to severe scoliosis. Early spinal fusion stiffens the thoracic wall and, along with early respiratory muscle weakness, causes severe restrictive pulmonary disease with inadequate growth and development of the

bronchial tree and respiratory exchange membrane. These patients tend to have paradoxic collapse of the chest wall during diaphragm activity. This situation decreases the efficiency of an already severely weakened diaphragm. Patients with mild type 2 disease and type 3 spinal muscular atrophy may tolerate mild GAH for many years before ongoing ventilatory assistance becomes necessary.[15]

Patients with myotonic dystrophy usually present with slowly progressive, generalized as well as respiratory and bulbar muscle weakness. GAH often results from a combination of inspiratory muscle weakness, altered central ventilatory control, and impaired ventilatory mechanics.[18] Interestingly, many patients hypoventilate despite relatively normal VC, and patients whose hypoventilation is corrected with assisted ventilation often experience no improvement in symptoms of GAH. Narcolepsylike excessive diurnal sleepiness appears characteristic of this disorder.[56] There is also a relatively reduced ventilatory response to carbon dioxide and hypoxemia,[17,18] which may be due to respiratory muscle myotonia[49,72] but is more likely due to central nervous system dysfunction,[72] perhaps of the hypothalamic-pituitary axis.[35] As for patients with nemaline myopathy, mitochondrial myopathies, and myasthenia gravis, the fact that the extent of ventilatory insufficiency is out of proportion to inspiratory muscle weakness or diminution in VC suggests that it may result more from a disturbance of the feedback required for normal control of breathing.[55]

Postpoliomyelitis patients have also been documented to lose VC at greater than normal rates, that is, at 1.7% to 1.9% per year.[9] Similar to spinal cord injury patients, they often required ventilatory support during their initial acute care. Some were never weaned from ventilator use. Most, however, were weaned within several years of acute poliomyelitis but developed late-onset GAH. Patients who required ventilatory support for acute poliomyelitis are at high risk of developing late-onset ventilatory insufficiency 20 years or more after acute poliomyelitis.[5] Virtually all can be managed without tracheostomy.

The VC of stable C-4 to C-7 tetraplegics in the sitting position range from 42% (range, 28% to 63%)[37] to 52% ± 11%[57] of predicted normal. Supine VC, however, which is usually greater than when sitting, may be significantly less than when sitting when the patient is adept at supplementing inspiratory volumes by accessory muscle use. Regardless of changes in VC, which can increase for 5 years or more after injury,[16] for patients with traumatic tetraplegia who may or may not have required ventilator use at onset, blood gases often deteriorate during sleep, and GAH can develop over time and necessitate late-onset ventilator use up to 24 hours a day.[4] Besides being inappropriately weaned from ventilator use during the initial injury recovery period, some patients are maintained on ventilatory support longer than needed.[4]

Patients with paralytic-restrictive syndromes are particularly susceptible to the development of sleep-disordered breathing.[43,79] Sleep-disordered breathing is a common entity that can develop into or complicate GAH and that may complicate chronic obstructive or restrictive pulmonary conditions. It refers to the occurrence of central, obstructive, or mixed apneas, hypopneas, or both during sleep. The obstructive apneas are most commonly due to hypopharyngeal collapse from a transluminal pressure gradient across the airway and failure of airway dilator muscles that are normally reflexly activated at the onset of inspiration. Obstructive apneas are often accompanied by central apneas. There may be a causative association between them. It is conceivable that for some patients with severe obstructive sleep apnea syndrome, central apneas result at least in part from central nervous system desensitivity to hypoxia. This desensitivity also occurs in the presence of the chronic respiratory muscle weakness.

For subjects over 62 years of age, Carskadon and Dement[29] found that 37.5% had apneas or hypopneas. Apneas were defined as cessation of airflow for 10 seconds or more and hypopneas were reductions in normal tidal volumes by greater than 30%. Many apneas and hypopneas are associated with oxyhemoglobin desaturation of 4% or greater.[38] At least 3% of the general population is symptomatic for this condition and has an average number of apneas and hypopneas per hour (apnea/hypopnea index) of five or more.[38] Obstructive sleep apnea syndrome is diagnosed when such individuals are symptomatic and have an apnea-hypopnea index of 10 or more.[38,44] Symptoms, which include hypersomnolence, morning headaches, fatigue, frequent nocturnal arousals with gasping or tachycardia, and nightmares, are similar to those of GAH.[4] The risk of symptomatic sleep-disordered breathing is higher in males and increases with age, androgen therapy, obesity, brain stem and spinal cord lesions, hypothyroidism, generalized neuromuscular diseases, and any conditions that obstruct the airway.[22,54]

Patients with neuromuscular disease may have a higher incidence of sleep-disordered breathing because of a higher incidence of bulbar muscle weakness and obesity.[14,46] This can increase susceptibility to hypopharyngeal collapse and obstructive apneas during sleep.[14,43] The extent of the presence of sleep-disordered breathing and its effect on exacerbating GAH or causing acute respiratory failure have not been adequately studied in this patient population. For postpoliomyelitis patients, damage to respiratory control centers might also have occurred from the encephalitic process of the primary viral infection.[45,46,66,68]

Sleep-disordered breathing alone can result in GAH, hypoxia, right ventricular strain, and, when severe, acute cardiopulmonary failure. It also occurs in most patients with ventilatory insufficiency using negative pressure body ventilators[51,53] or electrophrenic nerve pacing.[11] The potential complications of sleep-disordered breathing appear to derive predominantly from associated blood gas derangements and, when severe, there are potentially serious cardiovascular and neuropsychiatric sequelae.[25] Significant weight reduction can improve or completely resolve this condition for most patients whose sleep-disordered breathing is associated with obesity.[53] Obesity is rarely reversed indefinitely, however, and even when weight gain does not reoccur, the apnea/hypopnea index increases and symptoms often return.[67]

Continuous positive airway pressure (CPAP) is the standard treatment. It acts as a pneumatic splint to maintain airway patency so that the inspiratory muscles can ventilate the lungs. Prone positioning in bed can be helpful, and a convenient long-term solution for many patients with predominately obstructive sleep apneas is the use of an orthodontic splint that brings the mandible and tongue forward (Fig. 22–2).[23,25] This device can be effective and is generally preferred over CPAP. The use of nasopharyngeal tubes is poorly tolerated, and uvulopalatopharyngoplasty and mandibular advancement procedures are often ineffective and should be considered only as a last resort.[12,53,71] Surgery and splinting, even when relieving airway obstruction, often do not result in alleviation of GAH; thus, tracheostomy, which maintains airway patency and can be used for the delivery of IPPV, is conventionally considered the ultimate solution for this problem, especially when physical medicine alternatives are not tried.

Many patients with sleep-disordered breathing, however, particularly those who are obese, also have severe restrictive pulmonary syndromes and hypercapnia, VC under 1000 mL, and poor pulmonary compliance. As a result, their inspiratory muscles are inadequate to ventilate the lungs even with a patent airway, and CPAP fails to decrease hypercapnia. Conventionally, bilevel positive airway pressure (BiPAP) is then used, often at less than maximal inspiratory positive airway pressures (IPAP), and this, too, is usually found to be inadequate to reverse hypercapnia because it does not adequately assist inspiratory muscle function even when wide pressure spans, IPAP-EPAP (expiratory airway pressure) differences, are used because spans greater than 20 cm H_2O are usually needed but cannot be delivered by currently available equipment. Oxygen therapy is also commonly used for these patients. This therapy exacerbates hypercapnia and symptoms of GAH and may lead to respiratory arrest. Theophylline and other respiratory stimulants may be tried, but no clinically significant benefits have been reported with their use.

Congenital central alveolar hypoventilation is a congenital, but apparently not genetically determined[58] disorder of impaired control of ventilation of unknown cause. Typically, patients with this disorder maintain adequate ventilation when awake but hypoventilate severely during sleep and have absent or depressed ventilatory responses to hypercapnia and hypoxia when awake or asleep.[65] A similar ventilatory drive insensitivity to hypoxia and hypercapnia is seen in patients with familial dysautonomia and some patients with diabetic microangiopathy.[75]

SUMMARY

GAH and inability to clear airway secretions lead to intercurrent respiratory complications, hospitalizations, and, in many cases, premature mortality. The conventional management approaches are based on knowledge and experience gleaned from the evaluation and management of patients with intrinsic lung disease and are not optimal, and indeed are at times harmful, when managing this specific population. Physical medicine approaches that address the primary difficulties in ventilating the lungs and clearing airway secretions need to be more widely understood and used when treating individuals with paralytic-restrictive pulmonary syndrome.

References

1. Aisen M, Arlt G, Foster S: Diaphragmatic paralysis without bulbar or limb paralysis in multiple sclerosis. Chest 98:499–501, 1990.

2. Alba A, Pilkington LA, Schultheiss M, et al: Long-term pulmonary care in multiple sclerosis. Respir Ther 7:25–29, 1977.

3. Bach JR: Mechanical insufflation-exsufflation: Comparison of peak expiratory flows with manually assisted and

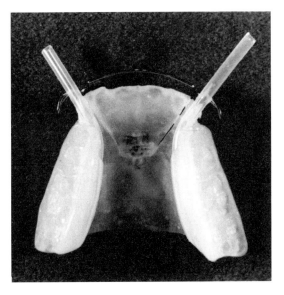

FIGURE 22–2. An intra-oral appliance used to treat obstructive sleep apnea. (Courtesy of Dr. John R. Haze, D.D.S., Montville, NJ.)

unassisted coughing techniques. Chest 104:1553–1562, 1993.

4. Bach JR: Inappropriate weaning and late onset ventilatory failure of individuals with traumatic quadriplegia. Paraplegia 31:430–438, 1993.

5. Bach JR: Management of post-polio respiratory sequelae. Ann N Y Acad Sci, 753:96–102, 1995.

6. Bach JR: Pulmonary assessment and management of the aging and older patient. In Felsenthal G, Garrison SJ, Steinberg FU (eds): Rehabilitation of the Aging and Elderly Patient. Baltimore, Williams & Wilkins, 1993, pp 263–273.

7. Bach JR: Neuromuscular and skeletal disorders leading to global alveolar hypoventilation. In Bach JR (ed): Pulmonary Rehabilitation: The Obstructive and Paralytic/Restrictive Pulmonary Syndromes. Philadelphia, Hanley & Belfus, 1996.

8. Bach JR, Alba AS: Management of chronic alveolar hypoventilation by nasal ventilation. Chest 97:52–57, 1990.

9. Bach JR, Alba AS, Bohatiuk G, et al: Mouth intermittent positive pressure ventilation in the management of post-polio respiratory insufficiency. Chest 91:859–864, 1987.

10. Bach JR, Alba AS, Mosher R, Delaubier A: Intermittent positive pressure ventilation via nasal access in the management of respiratory insufficiency. Chest 92:168–170, 1987.

11. Bach JR, O'Connor K: Electrophrenic ventilation: A different perspective. J Am Paraplegia Soc 14:9–17, 1991.

12. Bach JR, Penek J: Obstructive sleep apnea complicating negative pressure ventilatory support in patients with chronic paralytic/restrictive ventilatory dysfunction. Chest 99:1386–1393, 1991.

13. Bach JR, Robert D, Leger P, Langevin B: Sleep fragmentation in kyphoscoliotic individuals with alveolar hypoventilation treated by nasal IPPV. Chest, 107:1152–1158, 1995.

14. Bach JR, Tippett, DC, McCrary MM: Bulbar dysfunction and associated cardiopulmonary considerations in polio and neuromuscular disease. J Neuro Rehabil 6:121–128, 1992.

15. Bach JR, Wang TG: Noninvasive long-term ventilatory support for individuals with spinal muscular atrophy and functional bulbar musculature. Arch Phys Med Rehabil 76:213–217, 1995.

16. Bach JR, Wang TG: Pulmonary function and sleep disordered breathing in traumatic tetraplegics: A longitudinal study. Arch Phys Med Rehabil 75:279–284, 1994.

17. Begin R, Bureau MA, Lupien L, et al: Pathogenesis of respiratory insufficiency in myotonic dystrophy. Am Rev Respir Dis 125:312–318, 1982.

18. Begin R, Bureau MA, Lupien L, Lemieux B: Control and modulation of respiration in Steinert's myotonic dystrophy. Am Rev Respir Dis 121:281–289, 1980.

19. Begin R, Grassino A: Inspiratory muscle dysfunction and chronic hypercapnia in chronic obstructive pulmonary disease. Am Rev Respir Dis 143:905–912, 1983.

20. Bellemare F, Grassino A: Effect of pressure and timing of contraction on human diaphragm fatigue. J Appl Physiol 53:1190–1195, 1982.

21. Biering-Sorensen M, Biering-Sorensen F: Tracheostomy in spinal cord injured: Frequency and follow up. Paraplegia 30:656–660, 1992.

22. Bonekat HW, Andersen G, Squires J: Obstructive disorder breathing during sleep in patients with spinal cord injury. Paraplegia 28:392–398, 1990.

23. Bonham PE, Currier GF, Orr WC, et al: The effect of a modified functional appliance on obstructive sleep apnea. Am J Orthod Dentofac Orthop 94:384–392, 1988.

24. Boushy SF, Thompson HK Jr, North LB, et al: Prognosis in chronic obstructive pulmonary disease. Am Rev Respir Dis 108:1373–1383, 1973.

25. Bradley TD, Phillipson EA: Pathogenesis and pathophysiology of the obstructive sleep apnea syndrome. Med Clin North Am 69:1169–1185, 1985.

26. Braun NMT, Arora MS, Rochester DF: Respiratory muscle and pulmonary function in polymyositis and other proximal myopathies. Thorax 38:616–623, 1983.

27. Canny GJ, Szeinberg A, Koreska J, Levison H: Hypercapnia in relation to pulmonary function in Duchenne muscular dystrophy. Pediatr Pulmonol 6:169–171, 1989.

28. Caroscio JT, Mulvihill MN, Sterling R, Adrams B: Amyotrophic lateral sclerosis: Its natural course. Neurol Clin 5:1–8, 1987.

29. Carskadon M, Dement W: Respiration during sleep in the aged human. J Gerontol 36:420–425, 1981.

30. Same as Reference 32.

31. De Troyer A, Borenstein S, Cordier R: Analysis of lung volume restriction in patients with respiratory muscle weakness. Thorax 35:603–610, 1980.

32. De Troyer A, Deisser P: The effects of intermittent positive pressure breathing on patients with respiratory muscle weakness. Am Rev Respir Dis 124:132–137, 1981.

33. Enson Y, Giuntini C, Lewis ML, et al: The influence of hydrogen ion concentration and hypoxia on the pulmonary circulation. J Clin Invest 43:1146–1162, 1964.

34. Estenne M, De Troyer A: The effects of tetraplegia on chest wall statics. Am Rev Respir Dis 134:121–124, 1986.

35. Fernandez JM, Lara I, Gila L, et al: Disturbed hypothalamic-putuitary axis in idiopathic recurring hypersomnia syndrome. Acta Neurol Scand 82:361–363, 1990.

36. Fishburn MJ, Marino RJ, Ditunno JF: Atelectasis and pneumonia in acute spinal cord injury. Arch Phys Med Rehabil 71:197–200, 1990.

37. Fugl-Meyer AR: Effects of respiratory muscle paralysis in tetraplegic and paraplegic patients. Scand J Rehabil Med 3:141–150, 1971.

38. George CF, Millar TW, Kryger MH: Identification and quantification of apneas by computer-based analysis of oxygen saturation. Am Rev Respir Dis 137:1238–1240, 1988.

39. Gibson GJ, Pride NB, Newsom-Davis J, Loh LC: Pulmonary mechanics in patients with respiratory muscle weakness. Am Rev Respir Dis 115:389–395, 1977.

40. Gilgoff IS, Baydur A, Bach JR, et al: Tracheal intermittent positive pressure ventilation for patients with neuromuscular disease. J Neurol Rehabil 6:93–101, 1992.

41. Gracey DR, McMichan JC, Divertie MB, Howard FM: Respiratory failure in Guillain-Barré syndrome. Mayo Clin Proc 37:742–746, 1982.

42. Griggs RG, Donohoe KM, Utell MJ, et al: Evaluation of pulmonary function in neuromuscular disease. Arch Neurol 38:9–12, 1981.

43. Guilleminault C, Motta J: Sleep apnea syndrome as a long-term sequelae of poliomyelitis. In Guilleminault C (ed): Sleep Apnea Syndromes. New York, KROC Foundation, 1978, pp 309–315.

44. He J, Kryger MH, Zorick FJ, et al: Mortality and apnea index in obstructive sleep apnea. Chest 94:9–14, 1988.

45. Hill R, Robbins AW, Messing R, Arora NS: Sleep apnea syndrome after poliomyelitis. Am Rev Respir Dis 127:129–131, 1983.

46. Hodes HL: Treatment of respiratory difficulty in poliomyelitis. In Poliomyelitis: Papers and Discussions Presented at the Third International Poliomyelitis Conference. Philadelphia, JB Lippincott, 1955, pp 91–113.

47. Inkley SR, Oldenburg FC, Vignos PJ Jr: Pulmonary function in Duchenne muscular dystrophy related to stage of disease. Am J Med 56:297–306, 1974.

48. Jackson AB, Groomes TE: Incidence of respiratory complications following spinal cord injury. Arch Phys Med Rehabil 75:270–275, 1994.

49. Jammes Y, Pouget J, Grimaud C, Serratrice G: Pulmonary function and electromyographic study of respiratory muscles in myotonic dystrophy. Muscle Nerve 8:586–594, 1985.

50. Juan G, Calverley P, Talamo C: Effect of carbon dioxide on diaphragmatic function in human beings. N Engl J Med 310:874–879, 1984.

51. Katsantonis GP, Walsh JK, Schweitzer PK, Friedman WH: Further evaluation of uvulopalatopharyngoplasty in the treatment of obstructive sleep apnea syndrome. Otolaryngol Head Neck Surg 93:244–250, 1985.

52. Leith DE: Lung biology in health and desease: Respiratory defense mechanisms, part 2. In Brain JD, Proctor D, Reid L (eds): Cough. New York, Marcel Dekker, 1977, pp 545–592.

53. Levy RD, Bradley TD, Newman SL, et al: Negative pressure ventilation: Effects on ventilation during sleep in normal subjects. Chest 65:95–99, 1989.

54. Lombard R Jr, Zwillich CW: Medical therapy of obstructive sleep apnea. Med Clin North Am 69:1317–1335, 1985.

55. Maayan CH, Springer C, Armon Y, et al: Nemaline myopathy as a cause of sleep hypoventilation. Pediatrics 77:390–395, 1986.

56. Manni R, Zucca C, Martinetti M, et al: Hypersomnia in dystrophia myotonica: A neurophysiological and immunogenetic study. Acta Neurol Scand 84:498–502, 1991.

57. Mansel JK: Respiratory complications and management of spinal cord injuries. Chest 97:1446–1452, 1990.

58. Marcus CL, Livingston FR, Wood SE, Keens TG: Hypercapnic and hypoxic ventilatory responses in parents and siblings of children with congenital central hypoventilation syndrome. Am Rev Respir Dis 144:136–140, 1991.

59. McAlpine D, Comston N: Some aspects of the natural history of disseminated sclerosis. Q J Med 21:135–167, 1952.

60. McIntyre HD, McIntyre AP: Prognosis of multiple sclerosis. Arch Neurol Neurosurg Psychiatry 50:431–439, 1943.

61. Mier-Jedrzejowicz A, Brophy C, Green M: Respiratory muscle weakness during upper respiratory tract infections. Am Rev Respir Dis 138:5–7, 1988.

62. Miller WF: Rehabilitation of patients with chronic obstructive lung disease. Med Clin North Am 51:349–361, 1967.

63. Myllynen P, Kivioja A, Rokkanen P, Wilppula E: Cervical spinal cord injury: The correlations of initial clinical features and blood gas analyses with early prognosis. Paraplegia 27:19–26, 1989.

64. Ohtake S: Nocturnal blood gas disturbances and treatment of patients with Duchenne muscular dystrophy. Kokyu To Junkan 38:463–469, 1990.

65. Oren J, Kelly DH, Shannon DC: Long-term follow-up of children with congenital central hypoventilation syndrome. Pediatrics 80:375–380, 1987.

66. Petrén K, Ehrenberg L: Etudes cliniques sur la poliomyélite aigue. Nouv Inconog Salpètrière 22:373, 1909.

67. Pillar G, Peled R, Lavie P: Recurrence of sleep apnea without concomitant weight increase 7.5 years after weight reduction surgery. Chest 106:1702–1704, 1994.

68. Plum F, Swanson AG: Abnormalities in central regulation of respiration in acute and convalescent poliomyelitis. Arch Neurol Psychiatry 80:267–285, 1958.

69. Redding GJ, Okamoto GA, Guthrie RD, et al: Sleep patterns in nonambulatory boys with Duchenne muscular dystrophy, Arch Phys Med Rehabil 66:818–821, 1985.

70. Rideau Y, Jankowski LW, Grellet J: Respiratory function in the muscular dystrophies. Muscle Nerve 4:155–164, 1981.

71. Riley RW, Powell NB, Guilleminault C, Mino-Murcia G: Maxillary, mandibular, and hyoid advancement: An alternative to tracheostomy in obstructive sleep apnea syndrome. Otolaryngol Head Neck Surg 94:584–588, 1986.

72. Rimmer KP, Golar S, Lee MA, Whitelaw WA: Myotonia of the respiratory muscles in myotonic dystrophy. Am Rev Respir Dis 148:1018–1022, 1993.

73. Rochester DF, Braun NMT: Determinants of maximal inspiratory pressure in chronic obstructive pulmonary disease. Am Rev Respir Dis 132:42–47, 1985.

74. Shneerson J: Disorders of Ventilation. Boston, Blackwell Scientific Publications, 1988, p 43.

75. Silverstein D, Michlin B, Sobel HJ, Lavietes MH: Right ventricular failure in a patient with diabetic neuropathy (myopathy) and central alveolar hypoventilation. Respiration 44:460–465, 1983.

76. Smith PEM, Edwards RHT, Calverley PMA: Ventilation and breathing pattern during sleep in Duchenne muscular dystrophy. Chest 96:1346–1351, 1989.

77. Smith PEM, Edwards RHT, Calverley PMA: Oxygen treatment of sleep hypoxaemia in Duchenne muscular dystrophy. Thorax 44:997–1001, 1989.

78. Soudon P: Ventilation assistee au long cours dans les maladies neuro-musculaire: Expéience actuelle. Readaptation Revalidatie 3:45–65, 1987.

79. Steljes DG, Kryger MH, Kirk BW, Millar TW: Sleep in postpolio syndrome. Chest 98:133–140, 1990.

80. Strong MJ, Ferguson KA, Ahmad D: The pulmonary function testing as a predictor of survival in amyotrophic lateral sclerosis. Chest 102:180S, 1992.

81. Stubbing DG, Pengelly LD, Morse JLC, Jones NL: Pulmonary mechanics during exercise in subjects with chronic airflow obstruction. J Appl Physiol 49:511–515, 1980.

82. Tantucci C, Massucci M, Piperno R, et al: Control of breathing and respiratory muscle strength in patients with multiple sclerosis. Chest 105:1163–1170, 1994.

Conventional Approaches to Managing Neuromuscular Ventilatory Failure

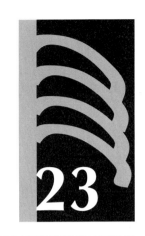

23

John R. Bach, MD

THE CONVENTIONAL STRATEGIES

Current strategies for managing progressive respiratory muscle insufficiency include:

1. Not treating global alveolar hypoventilation (GAH) and obtaining a "living will" or other decree of "informed consent" interdicting the use of ventilatory support.
2. Not treating GAH until an episode of acute respiratory failure leads to hospitalization and intubation, and tracheostomy becomes the ethical intervention.
3. Treating GAH and episodes of acute ventilatory failure like chronic obstructive pulmonary disease (COPD), with some combination of oxygen, bronchodilators, theophylline, and chest physical therapy.
4. "Prophylactic" tracheostomy.
5. Using nocturnal nasal intermittent positive pressure ventilation (IPPV) to delay tracheostomy.

Ignoring the Problem

The first two strategies for managing progressive respiratory muscle insufficiency, which are the most commonly used, essentially ignore the problem. In a survey of directors of Jerry Lewis Muscular Dystrophy Association clinics, 61% of 218 clinic directors ordered pulmonary function tests routinely, yet only 5 (3%) evaluated patients for GAH, and the great majority of patients were introduced to ventilator use only when acute respiratory failure necessitated endotracheal intubation and, subsequently, tracheostomy. More clinic directors reported being biased against the use of ventilators than being favorably disposed or impartial to their use. Sixty-four percent of clinic directors had never seen a patient use noninvasive ventilatory aids and in only 11% of clinics was there any familiarity with the more effective noninvasive IPPV methods.[2]

Thus, the great majority of patients are uninformed about noninvasive treatment options when consenting to or refusing endotracheal intubation or tracheostomy. Those who refuse "prophylactic" tracheostomy inevitably develop acute respiratory failure, and to survive, many change their minds and agree to be intubated and eventually undergo tracheostomy. It, then, is not surprising that only a small minority of patients with neuromuscular disease and GAH are introduced to ventilatory assistance in other than emergency situations (Table 23–1).

Medical Therapy

All conventional approaches often include medical therapy that is commonly used for COPD. The goals of medical therapy are to increase diaphragm contractility, facilitate airway secretion clearance, improve ventilatory drive, and decrease hypoxia without the use of ventilatory assistance. Unfortunately, no medical

TABLE 23–1
Guide to Abbreviations

BiPAP—bi-level positive airway pressure
CPAP—continuous positive airway pressure
DMD—Duchenne muscular dystrophy
EPAP—expiratory positive airway pressure
IPAP—inspiratory positive airway pressure
IPPV—intermittent positive pressure ventilation
MI-E—mechanical insufflation-exsufflation
NPBV—negative pressure body ventilator
PEEP—positive end-expiratory pressure
SaO$_2$—oxyhemoglobin saturation
SIMV—synchronized intermittent mandatory ventilation
SMA—spinal muscular atrophy
VC—vital capacity

therapy has been shown to be effective and safe for any of these goals. In a review of 25 studies of individuals with skeletal and neuromuscular respiratory insufficiency, methylxanthine administration was not found to alleviate diaphragm fatigue.[97] Indeed, in the presence of hypercapnia and hypoxia, theophylline appeared to increase or delay recovery from diaphragm fatigue, and side effects were common.[50] I have treated two patients who had generalized seizures from methylxanthine therapy from which they derived no benefit. Bronchodilators, too, are also often used on a long-term basis with no subjective or objective benefits for these patients. Bronchodilators often cause anxiety by increasing heart rate, and they can exacerbate cardiac dysfunction for many of these patients with cardiomyopathies or cor pulmonale.

Low-flow oxygen in combination with protriptyline[118] has been used to treat sleep hypoxia in this patient population. However, this approach appears to decrease hypoxia by suppressing rapid eye movement sleep.[118] Any resulting increase in fatigue may increase the risk of pulmonary complications. Furthermore, the anticholinergic effects of protriptyline preclude its regular use and may be hazardous for cardiomyopathy patients with decreased cardiac reserve and cardiac conduction defects. Other medications such as doxapram hydrochloride, acetazolamide, medroxyprogesterone, and almitrine, have been proposed as potential therapeutic agents but have not been adequately studied.[57,101]

Although first used to treat lung disease in 1924,[45] oxygen therapy only became widely accepted for treating hypoxia due to lung disease in the mid-1960s. Subsequently, oxygen therapy has been demonstrated to improve significantly the prognoses of hypoxic patients with COPD or other intrinsic lung diseases. This success has led to its use for treating hypoxia from ventilation impairment. However, considering the different pathophysiology underlying GAH,[9] it is not surprising that the preliminary results of our study of over 400 patients with respiratory muscle failure demonstrated a markedly greater incidence of pneumonias and hospitalizations for respiratory complications in patients who received oxygen therapy than in patients who were treated with respiratory muscle aids or who were not treated at all.

TRACHEOSTOMY FOR IPPV AND AIRWAY SUCTIONING

Development of Invasive Management Strategies

It is of interest that the evolution to tracheostomy stemmed from the use of negative pressure body ventilators (NPBVs), noninvasive approaches to ventilatory assistance. Body ventilators were the main devices used for both acute and long-term ventilatory support from 1929 until the late 1950s. They can provide normal alveolar ventilation for individuals with little or no vital capacity (VC). (A more indepth description of these devices appears in the next chapter.)

Trendelenburg was the first to describe the use of a tracheostomy tube with an inflated cuff for assisting ventilation during the anesthesia of a human in 1869.[122] The use of transoral intubation during anesthesia was described soon afterwards.[87] Tracheostomy and the use of a mechanical bellows for ventilatory support were popularized for anesthesia during World War I.[88] However, despite this and the fact that tracheostomies were often placed for managing airway secretions in patients ventilated continuously by body ventilators in the 1930s and 1940s (Fig. 23–1), tracheostomy tubes were not used for ongoing ventilatory support before an inadequate supply of body ventilators made this a necessity during the 1952 poliomyelitis epidemic in Denmark.[82]

During the Danish epidemic, 345 of 2300 acute poliomyelitis patients (15%) had ventilatory failure, impaired swallowing, or both. Lassen reported that the early mortality figures for ventilator-supported patients decreased from 80% to 41%, or to about 7% for the entire acute paralytic poliomyelitis population over-

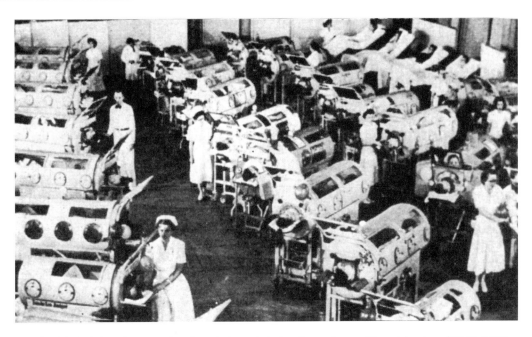

FIGURE 23–1. Iron lung use in a hospital ward during the poliomyelitis epidemics of 1948–1954.

all.[82] This decrease in mortality coincided with the use of tracheostomy for IPPV and the increased resort to tracheostomy for patients with severe bulbar involvement.[82] However, specialized centers in the United States also reported equally significant decreases in mortality by "individualizing" patient care. From 1948 to 1952, 3500 poliomyelitis patients were treated at Los Angeles General Hospital, where 15% to 20% required ventilatory support (Fig. 23–1). General mortality decreased from 12% to 15% in 1948 to 2% in 1952 without the use of tracheostomy for ventilatory support.[69] Although many patients at Los Angeles General Hospital, particularly those with bulbar polio, had tracheostomies placed for management of secretions while they were ventilated by NPBVs, in other centers where few tracheostomies were performed, mortality also decreased to about 2%.[69] It was concluded that the previously high fatality rate was not because of inadequacy of NPBVs but because of ineffective airway secretion clearance.[69] Better nursing care and attention to managing airway secretions, including the use of devices to eliminate them, were factors in decreasing mortality rates.

A long debate ensued as to whether tracheostomy or body ventilators were preferable for ventilatory support. In 1955, an International Consensus Symposium defined the indications for tracheostomy as the combination of respiratory insufficiency with swallowing insufficiency and disturbance in consciousness or vascular disturbances: "If a patient is going to be left a respirator cripple with a very low VC, a tracheotomy may be a great disadvantage. It is very difficult to get rid of a tracheotomy tube when the VC is only 500 or 600 cc and there is no power of coughing, whereas, as we all know, a patient who has been treated in a respirator from the first can survive and get out of all mechanical devices with a VC of that figure."[69] In 1958, Forbes wrote, "Tracheotomy, which is designed to provide a more efficient airway and access to the trachea in certain patients, does not materially assist in ridding the bronchi of secretions which must migrate to the upper bronchi and trachea before they become accessible to suction through the tracheotomy tube. The inaccessibility of these secretions in the lower bronchial tree even to bronchoscopy makes it necessary to provide indirect means for their mechanical expulsion."[52] Forbes noted that the published mortality figures in six studies among acute patients were lower with tank respiration than with tracheostomy IPPV, and that with tracheostomy in patients with respiratory paralysis without pharyngeal paralysis, tracheal damage, loss of capability for glossopharyngeal breathing, and loss of "the routine application of chest compression" and mechanical insufflation-exsufflation (MI-E) made for a worse prognosis in comparison to patients managed by noninvasive methods.[52]

NPBV users' lifestyles, however, were often greatly restricted, and elimination of respiratory tract secretions was often difficult for patients who were necessarily supine and to whose bodies caregivers had limited access for assisted coughing. Tracheostomy for IPPV permitted many patients to leave NPBVs and to use wheelchairs. Patients with severely affected bulbar muscle function required tracheostomy with cuff inflation to decrease aspiration of food and saliva. Intubation and tracheostomy also simplified intensive care nursing and equipment needs. They provided closed systems for ventilatory support that were amenable to precise monitoring of ventilation volumes and pressures, oxygen delivery, and the use of the high-technology respirators and alarm systems that were to follow.

As the use of endotracheal methods became widespread in the 1960s, manually assisted coughing was no longer taught in medical, nursing, and respiratory therapy curricula, and clinicians lost familiarity with body ventilators. Noninvasive IPPV methods, which are more effective than body ventilators and preferred over tracheostomy and over NPBVs,[3] were not to be described until 1969, and their use was not reported for a large population for 24-hour ventilatory support until the 1980s. Furthermore, the only studies of the use of MI-E devices had been for patients with acute poliomyelitis or with severe intrinsic pulmonary disease.[21] The polio group was felt to be a transient population, and the latter is a population for whom the use of noninvasive respiratory muscle aids is usually not ideal. Tracheostomy, thus, became the standard of care in the early 1960s.

Complications of Long-Term Tracheostomy

Because episodes of acute respiratory failure are inevitable for most conventionally managed patients with progressive generalized neuromuscular diseases, and because there is a higher rate of complications associated with emergency rather than elective tracheostomy, clinicians not uncommonly propose tracheostomy in anticipation of its presumed eventual need.[55] Whether performed under emergency or elective circumstances, and despite the proliferation of ventilation modes that include proportional assist, pressure support, jet, synchronized intermittent mandatory (SIMV), and assist-control ventilation as well as positive end-expiratory pressure (PEEP) and precise oxygen delivery systems, the hospital survival rates of patients with acute respiratory failure undergoing endotracheal intubation or tracheostomy have not improved over the last 20 years.[123] Likewise, our data on over 400 long-term ventilator-users indicated a greater incidence of pneumonias and hospitalizations for respiratory complications in patients receiving tracheostomy IPPV than in those assisted by noninvasive respiratory muscle aids.[11]

With widespread use of invasive endotracheal methods, reports of difficulties appeared.[22] These included infection associated with pathogenic bacterial colonization of the airway[37,75,76,100] and impaired mucociliary transport.[78] Four hours of tracheostomy cuff inflation was shown to affect ciliary appearance and function for 3 days.[114] Chronic purulent bronchitis, formation of granulation tissue, and development of sepsis from paranasal sinusitis were also associated with pathogenic bacterial colonization.[41,94] Sudden death was reported from mucus plugging,[35,38,39] cardiac arrhythmias,[24,91,129] accidental disconnections, and other related causes.[31,119] Swallowing was found to be impaired, and aspiration occurred because of the tracheostomy tube and, especially, inflated cuff restriction of the strap muscles in the neck.[42,48]

Interference with relaxation of the cricopharyngeal sphincter, compression of the esophagus, and changes in intratracheal pressure were shown to add to the problem.[85] Other reported complications included tracheomalacia and tracheal perforation, hemorrhage, and stenosis, with the latter occurring in up to 65%[105] of patients; tracheoesophageal fistula[66]; painful hemorrhagic tube changes; and psychosocial disturbances. Vocal cord paralysis, laryngeal strictures, hypopharyngeal muscle dysfunction, and airway collapse also resulted from endotracheal intubation.[36,67] Tracheostomy placement was shown to exacerbate endotracheal tube-associated laryngeal damage and increase the risk of laryngeal stenosis.[32] Even when not severely impairing ventilatory function, chronic upper airway obstruction decreases cough flows and thus can hamper tracheostomy tube removal.[17]

The presence of a tracheostomy tube increases airway secretions and mucus plugs that must be eliminated, and at the same time, adequate expiratory flows can no longer be generated by coughing or assisted coughing methods because of leak from or around the tube. Airway cilia are also destroyed by tracheal suctioning. Airway suctioning also appears to increase the production of secretions, and it may be accompanied by severe hypoxia. At best, suctioning clears only superficial airway secretions. Suctioning misses mucus adherent between the tube and tracheal wall, and routine suctioning misses the left mainstem bronchus 54% to 92% of the time. This leads to a high incidence of left lung pneumonias,[51] potentially fatal mucus plugging, and bronchoscopies. An indwelling tracheostomy tube also necessitates regular cleaning of the site and tube, tubing changes, and supplemental humidification. Ventilatory support by invasive methods also leads to chronic hyperventilation,[64] respiratory muscle deconditioning,[8] and often rapid loss of ventilator-free breathing capability. Appetite is decreased because the sense of smell is lost as air does not pass through the upper airway. In addition, in many states, a tracheostomy is considered an "open wound," which can prevent community living without prohibitively expensive nursing for suctioning and stoma care[8] and can restrict access to schools and places of employment.

Conventional Introduction of Tracheostomy

GAH is usually not treated until episodes of acute respiratory failure result from the patient's inability to clear airway secretions during otherwise benign upper respiratory tract infections.[2] For other patients, hypercapnia increases insidiously and results in respiratory arrest without an identifiable triggering event. When tracheostomy is offered electively to prevent respiratory failure, it is most often (appropriately) refused by the patient. As previously noted, medical interventions and intermittent positive pressure breathing, which is often used for inadequate periods and at inadequate pressures to support or rest inspiratory muscles, do not address the fundamental problems of significantly reducing the workload of breathing and effectively clearing airway secretions.

When acute respiratory failure occurs, these patients usually have intrinsic lung disease, most often gross atelectasis and pneumonia. The patient is then intubated, and when early ventilator weaning fails, tracheostomy is performed because "there is no alternative for IPPV and tracheal suctioning."

As the patient's condition stabilizes, ventilator weaning attempts are most often made using a combination of concomitant SIMV or assist-control ventilation, with pressure support, PEEP, and supplemental oxygen administration. Occasionally, periods of ventilator-free breathing are tried with the patient receiving continuous positive airway pressure (CPAP) and oxygen by T-piece. With these approaches, "weaning schedules" are imposed on the patient. These schedules often cause anxiety because the patient is not ready to breathe on his or her own, or the schedule is too conservative, delaying respiratory muscle reconditioning and function. The use of pulse oximetry, which effectively signals the presence of significant mucus plugging by the appearance of sudden decreases in oxyhemoglobin saturation (SaO_2), and monitors their clearance with treatment by the return of SaO_2 to baseline, is lost with the use of supplemental oxygen. In addition, intubated patients often develop malnutrition. These factors, along with a lack of use of or relative ineffectiveness of assisted coughing, pathogenic bacterial colonization, and loss of airway cilia in intubated patients, cause mucus plugs to form and linger and thus hamper ventilator weaning.

Because ventilator weaning eventually becomes impossible for many patients with progressive neuromuscular conditions, these patients are often discharged using tracheostomy IPPV. Although prolonged cuff inflation is virtually never necessary for stable patients with primarily ventilation impairment,[13] the cuff is often left inflated and the patient left with no ability to communicate verbally. Patients then experience the inevitable morbidity, swallowing difficulties, and, at times, fatal complications associated with tracheostomy and prolonged cuff inflation. This conventional approach to managing GAH can best be described as reactive, rather than proactive, or as "not-so-benign neglect."

Results of Long-term Tracheostomy

Spinal Cord Injury

There are an estimated 3000 ventilator-users with spinal cord injury (SCI) at any one time in the United States.[1] In a study of 435 SCI persons with a mean age at injury of 39.6 ± 22.6 years between 1973 and 1992, who were either ventilator-users at discharge from rehabilitation or who died prior to discharge while still using a ventilator daily, the overall survival rates were 25.4% at 1 year and 16.8% at 15 years. There was no indication of tracheostomy tube cuff status. For those who survived the first post-injury year, cumulative survival over the next 14 years was 61.4%. For those who survived the first 2 post-injury years, cumulative survival over the next 13 years was $70.7 \pm 6.0\%$. Among the 1-year survivors, the subsequent mortality rate was reduced by 39% for persons injured between 1980 and 1985 and 91% for those injured since 1986 relative to rates for those injured between 1973 and 1979.[43] In comparison with the general population, the annual death rate following the initial 2-year period was 20.86 times greater for the 1- to 30-year-olds, 8.87 times greater for the 31- to 60-year-olds, and 2.38 times greater for those over age 61. For example, the life expectancy for 15 ventilator-users with cord injury at 10 years of age and who survived the first 2 post-injury years was 43.2 years.[43] The mean survival for ventilator-users with SCI at age 30 who survived 1 and 2 post-injury years was another 15.9 and 23.6 years, respectively.

Although the overall mortality rate has been declining, the incidence of respiratory morbidity and mortality remains high. Respiratory complications accounted for 45.8% of deaths and contributed to the 24.6% of mortality listed as from probable heart disease.[43] Fifty-one percent of the latter was noted as sudden cardiac arrest, a condition with which sudden death from mucus plugging is often confused. An additional 16.7% of mortality was listed as unknown, which is also often due to bronchial mucus plugging and cardiac arrhythmias. Thus, by far the most common cause (>50%) of death for SCI ventilator-users in the immediate post-injury period and for at least 15 years thereafter is *respiratory complications*.[43] The common potentially fatal complications of pneumonia, mucus plugging, asphyxia from accidental tracheostomy tube disconnection, and cardiac arrhythmias are directly associated with failure of conventional management approaches.

Guillain-Barré Syndrome

Of 79 patients with acute Guillain-Barré syndrome, 21 were admitted to a respiratory intensive care unit for 58 ± 26 days. Thirteen underwent nasotracheal intubation followed by tracheostomy and IPPV. The tracheostomy remained for a mean of 50 ± 27 days. Two of the 13 patients receiving ventilatory support in this study died. Four patients had complications of tracheostomy, one of which was innominate artery hemorrhage and fatal sepsis.[61]

The duration of mechanical ventilation in this condition is usually 8 to 12 weeks. Although there apparently are no reports in the literature of the need for permanent ventilatory support from disease onset, I have treated one such pa-

tient who remained dependent on 24-hour tracheostomy IPPV for 14 years with no measurable VC until she had herself disconnected from the ventilator. In her case, bulbar muscle weakness precluded the use of alternative methods to tracheostomy.

Duchenne Muscular Dystrophy

An estimated 55%[27,98] to 90%[72,109,125] of ; patients with Duchenne muscular dystrophy (DMD) die from the pulmonary complications associated with untreated GAH between 16.2 and 19 years of age and uncommonly after age 25.[49,109] This is because most patients are not treated for GAH nor are expiratory muscle aids used to help them eliminate airway secretions during intercurrent upper respiratory tract infections. Most of the remaining patients succumb from cardiomyopathy. For the minority of patients who survive the initial episode of respiratory failure and who subsequently undergo tracheostomy, and for the even smaller number who are offered and agree to undergo prophylactic tracheostomy, a number of studies have reported success with long-term tracheostomy IPPV.

Gatin described the cases of eight tracheostomized patients.[55] Two patients died at 30 and 36 days following tracheostomy, one from accidental decannulation and the other from massive tracheal hemorrhage. The other six patients survived at least 38 months. None required more than 16 hours/day of IPPV. They experienced a total of four pneumonias, two near-respiratory arrests from tracheobronchial mucus plugging, and occurrences of tracheal stenosis, granulation, and pseudopolyp formation.[55] Splaingard et al. reported the cases of three patients with DMD who survived 3, 5, and 2 years, respectively, with tracheostomy tubes. The last patient apparently died from respiratory complications.[119] Baydur et al. reported on seven DMD patients who received full-time tracheostomy IPPV for 18.2, 4.2, 3, 4.2, 6.3, 3.5, and 3.2 years, respectively, from the mean age of 22.3 ± 6.5 (range, 17–36) to 28.5 ± 8.1 (range, 20.5–42.3) years.[20] Two of the seven died of pneumonia, and five of the seven patients were reported as having had pneumonia or recurrent pneumonias.[20] Fukunaga et al. reported on three DMD patients who received tracheostomy IPPV for 0.6, 1.5, and 2.5 years after using a chest shell ventilator overnight for 3.5, 4.5, and 2 years, respectively.[53] Complications were not reported. Bach et al. reported seven patients who received tracheostomy IPPV for a mean of 7.1 years, from 21.1 ± 3.8 to 28.1 ± 4.5 years of age. Two of the seven patients were still alive.[15] Complications were not reported. The Baydur and Bach study patients who had survived long enough after an episode of acute respiratory failure to be referred to a rehabilitation center had mean prolongations of survival of 6.2 and a bit more than 7.1 years, respectively, by tracheostomy IPPV.

Spinal Muscular Atrophy

Gilgoff et al. reported the cases of 15 patients with SMA, 13 with type 2 and 2 with type 1 disease, who received tracheostomy IPPV for an average of 8 years 10 months (range, 5 mos to 23 yrs 10 mos), from the average age of 12 years 5 months (range, 5 mos to 18 yrs 10 mos).[58] Three patients required 24-hour support from the point of their initial episode of ventilatory failure. The other 12 used only nocturnal support for an average of 8 years 7 months. All patients had VCs <20% of predicted normal when requiring IPPV. Six patients underwent tracheostomy to clear airway secretions before requiring ongoing assisted ventilation, and most of the patients had had multiple pneumonias before and while using aid. All patients had uncuffed tracheostomy tubes and could speak. Nine of them continued to receive only nocturnal aid. Two patients died after 5 and 14 years of support, respectively. One patient was institutionalized. Of the 10 patients over 18 years of age, 3 had college degrees, 2 were college students, 3 graduated from high school, and 2 completed eleventh grade. One patient is the mother of a healthy child. Two patients are employed, and 2 others do volunteer work.

In another study, six patients with SMA survived using IPPV via an indwelling tracheostomy tube 24 hours a day for a mean of 11.7 ± 17.7 years, despite frequent episodes of mucus plugging and pneumonia.[128] Four of the patients also received all nutrition via indwelling gastrostomy tubes because of severe bulbar muscle weakness. Four patients used tracheostomy IPPV with their tracheostomy cuffs deflated and could communicate verbally. Five of the six patients remained institutionalized from the onset of ventilator use. Two patients survived for 15 and 4 years, respectively, despite need for ventilatory support since early infancy. All four ventilator-users who could communicate remained socially active, and one was gainfully employed.

Although these are anecdotal reports that do not take into account SMA patients who died suddenly during an initial episode of respiratory failure, clearly, as for patients with other neuromuscular conditions, the survival of SMA patients with or without severe bulbar muscle involvement can be prolonged considerably by ventilatory support via an indwelling tracheostomy tube. Interestingly, however, even though bulbar muscle dysfunction was not so severe as to necessitate enteral nutrition and preclude verbal communication for a number of patients, there was a very high incidence of pneumonias and bronchial mucus plugging in these tracheostomized populations.

Amyotrophic Lateral Sclerosis

Pulmonary complications and respiratory failure account for at least 84% of mortality in amyotrophic lateral sclerosis (ALS).[26,99] Ventilatory failure and death can occur in as little as 2 months from onset of symptoms.[28] Because of ethical reservations about offering tracheostomy IPPV to these patients, many patients are never offered mechanical ventilatory support, even during episodes of acute respiratory failure. At least in some states, less than 10% of ALS patients undergo tracheostomy,[96] and the mean survival from onset of symptoms without the use of ventilatory support has been reported as 2.4,[120] 3.1,[74] and 4.1 years.[28] Jablecki et al. reported that about 20% of 194 patients survived 10 years without ventilatory support.[74]

Although relatively few ALS patients benefit from ventilatory assistance, 90% to 97% of ALS ventilator users are glad to have chosen mechanical ventilation and would do it over again.[7,96,102] However, from the point of undergoing tracheostomy, a mortality rate of 76% was reported at 12 months for 24 IPPV users.[113] For other tracheostomy IPPV user groups, mean survivals were reported as 20 months for 18 users,[54] 15 months (range, 3–48) for 12 users,[60] 26.6 months for 4 users,[102] 2.3 years for 3 users,[73] and 7 months for 3 users.[117] In another study, 89 ALS ventilator-users using 24-hour aid survived a mean of 4.4 ± 3.9 years (range, 1 mo to 26.5 yrs), with 37 of the patients still alive at the time of the study. Thirteen of the 89 patients had used only noninvasive methods of ventilatory support. The 76 ventilator-users who ultimately received tracheostomy IPPV survived using ventilatory support for a mean of 4.5 ± 4.0 years (range, 1 mo to 26.3 yrs). Six patients survived using tracheostomy IPPV for >10 years, including 3 patients for >14 years (Fig. 23–2). The 52 deceased

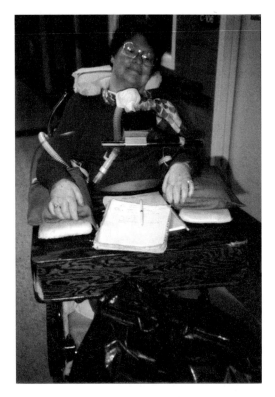

FIGURE 23–2. Seventy-six-year old woman with motor neuron disease, who had onset of disease at age 23, has been wheelchair-dependent since age 27, and is a 24-hour ventilator-user with no residual upper extremity function since age 47 in 1966. She continues to sell clothing (in the dark sack below her lap tray) and, with assistance, keep her accounts (open account book on her lap tray).

patients used ventilatory support for a mean of 3.8 ± 2.9 years (range, 3 mos to 14.5 yrs), including 4.1 ± 2.9 years (range, 1 mo to 14.5 yrs) of tracheostomy IPPV for the 45 deceased patients who were ultimately tracheostomized. In this study of 89 ALS patients, 42 of 74 patients (57%) with rapidly progressive disease and 11 of 15 (73%) with a slower form were managed predominantly in the community.[4]

Thus, resort to tracheostomy should not be taken lightly for ALS patients. Many of these patients can survive for >10 years using tracheostomy IPPV. However, deterioration in physical functioning and limited family resources often make it impractical, if not impossible, for them to be managed in the community. Although only about 5% of patients lose the ability to blink and therefore to operate augmentative communication systems,[4] communication can be lost when patients are placed into nursing facilities where their communication systems may not be set up or may be ignored. Institutionalization,

thus, can result in severe isolation and the loss of any meaningful interaction with the environment. Understanding the family's commitment to the patient, therefore, is essential before considering tracheostomy under any circumstances.

Non-Duchenne Myopathies

Robert et al. reported that of 18 *muscular dystrophy* patients, including those with DMD using tracheostomy IPPV in the home setting, 77% survived 1 year and 62% survived 5 years. No 10-year survival was reported.[110]

Three patients with *mitochondrial myopathies* had acute episodes of ventilatory failure. A 31-year-old woman was intubated and ultimately weaned from ventilatory support in 12 days. A 65-year-old woman had a history of multiple episodes of pneumonia, the last of which necessitated mechanical ventilation for which an indwelling tracheostomy tube was placed; 2 months later, she had another episode of pneumonia and sepsis from which she died. Another 37-year-old woman had had at least one episode of pneumonia per year for 12 years before presenting with atelectasis and a $PaCO_2$ of 89 mm Hg. She was intubated, bronchoscoped, and required ventilatory support for 7 days. Five months later, she presented with ventilatory failure with a $PaCO_2$ of 68 mm Hg, despite a VC of 2.1 liters, and underwent tracheostomy.[18]

Two patients with *nemaline myopathies* had episodes of ventilatory failure. One presented at age 9 with a $PaCO_2$ of 56 mm Hg when awake and 67 mm Hg when asleep. Oxygen therapy progressively exacerbated hypercapnia. Three months later, with severe symptoms of GAH, he developed acute ventilatory failure and underwent tracheostomy, which he continues to use for nocturnal IPPV. A second patient became symptomatic for GAH at 6.5 years of age, developed hypercapnic coma and underwent tracheostomy. She continues to require nocturnal ventilatory support 4 years after the initial admission.[86]

A 64-year-old patient with *acid maltase deficiency* presented with symptoms of hypersomnolence. He was treated with nocturnal oxygen administration and CPAP at 9 cm H_2O with "marked" symptomatic relief. "However, the next day the patient developed confusion and cyanosis . . . the lone preintubation blood gas measurement revealed a PaO_2 of 74 mm Hg, $PaCO_2$ of 102 mm Hg, and pH of 7.29 on 2-liters nasal oxygen. Nasotracheal intubation was performed and mechanical ventilation was instituted. Further pulmonary deterioration ensued and the patient died."[89]

These anecdotal cases typify the conventional approach of leaving GAH untreated, or worse, treating it with supplemental oxygen until hypercapnic coma, pneumonia, or other complications necessitate emergency intervention.

CONVENTIONAL NOCTURNAL NASAL IPPV

Nasal IPPV involves the delivery of IPPV via a nasal interface to assist inspiratory effort (Fig. 23–3). In this chapter, only nocturnal use of nasal IPPV is considered. When only nocturnal nasal IPPV is used, simple, commercially available CPAP masks are often adequate for delivery of IPPV because ventilatory assistance is usually delivered at less than ventilatory support pressures. Thus, little retention strap pressure may be necessary, and skin discomfort is not often a difficult problem.

Pressure-Cycled vs Volume-Cycled Ventilators

Although described much earlier, CPAP was rediscovered in 1976.[62] As the widespread prevalence of obstructive sleep apnea syndrome became appreciated in the 1980s, CPAP became the primary treatment to maintain upper airway patency. CPAP accomplishes this by increasing functional residual capacity and by its pneumatic splinting effect on the airway. CPAP, however, is ineffective for many patients who have severe concomitant restrictive pulmonary syndromes, as well as for others who have respiratory muscle dysfunction and hypercapnia, because CPAP does not directly assist inspiratory muscle function.

The first positive pressure ventilators used in the United States were the Monahan pressure-cycled ventilators. These ventilators permitted many post-poliomyelitis patients to return home using intermittent abdominal pressure ventilators and, occasionally, mouthpiece IPPV during daytime hours to complement their use of NPBVs overnight. Because they were smaller, simpler, and cheaper, blowers (Zephyrs) delivered a continuous stream of air that many patients used for mouthpiece IPPV. Except for blowers, pressure-cycled ventilators were the only options for home mechanical ventilation until portable volume-cycled ventilators became available in 1978. From 1978 until the advent of bi-level positive airway pressure (BiPAP) a few years ago,[115] virtually all new ventilator users were sent home using volume-cycled ventilators.

In 1987 nocturnal nasal IPPV delivered by portable volume-cycled ventilators was described.[14,46,77] Although 90% of subsequent reports of nocturnal nasal IPPV (Table 23–2) involved the use of ventilators without expiratory positive airway pressure (EPAP), clinicians continued to treat GAH due to neuromuscular disease with some combination of medications, oxygen, and CPAP. Because of the ineffectiveness of CPAP for patients with severe respiratory muscle dysfunction and difficulties tolerating high EPAP levels when CPAP is delivered at high pressures (often up to 15 cm H_2O), BiPAP was developed. Although pressure-cycled positive pressure ventilators like BiPAP had

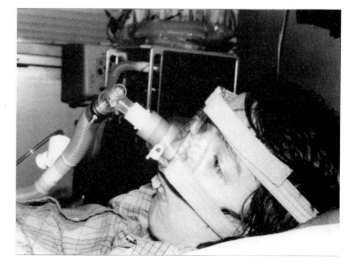

FIGURE 23–3. Woman with spinal muscular atrophy and chronic respiratory muscle insufficiency who was born in 1959. She used nasal IPPV via a volume ventilator and a standard CPAP mask (Respironics Inc., Murrysville, PA) for nocturnal ventilatory assistance from 1971 until March 1988. She required 24-hour ventilatory assistance only during intercurrent upper respiratory tract infections. She underwent tracheostomy when hospitalized for an upper respiratory tract infection in March 1988 and subsequently died from pneumonia in April 1990.

TABLE 23–2
Comparison of BiPAP and Portable Volume Ventilators

Volume Ventilators	BiPAP
Advantages	Advantages
1. Delivers higher volumes and at potentially higher pressures as needed for patients with poor lung compliance	1. No annoying alarms
2. Adjusts flow rates for comfort	2. Light weight
3. Uses 3 to 8 times less electricity for comparable air delivery, permitting greater patient mobility at same battery capacity	3. Less cost
4. Quieter	4. Can compensate to some extent for small insufflation leaks
5. Less mean thoracic pressures create less untoward hemodynamic effects on cardiac preload, which can be particularly hazardous for patients with cardiomyopathies	Disadvantages
6. Permits air stacking to obtain maximum insufflations and to increase dynamic pulmonary compliance by, as well as for, raising voice volume and increasing cough flows	1. Inability to air stack
7. Can operate intermittent abdominal pressure ventilators as well as noninvasive IPPV	2. Fixed, high initial flow rates can cause mouth drying, gaging (especially with insufflation leakage), and arousals from sleep
8. Has alarm systems that facilitate effective use of nocturnal noninvasive IPPV	3. High power utilization limits patient mobility
Disadvantages	4. Inadequate pressure generation capabilities for some patients
1. Heavier	5. Discomfort and increased thoracic pressures from unnecessary EPAP
2. Annoying alarms (low-pressure alarm can be eliminated by setting alarm to minimum and using flexed mouthpiece or a regenerative humidifier)	6. Gauge of pressure-cycled devices is less useful for feedback concerning insufflation leakages
3. Complicated (ventilators with fewer modes should be available)	7. No alarms to facilitate effective nocturnal IPPV for some patients
	8. Noisier
	9. EPAP unnecessary for most patients

been available since 1956, BiPAP's light weight, EPAP capabilities, and its similarity with CPAP lead to its quick acceptance and widespread use.

For volume-cycled ventilators, the volume is set and remains constant irrespective of the quantity of delivered air leaking out the nose or mouth rather than entering the lungs (insufflation leakage), and the peak airway pressures indicated on a ventilator gauge vary depending on ventilator-delivered volumes, insufflation leakage, interface leakage, and lung impedance. There are also low- and high-pressure alarms, sensitivity controls that permit the patient to trigger ventilator-delivered breaths, and flow rate adjustments. For pressure-cycled ventilators, the pressure is set and the ventilator delivers air volumes to achieve the set pressure. Insufflation leakage results in an increase in delivered volumes to achieve the set pressures. Increased airway resistance, such as from mucus plugging, results in a decrease in delivered volumes. Volume-cycled ventilators, such as the PLV-100 (Lifecare International Inc., Westmin-

ster, CO) and the LP-10 (Aequitron, Minneapolis, MN), can generally deliver up to 2500-ml volumes. The same is true of the traditional pressure-cycled ventilators, such as the Maxivent (J.H. Emerson Company, Cambridge, MA) and the Thompson Bantam (Lifecare International, Inc., Westminster, CO), for patients with normal lung impedance.

The BiPAP S/TD machine (Respironics, Murrysville, PA) and the PB335 Respiratory Support System (Puritan-Bennett Inc., Pickering, Ontario) are essentially pressure-limited blowers up to pressures of about 15 and 30 cm H_2O, respectively, with delivered volumes plateauing at greater pressures. Inspiratory positive airway pressures (IPAPs) and EPAPs can be adjusted separately. EPAP cannot be turned off completely. The IPAP-EPAP difference or span is essentially the amount of pressure support or inspiratory pressure assistance that the patient receives. The typically used BiPAP spans of 5 to 7 cm H_2O are more effective and comfortable than CPAP for most patients with obstructive sleep apneas, but such small spans only provide adequate inspiratory muscle assistance for patients with mild GAH. Instead of using high-span BiPAP or switching to volume-cycled ventilators for daytime aid via a mouthpiece or nosepiece when lowspan nocturnal BiPAP is no longer adequate, clinicians conventionally prescribe oxygen therapy or recommend tracheostomy. Ironically, once a tracheostomy tube is placed, the patient then receives appropriate tidal volumes at adequate peak pressures (usually 20 to 25 cm H_2O). Even when maximum spans are used, however, BiPAP units limited to IPAPs of ≤ 24 cm H_2O deliver <1200-ml volumes to many patients with normal lung impedance, and when lung impedance is increased, adequate ventilation cannot be achieved by BiPAP.

Volume-cycled and pressure-cycled ventilators including BiPAP units each have advantages and disadvantages (Table 2). BiPAP units weigh only 12 to 15 lbs. They are useful for air delivery without high- and low-pressure alarms, which can be an advantage or a disadvantage, depending on the particular patient. An adapter must be obtained if these units are to operate on direct current (DC). BiPAP devices and other pressure ventilators use three to eight times more electricity than volume-cycled ventilators. Depending on the external battery power source, they may run for about 2 hours in comparison with perhaps 10 hours or more for volume-cycled ventilators.

Air stacking to facilitate coughing, increase voice volume, and optimally expand the lungs is not possible with BiPAP devices.[10] Depending on the BiPAP unit, many patients may not even be able to obtain the 1.5-liter insufflation volumes needed for an effective assisted cough.[10] Air stacking is not possible with other pressure ventilators either, but they can generally be set to deliver much larger single breaths. Air stacking can be especially important for patients who require more than overnight ventilatory assistance and is a key reason that volume-cycled ventilators are more appropriate than BiPAP for patients with progressive ventilatory impairment. BiPAP use by clinicians with little experience treating patients with neuromuscular disorders leads to patient management errors.[8]

Indications for Nocturnal Nasal IPPV

There are many studies of the use of nasal IPPV, but, few attempt to define precise indications for its use (Table 23–3). For the most part, nasal IPPV is used nightly when patients become symptomatic from GAH and hypoxia, and blood gas abnormalities and symptoms are alleviated with its use. There is also often a history of frequent hospitalizations for respiratory complications.

The lack of consensus on indications for nocturnal nasal IPPV prompted a consensus conference on the subject in 1991.[111] It was agreed that nasal IPPV should be instituted when patients expressed symptoms of GAH, and that in the absence of symptoms, nocturnal nasal IPPV is indicated for DMD patients when $PaCO_2$ exceeds 45 mm Hg and/or PaO_2 is <60 mm Hg in blood gas samples taken early in the morning, late in the day, or during periods of oxyhemoglobin desaturation. It was also suggested that nocturnal SaO_2 <90% for 20% or more of the night might also be an indication for nasal IPPV.

In reality, asymptomatic patients, especially those with no history of respiratory complications, rarely tolerate using nasal IPPV. Likewise, use of nasal IPPV has not been shown to be effective for the treatment of respiratory failure associated with hypoxia alone.

It should also be understood that GAH develops insidiously. Symptoms are usually subtle and may be limited to fatigue or anxiety. After trying nasal IPPV, many patients report relief of fatigue and other symptoms of which they had been unaware. When such patients feel better the day after using nocturnal nasal IPPV, they usually do not need to be prompted to continue its use.

The consensus suggested the following indications and considerations for instituting nocturnal nasal IPPV for stable patients with DMD.[111] These are equally appropriate for other conditions:

1. The speed of progression of the illness,
2. The presence of hypercapnia or end-tidal $PaCO_2$ >50 mm Hg during sleep,
3. Nocturnal mean SaO_2 <95%, and
4. Symptoms of GAH.

Any patient with symptoms suggestive of GAH or sleep-disordered breathing[10] should undergo nocturnal SaO_2 monitoring and possibly capnography. Arterial blood gas monitoring is usually unnecessary. A VC in the supine position below 40% of predicted normal is indicative of nocturnal hypoventilation from inspiratory muscle weakness, whereas symptomatic patients with greater VCs may have predominantly central or obstructive sleep apneas without severe concomitant inspiratory muscle weakness. Although the use of volume-cycled

TABLE 23–3
Results of Nocturnal Nasal IPPV Studies on Patients with Neuromuscular Ventilatory Impairment[a]

Year	Author	Ventilator[b]	Settings	Users	Diagnosis[c]	Results[d]
1987	Kerby[77]	Volume	0.3–1.2 l	5	NMD	>3 mos
	DiMarco[44]	Pressure	?	1	Scoliosis	NR
1988	Ellis[47]	Volume	?	5	Scoliosis	>3 mos
	Carroll[30]	Volume	?	6	Various	>3–9 mos
1989	Guilleminault[63]	Volume	?	1	OSAS	NR
1990	Bach[12e]	Volume	CO_2<45[f]	43	Various[g]	>19.8 mos
	Heckmatt[65]	Volume	?	14	NMD	>2–34 mos
1991	Goldstein[59]	Volume	50% EMG[m]	6	NMD, scoliosis	>14 mos
	Gay[56]	Volume	Vt 0.6–1.5 l	21	NMD	up to 39 mos
	Laier-Groeneveld[80]	Volume	?	23	Restrictive PS	up to 33 mos
	Thommi[121]	Pressure	7 cm H_2O	1	OSAS	NR
1992	Hill[68]	BiPAP	12–18/0–6[h] cm H_2O	6	Scoliosis, DMD[i]	>12.7 mos
	Waldhorn[126]	BiPAP	16–18[h] cm H_2O	8	Restrictive PS	>3 mos
1993	Paulus[103]	Volume	?	34	NMD	>3.0 yrs
	Delguste[40]	Volume	Vt >20 ml/kg	9	NMD	NR
	Barois[19]	Volume	Vt >20 ml/kg	46	NMD	up to >3 yrs[j]
	Chetty[33]	BiPAP	CO_2<45mm Hg[f]	1	Phrenic neuropathy	NR
1994	Vianello[124]	Volume	?	5	DMD	>2 yrs
	Leger[83]	Volume	CO_2<45mm Hg	279	Various[k]	>2 yrs[l]
	Piper[107]	Volume	CO_2<45mm Hg	13	OSAS	NR

[a]In these studies, indications for nocturnal nasal IPPV included symptomatic global alveolar hypoventilation (GAH). All symptoms were alleviated and arterial blood gases improved with treatment.
[b]Ventilators included volume-cycled (volume), pressure-cycled (pressure), or bi-level positive airway pressure (BiPAP).
[c]Diagnoses: NMD, various neuromuscular diseases; OSAS, obstructive sleep apnea syndrome. DMD, Duchenne muscular dystrophy; restrictive PS, restrictive pulmonary syndromes (including 3 patients with OSAS).
[d]Results given as duration of clinical improvement, delay in resort to tracheostomy, or death. NR indicates successful for alleviating symptoms and arterial blood gases but duration of benefit not reported.
[e]Ten patients used conventional nocturnal-only nasal IPPV, and the others used nocturnal nasal IPPV in a regimen of up to 24-hour noninvasive ventilatory support.
[f]Settings that maintained $PaCO_2$ <45 mm Hg were used.
[g]Diagnoses included post-polio in 22 patients, Duchenne muscular dystrophy in 5, non-Duchenne myopathy in 5, traumatic tetraplegia in 5, motor neuron disease in 3, and spina bifida, COPD, and kyphoscoliosis in 1 each.
[h]IPAP/EPAP setting in cm H_2O.
[i]Includes 4 patients with kyphoscoliosis and 2 with muscular dystrophy.
[j]In this study of patients with congenital myopathies, congenital muscular dystrophy, and spinal muscular atrophy, at least 14 patients underwent tracheostomy after periods of nocturnal nasal IPPV for up to >3 years, and several patients died from cardiomyopathies.
[k]Diagnoses included scoliosis in 56, tuberculosis in 52, DMD in 75, COPD in 49, and bronchiectasis in 49.
[l]Tracheostomy was delayed for >2 years for 183 patients and 54 patients underwent tracheostomy or died in <2 years. Treatment populations included 155 patients with intrinsic lung disease.
[m]Tidal volumes increased until diaphragm electrical activity is reduced by 50% or more.

ventilators is more appropriate for the former, BiPAP may be advantageous when air trapping or obstructive sleep apneas predominate.[10]

Individuals with relatively stable neuromuscular conditions, such as SMA or certain congenital myopathies, can tolerate mild hypercapnia and mean nocturnal SaO_2 of 93% to 94% for years. They require ventilatory support only during upper respiratory tract infections. Patients with rapidly progressive conditions such as ALS or those who have frequent hospitalizations for respiratory difficulties may benefit from nocturnal noninvasive IPPV once nocturnal hypercapnia or prolonged oxyhemoglobin desaturation appears, whether or not symptoms are obvious;

however, expiratory muscle aids are usually more important.[5]

Use of Nasal IPPV for Acute Respiratory Failure

Most commonly, patients with slowly deteriorating respiratory muscle function breathe without assistance despite varying degrees of hypercapnia until an intercurrent upper respiratory tract infection or surgical intervention necessitating general anesthesia triggers acute respiratory failure. There are many recent reports on the use of nasal or oral-nasal interface IPPV, for both patients with primarily ventilatory impairment as well as for patients with intrinsic lung disease, as alternatives to intubation for short-term IPPV.[23,25,34,70,79,81,90,92,93,104,106,107,127,130] There is little evidence, however, that the use of these methods benefits patients whose respiratory failure is due to hypoxia alone.[130] Indeed, high supplemental oxygen requirement may decrease the efficacy of nocturnal nasal IPPV.[16]

Mechanisms of Action

Although hypercapnia is apparently not an indication of respiratory muscle fatigue, it is evidence of limited reserve before the appearance of overt fatigue. Respiratory muscle rest by the use of nasal IPPV and the alleviation of nocturnal hypoventilation are probably the most important mechanisms for improving daytime symptoms and gas exchange.[68] Diaphragm and accessory muscle activity has been shown to decrease when patients are ventilated by NPBVs,[112] or by nasal IPPV,[29] when patients are awake. Although this has not yet been studied, nasal IPPV, which improves blood gases during sleep,[12] also probably permits a decrease in respiratory muscle activity during sleep. Furthermore, by maintaining more normal blood pH during sleep, nocturnal ventilatory assistance also decreases the tendency to develop a compensatory metabolic alkalosis with bicarbonate retention that blunts central respiratory sensitivity to carbon dioxide tensions and permits worsening of hypercapnia. Reversal of sleep-induced hypoventilation by nocturnal nasal IPPV, partial loss of the reversal during the first night,[59] and the increasing losses that we have seen on subsequent nights without assisted ventilation are consistent with these mechanisms. In addition, functional residual capacity, or at least dynamic lung compliance, may be increased by IPPV in GAH patients.[71,116] This may reduce the work of breathing and further improve daytime ventilation. Nocturnal nasal IPPV may also improve daytime pulmonary function for some patients.[47,59] Thus, the benefits of nasal IPPV appear to be largely due to some combination of respiratory muscle rest and improvements in lung compliance and chemotaxic sensitivity.

Results of Long-Term Nocturnal Nasal IPPV

The use of nocturnal nasal IPPV has been reported to increase maximum inspiratory pressures[46] and may transiently increase or stabilize VC for patients with GAH.[124] More importantly, ongoing use alleviates symptoms, normalizes blood gases, increases respiratory muscle endurance,[59] decreases the risk of respiratory complications and hospitalizations, and postpones resort to tracheostomy for months to years depending on the rate of progression of the primary neuromuscular conditions of these patients (Table 2).

Failure of nasal IPPV has been described as occurring when symptoms and signs of hypoventilation persist or recur or when its use becomes necessary for >15 hours/day.[84] In reality, failure occurs only when the contraindications for using noninvasive IPPV, in general, are not respected,[10] when insufficient effort is made to find or fabricate comfortable IPPV interfaces for nasal IPPV users, and when inadequate attention is made to clearing airway secretions. As with nocturnal-only ventilatory assistance of any kind,[95] nocturnal-only use of nasal IPPV must eventually fail for patients with progressive disease who will eventually require the use of daytime ventilatory aid and expiratory muscle aids as well. Once daytime hypercapnia develops despite nocturnal aid, signs and symptoms of GAH reoccur, expiratory muscles are usually very dysfunctional, and conventional approaches inevitably result in respiratory failure and tracheostomy or death.

A classic example of the inadequacy of conventional thinking and approaches toward nocturnal nasal IPPV was recently published in an otherwise reputable medical journal.[108] In a poorly designed and executed study, nocturnal nasal IPPV was prescribed for DMD patients without attention to daytime $PaCO_2$ levels, patient compliance with the prescription, patient training or interface optimization, consideration of airway secretion clearance, or consideration of need for daytime aid.[6] Obviously, patients treated in this manner would have higher mortality than those receiving up to 24-hour ventilatory support. The apparently logical recommendations derived from such inadequate patient management was, naturally, for earlier resort to tracheostomy![108]

CONCLUSION

The use of nocturnal-only nasal IPPV, whether by volume ventilator or BiPAP, can temporarily improve daytime blood gases and alleviate symptoms for patients with GAH; it can delay tracheostomy by months to years depending on the rate of progression of respiratory muscle dysfunction; and it can prolong survival for some patients[124] provided that episodes of hypoxic respiratory failure are avoided (Table 23–2).

References

1. Bach JR: Alternative methods of ventilatory support for the patient with ventilatory failure due to spinal cord injury. J Am Paraplegia Soc 14:158–174, 1991.
2. Bach JR: Ventilator use by Muscular Dystrophy Association patients: An update. Arch Phys Med Rehabil 73: 179–183, 1992.
3. Bach JR: A comparison of long-term ventilatory support alternatives from the perspective of the patient and care giver. Chest 104:1702–1706, 1993.
4. Bach JR: Amyotrophic lateral sclerosis: Communication status and survival with ventilatory support. Am J Phys Med Rehabil 72:343–349, 1993.
5. Bach JR: Mechanical insufflation-exsufflation: Comparison of peak expiratory flows with manually assisted and unassisted coughing techniques. Chest 104:1553–1562, 1993.
6. Bach JR: Misconceptions concerning nasal ventilation [letter]. Lancet 344:752, 1994.
7. Bach JR: Amyotrophic lateral sclerosis: Predictors for prolongation of life by noninvasive respiratory aids. Arch Phys Med Rehabil 76:828–832, 1995..
8. Bach JR: Case studies of respiratory management. In Bach JR (ed): Pulmonary Rehabilitation: The Obstructive and Paralytic/Restrictive Pulmonary Syndromes. Philadelphia, Hanley & Belfus, 1995.
9. Bach JR: Pathophysiology of paralytic/restrictive pulmonary syndromes. In Bach JR (ed): Pulmonary Rehabilitation: The Obstructive and Paralytic/Restrictive Pulmonary Syndromes. Philadelphia, Hanley & Belfus, 1995.
10. Bach JR: Prevention of morbidity and mortality with the use of physical medicine aids. In Bach JR (ed): Pulmonary Rehabilitation: The Obstructive and Paralytic/Restrictive Pulmonary Syndromes. Philadelphia, Hanley & Belfus, 1995.
11. Bach JR: Psychosocial, vocational, quality of life and ethical issues. In Bach JR (ed): Pulmonary Rehabilitation: The Obstructive and Paralytic/Restrictive Pulmonary Syndromes. Philadelphia, Hanley & Belfus, 1995.
12. Bach JR, Alba AS: Management of chronic alveolar hypoventilation by nasal ventilation. Chest 97:52–57, 1990.
13. Bach JR, Alba AS: Tracheostomy ventilation: A study of efficacy with deflated cuffs and cuffless tubes. Chest 97:679–683, 1990.
14. Bach JR, Alba AS, Mosher R, Delaubier A: Intermittent positive pressure ventilation via nasal access in the management of respiratory insufficiency. Chest 92:168–170, 1987.
15. Bach JR, O'Brien J, Krotenberg R, Alba A: Management of end stage respiratory failure in Duchenne muscular dystrophy. Muscle Nerve 10:177–182, 1987.
16. Bach JR, Robert D, Leger P, Langevin B: Sleep fragmentation in kyphoscoliotic individuals with alveolar hypoventilation treated by nasal IPPV. Chest 107:1552–1558, 1995.
17. Bach JR, Saporito LS: Indications and criteria for decannulation and transition from invasive to noninvasive long-term ventilatory support. Respir Care 39:515–531, 1994.
18. Barohn RJ, Clanton T, Sahenk Z, Mendell JR: Recurrent respiratory insufficiency and depressed ventilatory drive complicating mitochondrial myopathies. Neurology 40:103–106, 1990.
19. Barois A, Estournet-Mathiaud B: Nasal ventilation in congenital myopathies and spinal muscular atrophies. Eur Respir R 3:275–278, 1993.
20. Baydur A, Gilgoff I, Prentice W, et al: Decline in respiratory function and experience with long-term assisted ventilation in advanced Duchenne's muscular dystrophy. Chest 97:884–889, 1990.
21. Beck GJ, Barach AL: Value of mechanical aids in the management of a patient with poliomyelitis. Ann Intern Med 40:1081–1094, 1943.
22. Bellamy R, Pitts FW, Stauffer S: Respiratory complications in traumatic quadriplegia. J Neurosurg 39:596–600, 1973.
23. Benhamou D, Girault C, Faure C, et al: Nasal mask ventilation in acute respiratory failure: Experience in elderly patients. Chest 102:912–917, 1992.
24. Berk JL, Levy MN: Profound reflex bradycardia produced by transient hypoxia or hypercapnia in man. Eur Surg Res 9:75–84, 1977.
25. Bott J, Baudouin SV, Moxham J: Nasal intermittent positive pressure ventilation in the treatment of respiratory failure in obstructive sleep apnoea. Thorax 46:457–458, 1991.
26. Bowman K, Meurman T: Prognosis of amyotrophic lateral sclerosis. Acta Neurol Scand 43:489–498, 1967.
27. Brooke MH, Fenichel GM, Griggs RC, et al: Duchenne muscular dystrophy: Patterns of clinical progression and effects of supportive therapy. Neurology 39:475–480, 1989.
28. Caroscio JT, Mulvihill MN, Sterling R, Adrams B: Amyotrophic lateral sclerosis: Its natural course. Neurol Clin 5:1–8, 1987.
29. Carrey Z, Gottfried SB, Levy RD: Ventilatory muscle support in respiratory failure with nasal positive pressure ventilation. Chest 93:150–158, 1990.
30. Carroll N, Branthwaite MA: Control of nocturnal hypoventilation by nasal intermittent positive pressure ventilation. Thorax 43:349–353, 1988.
31. Carter RE, Donovan WH, Halstead L, Wilkerson MA: Comparative study of electrophrenic nerve stimulation and mechanical ventilatory support in traumatic spinal cord injury. Paraplegia 25:86–91, 1987.
32. Castella X, Gilbert J, Torner F: [Letter.] Chest 98:776–777, 1990.
33. Chetty KG, McDonald RL, Berry RB, Mahutte CK: Chronic respiratory failure due to bilateral vocal cord paralysis managed with nocturnal nasal positive pressure ventilation. Chest 103:1270–1271, 1993.
34. Chevrolet JC, Joliet P, Abajo B, et al: Nasal positive pressure ventilation in patients with acute respiratory failure. Chest 100:775–782, 1991.
35. Cohn JR, Steiner RM, Posuniak E, Northrup BE: Obstructive emphysema due to mucus plugging in quadriplegia. Arch Phys Med Rehabil 68:315–317, 1987.
36. Colice GL: Resolution of laryngeal injury following translaryngeal intubation. Am Rev Respir Dis 145:361–364, 1992.
37. Craven DE, Kunches LM, Kilinsky V, et al: Risk factors for pneumonia and fatality in patients receiving continuous mechanical ventilation. Am Rev Respir Dis 133: 792–796, 1986.
38. de Groot REB, Dik H, Groot HGW, Bakker W: A nearly fatal tracheal obstruction resulting from a transtracheal oxygen catheter. Chest 104:1634–1635, 1993.
39. Dee PM, Suratt PM, Bray ST, Rose CE: Mucous plugging simulating pulmonary embolism in patients with quadriplegia. Chest 85:363–366, 1984.
40. Delguste P, Rodenstein: Implementation and monitor-

ing of mechanical ventilation via nasal access. Eur Respir Rev 3:266–269, 1993.

41. Deutschman CS, Wilton P, Sinow J, et al: Paranasal sinusitis associated with nasotracheal intubation: A frequently unrecognized and treatable source of sepsis. Crit Care Med 14:111–114, 1986.

42. DeVita MA, Spierer-Rundback L: Swallowing disorders in patients with prolonged orotracheal intubation or tracheostomy tubes. Crit Care Med 18:1328–1330, 1990.

43. DeVivo MJ, Ivie CS: Life expectancy of ventilator-dependent persons with spinal cord injuries. Chest 108:226–232, 1995.

44. DiMarco AF, Connors AF, Altose MD: Management of chronic alveolar hypoventilation with nasal positive pressure breathing. Chest 92:952–954, 1987.

45. Elliott LS: Steps toward effective pulmonary therapy: Alvan L. Barach, MD. Respir Ther 9:13–18, 1979.

46. Ellis ER, Bye PTP, Bruderer JW, Sullivan CE: Treatment of respiratory failure during sleep in patients with neuromuscular disease: Positive-pressure ventilation through a nose mask. Am Rev Respir Dis 135:148–152, 1987.

47. Ellis ER, Grunstein RR, Chan RR, et al: Noninvasive ventilatory support during sleep improves respiratory failure in kyphoscoliosis. Chest 94:811–815, 1988.

48. Elpern EH, Scott MG, Petro L, Ries MH: Pulmonary aspiration in mechanically ventilated patients with tracheostomies. Chest 105:563–566, 1994.

49. Emery AEH: Duchenne muscular dystrophy: Genetic aspects, carrier detection and antenatal diagnosis. Br Med Bull 36:117–122, 1980.

50. Esau SA: The effect of theophylline on hypoxic, hypercapnic hamster diaphragm muscle in vitro. Am Rev Respir Dis 143:954–959, 1991.

51. Fishburn MJ, Marino RJ, Ditunno JF: Atelectasis and pneumonia in acute spinal cord injury. Arch Phys Med Rehabil 71:197–200, 1990.

52. Forbes JA: Management of respiratory paralysis using a "mechanical cough" respirator. BMJ 1:798–802, 1958.

53. Fukunaga H, Okubo R, Moritoyo T, et al: Long-term follow-up of patients with Duchenne muscular dystrophy receiving ventilatory support. Muscle Nerve 16:554–558, 1993.

54. Gabinski CL, Barthe A, Castaing Y, Favarel-Garrigues JC: Sclerose laterale amyotrophique et reanimation. Concours Med 105:249–252, 1983.

55. Gatin G: Intêret de la ventilation assistée dans les dystrophies musculaires. Ann Readapt Med Phys 26:111–128, 1983.

56. Gay PC, Patel AM, Viggiano RW, Hubmayr RD: Nocturnal nasal ventilation for treatment of patients with hypercapnic respiratory failure. Mayo Clin Proc 66:695–703, 1991.

57. George CF, Kryger MH: Sleep in restrictive lung disease. Sleep 10:409–418, 1987.

58. Gilgoff IS, Kahlstrom E, MacLaughlin E, Keens TG: Long-term ventilatory support in spinal muscular atrophy. J Pediatr 115:904–909, 1989.

59. Goldstein RS, DeRosie JA, Avendano MA, Dolmage TE: Influence of noninvasive positive pressure ventilation on inspiratory muscles. Chest 99:408–415, 1991.

60. Goulon M, Goulon-Goeau C: Sclérose latérale amyotrophique et assistance respiratoire. Rev Neurol (Paris) 145:293–298, 1989.

61. Gracy DR, McMichan JC, Divertie MB, Howard FM Jr: Respiratory failure in Guillain-Barré syndrome: A 6-year experience. Mayo Clin Proc 57:742–746, 1982.

62. Greenbaum DM, Miller JE, Eross B, et al: Continuous positive airway pressure without tracheal intubation in spontaneously-breathing patients. Chest 69:615–619, 1976.

63. Guilleminault C, Stoohs R, Schneider H, et al: Central alveolar hypoventilation and sleep: Treatment by intermittent positive pressure ventilation through nasal mask in an adult. Chest 96:1210–1212, 1989.

64. Haber II, Bach JR: Normalization of blood carbon dioxide levels by transition from conventional ventilatory support to noninvasive inspiratory aids. Arch Phys Med Rehabil 75:1145–1150, 1994.

65. Heckmatt JZ, Loh L, Dubowitz V: Night-time nasal ventilation in neuromuscular disease. Lancet 335:579–582, 1990.

66. Hedden M, Ersoz C, Safar P: Tracheoesophageal fistulas following prolonged artificial ventilation via cuffed tracheostomy tubes. Anesthesiology 31:281–289, 1969.

67. Heffner JE: Timing of tracheotomy in mechanically ventilated patients. Am Rev Respir Dis 147:768–771, 1993.

68. Hill NS, Eveloff SE, Carlisle CC, Goff SG: Efficacy of nocturnal nasal ventilation in patients with restrictive thoracic disease. Am Rev Respir Dis 145:365–371, 1992.

69. Hodes HL: Treatment of respiratory difficulty in poliomyelitis. In Poliomyelitis: Papers and Discussions Presented at the Third International Poliomyelitis Conference. Philadelphia, JB Lippincott, 1955, pp 91–113.

70. Hodson ME, Madden BP, Steven MH, et al: Non-invasive mechanical ventilation for cystic fibrosis patients—A potential bridge to transplantation. Eur Respir J 4:524–527, 1991.

71. Hoeppner VH, Cockcroft DW, Dosman JA, Cotton DJ: Nighttime ventilation improves respiratory failure in secondary kyphoscoliosis. Am Rev Respir Dis 129:240–243, 1984.

72. Inkley SR, Oldenburg FC, Vignos PJ Jr: Pulmonary function in Duchenne muscular dystrophy related to stage of disease. Am J Med 56:297–306, 1974.

73. Iwata M: Clinico-pathological studies of long survival ALS cases maintained by active life support. Adv Exper Med Biol 209:223–225, 1987.

74. Jablecki CK, Berry C, Leach J: Survival prediction in amyotrophic lateral sclerosis. Muscle Nerve 12:833–841, 1989.

75. Johanson WG, Pierce AK, Sanford JP, Thomas GD: Nosocomial respiratory infections with gram-negative bacilli: The significance of colonization of the respiratory tract. Ann Intern Med 77:701–706, 1972.

76. Johanson WG, Seidenfeld JJ, Gomez P, et al: Bacteriologic diagnosis of nosocomial pneumonia following prolonged mechanical ventilation. Am Rev Respir Dis 137:259–264, 1988.

77. Kerby GR, Mayer LS, Pingleton SK: Nocturnal positive pressure ventilation via nasal mask. Am Rev Respir Dis 135:738–740, 1987.

78. Konrad F, Schreiber T, Brecht-Kraus D, Georgieff M: Mucociliary transport in ICU patients. Chest 105:237–241, 1994.

79. Laier-Groeneveld G, Huttemann U, Criee C-P: Noninvasive nasal ventilation in acute and chronic ventilatory insufficiency [abstract]. Am Rev Respir Dis 141:237, 1990.

80. Laier-Groeneveld G, Huttemann V, Criee C-P: Nasal ventilation can reverse chronic ventilatory failure in both chest wall diseases and COPD. In Proceedings of the International Conference on Pulmonary Rehabilitation and Home Ventilation. Denver, National Jewish Center for Immunology and Respiratory Medicine, 1991, p 104.

81. Lapinsky SE, Mount DB, Mackey D, Grossman RF: Management of acute respiratory failure due to pulmonary edema with nasal positive pressure support. Chest 105:229–231, 1994.

82. Lassen HCA: The epidemic of poliomyelitis in Copenhagen, 1952. Proc R Soc Med 47:67–71, 1954.

83. Leger P, Bedicam JM, Cornette A, et al: Nasal intermittent positive pressure ventilation: Long-term follow-up in patients with severe chronic respiratory insufficiency. Chest 105:100–105, 1994.

84. Leger P, Langevin B, Guez A, et al: What to do when nasal ventilation fails for neuromuscular patients. Eur Respir Rev 3:279–283, 1993.

85. Logemann JA: Evaluation and Treatment of Swallowing Disorders. San Diego, College-Hill Press, 1983, p 119.

86. Maayan Ch, Springer C, Armon Y, et al: Nemaline myopathy as a cause of sleep hypoventilation. Pediatrics 77:390–395, 1986.

87. MacEwen W: Clinical observations on the introduction of tracheal tubes by the mouth instead of performing tracheotomy or laryngotomy. BMJ 2:122–124, 1880.

88. Magill IW: Development of endotracheal anesthesia. Proc R Soc Med 22:83–88, 1928.

89. Margolis ML, Howlett P, Goldberg R, et al: Obstructive sleep apnea syndrome in acid maltase deficiency. Chest 105:947–949, 1994.

90. Marino W: Intermittent volume cycled mechanical ventilation via nasal mask in patients with respiratory failure due to COPD. Chest 99:681–684, 1991.

91. Mathias CJ: Bradycardia and cardiac arrest during tracheal suction—Mechanisms in tetraplegic patients. Eur J Intens Care Med 2:147–156, 1976.

92. Meduri GU, Abou-Shala N, Fox RC, et al: Noninvasive face mask mechanical ventilation in patients with acute hypercapnic respiratory failure. Chest 100:445–454, 1991.

93. Meduri GU, Conoscenti CC, Menashe P, Nair S: Noninvasive face mask ventilation in patients with acute respiratory failure. Chest 95:865–870, 1989.

94. Moar JJ, Lello GE, Miller SD: Stomal sepsis and fatal haemorrhage following tracheostomy. Int J Oral Maxillofac Surg 15:339–341, 1986.

95. Mohn CH, Hill NS: Long-term follow-up of nocturnal ventilatory assistance in patients with respiratory failure due to Duchenne-type muscular dystrophy. Chest 97:91–96, 1990.

96. Moss AH, Casey P, Stocking CB, et al: Home ventilation for amyotrophic lateral sclerosis patients: Outcomes, costs, and patient, family, and physician attitudes. Neurology 43:438–43, 1993.

97. Moxham J: Aminophylline and the respiratory muscles: An alternative view. Clin Chest Med 9:325–336, 1988.

98. Mukoyama M, Kondo K, Hizawa K, et al: Life spans of Duchenne muscular dystrophy patients in the hospital care program in Japan. J Neurol Sci 81:155–158, 1987.

99. Mulder DW, Howard FM: Patient resistance and prognosis in amyotrophic lateral sclerosis. Mayo Clin Proc 51:537–541, 1976.

100. Niederman MS, Ferranti RD, Ziegler A, et al: Respiratory infection complicating long-term tracheostomy: The implication of persistent gram-negative tracheobronchial colonization. Chest 85:39–44, 1984.

101. Ohi M, Nakashima M, Heki S, et al: Doxapram hydrochloride in the treatment of acute exacerbation of chronic respiratory failure: A patient with four episodes treated without use of a respirator. Chest 74:453–454, 1978.

102. Oppenheimer EA, Baldwin-Myers A, Tanquary P: Ventilator use by patients with amyotrophic lateral sclerosis. In Proceedings of the International Conference on Pulmonary Rehabilitation and Home Ventilation. Denver, National Jewish Center, 1991, p 49.

103. Paulus J, Willig T-N: Nasal ventilation in neuromuscular disorders: Respiratory management and patients' experience. Eur Respir Rev 3:245–249, 1993.

104. Pennock B, Kaplan PD, Carlin BW, et al: Pressure support ventilation with a simplified ventilatory support system administered with a nasal mask in patients with respiratory failure. Chest 100:1371–1376, 1991.

105. Pingleton SK: Complications of acute respiratory failure. Am Rev Respir Dis 37:1463–1493, 1988.

106. Piper AJ, Parker S, Torzillo PJ, et al: Nocturnal nasal IPPV stabilizes patients with cystic fibrosis and hypercapnic respiratory failure. Chest 102:846–850, 1992.

107. Piper AM, Sullivan CE: Effects of short-term NIPPV in the treatment of patients with severe obstructive sleep apnea and hypercapnia. Chest 105:434–440, 1994.

108. Raphael J-C, Chevret S, Chastang C, Bouvet F: Randomised trial of preventive nasal ventilation in Duchenne muscular dystrophy. Lancet 343:1600–1604, 1994.

109. Rideau Y, Gatin G, Bach J, Gines G: Prolongation of life in Duchenne muscular dystrophy. Acta Neurol 5:118–124, 1983.

110. Robert D, Laier-Groeneveld G, Leger P: Mechanical assistance. Prax Klin Pneumol 42:846–849, 1988.

111. Robert D, Willig TN, Paulus J, Leger P: Long-term nasal ventilation in neuromuscular disorders: Report of a consensus conference. Eur Respir J 6:599–606, 1993.

112. Rochester DF, Braun NMT, Laine S: Diaphragmatic energy expenditure in chronic respiratory failure: The effect of assisted ventilation with body respirators. Am J Med 63:223–232, 1977.

113. Salamand J, Robert D, Leger P, et al: Definitive mechanical ventilation via tracheostomy in end stage amyotrophic lateral sclerosis. In Proceedings of the International Conference on Pulmonary Rehabilitation and Home Ventilation. Denver, National Jewish Center, 1991, p 51.

114. Sanada Y, Kohima Y, Fonkalsrud EW: Injury of cilia induced by tracheal tube cuffs. Surg Gynecol Obstet 154:648–652, 1982.

115. Sanders MH, Kern N: Obstructive sleep apnea treated by independently adjusted inspiratory and expiratory positive airway pressure via nasal mask: Physiologic and clinical implications. Chest 98:317–324, 1990.

116. Sinha R, Bergofsky EG: Prolonged alteration of lung mechanics in kyphoscoliosis by positive hyperinflation. Am Rev Respir Dis 106:47–57, 1972.

117. Sivak ED, Gipson WT, Hanson MR: Long-term management of respiratory failure in amyotrophic lateral sclerosis. Ann Neurol 12:18–23, 1982.

118. Smith PEM, Edwards RHT, Calverley PMA: Protriptyline treatment of sleep hypoxaemia in Duchenne muscular dystrophy. Thorax 44:1002–1005, 1989.

119. Splaingard ML, Frates RC, Harrison GM, et al: Home positive-pressure ventilation: Twenty years' experience. Chest 4:376–382, 1984.

120. Strong MJ, Ferguson KA, Ahmad D: The pulmonary function testing as a predictor of survival in amyotrophic lateral sclerosis [abstract]. Chest 102:180S, 1992.

121. Thommi G, Nugent K, Bell GM, Liu J: Termination of central sleep apnea episodes by upper airway stimulation using intermittent positive pressure ventilation. Chest 99:1527–1529, 1991.

122. Trendelenburg F: Beitrage zur den operationen an

den luftwagen 2. Tamponnade der trachea. Arch Klin Chir 12:121–233, 1871.

123. Vasilyev S, Schaap RN, Mortensen JD: Hospital survival rates of patients with acute respiratory failure in modern respiratory intensive care units: An international, multicenter, prospective survey. Chest 107:1083–1088, 1995.

124. Vianello A, Bevilacqua M, Salvador V, et al: Long-term nasal intermittent positive pressure ventilation in advanced Duchenne's muscular dystrophy. Chest 105:445–448, 1994.

125. Vignos PJ: Respiratory function and pulmonary infection in Duchenne muscular dystrophy. Isr J Med Sci 13:207–214, 1977.

126. Waldhorn RE: Nocturnal nasal intermittent positive pressure ventilation with bi-level positive airway pressure in respiratory failure. Chest 101:516–521, 1992.

127. Waldhorn RE, Robinson R, Murthy R, Jennings C: Nasal intermittent positive pressure ventilation with bi-level positive airway pressure in acute and chronic respiratory failure. Am Rev Respir Dis 141:238–241, 1990.

128. Wang TG, Bach JR, Avilez C, et al: Survival of individuals with spinal muscular atrophy on ventilatory support. Am J Phys Med Rehabil 73:207–211, 1994.

129. Welply NC, Mathias CJ, Frankel HL: Circulatory reflexes in tetraplegics during artificial ventilation and general anesthesia. Paraplegia 13:172–182, 1975.

130. Wysocki M, Tric L, Wolff MA, et al: Noninvasive pressure support ventilation in patients with acute respiratory failure. Chest 103:907–913, 1993.

Prevention of Morbidity and Mortality with the Use of Physical Medicine Aids

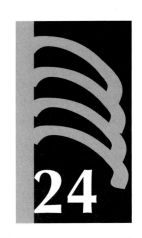

24

John R. Bach, MD

Although in some centers, the use of bi-level positive-airway pressure (BiPAP) or volume-cycled ventilators for nocturnal nasal intermittent positive-pressure ventilation (IPPV) has become accepted conventional care, the patient with progressive global alveolar hypoventilation (GAH) will not be spared eventual tracheostomy or death from respiratory failure by this approach. Currently orthodox approaches to managing neuromuscular ventilatory failure do not take into account the facts that alveolar ventilation can be maintained by noninvasive means, irrespective of the extent of respiratory muscle dysfunction, and that for most patients it is possible to generate sufficient cough flows to clear airway secretions effectively without resorting to tracheal intubation. The three goals of optimal respiratory management for patients with GAH are:

1. To maintain alveolar ventilation as normal as possible around-the-clock,
2. To expand the lungs to maintain pulmonary compliance,
3. To maximize peak cough flows (PCF) to clear airway secretions when necessary.

Physical medicine respiratory muscle aids are used to accomplish these goals and, in doing so, to prevent pulmonary morbidity and mortality without resort to tracheostomy. When these aids used correctly, many patients eventually require 24-hour ventilator use with no significant venti-

lator-free breathing time (VFBT) but without ever being hospitalized (Table 24–1).

WHAT ARE PHYSICAL MEDICINE RESPIRATORY MUSCLE AIDS?

Inspiratory and expiratory muscle aids are devices and techniques that involve the manual or mechanical application of forces to the body or intermittent pressure changes to the airway to assist inspiratory or expiratory muscle function. The devices that act on the body include the negative-pressure body ventilators (NPBVs) and oscillators that create atmospheric pressure changes around the thorax and abdomen, body ventilators and exsufflation devices that apply force directly to the body to mechanically displace respiratory muscles, and devices that apply intermittent pressure changes directly to the airway.

Certain positive-pressure ventilators or blowers have the capacity to deliver continuous positive airway pressure (CPAP). Likewise, certain negative-pressure generators or ventilators that can be used to operate a chest shell or tank-style ventilator can create continuous negative extrathoracic pressure (CNEP). CPAP and CNEP, both described in the 1870s,[109] act as pneumatic splints to help maintain airway and alveolar patency and to increase functional residual capacity. They do not directly assist respiratory muscle activity. For patients with GAH, these

303

TABLE 24–1
Guide to Abbreviations

BiPAP—bi-level positive airway pressure
CNEP—continuous negative extrathoracic pressure
COPD—chronic obstructive pulmonary disease
CPAP—continuous positive airway pressure
DMD—Duchenne muscular dystrophy
dSaO2—oxyhemoglobin desaturation
EPAP—expiratory positive airway pressure
EPR—electrophrenic respiration
GAH—global alveolar hypoventilation
GPB—glossopharyngeal breathing
IAPV—intermittent abdominal pressure ventilator
IPPB—intermittent positive pressure breathing
IPPV—intermittent positive pressure ventilation
MIC—maximum insufflation capacity
MI-E—mechanical insufflation-exsufflation
NPBV—negative pressure body ventilator
PCF—peak cough flows
S_aO_2—oxyhemoglobin saturation
SONI—strapless oral-nasal interface
VC—vital capacity
VFBT—ventilator-free breathing time (maximum tolerable)

techniques are usually ineffective or inadequate.

INSPIRATORY MUSCLE AIDS

Body Ventilators: An Historical Perspective

In 1852, Meryon described how a 16-year-old boy with what was to become known as Duchenne muscular dystrophy (DMD) died from acute respiratory failure during a febrile episode with "profuse secretion of mucus from the trachea and larynx."[89] One hundred fifty years later, most patients with progressive neuromuscular disorders still die prematurely, or are hospitalized and needlessly undergo tracheostomy, because of failure to assist their respiratory muscles.

Negative Pressure Body Ventilators

NPBVs intermittently create subatmospheric pressure around the thorax and abdomen to assist or support the inspiratory effort.[11] *Tank ventilators* consist of either a tank or cylinder (e.g., the iron lung) that envelopes the body up to the neck. The first tank ventilator was described by the Scottish physician, John Dalziel, in 1832.[109] Negative pressure was created in the tank by manually operating a piston rod (Fig. 24–1) or, later, by motorized bellows (Fig. 24–2 and 24–3).

The *iron lung*, which was perfected in 1928,[61] was the first body ventilator to receive widespread use. It became the main device used for both acute and long-term ventilatory support from 1931 until the mid-1950s (Fig. 24–4). Iron lungs continue to be manufactured and used in the United States, England, Germany, and Italy. In centers in northern Italy, and possibly elsewhere, iron lungs are the mainstay of ventilatory support in the intensive care unit.[50] Currently, however, for portable iron lungs (PortaLung, Lifecare International Inc, Westminster, CO) as well as for most other NPBVs, the negative pressure is not created by a motorized bellows but by pumps or ventilators that can provide negative and, at times, positive pressures.

The *chest shell-style ventilators* consist of a firm shell that covers the chest and abdomen (*see* Fig. 25–5 in Chapter 25). They were first described shortly after the Dalziel apparatus.[61,109] Negative pressure is cycled under the shell. The Fairchild-Huxley chest respirator[52] and Monaghan Portable Respirator,[51] which were introduced in 1949, became the first mass-produced chest shell ventilators. They can support ventilation with the patient sitting or supine but are only optimal for the latter. Their use for daytime aid has been largely supplanted by the more practical intermittent abdominal pressure ventilator (IAPV), noninvasive IPPV methods, and glossopharyngeal breathing (GPB).[19]

The *wrap-style ventilators,* similar in principle and function to the chest shell ventilator, are the most recently developed NPBVs. The prototype wrap ventilator was the Tunnicliffe breathing jacket, which was described in 1955 and continues to be used in England.[103] All wrap ventilators consist of a firm plastic grid that covers the thorax and abdomen. The grid and the body under it are covered by a wind-proof jacket that is sealed around the neck and extremities. Negative pressure ventilators cycle subatmospheric pressure under the wrap and grid. Although more time-consuming to don, wrap ventilators can be more effective than chest shell ventilators because of their more complete covering of the thorax and abdomen.

The evolution of NPBVs was summarized by Woollam in 1976.[109,110] Since 1976 the major advancements have been in the materials used in the shells and wraps, the length and form of the wrap sleeves, and the negative pressure generators themselves.[11] A wrap with its caudal end sealed over the lower abdomen or pelvis has the

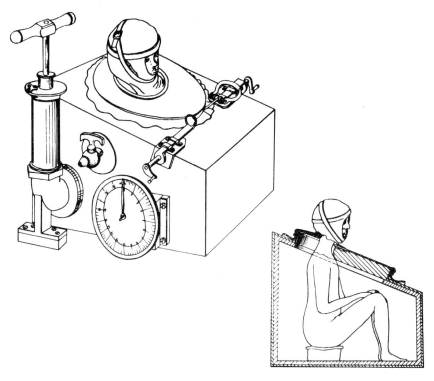

FIGURE 24–1. Body-enclosing iron lung described by Alfred F. Jones of Lexington, Kentucky, in 1864. With it, he "cured paralysis, neuralgia, rheumatism, seminal weakness, asthma, bronchitis, and dyspepsia. Also deafness. When properly and judiciously applied, many other diseases may be cured . . . "[61]

advantage of easier patient access for perineal care and greater lower extremity mobility, but there is a tendency for the wrap to slip up and under the grid. This decreases comfort and causes air leak, especially at pressures exceeding -45 cm H_2O. Wraps that extend down the legs and are sealed at the thighs or ankles are easier to seal but some patients complain of the fabric squeezing the legs during use. A Pulmobag (Lifecare International Inc., Westminster, CO) or Pneumobag (New Tech, Palisades Park, NJ) is essentially a full-length wrap ventilator that completely seals the lower extremities. This design decreases leak and facilitates donning, but the dorsiflexion of the feet and the "squeezing" of the legs that occur during use can be uncomfortable. A wind-impermeable cloth that permits the escape of humidity (Gortex, W.C. Gore & Assoc., Elkton, MD) is now an alternative to nylon in the fabrication of the wrap. Gortex makes for a cooler, more flexible wrap and increases both comfort and expense. For the Red Poncho (J.H. Emerson Co., Cambridge, MA), Pneumosuit (New Tech), or NuMo Suit (Lifecare International Inc.), the wrap is formed into arms and pants legs that separately seal each extremity, and there is a long anterior air-tight zip-

per closure. This design optimizes lower extremity mobility and may discourage venous stasis in the lower extremities, but it is inconvenient for toileting.

Negative-pressure generators include the 33-CR (J.H. Emerson Co.), NEV-100 (Lifecare Inc.), and Maxivent (Puritan-Bennett Inc., Pickering, Ontario). The latter two ventilators can alternately deliver both negative and positive pressures, which is especially useful for patients who depend on both NPBVs and noninvasive IPPV methods at different times during the day. The NEV-100 and 33-CR permit the use of CNEP. The ventilation modes, alarms, and other options available on these ventilators have been described.[11]

In 1939, it was recognized that alveolar ventilation could be assisted and circulation supported by rapidly alternating negative and positive pressure under a chest shell.[59] The Hayek *Oscillator* (Breasy Medical Equipment Inc., Stamford, CN) is an NPBV that can operate as a standard chest shell ventilator at normal respiratory rates, but it incorporates the capacity to provide CNEP and oscillation at up to 17 Hz around a negative pressure, positive pressure, or atmospheric pressure baseline. It can provide al-

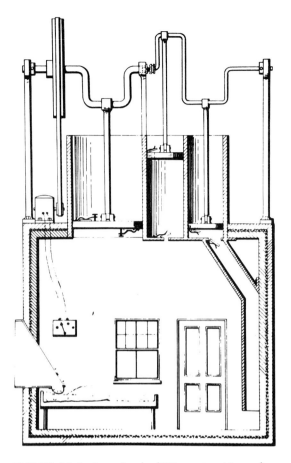

FIGURE 24–2. Peter Lord of Worcester, Massachusetts, patented this iron lung room in 1908. Huge pistons would create the pressure changes and supply fresh air. This could not only facilitate nursing care but reduce housing costs!

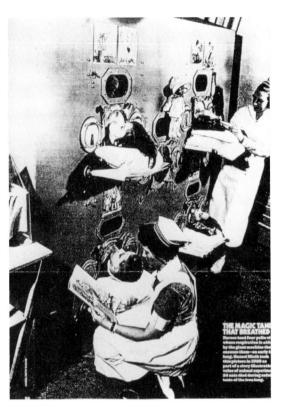

FIGURE 24–3. Thirty-five years later, an iron lung room ventilates four patients.

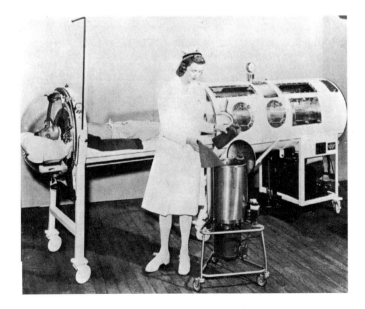

FIGURE 24–4. The Emerson iron lung, the standard ventilator for both acute and long-term respiratory support from 1931 to 1956. It had a dome to enclose the head for positive pressure ventilation when the body-enclosing cylinder was open.

ternating positive-negative pressure cycles or oscillations with pressures from +70 to −70 cm H_2O. By adjustments in the inspiratory/expiratory (I:E) ratio, an expiratory bias may be created to assist in airway secretion elimination. For example, an I:E ratio of 2:1 can create airway pressures of +6 to −3 cm H_2O that should favor the movement of airway secretions up the airways toward the mouth. The chest shell of the Hayek Oscillator is a light, moldable, clear plastic, flexible cuirass with soft foam rubber and Velcro closures that comfortably form a tight seal. Although the Hayek Oscillator has been reported to be effective in assisting alveolar ventilation in humans for short periods of time at the high frequencies of 1 to 5 Hz,[56] in this author's experience, high-frequency chest wall oscillation is uncomfortable for the patient and not reliable for maintaining alveolar ventilation when inspiratory muscle impairment is severe.

NPBVs are suitable for overnight ventilatory support and have been used to ventilate the lungs of patients with little or no vital capacity (VC) for decades, despite frequent transient oxyhemoglobin desaturations ($dSaO_2$) due to apparent episodes of airway collapse.[29] As patients age and pulmonary compliance decreases, NPBVs can become ineffective, associated with the development of systemic hypertension, and patients must be switched to the use of more effective inspiratory muscle aids.[8,22] Furthermore, except for the iron lung and PortaLung, NPBVs are generally not useful in the presence of severe scoliosis or extreme obesity. Back discomfort is also common when negative pressures must exceed −60 cm H_2O, as is often the case when using a chest shell or wrap ventilator, particularly for the patient with back deformity.

Other Body Ventilators

One of two types of body ventilators that applies force directly to the body is the *rocking-bed ventilator* (J.H. Emerson Company). It rocks the patient in an arc of 15° to 30°, allowing gravity to displace the abdominal contents cyclically. This causes diaphragmatic excursion and assists ventilation. It has been used since 1932 by predominantly poliomyelitis and muscular dystrophy patients. Although it is still being used for ventilatory support and can provide as much as 1000-ml tidal volumes for some patients with no measurable VC or VFBT, as with the NPBVs, it is mostly of historical interest. It is generally not as effective as NPBVs or noninvasive IPPV.[68]

NPBVs and the rocking-bed ventilator were the predominant methods of ventilatory support until the mid-1950s. Largely because these devices were only practical and effective with the user recumbent and because tracheostomy tubes could facilitate airway secretion management, particularly during episodes of acute respiratory failure, there has been widespread resort to tracheostomy and translaryngeal delivery of IPPV and suctioning since the late 1950s.[14] Because of the many difficulties, complications, and the expense associated with maintaining an indwelling tracheostomy tube,[14] and because of recent advances in noninvasive IPPV and airway secretion elimination, it has become clear that resort to tracheostomy is both unnecessary[31] and undesirable[7] for the majority of patients with neuromuscular GAH.

Noninvasive IPPV

Noninvasive IPPV methods, which are more effective than body ventilators and preferred over tracheostomy and body ventilator methods,[7] were not described until 1969, and their use was not reported for a significant population for 24-hour ventilatory support until the 1980s. Furthermore, the long-term use of noninvasive IPPV is permitted by effective airway secretion management. However, mechanical insufflation-exsufflation (MI-E) had only been used over the last 40 years by the few patients with poliomyelitis or patients with severe intrinsic pulmonary disease who had access to these machines to clear airway secretions.[22] The polio patients were felt to be a transient population, and the latter group is a population for which the use of noninvasive respiratory muscle aids is problematic. The recent availability of devices for MI-E and new noninvasive IPPV methods now make it practical to manage long-term ventilatory insufficiency by strictly noninvasive approaches.

Daytime Inspiratory Muscle Aids

Body Ventilators

Although the chest shell ventilator can be used for ventilatory assistance with the user sitting, it is cumbersome, inconvenient, and often not very effective. The intermittent abdominal pressure ventilator (IAPV), on the other hand, can be very effective. It was first described by McSweeney in 1938[88] and involves the intermittent inflation of an elastic air sac that is contained in a corset or belt worn beneath the patient's outer clothing (Fig. 24–5) (Exsufflation Belt, Lifecare International Inc.). The sac is in-

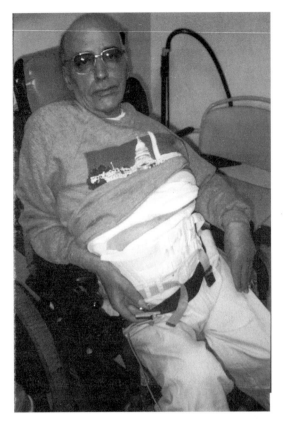

FIGURE 24–5. A 51-year-old man with muscular dystrophy who has been a 24-hour/day ventilator-user using the intermittent abdominal pressure ventilator (Exsufflation Belt, Lifecare International Inc.) during daytime hours and lipseal IPPV nightly since 1979.

flated by a positive-pressure ventilator. Bladder action moves the diaphragm upward, causing a forced exsufflation. During bladder deflation, the abdominal contents and diaphragm return to the resting position and inspiration occurs passively. A trunk angle of 30° or more from horizontal is necessary for its effectiveness. If the patient has any inspiratory capacity or is capable of GPB, he or she can add autonomous tidal volume to the mechanically assisted inspirations. The IAPV generally augments tidal volumes by about 300 ml, but volumes as high as 1200 ml have been reported.[19] Patients with 1 hour of VFBT usually prefer to use the IAPV rather than noninvasive methods of IPPV when sitting.[19] The IAPV is often inadequate in the presence of scoliosis or obesity.

Mouthpiece IPPV

Mouthpiece IPPV may have first been attempted with a mechanical device by Paracelsus,

who ventilated lungs using a chimney bellows in 1530. His technique was used in Europe through the 19th century.[70]

From 1931 until the mid-1950s, when iron lungs had to be opened to permit nursing care to the body, patients with no VFBT received IPPV via a hood that enclosed their heads (Fig. 24–4). This is ironic when one considers that these patients simply could have received IPPV via mouthpieces; however, there is no evidence that this mode was tried until 1956, when positive-pressure ventilators separate from the iron lung became available.

As early as 1952, many post-poliomyelitis ventilator-users with little VC or VFBT refused the advice of their physicians to undergo tracheostomy and continued to use body ventilators up to 24 hours a day. Many learned how to receive IPPV via a mouthpiece held between their lips and teeth. Others preferred to have the mouthpiece held near the mouth by either a metal clamp attached to the wheelchair or fixed onto motorized wheelchair controls (sip-and-puff, chin, or tongue control) (Fig. 24–6), from where they used the mouthpiece for IPPV as necessary.[22] The Monaghan positive-pressure ventilator was placed on wheels and rolled behind the wheelchair. Patients thus, were freed from their body ventilators during daytime hours without resort to tracheostomy.

To learn mouthpiece IPPV, the patient learns palatal movements to prevent insufflation leakage out the nose and learns to open the glottis with each assisted breath. This maneuver can be difficult to learn for patients who are being transferred from tracheostomy IPPV, especially with an inflated cuff, to noninvasive IPPV, because the normal inspiratory-onset reflex abduction of the vocal cords and hypopharynx is lost. Often patients are thought to have laryngotracheal stenosis until learning to reopen the glottis to permit IPPV. This is not usually a problem following translaryngeal tracheal intubation.

Dr. Augusta Alba recognized that patients would occasionally nap while sitting in their wheelchairs using mouthpiece IPPV without the mouthpiece falling out of their mouths. By 1964, a number of patients had left their body ventilators to use up to 24-hour mouthpiece IPPV.[7,21,24] Ultimately, several hundred of her patients relied on this technique alone or in combination with body ventilators for up to 24-hour ventilatory support for over 40 years (Fig. 24–6).[17,21,24,27] Simple mouthpiece IPPV continues to be the most convenient, reliable, effective, and patient-preferred method of daytime

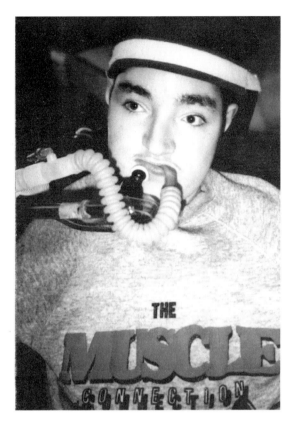

FIGURE 24–6. Patient with Duchenne muscular dystrophy who has used 24-hour mouth piece IPPV for 11 years, now with <5 minutes of ventilator-free breathing time. The mouthpiece is fixed adjacent to the chin controls for his motorized wheelchair.

ventilatory support for most wheelchair users with GAH. It is the most important noninvasive method of daytime ventilatory support.

During daytime use, in addition to using mouthpiece IPPV for normal minute ventilation, patients are taught to air stack by taking breaths consecutively without exhaling. The goal is to approach the predicted inspiratory capacity. The maximum volume of air that can be held is the maximum insufflation capacity (MIC). Air stacking may not only help maintain static lung compliance but also, at least temporarily, improve dynamic pulmonary compliance.[91] Most importantly, the higher volumes increase both unassisted and assisted peak cough flow (PCF) and permit the patient to raise voice volume as needed.

Besides opening the glottis and vocal cords to receive the air, to use mouthpiece IPPV effectively and conveniently, the patient must have adequate neck rotation and oral motor function to grab the mouthpiece and receive

IPPV without insufflation leakage from the mouth or nose (Fig. 24–6). To prevent leakage from the nose, the soft palate must have sufficient function to seal off the nasopharynx.

Ventilator styles have been discussed elsewhere.[14] In general, because of the importance of air stacking, any GAH patient without significant air trapping, documented obstructive sleep apneas despite noninvasive IPPV, or other specific need to increase functional residual capacity uses volume-cycled ventilators rather than pressure-cycled ventilators or BiPAP, unless the pressure-cycled ventilator can attain pressures sufficient to provide insufflations to the patient's MIC and expiratory positive airway pressure (EPAP), if present, can be turned completely off. In addition, some patients benefit from the use of the low-pressure alarm to help them develop conditioned reflexes during sleep to maintain adequate alveolar ventilation despite the use of these "open systems" of ventilatory support (*see* later discussion).

Nocturnal Inspiratory Muscle Aids

Although NPBVs continue to be used by many, noninvasive IPPV methods are more effective and are preferred for nocturnal ventilatory support. Contraindications to their use are listed in Table 24–2.[11]

Lipseal IPPV

From the mid-1960s until nocturnal nasal IPPV was described in 1987, mouthpiece IPPV was the only method of noninvasive IPPV. Many patients with little or no measurable VC maintained alveolar ventilation during sleep using

TABLE 24–2
Contraindications for Long-Term Noninvasive IPPV

1. Lack of cooperation or use of heavy sedation or narcotics
2. High levels of supplemental oxygen therapy
3. SaO_2 cannot be maintained above 90% by IPPV and assisted coughing
4. Bulbar muscle function is inadequate for swallowing without severe aspiration
5. History of substance abuse or uncontrollable seizures
6. Unassisted or assisted PCFs cannot exceed 3 l/sec
7. Conditions that interfere with use of IPPV interfaces: e.g., facial fractures, inadequate bite for mouthpiece entry, nasogastric tube, or beards that hamper seal with IPPV interfaces

simple mouthpiece IPPV. It was not until oximeters became widely available in the early 1980s, however, that it was discovered that these patients experienced frequent, and at times, severe $dSaO_2$ associated with periods of insufflation leakage (Fig. 24–7 A and B). In 1972, the lipseal (Puritan-Bennett Inc.) became available,[11] which sealed the mouth and firmly retained the mouthpiece in the mouth. Lipseal IPPV (*see* Fig. 25–2 in Chapter 25) could then be delivered during sleep with little insufflation leakage from the mouth and with virtually no risk of the mouthpiece falling from the mouth (Fig. 24–7C). Orthodontic bite plates and custom-fabricated acrylic lipseals (Fig. 24–8) can also increase comfort and efficacy and eliminate the risk of orthodontic deformity, which occurs in about 10% to 15% of 24-hour long-term mouthpiece IPPV users (Fig. 24–9).

For the 3% of patients with no VFBT (5 of 161)[24] who have excessive insufflation leakage and redevelop symptoms of GAH despite nocturnal lipseal IPPV, the nose can be clipped or plugged. Generally, however, nasal insufflation leakage during lipseal IPPV is not a clinical problem because high ventilator insufflation volumes, 1200 up to 2000 ml, can be used to compensate for nasal leakage. The use of the low-pressure alarm and conditioned reflexes also prevent excessive leak-associated $dSaO_2$ and hypoventilation.

Besides orthodontic deformities, other potential difficulties include allergy to the plastic lipseal and aerophagia. Although we have never had to discontinue noninvasive IPPV for any patient because of de novo aerophagia, one patient with a 35-year history of severe abdominal distention did have it exacerbated by noninva-

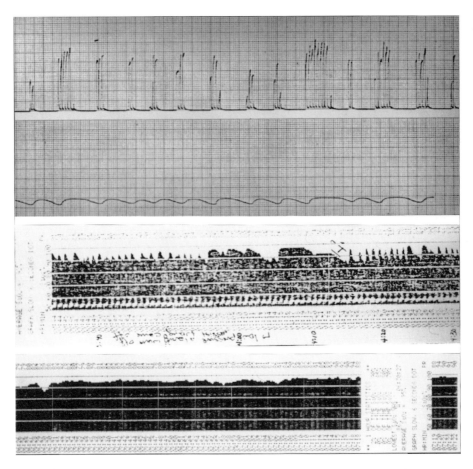

FIGURE 24–7. *A,* Capnograph recording of a sleeping patient. This patient is using mouthpiece IPPV without a lipseal. Although the mouthpiece remains in the mouth, insufflation leakage occurs until there is an oxyhemoglobin desaturation. This triggers the patient to grasp the mouthpiece firmly for several deep insufflations that once again normalize the SaO_2 until the next leak episode. *B,* Oxyhemoglobin desaturations can become severe. *C,* Severe desaturations can be eliminated by using lipseal retention for nocturnal IPPV.

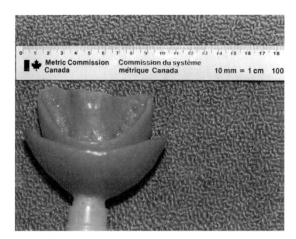

FIGURE 24–8. Custom acrylic mouthpiece with orthodontic biteplate and lipseal. (Courtesy of Mr. G. McPherson.)

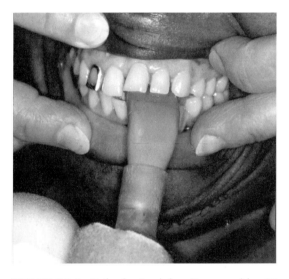

FIGURE 24–9. Orthodontic deformity caused by 15 years of 24-hour mouthpiece IPPV without a custom biteplate. (Courtesy of Dr. Augusta Alba.)

sive IPPV and could not tolerate using this technique. This patient used a NPBV for 10 years and ultimately underwent a colostomy to relieve the distention. Normally, the gastroesophageal spincter can withstand usual peak IPPV airway pressures without leak. Aerophagia tends to occur when ventilator-delivered volumes result in peak pressures >about 25 cm H_2O. Abdominal distention often occurs sporadically. The air passes as flatus once the patient gets up or is placed in a wheelchair in the morning. When severe, a rectal tube can usually decompress the colon.

Nasal IPPV

In January 1982, as an alternative to mouth-piece IPPV for "resting" the inspiratory muscles of muscular dystrophy patients, Rideau suggested delivering IPPV through the nostrils. Delaubier delivered nasal IPPV via urinary drainage catheters with the cuffs inflated in each nostril.[56] Although nocturnal nasal IPPV has become a conventional approach to temporarily relieving nocturnal hypoventilation, there is only one description of its use for 24-hour ventilatory support before 1989. In 1984 it was used for a multiple sclerosis patient with a VC of 100 ml and no VFBT.[23] A nasal CPAP mask was used as the nasal interface. There are now commercially available CPAP masks from Lifecare (Westminster, CO), Respironics (Murrysville, PA), Healthdyne (Cedar Grove, NJ), Puritan-Bennett (Pickering, Ontario), and Res Care, Inc. (San Diego, CA), that can be used for IPPV. Each design applies pressure differently to the paranasal area. It is impossible to predict which model will be most effective and preferred by any particular patient. Many patients use different styles on alternate nights to vary skin contact pressure. Nasal bridge pressure and insufflation leakage into the eyes are common complaints with several of these generic models. Such difficulties resulted in the development of custom-molded nasal interfaces[17,23,81,86] which can now be obtained both commercially (SEFAM Co., distributed by Lifecare Inc.) (Fig. 24–10) and individually in New Jersey (Fig. 24–11).[86]

Because patients generally prefer to use mouthpiece IPPV or the IAPV for daytime use,[17,19] nasal IPPV is most practical only for nocturnal use. Daytime nasal IPPV is indicated for those who can not grab or retain a mouthpiece because of oral muscle weakness, inadequate jaw opening, or insufficient neck movement. Twenty-four hour nasal IPPV can, nevertheless, be a viable alternative to tracheostomy even for some patients with severe lip and oropharyngeal muscle weakness.[17]

Oral-Nasal Interfaces

Oral-nasal interfaces were described for long-term ventilatory support in 1989.[95] These interfaces used strap retention systems like those for lipseal or nasal IPPV. However, because effective ventilatory support can be provided by either nasal or lipseal IPPV, or when necessary, lipseal IPPV with the nose clipped or plugged by cotton pledgets and tape, strap-retained oral-nasal in-

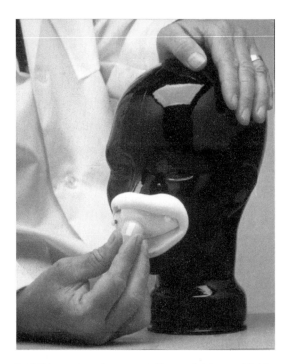

FIGURE 24–10. Commercially available, moldable, custom nasal interface (available from Lifecare International Inc.).

terfaces have not been widely used. Strapless oral-nasal interfaces (SONIs) with biteplate retention have been used in Europe since 1985 and were described in 1989.[86] Although 10 hours or more are required for their construction, these interfaces not only provide an essentially airtight seal for the delivery of IPPV, but simple tongue thrust is all that is necessary to expel them.[106] The biteplate retention is also important for patients living alone who are unable to don straps independently (Fig. 24–12).[27] Adequate and stable dentition is necessary to use them.

Although mouthpiece and nasal IPPV are generally open systems that rely in large part on central nervous system reflexes to prevent excessive insufflation leakage during sleep,[17,20,30] IPPV can be delivered via a SONI with very little insufflation leakage. To provide a closed, essentially leakless system, their use needs to be observed while the user sleeps, and the final touches applied to the acrylic shell and biteplate to eliminate residual insufflation leakage.[86]

EXPIRATORY MUSCLE AIDS

Why Are Expiratory Muscle Aids Needed?

Although the ability to inspire deeply is very important, the primary muscles for effective coughing are the muscles of expiration or the abdominal muscles. Clearing airway secretions and bronchial mucus plugs may be a continual problem for patients with airway or lung disease and for those who cannot swallow saliva without aspiration. For patients with GAH and functional bulbar musculature it becomes a problem during upper respiratory tract infections, following general anesthesia, and during other periods of bronchial hypersecretion.

A normal cough requires a pre-cough inspiration or insufflation to about 85% to 90% of total lung capacity.[84] Glottic closure follows for about 0.2 seconds, and sufficient intrathoracic pressures are generated to obtain peak transient

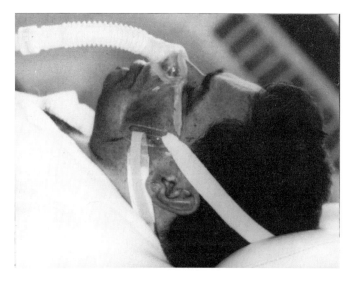

FIGURE 24–11. Patient with severe chronic alveolar hypoventilation due to kyphoscoliosis who uses a low-profile, custom, acrylic nasal interface for nocturnal nasal IPPV.[86]

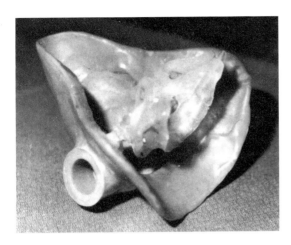

FIGURE 24–12. Strapless oral-nasal interface for IPPV.

expiratory flows or PCF exceeding 6 l/sec upon glottic opening.[32,64] Total expiratory volume during normal coughing is about 2.3 ± 0.5 liters.[84]

For patients with restrictive pulmonary syndromes, the VC, forced vital capacity, and ability to cough or PCF are diminished following general anesthesia and during upper respiratory tract infections because of fatigue, temporary weakening of both inspiratory and expiratory muscles,[90] and bronchial mucus plugging. Concomitant weakness of oropharyngeal muscles exacerbates the problem. The attainment of adequate PCF is extremely important for preventing pulmonary complications in these patients.[77]

Evaluation

Both inspiratory and expiratory muscle function is important for effective coughing. If the VC is under 1.5 liters, attaining higher insufflation capacities becomes critical for effective assisted coughing. Although it is useful to measure unassisted PCF (Access Peak Flow Meter, Health Scan, Inc., Cedar Grove, N.J.) as well as PCF from an insufflation to the MIC, the most important PCF is the cough flow from the MIC with a manual thrust timed to the cough (exsufflation or assisted PCF). When the PCF is >3 l/sec, safe tracheostomy tube removal and conversion to noninvasive ventilatory support is possible, irrespective of the extent of respiratory muscle dysfunction,[31] and noninvasive ventilatory support methods can be used to greatly prolong survival with minimal risk of respiratory complications.[16]

The inability to generate >3 l/sec of assisted PCF despite having an MIC >1 liter usually indicates fixed upper airway obstruction or severe bulbar muscle weakness and hypopharyngeal collapse occurs during MI-E (as described later). Vocal cord adhesions or laryngotracheal stenosis may have resulted from a previous transtracheal intubation and subsequent tracheostomy.[97] Because some lesions, especially the presence of obstructing granulation tissue, are amenable to surgical correction, laryngoscopic examination is warranted.

Patients with severe scoliosis may have poor assisted PCF because of a combination of restricted lung capacity and the inability to effect adequate diaphragm movement by abdominal thrusting because of rib cage deformity. Unlike patients with fixed upper airway obstruction, these patients can often benefit considerably from the use of MI-E.

Manually Assisted Coughing

As the use of endotracheal methods became widespread in the 1960s, manually assisted coughing was no longer taught in medical, nursing, and respiratory therapy curricula. Techniques of manually assisted coughing involve different hand and arm placements for expiratory cycle thrusts (Fig. 24–13). For patients with <1.5 liters of VC, efficacy is enhanced by preceding the assisted exsufflation with a deep insufflation.[10] A manual resuscitator, positive-pressure blower, intermittent positive-pressure breathing (IPPB) machine, or portable ventilator can be used to deliver the deep insufflations. Manually assisted coughing requires a cooperative patient, good coordination between the patient and caregiver, and adequate physical effort and often frequent application by the caregiver.

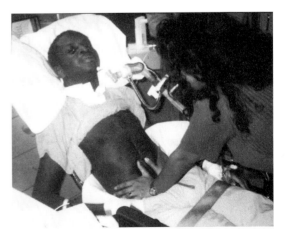

FIGURE 24–13. Hand placement for manually assisted coughing.

It is usually ineffective in the presence of significant scoliosis. Certain techniques must be performed with caution in a patient with an osteoporotic rib cage, and it should not be used for 2 hours following a meal. Unfortunately, because it is no longer widely taught to health care professionals[32] manually assisted coughing is greatly underutilized.[102] When this technique is inadequate, the most effective alternative for generating optimal PCF and clearing airway secretions is the use of MI-E.

Mechanical Insufflation-Exsufflation

"The life-saving value of exsufflation with negative pressure was made clear through the relief of obstructive dyspnea as a result of immediate elimination of large amounts of purulent sputum and, in a second episode, by the substantial clearing of pulmonary atelectasis after 12 hours' treatment."[41]

MI-E Devices and Use

In 1951, Barach et al. described an exsufflator attachment for iron lungs. The device used a vacuum-cleaner motor with a 5-inch solenoid valve attachment to an iron lung portal. With the valve closed, the motor developed a negative intratank pressure to −40 mm Hg. At peak negative pressure, the valve opened, triggering a return to atmospheric pressure in 0.06 seconds, and causing a passive exsufflation.[36] This increased the PCF in six ventilator-supported poliomyelitis patients from 1.2 l/sec unassisted to 1.6 l/sec, or by 45%. An additional increase was obtained by timing an abdominal compression with valve opening.[37] These techniques were sufficiently effective for the investigators to report that the exsufflation produced by this device "completely replaced bronchoscopy as a means of keeping the airway clear of thick tenacious secretions." Another "patient would have required bronchoscopy or re-opening of the tracheotomy if the exsufflator had not been successful in clearing the airway."[36]

In 1952, Barach and colleagues reported their "mechanical cough chamber." A pressure change of 110 mm Hg was induced 25 times/minute. A close-fitted baffle around the neck split the chamber into two. A blower applied positive pressure to the head chamber, which resulted in a higher pressure in the head chamber than in the body end of the chamber. When the pressure rose 110 mm Hg above the atmosphere

in the head chamber, a differential head-body pressure gradient of up to 40 mm Hg caused air to enter the lungs. The sudden opening of the 5-inch valve in the head compartment resulted in a 100-mm Hg explosive decompression there and a head-body pressure differential shift from +40 to about −40 mm Hg, thereby creating a forced exsufflation. The expiratory flows were enhanced by the perceptible forward shift of the body that occurred as the positive differential pressure in the body compartment dropped to 0 mm Hg with the return of atmospheric pressure on both sides of the baffle. This approach created PCF comparable to that of currently used portable MI-E devices.[4,32]

In 1953, various portable devices were manufactured to deliver MI-E directly to the airway via a mouthpiece, mask, or endotracheal tube.[93,100] Insufflation and exsufflation pressures were independently adjusted for comfort and efficacy. The best known of these devices and one that many of my patients have been using for over 40 years, although it was no longer commercially available, is the Cof-Flator (OEM Co., Norwalk, CT).[93] The Cof-Flator consisted of a two-stage axial compressor that gradually inflated the lungs with positive pressures of 50 cm H_2O over a 2-second period. The pressure in the upper respiratory passageway was then dropped to −30 to −50 cm H_2O in 0.02 seconds by the swift opening of a solenoid valve connected to a negative-pressure blower. The negative pressure was maintained for 1 to 3 seconds.[38,44]

In February 1993, an MI-E device (In-Exsufflator, J.H. Emerson Co.; Fig. 24–14) that operated like the Cof-Flator, except that cycling between positive and negative pressure had to be done manually, was approved by the Federal

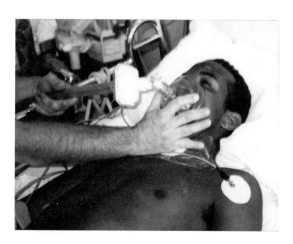

FIGURE 24–14. Mechanical insufflation-exsufflation.

Food and Drug Administration. The manual cycling feature facilitates caregiver–patient coordination of inspiration and expiration with insufflation and exsufflation but requires an additional hand if an abdominal thrust is to be given in conjunction with exsufflation or if one hand is inadequate to hold the mask. As with the Cof-Flator, one treatment consists of about five cycles of MI-E, followed by a period of normal breathing or ventilator use for 20 to 30 seconds to avoid hyperventilation. Five or more treatments are given in one sitting, and the treatments are repeated until no further secretions are expulsed and any mucus plug-induced dSaO$_2$ is reversed. Use can be required as frequently as every 10 to 60 minutes during upper respiratory tract infections. An abdominal thrust applied during the exsufflation cycle further increases PCF and airway secretion expulsion.[10] Although no medications are usually required for effective MI-E in neuromuscular ventilator-users with upper respiratory infections, liquefaction of sputum using heated aerosol treatments can facilitate exsufflation when secretions are inspissated.

MI-E is also extremely effective via a tracheostomy tube. When used in this manner, the tube cuff should be inflated. A concomitant abdominal thrust is unnecessary. Because effective flows are created in both right and left airways without the discomfort or airway trauma of tracheal suctioning (*see* Case 14, Chapter 25), patients invariably prefer MI-E to suctioning, and suctioning can be discontinued entirely for most patients.

Efficacy of MI-E

The efficacy of MI-E was demonstrated both clinically and on animal models.[44] Flow generation is adequate in both proximal and distal airways to eliminate respiratory tract debris.[83,101] VC, pulmonary flow rates, and SaO$_2$ (when abnormal) improve immediately with clearing of mucus plugs by MI-E.[4,5,32] An increase in VC of 15% to 42% was noted immediately following treatment in 67 patients with "obstructive dyspnea," and a 55% increase in VC was noted following MI-E in patients with neuromuscular conditions.[35] We have observed 15% to 50% improvements in FVC and normalization of SaO$_2$ as MI-E eliminates mucus plugs for acutely ill ventilator-assisted neuromuscular patients.[10]

Significant increases in PCF were also demonstrated by MI-E in patients with poliomyelitis, bronchiectasis, asthma, and pulmonary emphysema.[38] Following instillation of a mucin-thorium dioxide suspension into the lungs of anesthetized dogs, bronchograms revealed virtually complete elimination of the suspension after 6 minutes of MI-E.[44] The technique was shown to be equally effective in expulsing bronchoscopically inserted foreign bodies.[44] The use of MI-E through an indwelling tracheostomy tube was demonstrated in 1954 to be effective in reversing acute atelectasis associated with productive airway secretions[41]; however, PCFs were noted to be greater when MI-E was applied via a mask.[42] Barach and Beck demonstrated clinical and radiographic improvement with the use of MI-E in 92 of 103 acutely ill bronchopulmonary and neuromuscular patients with upper respiratory tract infections[35] including 72 patients with bronchopulmonary disease and 27 with skeletal or neuromuscular conditions including poliomyelitis[41]; however, it was more effective for the latter than for the former.[35]

Colebatch observed that applying negative pressure of 40 to 50 mm Hg is unlikely to have any deleterious effects on pulmonary tissues.[49] He noted that because the negative pressure applied to the airways is analogous to positive pressure on the surface of the lungs during a normal cough, it is improbable that this negative pressure can be more detrimental to the lungs than the normal cough pressure gradient. Bickerman found no evidence of parenchymal damage, hemorrhage, alveolar tears, or emphysematous blebs in the lungs of animals treated with MI-E.[44] Barach and Beck reported no serious complications in the 103 patients they treated with over 2000 courses of MI-E, and for no patient did MI-E have to be discontinued.[35] They noted that the initial transient appearance of blood-streaked sputum seen in a few patients probably originated from the bronchial wall sites of detachment of mucus plugs. Immediately following the initial elimination of blood-streaked sputum, the profuse outpouring of mucopurulent sputum indicated that "obstruction of the atelectatic area had been relieved." In one study, 1 of 19 patients complained of transient nausea associated with the onset of MI-E, but this passed with continued use.[48] Patients with wounds of the abdomen or chest reported less wound pain during MI-E than during spontaneous coughing, and no incidence of aspiration of gastric contents has been observed in either humans[108] or anesthetized dogs.[44] No reports of damaging side effects were disclosed in more than 6000 treatments in over 400 patients with MI-E, most of whom had primarily lung disease.[34,49] We continue to be unable to find literature contradicting the reports of effectiveness or describing significant complications of MI-E. Even when MI-E was used following abdominal surgery and following extensive chest wall surgery, no disruption of recently sutured wounds was noted.[108]

Consistent with these findings is the fact that in over 650 patient-years and thousands of applications of MI-E by our neuromuscular ventilator-users, no episodes of acute pneumothorax, aspiration of gastric contents, or blood-streaking of sputum were observed. Borborygmus and abdominal distention are infrequent and eliminated by decreasing insufflation (not exsufflation) pressures. The absence of any decrease and, indeed, the consistent increase in forced expiratory flows in the immediate post-exsufflation period indicated that no sustained airway obstruction resulted from MI-E.[10] Because, as with tracheal suctioning, MI-E can be associated with bradycardias for spinal-cord-injured patients in spinal shock, caution must be observed, and insufflation and exsufflation increased gradually when MI-E is used for these patients. Premedication with anticholinergic agents can be used when necessary. The use of high insufflation pressures can cause acute rib cage muscle pulls for patients with low VCs who do not routinely receive maximal insufflations. Insufflation pressures should be increased gradually for these patients.

Physiologic effects of MI-E were studied in depth in the early 1950s.[43] Peripheral venous pressures measured in the anterior cubital vein are slightly raised, i.e., 5.8 cm H_2O, during exsufflation. This is about one-third of the increase seen during normal coughing. Blood pressure is increased an average of 8 mm Hg in systole and 4 mm Hg in diastole. The pulse can increase or decrease during MI-E, and electrocardiographic changes reflect the rotation of the heart at peak inspiratory volumes. The increase in intragastric pressure is 26 mm Hg during MI-E and 85 mm Hg during normal coughing.[63]

Dayman found that in patients with emphysema, the production of high intrathoracic pressures during the glottic-closure phase of unassisted coughing and the subsequent pressure drop may result in an even greater pressure difference between the alveoli and lumen of the bronchioles than is normally present.[55] The resulting high alveolar-bronchial pressure gradient may result in closure of bronchioles and obstruction to air exiting the alveoli. Coughing is, thus, often ineffective. Part of the benefit of MI-E for chronic obstructive pulmonary disease (COPD) patients was that high expiratory flows occur with lower intrathoracic pressures.[35] It was suggested that COPD patients and others with severe intrinsic disease should practice passive MI-E[34]—i.e., they should leave their airways passively open and not attempt to cough with the exsufflation.

MI-E has been noted to be effective in eliminating tenacious sputum before, and of contrast medium after, bronchography in patients with bronchial asthma and bronchiectasis, and it has been suggested that MI-E may improve the results of bronchoscopy.[35] Williams and Holaday reported that MI-E could effectively eliminate airway secretions and ventilate patients in the minutes following generalized anesthesia.[108] They applied MI-E to both cooperative and unconscious patients and reported normalization of blood gases in all seven patients studied, including two with advanced pulmonary emphysema. In addition, improved breath sounds, increased percussion resonance, reduced respiratory rate, clearing of cyanosis, and reversal of right lower lobe collapse were reported for individual patients as a direct result of MI-E.

The use of MI-E has permitted us to consistently extubate elective surgical neuromuscular patients immediately following general anesthesia, despite their having no VFBT, and to convert them to the use of noninvasive IPPV. It has also permitted us to avoid intubation or to extubate neuromuscular patients quickly despite acute respiratory failure due to intercurrent upper respiratory tract infections with profuse airway secretions. MI-E is not helpful if the patient cannot cooperate sufficiently to keep the airway open, if there is a fixed upper airway obstruction, or if upper airway dilators cannot maintain sufficient patency to allow for adequate PCF.[79] This is most often seen in patients with advanced amyotrophic lateral sclerosis and severe infantile spinal muscular atrophy.

Mechanical Oscillation Techniques

Beck first described the use of high-frequency chest wall oscillation to facilitate bronchial secretion clearance in patients with chronic bronchial asthma and emphysema in 1966.[40] Oscillation can be applied externally to the chest wall or abdomen or directly to the airway as high-frequency positive-pressure ventilation, jet ventilation, or oscillation in which there are rapid small-amplitude pressure swings above and below atmospheric pressure.[47] Intrapulmonary percussive ventilation, or the delivery of high-flow minibursts of air to the lungs at 2 to 7 Hz, has also been proposed.[105] All of these techniques have been shown to benefit mucociliary transport in animal models. Although they have not yet been shown to be clinically effective in facilitating elimination of airway secretions in patients with COPD, they should, in theory, be useful for these patients. There is, however, no reason to use them for patients with GAH, because for these patients, the primary impediment to eliminating airway secretions is the inability to achieve adequate PCF. Because the airways are stable for most of these patients, assisted coughing is in both theory, and practice most effective.

Other Techniques to Assist Respiratory Muscle Effort

For patients with paralyzed abdominal musculature from spinal cord injury or any other reason, a thoracoabdominal corset limits the increase in functional residual capacity that occurs when the patient assumes the upright position. The mildly increased VC that results when sitting can increase PCF in this position. It can also help to maintain blood pressure and trunk stability for these patients when sitting.[78] Use of an abdominal binder has also been reported to decrease the subjective effort of breathing, relieve accessory neck and upper intercostal muscle activity, decrease the respiratory rate, and increase tidal air with a lowering of the total pulmonary ventilation for patients with neuromuscular disease or pulmonary emphysema.[41]

A 4-inch-wide abdominal belt with handgrips or handles has been designed as a postoperative coughing aid.[96] When the patient needs to cough, he or she passes one handle through the other and pulls with both hands. This instantaneously applies pressure to the abdomen and facilitates a pain-free cough.

An abdominal binder with functional electrical stimulation electrodes has become available to enhance the coughs of patients with spinal cord tetraplegia (Quik Coff Belt Company, Sunnyvale, CA). It increases maximum expiratory pressure at the mouth during coughing from 30 cm H_2O for spontaneous coughing to 60 cm H_2O with assisted coughing and compares favorably with the 80 cm H_2O obtained during manually assisted coughing. Its use can be triggered by the patient, and stimulation can be provided at regular intervals without the need for personal assistance. Further studies are needed to determine if adequate PCF can be generated to establish clinical utility for this apparatus.[85]

CLINICAL SETTINGS FOR THE USE OF RESPIRATORY MUSCLE AIDS

For most patients, respiratory muscle aids are first used during periods of acute ventilatory failure that are triggered by upper respiratory tract infections or elective surgery. During these episodes, fatigue occurs and respiratory muscle weakness is exacerbated.[90] These factors, in combination with the presence of airway secretions and impaired airway clearance mechanisms, cause ventilatory function and VC to decrease sharply.

Respiratory muscle aids can be used as alternatives to translaryngeal intubation for patients in acute respiratory failure and as alternatives to long-term tracheostomy IPPV. If the criteria for introduction of nocturnal noninvasive IPPV are met,[14] then the patient is offered trials of various nasal interfaces for nocturnal nasal IPPV (Fig. 24–15) and the lipseal for nocturnal lipseal IPPV (see Fig. 25–2 in Chapter 25) and allowed to choose between them. Interface use is evaluated for comfort and seal around the nose. If a comfortable, commercially available interface (CPAP mask) cannot be found, custom-molded

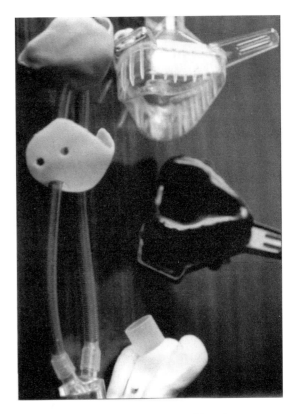

FIGURE 24–15. Various nasal interfaces.

varieties are tried (Fig. 25–9 to 25–11). No patient should be offered and expected to use only one CPAP mask for nasal IPPV. Alternating IPPV interfaces nightly should be encouraged.

Volume-cycled ventilators are generally used because these patients are likely eventually to require daytime IPPV and air stacking. Sufficiently powerful pressure-cycled ventilators can also be tried and the patient can choose the ventilator style as well as the IPPV interface. Oximetry feedback becomes very useful as daytime aid becomes necessary and during upper respiratory tract infections.

The evaluation of patients with GAH includes the measurements of VC (in sitting and recumbent positions), MIC, PCF, SaO_2, and, at times, end-tidal CO_2 or $PaCO_2$.

Oximetry Biofeedback and Capnography

Although $PaCO_2$ levels can exceed 50 mm Hg despite SaO_2 levels š95%, provided that oxygen therapy is avoided, symptomatic hypercapnia is usually minimal, and hypercapnia is often well tolerated when SaO_2 levels are maintained within normal limits. For a patient with GAH who has not been using ventilatory support, introduction to and use of mouthpiece or nasal IPPV is facilitated by oximetry biofeedback. Because these patients do not receive oxygen therapy unless critically ill and receiving intensive care, the patient and care providers are instructed that once artifact is ruled out,[107] any SaO_2 decrease below 95% is due to hypoventilation, bronchial mucus plugging, or intrinsic lung disease, usually pneumonia. End-tidal CO_2 monitoring can be used to document hypoventilation. However, GAH patients with upper respiratory infections usually require 24-hour noninvasive IPPV for alveolar ventilation and for air stacking. When using IPPV, $dSaO_2$s are not due to hypoventilation. Therefore, if not using IPPV, PaO_2 and SaO_2 should always first be increased by normalizing alveolar ventilation by noninvasive IPPV.

For patients already using noninvasive IPPV continuously, $dSaO_2$s are usually due to bronchial mucus plugging. PCF should be assessed, and both manually assisted coughing and MI-E used until SaO_2 returns to normal or baseline levels. If the baseline is 92% to 94%, the chest radiograph is usually clear and the hypoxia is often due to microscopic atelectasis. Despite hyperpyrexia and elevated leukocyte counts, baseline SaO_2 returns to normal and pneumonia and hospitalization are avoided when patients use noninvasive IPPV and conscientiously eliminate airway secretions by assisted coughing as needed. As the SaO_2 returns to normal, patients may wean to nocturnal only use or, at times, to no daily use of respiratory muscle aids until the next upper respiratory tract infection.

When patients do not use or have access to oximetry feedback, and therefore do not maintain adequate SaO_2 by effective assisted coughing and IPPV, they often present with baseline SaO_2 levels <90% and macroscopic atelectasis or pneumonia that has usually been triggered by an otherwise benign upper respiratory tract infection. At this point, oxygen therapy is indicated, and the patient will most likely require translaryngeal intubation because noninvasive IPPV is not very effective with concomitant oxygen therapy.

Oximetry biofeedback can serve as a guide to indicate how much noninvasive IPPV is required per day to maintain normal SaO_2. Patients are instructed to maintain SaO_2 >94% by autonomous breathing and to take mouthpiece-assisted breaths only when necessary to maintain normal SaO_2. An oximetry alarm may be set from 93% to 94% to remind the patient to take assisted breaths. The patient sees that by taking slightly deeper or assisted breaths, the SaO_2 goes above 94% within seconds. Usually, the patient maintains normal SaO_2 by unassisted breathing for a period of time and, once tiring, uses noninvasive IPPV as needed. Eventually noninvasive IPPV use becomes continuous, and all VFBT is lost with advancing disease. The use of oximetry in this manner can help to reset central ventilatory drive by reversing compensatory metabolic alkalosis and can virtually guarantee the effectiveness of noninvasive IPPV during sleep as well as during waking hours.

Oximetry is also very useful for monitoring the effectiveness of nocturnal noninvasive IPPV. Patients who benefit from nocturnal nasal or mouthpiece/lipseal IPPV should have a higher mean nocturnal SaO_2 using IPPV than when breathing on their own. For patients who benefit from nocturnal nasal IPPV, withdrawing nasal IPPV results in decreases in mean nocturnal SaO_2 and possibly increasing daytime symptoms and worsening blood gases[71,74] until nocturnal nasal IPPV is reinstituted. If there is no improvement observed in the mean nocturnal SaO_2 using nasal IPPV, there is usually no reason to think that its nocturnal use is benefiting the patient.

Decannulation and Conversion to Noninvasive Respiratory Aids

Ideally, patients for whom upper respiratory infections are likely to develop into acute respiratory failure should be equipped with an oximeter and have rapid access to an In-Exsufflator and, if not already using one, a portable volume ventilator. If the patient has at least been using occasional deep insufflations and therefore knows how to use mouthpiece or nasal IPPV, even when transtracheally intubated and with no VFBT, he or she can be extubated and converted directly to noninvasive IPPV. MI-E and manually assisted coughing remain critical for successful transition to noninvasive IPPV. Upper airway obstruction or failure to open the glottis with IPPV is usually not a problem for translaryngeally intubated patients.

When patients are being converted from tracheostomy to noninvasive IPPV, however, the patient may have to relearn how to open the vocal cords and glottis to receive the IPPV. A cuffed, fenestrated tracheostomy tube is placed (the cuff is needed for MI-E), and the patient practices receiving IPPV via a mouthpiece or nasal interface. It must be realized that obstruction from an indwelling tracheostomy tube, even one with a fenestration, can make if difficult for patients to be adequately ventilated in this manner, and the high oropharyngeal pressures generated by the ventilator-delivered volumes can make using noninvasive IPPV difficult. Although earlier, NPBVs were often used as a bridge to ventilate the patient's lungs while the tracheostomy site was closing,[2] we currently decannulate and convert patients directly to noninvasive IPPV. After the patient has become accustomed to using mouthpiece and nasal IPPV for at least brief periods with the tracheostomy tube in place, the tube is removed, and ideally, a tracheostomy button is placed for 24 hours to keep the site open so that the tracheostomy tube can be replaced in the event of tracheal edema or other unexpected airway obstruction and respiratory distress. Once the tracheostomy site is buttoned, and later when it is ultimately closed, PCF can be measured accurately. If assisted PCF cannot exceed 3 l/sec with the site buttoned, the tracheostomy tube should not be removed.[31] Otherwise, after 24 hours of noninvasive IPPV, the button is removed. A flexible silicon tracheostomy site cover (Respironics Inc., Murrysville, PA) and an elastic figure-of-8 dressing over that (*see* Clinical Tips at the end of this

chapter) can prevent IPPV insufflation leakage from the site,[31] despite the IPPV pressures, while the site is closing. Although the tracheostomy site usually closes in 24 to 78 hours, if it does not close in 7 days, it can be sutured closed. Besides relying on noninvasive IPPV for their predominant ventilatory support methods, patients with little or no VFBT try, and may decide to use, IAPVs as their predominant method of daytime support. Once the tracheostomy site is closed, the patient is taught GPB.

Glossopharyngeal Breathing

Both inspiratory and, indirectly, expiratory muscle function can be assisted by GPB.[21] This technique, first recognized and described in the early 1950s as an aid for coughing,[53,62] involves the use of the tongue and pharyngeal muscles to add to inspiratory efforts by projecting (gulping) boluses of air past the glottis. The glottis closes with each "gulp." One breath usually consists of six to nine gulps of 60- to 100-ml each (Fig. 24–16). During the training period, the efficiency of GPB can be monitored by spirometrically measuring the milliliters of air per gulp, gulps per breath, and breaths per minute (Fig. 24–16). An excellent training manual and video are available.[53,55] GPB can provide an individual

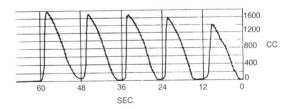

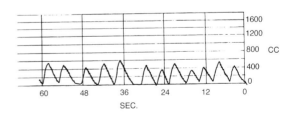

FIGURE 24–16. *A,* Maximal GPB minute ventilation is 8.39 l/min; GPB inspirations average 1.67 liters, 20 gulps, 84 ml/gulp for each breath in a patient with a vital capacity of 0 ml. *B,* Same patient with regular GPB minute ventilation of 4.76 l/min, 12.5 breaths, average of 8 gulps/breath, 47.5 ml/gulp, performed over a 1-minute period. (Courtesy of March of Dimes.)[21]

with weak inspiratory muscles and no VC or VFBT with normal alveolar ventilation for hours and perfect safety when not using a ventilator or in the event of sudden ventilator failure day or night.[3,21]

Although severe oropharyngeal muscle weakness can limit the usefulness of GPB. Baydur et al. described two DMD ventilator-users who were very successful at GPB.[39] We have managed four DMD ventilator-users who had no VFBT other than by using GPB. Approximately 60% of ventilator-users with no VFBT and good bulbar muscle function can use GPB for VFBT.[3,18] Although potentially extremely useful, GPB is rarely taught since there are few health care professionals familiar with the technique. GPB is also rarely useful in the presence of an indwelling tracheostomy tube. It cannot be used when the tube is uncapped, as it is during tracheostomy IPPV, and even when capped, the gulped air tends to leak around the outer walls of the tube and out the tracheostomy site as airway volumes and pressures increase during the air stacking process of GPB. The safety and versatility afforded by effective GPB are key reasons to eliminate tracheostomy in favor of noninvasive aids (Table 24–3).

Electrophrenic Respiration

Although electrophrenic respiration (EPR) is not a noninvasive aid and it generally obliges maintenance of an indwelling tracheostomy tube, it can serve as a complement to noninvasive methods for certain patients. The effect of electrical stimulation of the phrenic nerve on diaphragm motion was first recorded over 200 years ago by Caldani.[45] There were numerous reports of resuscitation by EPR.[58,67] Despite this, studies in EPR were discontinued when NPBVs became available.[67] Then, in 1948, Sarnoff and associates demonstrated that adequate ventilation could be obtained by unilateral phrenic

nerve stimulation.[99] In 1968, Judson and Glenn reported a case in which they used a permanently implantable system for intermittent electrical stimulation of the phrenic nerve of a patient with primary hypoventilation.[75] Since 1972, over 800 phrenic nerve pacers have been implanted into patients with central hypoventilation, COPD, and spinal cord tetraplegia with generally unfavorable results.[66]

EPR involves the transmission of a radiowave signal by an antenna placed on the skin to an implanted receiver. The signal is converted to electrical impulses that are carried to electrodes in contact with the phrenic nerves. The impulses can be delivered in a manner that simulates the natural recruitment of phrenic nerve fibers to stimulate the diaphragm.

The inhospital training period is at least 4 to 6 weeks, often much longer, and total initial costs exceed $300,000. Problems include operative risks, infection, and trauma to the easily damaged phrenic nerves. Unilateral pacing causes paradoxical diaphragmatic movement and microatelectasis. Tidal volumes cannot be routinely modified or precisely controlled, and voice quality is poorer than for patients using noninvasive methods of support complemented by GPB. EPR patients are also subject to potential complications from their tracheostomy. A tracheostomy is maintained in at least 90% of EPR patients[66] because of the upper airway collapse that occurs during sleep on EPR and because of not uncommon sudden operational failure.[92] This failure is particularly dangerous because of the lack of internal alarms and the inability to use GPB effectively. Neuromuscular fatigue can also lead to irreparable phrenic nerve and diaphragm damage.[87,97]

Despite the fact that EPR has few indications and is invasive, extremely expensive, suboptimally effective or ineffective for over 60% of patients,[28] and entails complications associated with having an indwelling tracheostomy (thus negating the advantage of increased portability with this approach), it may be indicated for some C1–2 traumatic tetraplegic patients who have no measurable VC and inadequate neck rotation or labial strength to use mouthpiece IPPV. Such patients could, for example, use EPR for daytime aid and nasal IPPV overnight. This would permit decannulation and GPB training for VFBT. EPR can also be useful during tracheostomy site closure for transition to nocturnal nasal IPPV for these patients. Considering the difficulties with EPR and the fact that virtually all patients with pacemakers who learn noninvasive aids discontinue use of their pacemak-

---

TABLE 24–3
Uses of Glossopharyngeal Breathing

Backup in the event of ventilator failure
Increased ventilator-free breathing time
Ventilatory support during transfer between different methods of noninvasive ventilatory support
Deeper breath to improve cough effectiveness
Increase speech volume or shout
Normalize the volume and rhythm of speech
Improve or maintain pulmonary compliance
Prevent microatelectasis

ers, there are no other indications for EPR in the adult population.

BENEFITS OF NONINVASIVE AIDS OVER TRACHEOSTOMY

The advantages of using noninvasive aids over tracheostomy have been discussed elsewhere in this volume[15] and include safety, convenience, comfort, and improved speech, swallowing, sleep, and appearance. In addition, patients receiving tracheostomy IPPV are generally hyperventilated, which can exacerbate respiratory muscle deconditioning,[13] and the resulting chronic hypocapnia may result in bone decalcification.[25]

Experience in Use of Noninvasive Respiratory Muscle Aids

Since 1977, the author has managed 536 long-term ventilator-dependent noninvasive IPPV users with a wide range of diagnoses (Table 24–4). The pulmonary function, extent

TABLE 24–4
Diagnoses of Long-Term Noninvasive IPPV Users at One Center

Poliomyelitis	209 patients
Duchenne muscular dystrophy	77
Spinal cord injury	66
Non-Duchenne myopathies*	65
Amyotrophic lateral sclerosis	33
Diagnosis not confirmed	19
Spinal muscular atrophy	14
Chronic obstructive pulmonary disease	10
Scoliosis	10
Obesity/hypoventilation	5
Multiple sclerosis	4
Phrenic neuropathy	4
Polymyositis	3
Myasthenia gravis	3
Other respiratory disease†	3
Myelopathy other than traumatic	2
Charcot-Marie-Tooth disease	2
Miscellaneous‡	7
TOTAL	536

*Includes Emery-Dreifuss, limb-girdle, and myotonic muscular dystrophies and generalized myopathies including acid maltase deficiency.
†Includes pulmonary fibrosis, Milroy's disease, and tuberculosis
‡Includes Friedreich's ataxia, neuropathy associated with cancer, osteogenesis imperfecta, Guillain-Barré syndrome, central alveolar hypoventilation, brainstem astrocytoma, and post-curarization paralysis (in 1 each).

of ventilator need, duration of use, and prolongation of survival for many of these patients have been published previously.[9,16,17,24,33] Numerous other patients with many other diagnoses have also used this respiratory muscle aid protocol on many occasions to avoid hospitalizations and intubations and, with the successful prevention of acute respiratory failure, were weaned from ventilator use until their next episodes requiring ventilator use. Over 80 patients, mostly high-level spinal-cord-injured individuals but occasionally patients with amyotrophic lateral sclerosis, non-Duchenne myopathies, or post-polio, have had their tracheostomy tubes removed and been switched to 24-hour noninvasive IPPV. The risk of pulmonary morbidity and hospitalization rates for patients using noninvasive IPPV are less than those for comparable tracheostomy IPPV users.[15]

Although certain other groups have reported isolated cases of the use of up to 24-hour noninvasive ventilatory support,[46] thus far, this has been mostly as a result of the patients refusing tracheostomy, and the use of noninvasive expiratory muscle aids has not been cited.[80] Long-term noninvasive ventilatory support cannot be successful without appropriate resort to assisted coughing techniques.

Two other centers have reported tracheostomy tube removal for conversion to noninvasive respiratory muscle aids. One center has wide experience in this regard, particularly for high-level spinal-cord-injured ventilator-users.[106] The other group reported transition from tracheostomy to noninvasive IPPV and site closure for one post-polio nocturnal ventilator-user.[69]

Why Does Noninvasive IPPV Work?

Although users of mouthpiece or nasal IPPV risk underventilation and $dSaO_2$ because of excessive insufflation air leakage during sleep, this appears to be prevented by reflex oromotor activity that decreases insufflation leakage.[17,20,30] Patients with no measurable VC can maintain normal nocturnal SaO_2 by using these open systems. For patients with GAH and milder respiratory muscle dysfunction, noninvasive IPPV improves sleep SaO_2[17,71] and daytime arterial blood gases,[17,60,76] and it decreases the risk of pulmonary complications requiring hospitalization, despite varying degrees of insufflation leakage during the majority of sleep.[30,80]

The neurophysiologic mechanisms by which noninvasive IPPV can be effective during sleep must include mechanical sealing of the oropharynx by the soft palate or lip closure. Bach and Alba noted that some patients maintained a predominant passive mechanical seal and normal SaO_2, but most nasal IPPV users demonstrated a "sawtooth" pattern of $dSaO_2$ throughout the night with arousal-associated tongue and pharyngeal movements to decrease leakage.[17] It has been noted that insufflation leakage can occasionally be so severe as to warrant the user switching to other methods of noninvasive ventilatory assistance,[17] usually in patients using only nocturnal noninvasive IPPV despite daytime hypercapnia and $dSaO_2$.[82,95,98]

In another study of nocturnal nasal IPPV, $dSaO_2$s of š4% were common and were reversed by brief arousal 71% of the time, by lightening of sleep stage or arousal 76% of the time, and without apparent sleep stage change 24% of the time (Fig. 24–17).[30] Infrequently, $dSaO_2$s were reversed at the point of entering a deeper stage of sleep (Fig. 24–17) and occasionally leakage and $dSaO_2$ occurred suddenly without a sleep stage change (Fig. 24–18).

With or without sleep stage changes, all recoveries in SaO_2 were accompanied by changes in the configuration of the pneumotachograph flows or mask pressure patterns, indicating decreased insufflation leakage. The oxyhemoglobin desaturation initiated specific oromotor activity to decrease or eliminate leakage, which was clearly observed to occur at the nadir of many of the $dSaO_2$s. The oromotor activity resulted in a return of the SaO_2 to baseline prior to the next leak episode. Repeated episodes of leakage and recovery resulted in the "sawtooth" pattern of $dSaO_2$ also seen during nocturnal mouthpiece IPPV use when not using a lipseal.[24] When nocturnal mouthpiece IPPV is used with lipseal retention, paraoral air leakage is decreased passively, and the use of pressure-triggered ventilators or volume-triggered ventilators with high delivered volumes compensates for paranasal leakage.[20] Thus, nocturnal lipseal IPPV can normalize mean nocturnal SaO_2 and probably improve sleep quality since arousals may not be necessary to normalize SaO_2.[20]

As during nocturnal mouthpiece IPPV use without a lipseal, the central nervous system, probably through chemotactic sensitivity, triggers the muscular activity needed to prevent life-threatening air leakage. This is not surprising because it is unlikely that open systems of ventilatory support, such as nasal or mouthpiece IPPV, could sustain individuals with no VFBT 24 hours a day by postural or passive mechanisms alone.[17] The centrally triggered activity occurs at the nadir of the $dSaO_2$, with sensitivity to

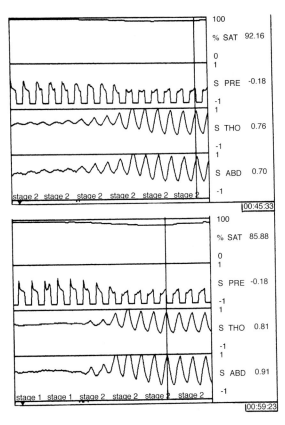

FIGURE 24–17. Normalization of tidal volumes and oxyhemoglobin saturation with reduction of insufflation leakage without apparent sleep stage change (*panel A*) and with deepening in sleep to stage 2 (*panel B*). The parameters include oxyhemoglobin saturation (SAT), nasal interface pressure (PRE), and thoracoabdominal movement (THO and ABD). (From Bach JR, Robert D, Leger P, Langevin B: Sleep fragmentation in kyphoscoliotic individuals with alveolar hypoventilation treated by nasal IPPV. Chest 107: 1552–1558, 1995; with permission of the American College of Chest Physicians.)

$dSaO_2$ differing in all sleep stages (Figs. 24–19 and 24–20). The fact that some patients also have long and variable periods of insufflation leakage without significant changes in SaO_2, and that this can happen during any sleep stage,[30] implies that passive mechanisms such as lip plugging by the tongue or apposition of the tongue and soft palate may also be at work in some instances.[2] Although obstruction to air occasionally occurs, whether by vocal cord or glottic closure or palatal seal of the nasopharynx (Fig. 24–18), these events do not appear to be frequent.[30] Their occurrence at times can be useful to prevent hyperventilation.

There is evidence that nasal IPPV is less effective in the acute setting for ventilator-users

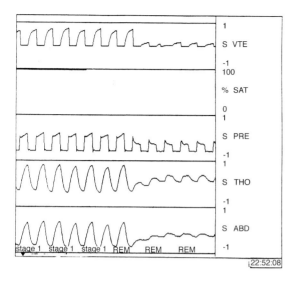

FIGURE 24–18. Assisted insufflations in stage 1 sleep indicated by high mask pressures (PRE) and expiratory flows (VTE) and good thoracoabdominal movement (THO and ABD). With change into rapid eye movement sleep, all parameters indicate massive insufflation leakage. Once the oxyhemoglobin saturation (SAT) decreased to 87%, this patient had a brief arousal (of which he was unaware), which returned insufflation parameters and SaO_2 to normal levels. (From Bach JR, Robert D, Leger P, Langevin B: Sleep fragmentation in kyphoscoliotic individuals with alveolar hypoventilation treated by nasal IPPV. Chest 107:1552–1558, 1995; with permission of the American College of Chest Physicians.)

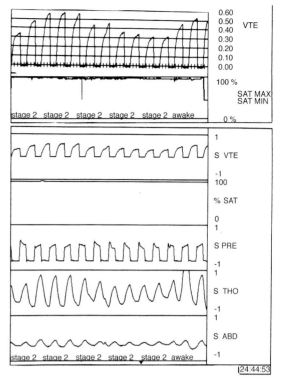

FIGURE 24–19. Alternating optimal insufflations with variable insufflation leak with oxyhemoglobin saturation oscillating in 8 breath cycles between 94% and 95% in stage 2 sleep. Parameters include expired flow (VTE), oxyhemoglobin saturation (SAT), nasal mask pressure (PRE), and thoracoabdominal movement (THO and ABD). (From Bach JR, Robert D, Leger P, Langevin B: Sleep fragmentation in kyphoscoliotic individuals with alveolar hypoventilation treated by nasal IPPV. Chest 107:1552–1558, 1995; with permission of the American College of Chest Physicians.)

requiring oxygen supplementation, particularly during sleep.[17,111] We have also noted nocturnal nasal IPPV to be ineffective in ventilator-users receiving heavy sedation or narcotics. This loss of effectiveness can be explained by failure of central-mediated activity to decrease insufflation leakage when blood oxygenation is maintained by oxygen supplementation.

Periods of insufflation leakage and $dSaO_2$ alternate with effective insufflations during all sleep stages. In particular, this pattern often occurred as SaO_2 oscillated between 94% to 95%,[30] which may represent an activation threshold for central neural mechanisms (Figs. 24–19 and 24–20). Ventilator-users who use daytime as well as nocturnal ventilatory support and who have intact chemotactic drive use nasal or mouthpiece IPPV during sleep with few $dSaO_2$s, whereas individuals with daytime hypercapnia appear to have less improvement in nocturnal ventilation by nasal IPPV.[17,25] Therefore, ventilator use should be extended into daytime hours for individuals with advanced respiratory muscle

dysfunction to prevent the bicarbonate retention that can suppress the chemotactic response to insufflation leakage and $dSaO_2$. In one study,[17] 16 patients with <400 ml of supine VC and <15 minutes of VFBT, who maintained normal alveolar ventilation by ventilator use up to 24 hours a day, had a mean nocturnal SaO_2 of $95.9 \pm 2.6\%$ using nasal IPPV, whereas 17 others who were hypercapnic during daytime hours and used only nocturnal nasal IPPV did not normalize their nocturnal SaO_2. Thus, nocturnal use of open systems of noninvasive IPPV may not be adequate, and either closing the system by lipseal IPPV and, possibly, nasal plugs or extending ventilatory assistance into daytime hours may become necessary.[24]

The fact that open systems of ventilatory support are being used during sleep by individuals with no upper extremity function and no VFBT

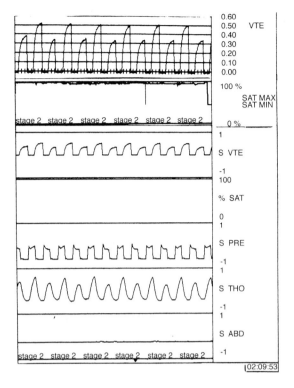

FIGURE 24–20. Alternating optimal insufflations with variable insufflation leak with oxyhemoglobin saturation oscillating between 94% and 95% in stage 2 sleep. In this example, the cycles are 2 breaths. Parameters include expired flow (VTE), oxyhemoglobin saturation (SAT), nasal mask pressure (PRE), and thoracoabdominal movement (THO and ABD).

makes it imperative that their safety be established and their functioning understood. Such individuals cannot adjust a poorly fitting, leaking nasal interface in the event of leakage-associated dyspnea. The mechanisms by which nasal IPPV can improve the clinical picture include:

1. Resting respiratory muscles and decreasing metabolic demand
2. Resetting chemoreceptors
3. Opening atelectatic airways
4. Maintaining airway patency
5. Improving ventilation/perfusion matching
6. Most importantly, by assisting, supporting, and substituting for inspiratory muscle function[30]

DIFFICULTIES IN INITIATING THE USE OF NONINVASIVE AIDS AND CONCLUSION

Despite patient and caregiver preferences for noninvasive approaches,[7] the ability of these methods to lower the cost of home mechanical ventilation;[26] their ability to eliminate the need for hospitalization, intubation, and bronchoscopy, particularly for patients with GAH; and their safety and efficacy for long-term ventilatory support and secretion management, they are not being used widely. They are not a part of medical or other health professional school curricula, and use of current invasive approaches is consistent with the general tendency to resort to the highest available and most costly technology. Physician and hospital reimbursement is procedure-based and directed toward inpatient management rather than preventive care. One can be remunerated for hospitalizing a patient for respiratory failure, intubating or placing a tracheostomy, and performing bronchoscopy, but outpatient management that prevents hospitalization by using noninvasive IPPV, oximetry, and MI-E is not recognized and often not fully reimbursed by third-party payers, even though it costs only a fraction of the alternative's price. Furthermore, the initial use of noninvasive aids requires a significant time commitment for evaluating the use of various IPPV interfaces to optimize comfort and effectiveness and for training the patient and care provider.

Even more important than using inspiratory muscle aids is the evaluation of PCF and using methods for increasing them. In none of the studies in which the use of nocturnal-only nasal IPPV ultimately resulted in acute respiratory failure and thus resort to tracheostomy was cough evaluated or the use of expiratory muscle aids considered.[39,65,80,81,95] Thus, instead of the common practice of providing supplemental oxygen for the underventilated or airway secretion–encumbered patient, noninvasive IPPV methods and assisted coughing should be used to normalize blood gases and prevent mucus plug–induced pneumonia, respiratory failure, and the need for tracheal intubation.

Yet another difficulty is the low number of GAH patients seen by pulmonologists and physiatrist pulmonary specialists. Neuromuscular patients are rarely referred before an episode of acute respiratory failure has led to emergency care and intubation. Part of this low referral rate is because less than 1% of over 220 Muscular Dystrophy Association clinics in the United States have pulmonary specialists as codirectors. Neurologists and other physicians who usually direct these clinics are rarely experienced in the use of noninvasive respiratory muscle aids, and mucus plugging inevitably leads to pneumonias, respiratory failure, and bronchoscopies.[6] Certainly, our experience with the neuromuscular patient has been consistent with the following statement, from Colebatch in 1961:

"As experience with exsufflation with negative pressure increased, bronchoscopy was performed less frequently for the removal of bronchial secretions. At times, bronchoscopic aspiration did relieve acute obstructive anoxia, but it is clear from the case reports that bronchoscopy contributed little to the overall control of bronchial secretions. . . . Had not artificial coughing been available, death might well have followed bronchoscopy in [several cases]. The only possible value of bronchoscopy is to relieve obstruction due to secretions in the trachea and main bronchi. This is usually only of transient benefit, and as the relief can be more easily achieved with exsufflation with negative pressure, bronchoscopic aspiration should rarely, if ever, be performed in patients undergoing artificial respiration."[49]

CLINICAL TIPS

Maximum Insufflation Capacity

The MIC is the maximum air-stacked or single-breath insufflation that the patient can hold with a closed glottis. It also can be attained by using GPB or some combination of GPB and air stacking. The extent to which it is greater than the patient's VC predicts the capacity of the patient to be maintained by noninvasive rather than tracheostomy ventilatory support.[16] This is because the MIC–VC difference, like the extent of the PCF, is a function of bulbar muscle function. Therefore, even before requiring ongoing daytime ventilator use, patients whose VCs have been decreasing (we use 50% of predicted normal VC as a rule of thumb) are instructed to receive multiple maximum insufflations via mouthpiece or nasal interface to the MIC two or three times daily. A manual resuscitator can be used for this insufflation. Successful use of insufflations indicates to the clinician that the patient has mastered the techniques of mouthpiece and nasal IPPV. This approach has permitted us to extubate patients in acute respiratory failure and convert them to continuous noninvasive IPPV despite absence of VFBT. Extubation of such a patient who has not been trained to receive noninvasive IPPV would otherwise result in panic, glottic closure, apnea, and reintubation.

Low-Pressure Alarm: Utility and Elimination

Because the low-pressure alarms of volume-cycled ventilators often cannot be turned off, their sounding during routine daytime use when not every delivered breath is taken by the patient can be prevented by using a flexed mouthpiece for IPPV or an in-line regenerative humidifier. These devices create 2 or 3 cm H_2O of back-pressure, which is adequate to prevent the low-pressure alarm from sounding.

Despite the use of 24-hour noninvasive IPPV and maintenance of normal daytime alveolar ventilation, some patients permit excessive insufflation leakage during sleep using nasal or mouthpiece IPPV. This can cause transient $dSaO_2$s and periods of hypercapnia. Often, the patient complains of recurrence of morning headaches, fatigue, and perhaps nightmares and anxiety. Although this problem can be relieved by "closing" the air-delivery system by resorting to lipseal IPPV and plugging the nose during sleep, another possible solution is to set the low-pressure alarm at a level that, by its prolonged sounding, stimulates the patient sufficiently to shorten periods of excessive insufflation leakage. Commonly, a low-pressure alarm setting of 10 to 20 cm H_2O is used for this purpose.

Nasal Congestion

NPBV use has been helpful during tracheostomy site closure when transferring patients from endotracheal IPPV to noninvasive support methods.[2,18] NPBVs can also be used when nasal congestion renders nasal IPPV ineffective. More often, however, patients either continue nasal IPPV with frequent use of nasal decongestants, or they switch to lipseal IPPV until the upper respiratory tract infection has resolved.

ICU Ventilators

The expiratory-volume alarm of intensive care volume ventilators makes it impractical to introduce or use IPPV via a mouth- or nosepiece. Patients must use portable volume or pressure-cycled ventilators when being introduced to noninvasive IPPV.

Pressure Dressing to Permit Tracheostomy Site Closure Despite IPPV

Soft 2-inch-diameter silicon material in the form of a plugged donut (Respironics Inc., Murrysville, PA) is placed over an occlusive tracheostomy site dressing (Tegaderm; 3M Company, St. Paul, MN). The Tegaderm dressing decreases any tendency for silicon slippage and prevents airway secretions from wetting and loosening the overlying gauze and elastic dressing. A layer or two of 4 × 4-inch sterile gauze is placed over the silicon donut, which is then covered and fixed in place by adhesive tape. IPPV leaking through the site must then be countered by placing an elastic figure-of-8 strap or Ace bandage. The strap descends, crosses anteriorly under the neck, goes under the axillae, ascends to cross over the back, runs over the shoulders, and reinserts into an elastic band in front.[31] This approach minimizes skin maceration from secretions leaking through the tracheostomy site and minimizes the amount of adhesive tape applied to the skin.

Nasal IPPV Misinformation

Noted briefly in Chapter 23, misinformation concerning nasal IPPV is perhaps best exemplified by a recent publication.[94] In this work, 70 DMD patients, aged 15 to 16 years, were randomized to receive nocturnal nasal IPPV or to a control group that did not use nasal IPPV. The patients were reported to have VCs of 20% to 50% of predicted normal, but they had neither hypercapnia nor hypoxia (PaO$_2$ >60 mm Hg). The 70 subjects came from 17 centers. There was no standardization in ventilator use, nasal interface use, caregiver or patient training, or follow-up. The authors stated that 15 of the 35 nasal IPPV subjects claimed to use nasal ventilation less than the minimum 6 hours/night, and so the authors concluded by history only, that 20 subjects were "effectively ventilated." However, the authors made no effort to substantiate this finding by using ventilators that indicate hours of use. Historical claims tend to overestimate ventilator utilization, especially when the claims are by users who do not need them. Furthermore, it is also very difficult to convince asymptomatic individuals to use any form of ventilatory support, especially when told to do so by clinicians with little or no experience in their use, and with no effort made to optimize comfort for any patient. In our experience, no interface, not even our own,[86] is tolerated by all patients. The stated goal of lowering the PaCO$_2$ by 10%, or to decrease it by "at least 10% of recorded daytime value(s)," is interesting when one considers that daytime values were already normal, and it shows that the authors did not recognize the importance monitoring noctur-

nal PaCO$_2$ and improving nocturnal blood gas levels when abnormal. Furthermore, no effort was made to determine whether the nasal interfaces were worn sufficiently snugly to provide effective insufflations during sleep. Rather than performing useless daytime arterial blood gases and other testing, improvements in nocturnal oximetry or transcutaneous or end-tidal CO$_2$ could have monitored efficacy.[17,73]

The tragedy of publishing such a report is in the perpetration of misconceptions that may dissuade clinicians from appropriate use of nasal IPPV.[94] The authors reported that the mortality of their "nasal IPPV users" may have actually been increased. However, although the predominant cause of death was mucus plugging during upper respiratory tract infections, the subjects were not offered effective means of noninvasive ventilatory support during these episodes. Furthermore, neither manually nor mechanically assisted coughing was used,[10,12] and so it is no surprise that the patients died, both subjects and controls. For those with "left ventricular hypokinesis," cardiac ejection fractions <20% would be predictive of early mortality,[104] but this, too, was not taken into account.

Thus, this "study" succeeded in perpetrating the following *misconceptions* about noninvasive IPPV:

1. That nasal ventilation is the only method to be considered, thereby ignoring IPPV via mouthpieces, lipseals, oral-nasal interfaces, and body ventilator use;
2. That when nocturnal use of nasal ventilation is no longer adequate, one must resort to tracheostomy;
3. That simple prescription of nasal ventilation can be enough without the participation of a specifically trained respiratory therapist to evaluate trials with various interfaces and to train in assisted coughing and oximetry biofeedback;
4. That the primary difficulty in preventing mortality in DMD patients is in assisting ventilation rather than in effective evacuation of airway secretions and treating any complicating cardiomyopathy.[72]

Acknowledgment

The author thanks the American College of Chest Physicians for permitting republication of passages from references 11 and 12; and Mr. Jack Emerson for permitting use of Figures 1 through 4.

References

1. Alba A, Solomon M, Trainor FS: Management of respiratory insufficiency in spinal cord lesions. In Proceedings of the 17th Veteran's Administration Spinal Cord Injury Conference, 1969. Washington, DC, Government Printing Office, 1971; pp 200–213. [Publ. no. 0-436-398.]
2. Bach JR: Alternative methods of ventilatory support for the patient with ventilatory failure due to spinal cord injury. J Am Paraplegia Soc 14:158–174, 1991.
3. Bach JR: New approaches in the rehabilitation of the traumatic high level quadriplegic. Am J Phys Med Rehabil 70:13–20, 1991.
4. Bach JR: Mechanical exsufflation, noninvasive ventilation and new strategies for pulmonary rehabilitation and sleep disordered breathing. Bull N Y Acad Med 68:321–340, 1992.
5. Bach JR: Pulmonary rehabilitation considerations for Duchenne muscular dystrophy: The prolongation of life by respiratory muscle aids. Crit Rev Phys Rehabil Med 3:239–269, 1992.
6. Bach JR: Ventilator use by Muscular Dystrophy Association patients: An update. Arch Phys Med Rehabil 73:179–183, 1992.
7. Bach JR: A comparison of long-term ventilatory support alternatives from the perspective of the patient and care giver. Chest 104:1702–1706, 1993.
8. Bach JR: Inappropriate weaning and late onset ventilatory failure of individuals with traumatic quadriplegia. Paraplegia 31:430–438, 1993.
9. Bach JR: Management of neuromuscular ventilatory failure by 24-hour noninvasive intermittent positive pressure ventilation. Eur Respir Rev 3:284–291, 1993.
10. Bach JR: Mechanical insufflation-exsufflation: Comparison of peak expiratory flows with manually assisted and unassisted coughing techniques. Chest 104:1553–1562, 1993.
11. Bach JR: Update and perspectives on noninvasive respiratory muscle aids: Pt 1—The inspiratory muscle aids. Chest 105:1230–1240, 1994.
12. Bach JR: Update and perspectives on noninvasive respiratory muscle aids: Pt 2—The expiratory muscle aids. Chest 105:1538–1544, 1994.
13. Bach JR: Case studies of respiratory management. In Bach JR (ed): Pulmonary Rehabilitation: The Obstructive and Paralytic/Restrictive Pulmonary Syndromes. Philadelphia, Hanley & Belfus, 1996.
14. Bach JR: Conventional approaches to managing neuromuscular ventilatory failure. In Bach JR (ed): Pulmonary Rehabilitation: The Obstructive and Paralytic/Restrictive Pulmonary Syndromes. Philadelphia, Hanley & Belfus, 1996.
15. Bach JR, Barnett VA: Psychosocial, vocational, quality of life, and ethical issues. In Bach JR (ed): Pulmonary Rehabilitation: The Obstructive and Paralytic/Restrictive Pulmonary Syndromes. Philadelphia, Hanley & Belfus, 1996.
16. Bach JR: Amyotrophic lateral sclerosis: Predictors for prolongation of life by noninvasive respiratory aids. Arch Phys Med Rehabil 76:828–832, 1995.
17. Bach JR, Alba AS: Management of chronic alveolar hypoventilation by nasal ventilation. Chest 97:52–57, 1990.
18. Bach JR, Alba AS: Noninvasive options for ventilatory support of the traumatic high level quadriplegic. Chest 98:613–619, 1990.
19. Bach JR, Alba AS: Total ventilatory support by the intermittent abdominal pressure ventilator. Chest 99:630–636, 1991.
20. Bach JR, Alba AS: Sleep and nocturnal mouthpiece IPPV efficiency in post-poliomyelitis ventilator users. Chest 106:1705–1710, 1994.
21. Bach JR, Alba AS, Bodofsky E, et al: Glossopharyngeal breathing and non-invasive aids in the management of post-polio respiratory insufficiency. Birth Defects 23:99–113, 1987.
22. Bach JR, Alba AS, Bohatiuk G, et al: Mouth intermittent positive pressure ventilation in the management of post-polio respiratory insufficiency. Chest 91:859–864, 1987.
23. Bach JF, Alba A, Mosher R, Delaubier A: Intermittent positive pressure ventilation via nasal access in the management of respiratory insufficiency. Chest 92:168–170, 1987.
24. Bach JR, Alba AS, Saporito LR: Intermittent positive pressure ventilation via the mouth as an alternative to tracheostomy for 257 ventilator users. Chest 103:174–182, 1993.
25. Bach JR, Haber II, Wang TG, Alba AS: Alveolar ventilation as a function of ventilatory support method. Eur J Phys Med Rehabil 5:80–84, 1995.
26. Bach JR, Intintola P, Alba AS, Holland I: The ventilator individual: Cost analysis of institutionalization versus rehabilitation and in-home management. Chest 101:26–30, 1992.
27. Bach JR, McDermott I: Strapless oral-nasal interfaces for positive pressure ventilation. Arch Phys Med Rehabil 71:908–911, 1990.
28. Bach JR, O'Connor K: Electrophrenic ventilation: A different perspective. J Am Paraplegia Soc 14:9–17, 1991.
29. Bach JR, Penek J: Obstructive sleep apnea complicating negative pressure ventilatory support in patients with chronic paralytic/restrictive ventilatory dysfunction. Chest 99:1386–1393, 1991.
30. Bach JR, Robert D, Leger P, Langevin B: Sleep fragmentation in kyphoscoliotic individuals with alveolar hypoventilation treated by nasal IPPV. Chest 107:1552–1558, 1995.
31. Bach JR, Saporito LS: Indications and criteria for decannulation and transition from invasive to noninvasive long-term ventilatory support. Respir Care 39:515–531, 1994.
32. Bach JR, Smith WH, Michaels J, et al: Airway secretion clearance by mechanical exsufflation for post-poliomyelitis ventilator assisted individuals. Arch Phys Med Rehabil 74:170–177, 1993.
33. Bach JR, Wang TG: Noninvasive long-term ventilatory support for individuals with spinal muscular atrophy and functional bulbar musculature. Arch Phys Med Rehabil 76:213–217, 1995.
34. Barach AL: The application of pressure, including exsufflation, in pulmonary emphysema. Am J Surg 89:372–382, 1955.
35. Barach AL, Beck GJ: Exsufflation with negative pressure: Physiologic and clinical studies in poliomyelitis, bronchial asthma, pulmonary emphysema and bronchiectasis. Arch Intern Med 93:825–841, 1954.
36. Barach AL, Beck GJ, Bickerman HA, Seanor HE: Mechanical coughing: Studies on physical methods of producing high velocity flow rates during the expiratory cycle. Trans Assoc Am Physicians 64:360–363, 1951.
37. Barach AL, Beck GJ, Bickerman HA, et al: Physical methods simulating mechanisms of the human cough. J Appl Physiol 5:85–91, 1952.
38. Barach AL, Beck GJ, Smith RH: Mechanical production of expiratory flow rates surpassing the capacity of human coughing. Am J Med Sci 226:241–248, 1953.
39. Baydur A, Gilgoff I, Prentice W, et al: Decline in respi-

ratory function and experience with long-term assisted ventilation in advanced Duchenne's muscular dystrophy. Chest 97:884–889, 1990.

40. Beck GJ: Chronic bronchial asthma and emphysema rehabilitation and use of thoracic vibrocompression. Geriatrics 21:139–158, 1966.

41. Beck GJ, Barach AL: Value of mechanical aids in the management of a patient with poliomyelitis. Ann Intern Med 40:1081–1094, 1954.

42. Beck GJ, Graham GC, Barach AL: Effect of physical methods on the mechanics of breathing in poliomyelitis. Ann Intern Med 43:549–566, 1955.

43. Beck GJ, Scarrone LA: Physiological effects of exsufflation with negative pressure. Dis Chest 29:1–16, 1956.

44. Bickerman HA: Exsufflation with negative pressure: elimination of radiopaque material and foreign bodies from bronchi of anesthetized dogs. Arch Intern Med 93:698–704, 1954.

45. Caldani LMA: Institutiones Physiologicae. Venezia, Pezzana, 1786. [Cited by Schecter DC: Application of electrotherapy to non-cardiac disorders. Bull N Y Acad Med 46:932–951, 1970.]

46. Cantas-Yamsuan M, Sanchez I, Kesselman M, Chernick V: Morbidity and mortality patterns of ventilator-dependent children in a home care program. Clin Pediatr 32:706–713, 1993.

47. Chang HK, Harf A: High-frequency ventilation: A review. Respir Physiol 57:135–152, 1984.

48. Cherniack RM, Hildes JA, Alcock AJW: The clinical use of the exsufflator attachment for tank respirators in poliomyelitis. Ann Intern Med 40:540–548, 1954.

49. Colebatch HJH: Artificial coughing for patients with respiratory paralysis. Australas J Med 10:201–212, 1961.

50. Corrado A, Gorini M, De Paola E: Alternative techniques for managing acute neuromuscular respiratory failure. Semin Neurol 15:84–89, 1995.

51. Council on Physical Medicine: The Monaghan Portable Respirator acceptance report. JAMA 139:1273, 1949.

52. Council on Physical Medicine: Acceptability of the Fairchild-Huxley cuirass respirator. JAMA 143:1157, 1950.

53. Dail CW, Affeldt JE: Glossopharyngeal Breathing [video]. Los Angeles, College of Medical Evangelists, 1954.

54. Dail C, Rodgers M, Guess V, Adkins HV: Glossopharyngeal breathing manual. Downey, CA, Rancho Los Amigos Hospital, 1979.

55. Dayman HG: Mechanics of airflow in health and emphysema. J Clin Invest 30:1175–1190, 1951.

56. Delaubier A: Traitement de l'insuffisance respiratoire chronique dans les dystrophies musculaires. In Memoires de Certificat d'etudes Superieures de Reeducation et Readaptation Fonctionnelles. Paris, Universite R Descarte, 1984, pp 1–124.

57. Dolmage TE, Hayek Z, De Rosie JA, Goldstein RS: Effect of external high frequency oscillation at 1–5 Hz on gas exchange in normal lung. Am Rev Respir Dis 145:A528, 1992.

58. Duchenne G: De l'electrisation Localisée et de son Application à la Pathologie et à la Therapeutique. Paris, Bailliere, 1872, p 914.

59. Eisenmenger R: Suction and pressure over the belly: Its action and application [in German]. Wien Med Wochenschr 31:807–812, 1939.

60. Ellis ER, Bye PTP, Bruderer JW, Sullivan CE: Treatment of respiratory failure during sleep in patients with neuromuscular disease, positive-pressure ventilation through a nose mask. Am Rev Respir Dis 135:148–152, 1987.

61. Emerson JH, Loynes JA: The Evolution of Iron Lungs: Respirators of the Body-Encasing Type. Cambridge, MA, J.H. Emerson Co., 1978.

62. Feigelson CI, Dickinson DG, Talner NS, Wilson JL: Glossopharyngeal breathing as an aid to the coughing mechanism in the patient with chronic poliomyelitis in a respirator. N Engl J Med 254:611–613, 1956.

63. Freitag L, Long WM, Kim CS, Wanner A: Removal of excessive bronchial secretions by asymmetric high-frequency oscillations. J Appl Physiol 67:614–619, 1989.

64. Fugl-Meyer AR, Grimby G: Ventilatory function in tetraplegic patients. Scand J Rehabil Med 3:151–160, 1971.

65. Gay PC, Patel AM, Viggiano RW, Hubmayr RD: Nocturnal nasal ventilation for treatment of patients with hypercapnic respiratory failure. Mayo Clin Proc 66:695–703, 1991.

66. Glenn WWL, Brouillette RT, Dentz B, et al: Fundamental considerations in pacing of the diaphragm for chronic ventilatory insufficiency: A multicenter study. PACE 11:2121–2127, 1988.

67. Glenn WWL, Phelps ML: Diaphragmatic pacing by electrical stimulation of the phrenic nerve. Neurosurgery 17:974–984, 1985.

68. Goldstein RS, Molotiu N, Skrastins R, et al: Assisting ventilation in respiratory failure by negative pressure ventilation and by rocking bed. Chest 92:470–474, 1987.

69. Goodenberger DM, Couser JI Jr, May JJ: Successful discontinuation of ventilation via tracheostomy by substitution of nasal positive pressure ventilation. Chest 102:1277–1279, 1992.

70. Gordon AS: History and evolution of modern resuscitation techniques. In Gordon AS (ed): Cardiopulmonary Resuscitation Conference Proceedings. Washington, DC, National Academy of Sciences, 1966, pp 7–32.

71. Hill NS, Eveloff SE, Carlisle CC, Goff SG: Efficacy of nocturnal nasal ventilation in patients with restrictive thoracic disease. Am Rev Respir Dis 145:365–371, 1992.

72. Ishikawa Y, Bach JR, Sarma RJ, et al: Cardiovascular considerations in the management of neuromuscular disease. Semin Neurol 15:93–108, 1995.

73. Ishikawa Y, Ishikawa Y, Minami R: The effect of nasal IPPV on patients with respiratory failure during sleep due to Duchenne muscular dystrophy. Clin Neurol 33:856–861, 1993.

74. Jimenez JFM, Sanchez de Cos Escuin J, Vicente CD, et al: Nasal intermittent positive pressure ventilation: Analysis of its withdrawal. Chest 107:382–388, 1995.

75. Judson JP, Glenn WWL: Radiofrequency electrophrenic respiration: Long-term application to a patient with primary hypoventilation. JAMA 203:1033–1037, 1968.

76. Kerby GR, Mayer LS, Pingleton SK: Nocturnal positive pressure ventilation via nasal mask. Am Rev Respir Dis 135:738–740, 1987.

77. King M, Brock G, Lundell C: Clearance of mucus by simulated cough. J Appl Physiol 58:1776–1785, 1985.

78. Kirby NA, Barnerias MJ, Siebens AA: An evaluation of assisted cough in quadriparetic patients. Arch Phys Med Rehabil 47:705–710, 1966.

79. Kobayashi I, Perry A, Rhymer J, et al: Relationships between the electrical activity of genioglossus muscle and the upper airway patency: A study in laryngectomised subjects. Respir Crit Care Med 149:A148, 1994.

80. Leger P, Bedicam JM, Cornette A, et al: Nasal intermittent positive pressure ventilation: Long-term follow-up in patients with severe chronic respiratory insufficiency. Chest 105:100–105, 1994.

81. Leger P, Jennequin J, Gerard M, Robert D: Home positive pressure ventilation via nasal mask for patients with neuromuscular weakness or restrictive lung or chest-wall disease. Respir Care 34:73–79, 1989.

82. Leger P, Langevin B, Guez A, et al: What to do when

nasal ventilation fails for neuromuscular patients. Eur Respir Rev 3:279–283, 1993.

83. Leiner GC, Abramowitz S, Small MJ, et al: Expiratory peak flow rate: Standard values for normal subjects. Am Rev Respir Dis 88:644, 1963.

84. Leith DE: Cough. In Brain JD, Proctor D, Reid L (eds): Lung Biology in Health and Disease: Respiratory Defense Mechanisms, Pt 2. New York, Marcel Dekker, 1977, pp 545–592.

85. Linder SH: Functional electrical stimulation to enhance cough in quadriplegia. Chest 103:166–169, 1993.

86. McDermott I, Bach JR, Parker C, Sortor S: Custom-fabricated interfaces for intermittent positive pressure ventilation. Int J Prosthod 2:224–233, 1989.

87. McMichan JC, Piepgras DG, Gracey DR, et al: Electrophrenic respiration. Mayo Clin Proc 54:662–668, 1979.

88. McSweeney CJ: The Bragg-Paul pulsator in treatment of respiratory paralysis. BMJ 1:1206–1207, 1938.

89. Meryon E: On granular or fatty degeneration of the voluntary muscles. Medi-Chir Trans 35:73–85, 1852.

90. Mier-Jedrzejowicz A, Brophy C, Green M: Respiratory muscle weakness during upper respiratory tract infections. Am Rev Respir Dis 138:5–7, 1988.

91. Miller WF: Rehabilitation of patients with chronic obstructive lung disease. Med Clin North Am 51:349–361, 1967.

92. Oakes DD, Wilmot CB, Halverson D, Hamilton RD: Neurogenic respiratory failure: A 5-year experience using implantable phrenic nerve stimulators. Ann Thorac Surg 30:118–122, 1980.

93. [Reference deleted.]

94. Raphael J-C, Chevret S, Chastang C, Bouvet F: Randomised trial of preventive nasal ventilation in Duchenne muscular dystrophy. Lancet 343:1600–1604, 1994.

95. Ratzka A: Uberdruckbeatmung durch Mundstuck. In Frehse U (ed): Spatfolgen nach Poliomyelitis: Chronische Unterbeatmung und Moglichkeiten selbstbestimmter Lebensfuhrung Schwerbehinderter. Munchen, Pfennigparade eV, 1989, p 149.

96. Rennie H, Wilson JAC: A coughing-belt. Lancet 1:138–139, 1983.

97. Richard I, Giraud M, Perrouin-Verbe B, et al: Laryngotracheal stenosis after intubation or tracheostomy in neurological patients. Arch Phys Med Rehabil (in press).

98. Robert D, Willig TN, Paulus J, Leger P: Long-term nasal ventilation in neuromuscular disorders: Report of a consensus conference. Eur Respir J 6:599–606, 1993.

99. Sarnoff SJ, Hardenbergh E, Whittenberger JL: Electrophrenic respiration. Am J Physiol 155:1–9, 1948.

100. Segal MS, Salomon A, Herschfus JA: Alternating positive-negative pressures in mechanical respiration (the cycling valve device employing air pressures). Dis Chest 25:640–648, 1954.

101. Siebens AA, Kirby NA, Poulos DA: Cough following transection of spinal cord at C-6. Arch Phys Med Rehabil 45:1–8, 1964.

102. Sortor S, McKenzie M: Toward Independence: Assisted Cough [video]. Dallas, BioScience Communications of Dallas, 1986.

103. Spalding JMK, Opiel L: Artificial respiration with the Tunnicliffe breathing jacket. Lancet 274:613–615, 1958.

104. Stewart CA, Gilgoff I, Baydur A, et al: Gated radionuclide ventriculography in the evaluation of cardiac function in Duchenne's muscular dystrophy. Chest 94:1245–1248, 1988.

105. Toussaint M, De Win H, Steens M, Soudon P: A new technique in secretion clearance by the percussionaire for patients with neuromuscular disease [abstract]. In Programme des Journées Internationales de Ventilationà Domicile. Lyon, France, Hopital de la Croix Rousse, 1993, p 27.

106. Viroslav J, Sortor S, Rosenblatt R: Alternatives to tracheostomy ventilation in high level SCI [abstract]. J Am Paraplegia Soc 14:87, 1991.

107. Welch JR, DeCesare R, Hess D: Pulse oximetry: Instrumentation and clinical applications. Respir Care 35:584–594, 1990.

108. Williams EK, Holaday DA: The use of exsufflation with negative pressure in postoperative patients. Am J Surg 90:637–640, 1955.

109. Woollam CHM: The development of apparatus for intermittent negative pressure respiration: (pt 1) 1832–1918. Anaesthesia 31:537–547, 1976.

110. Woollam CHM: The development of apparatus for intermittent negative pressure respiration: (pt 2) 1919–1976. Anaesthesia 31:666–686, 1976.

111. Wysocki M, Tric L, Wolff MA, et al: Noninvasive pressure support ventilation in patients with acute respiratory failure. Chest 103:907–913, 1993.

Case Studies of Respiratory Management

25

John R. Bach, MD

Two basic principles guide the use of noninvasive alternatives to endotracheal methods of ventilatory support and airway secretion elimination: (1) Noninvasive approaches can be used by any patient without primarily intrinsic lung disease or severely decreased pulmonary compliance irrespective of the extent or duration of respiratory muscle failure, and (2) airway secretions can be eliminated whenever peak cough flows (PCF) of at least 3 l/sec can be generated.[3]

In large part because of the failure to recognize these principles and of the lack of familiarity with noninvasive approaches, clinicians have evaluated and treated patients with primarily mechanical impairment of alveolar ventilation in the same manner as patients with intrinsic lung disease and primarily oxygenation impairment. The following are the most common errors in the management of patients with respiratory muscle dysfunction:

1. Misinterpretation of symptoms
2. Failure to perform spirometry with the patient in various positions
3. Failure to evaluate PCF
4. Use of arterial blood gas analyses rather than noninvasive monitoring of oxyhemoglobin saturation (SaO_2) and carbon dioxide tensions
5. Unnecessary resort to endotracheal intubation and tracheostomy
6. Failure to deflate or eliminate tracheostomy tube cuffs
7. Over-reliance on tracheal suctioning
8. Administration of oxygen, bronchodilators, and chest physical therapy
9. Use of negative pressure body ventilators as alternatives to noninvasive intermittent positive pressure ventilation (IPPV)
10. Use of continuous positive airway pressure (CPAP) or bilevel positive airway pressure (BiPAP) at inadequate pressures
11. Use of BiPAP rather than volume-cycled ventilators during waking hours
12. Failure to evaluate various IPPV interfaces for fit, comfort, and efficacy for each patient
13. Failure to extend noninvasive IPPV use into daytime hours
14. Unnecessary ventilator use
15. Inappropriate ventilator weaning
16. Failure to train in glossopharyngeal breathing
17. Inappropriate resort to electrophrenic pacing

Case 1: Misinterpretation of Symptoms and Lack of Utility of Arterial Blood Gases

In February 1986, a 36-year-old woman with a 19-year history of multiple sclerosis and a baseline vital capacity (VC) of 1500 ml developed rapidly progressive tetraplegia. She was hospitalized and became increasingly anxious and tachypneic. On the fourth hospital day, an arterial blood sample had a pH, 7.38; PaO_2, 86 mm Hg; and $PaCO_2$, 46 mm Hg. Upon consultation

331

that evening, she complained of extreme fatigue and 3 days of sleeplessness because of anxiety and inability to breathe when lying down. She had a VC of 180 ml when supine and 250 ml when sitting (6% of predicted normal). Because of hypercapnia and impending ventilatory failure, we placed her on nasal IPPV, using the synchronized intermittent mandatory ventilation mode at 900 ml and at a rate of 14/min. Expiratory volumes measured at the expiratory valve were 750 ml with her awake and, later, asleep and with the mouth open or closed. On direct observation, the insufflated air mechanically sealed the soft palate against the posterior aspect of the tongue with each breath, thereby preventing significant oral air (insufflation) leakage. $PaCO_2$ was 29 mm Hg while she used nasal IPPV, and she almost immediately fell asleep. At no time overnight did her end-tidal pCO_2 ($EtCO_2$) exceed 36 mm Hg. The next morning her VC had decreased to 100 ml, and she was dependent on nasal IPPV with no ventilator-free breathing time (VFBT). This continued for the next 72 hours, at which point her VC began to increase as she responded to treatment with adrenocorticotrophic hormone, and after 5 days she no longer required ventilatory support.

This was the first reported use of nasal IPPV for 24-hour ventilatory support for a patient with no VFBT and negligible VC. For 3 days her fatigue, anxiety, and sleeplessness, common in wheelchair users with global alveolar hypoventilation (GAH), had not been recognized as signaling impending ventilatory failure. Other symptoms of GAH, such as headaches, frequent arousals from sleep, and nightmares, are also often incorrectly ascribed to conditions other than ventilatory insufficiency. The arterial blood gas measurements also did not alert the clinicians to intervene. $EtCO_2$ monitoring and oximetry are often more useful.

Case 2: Misinterpretation of Symptoms and Inappropriate Ventilator Weaning

In November 1989, a 53-year-old man with primary congenital lymph edema was hospitalized for shortness of breath, fatigue, and headaches. He reported having had extreme daytime drowsiness for 10 years. He also had a history of "asthma" with daily wheezing since adolescence and had been taking bronchodilators for 12 years without objective or subjective relief. His VC was 1.15 liters (20% of predicted normal); FEV_1, 0.94 liters (23%); and FEV_1/forced vital capacity (FVC) ratio, 103%. He was intubated and required ventilatory support and hospitalization for 3 weeks. He was subsequently rehospitalized, intubated, and required mechanical ventilation and chest tube placement for respiratory failure and pleural effusions three times during the next 2 years.

During the last of these admissions, an arterial blood gas sample had a pH 7.43; $PaCO_2$, 50 mm Hg; PaO_2, 61 mm Hg; and bicarbonate, 33.7 meq/l. He developed progressive respiratory failure and was nasotracheally intubated 2 weeks after admission. Chest tubes were placed bilaterally, and a thoracocentesis biopsy showed pulmonary fibrosis. Because of failure to wean, a tracheostomy tube was placed on the 52nd hospital day, and his nasotracheal tube was removed. He lost all VFBT while using tracheostomy IPPV. Four days following tracheostomy, he became septic. He subsequently developed right lower lobe *Klebsiella* pneumonia, and a right lower lobe abscess was drained. Atelectasis, lobar collapse, and bronchial mucus plugging became persistent problems. Episodes of respiratory arrest during weaning attempts and septic shock necessitated pressor support. Although the effusion and infiltrate eventually cleared and his chest tubes were removed, weaning attempts continued to fail over a period of 3 additional months with $PaCO_2$ levels quickly exceeding 60 mm Hg. Weaning was attempted in the conventional manner of gradually decreasing rates and volumes of synchronized intermittent mandatory ventilation while providing pressure support ventilation, positive end-expiratory pressure, and oxygen therapy. These attempts continued despite the fact that his maximum effort VC was 570 ml, he had no VFBT, and he had extremely hypersecretory airways. He also continued to require full alimentation via a nasogastric tube.

We were consulted during the sixth month of hospitalization. A fenestrated tracheostomy tube was placed, and it was capped to permit him to practice receiving mouthpiece IPPV. After several days, he was able to tolerate mouthpiece IPPV for most of the day and nasal IPPV overnight. Oxygen therapy was discontinued. As he breathed room air, SaO_2 was 90% to 95% during daytime hours, and at night, mean SaO_2 was 93% with typical "sawtooth" oxyhemoglobin desaturations.[9] The tracheostomy tube was then removed and the site buttoned for 5 days before being allowed to close (Fig. 25–1). Thus, despite absence of any ability to breathe without a ventilator, he was converted directly from continuous tracheostomy IPPV to daytime mouthpiece

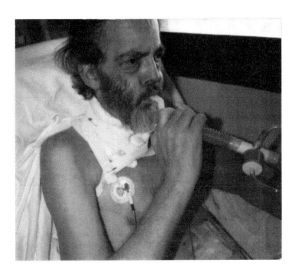

FIGURE 25–1. Patient with severe restrictive pulmonary impairment and no ventilator-free breathing ability being switched from tracheostomy to noninvasive IPPV. The tracheostomy button was removed, and the site is seen closing under a pressure dressing as the patient ventilates his lungs using mouthpiece IPPV.

and nocturnal nasal IPPV. PaO_2 was maintained over 60 mm Hg by providing adequate ventilatory support and assisting coughing by air stacking. Since his abdominal muscles were functional, manually assisted coughing techniques were not useful. PCF increased from 1.3 to 4.4 l/s, however, when he maximally air stacked via a mouthpiece. Transition to noninvasive IPPV and tracheostomy site closure took 2 weeks. VFBT remained under 5 minutes despite an increase in VC to 640 ml and the alleviation of airway hypersecretion by tracheostomy site closure.

During the 6 months before this hospitalization, the patient was unable to walk 200 ft without assistance, and he had not been able to climb more than five steps because of dyspnea. At the initiation of his rehabilitation program, he was able to ambulate only a few feet with a walker while using IPPV, and he was dependent in all activities of daily living.

His rehabilitation included training in glossopharyngeal breathing, general strengthening, mobility, and endurance exercises. His ability to walk increased, but his VC remained <700 ml and he still had no VFBT. With inadequate strength to propel himself in a standard wheelchair carrying a ventilator and not wishing to use a motorized wheelchair, the patient was given a rolling walker with a tray.

After a rehabilitation stay of 60 days, the patient was discharged home independent in activities of daily living, transfers, and automobile use, and he could ambulate >400 ft using mouthpiece IPPV with the rolling walker. He maintained normal ventilation and SaO_2 only while using his ventilator, but he returned to full-time employment as an accountant despite using noninvasive IPPV continuously. He has now been working and living at home for the last 4.5 years. He has had no further hospitalizations, pleural effusions, or "asthmatic" episodes and has discontinued all medications. His VC has increased to 1050 ml, and he now can tolerate 15- to 180-minute periods of VFBT before becoming dyspneic and hypercapnic.

This patient demonstrated that:

1. Noninvasive IPPV can be used as an alternative to tracheostomy IPPV for long-term 24-hour ventilatory support.
2. Except when there is premorbid chronic bronchitis, chronic aspiration, or other reasons for chronic airway hypersecretion, the hypersecretory state of the airways associated with tracheal intubation is reversed by decanulation and site closure.
3. Noninvasive IPPV and oximetry biofeedback can be used as an alternative to conventional ventilator weaning strategies, provided that ventilatory drive is not suppressed by oxygen therapy, sedatives, or narcotics. The patient simply takes fewer and fewer assisted breaths as needed rather than following a more constraining and imprecisely derived clinician's schedule.
4. Although the conversion to noninvasive IPPV was made with a nasogastric tube in place, such a tube interferes with nasal interface placement, increases air leakage during mouthpiece or nasal IPPV, and lends to gastric insufflation and abdominal distention by opening the gastroesophageal sphincter. In general, nasogastric tubes should be removed before transition to noninvasive IPPV.
5. Despite failure to benefit from abdominal thrusts, PCF can be greatly increased by air stacking.
6. A rolling walker can be useful for ventilator-users who can walk.
7. Under certain circumstances, wheezing that is mistaken for asthma may be due to peribronchial edema that is reversible by increasing thoracic pressures by IPPV.
8. Despite having GAH for over 10 years, he was inappropriately weaned from ventilator use on three previous occasions. Hypoventilation was permitted because his clinicians were unfamiliar with noninvasive alternatives to tra-

cheostomy, an option the patient had repeatedly refused.

9. VFBT can decrease rapidly following tracheostomy because of inspiratory muscle deconditioning; induction of airway hypersecretion and bronchial mucus plugging; the tendency for respiratory chemotaxic centers to reset and bicarbonate levels to decrease; and frequent patient requests to increase ventilation despite having low $PaCO_2$.[11]

10. Gradual improvements in pulmonary volumes and VFBT can result from effective use of inspiratory muscle aids. Noninvasive IPPV reversed the chronic hypercapnia that in itself has been shown to exacerbate respiratory muscle weakness.[14]

Case 3: Failure to Evaluate Spirometry with Patient Supine, Inappropriate Oxygen Therapy, and Failure to Offer Various IPPV Interfaces

A man born in 1951 with scoliosis and an undifferentiated myopathy complained of increasing dyspnea, headaches, orthopnea, and leg edema and decreased ability to concentrate since 1975, from which time he slept sitting. By 1984 he had severe continuous headaches, sleep and arousal dysfunction, violent nightmares, obtundation, and massive pretibial edema despite taking 120 mg of furosemide daily for 2 years. He described feeling "like I was dreaming when I was awake, and I did things without being aware of what I was doing." Falling asleep at 5- to 15-minute intervals, he burned his arm twice on his stove.

He developed pneumonia in May 1984 and was intubated for 5 weeks. From 19 August 1984 to 6 May 1985, his $PaCO_2$ ranged from 40 to 51 mm Hg, his SaO_2 ranged from 85% to 92% during daytime hours, and $EtCO_2$ was between 60 and 80 mm Hg with a maximum of 90 mm Hg during four sleep studies.

In December 1985, he had jugular distention at 45°, massive pretibial edema with severe chronic stasis dermatitis, anasarca, cardiomegaly, tender and enlarged liver with elevated liver function enzymes, pulmonary congestion, and polycythemia (hematocrit of 52.6%). His VC (sitting) was 1410 ml (31% of normal) and his FEV_1/FVC was 90%. SaO_2 was 87%, and $PaCO_2$ was 57 and increased to 63 mm Hg when he received 0.5 l/min of supplemental oxygen by nasal cannula. He refused to use nocturnal lipseal IPPV and, despite his hypercapnia, was treated with nocturnal oxygen delivered at

0.5 l/min by nasal cannula. However, obtundation and cor pulmonale worsened, and he developed pneumonia for which he was hospitalized, intubated, and mechanically ventilated on two occasions through June 1986.

In June 1986, polysomnography and capnography were performed with the patient semisupine (Grass Model 78 D polysomnograph, Grass Instruments Co., Quincy, MA). He had 118 hypopneas/hour, a mean SaO_2 of 55.2%, and $EtCO_2$ levels to 91 mm Hg. He had neither rapid eye movement (REM) nor slow-wave sleep.

In August 1986, he was hospitalized for dyspnea and obtundation and further elevations of plasma liver function enzymes. Furosemide therapy was increased to 160 mg daily, and he was placed on nocturnal nasal IPPV which he used supine. Two weeks later, polysomnography was repeated while he used nasal IPPV and breathed room air. There was normal total sleep and sleep efficiency and normal sleep latency, sleep onset, and REM sleep. He had 13 apneas/hypopneas per hour. SaO_2 was 48% to 63% during the first hour (12–1AM) and then 70% to 96% for the rest of the night. He was discharged home using nasal IPPV and slept supine. His furosemide dosage was gradually lowered to 60 mg once a week.

In January 1987, after 5 months of nocturnal nasal IPPV, he had only minimal residual dependent lower-extremity edema. His former symptoms of headaches, hypersomnolence, sleep dysfunction, and nightmares had been completely relieved for months. Liver size and enzymes were normal, and his hematocrit was 40%. His VC was 1300 ml sitting and 600 ml supine. His VFBT while supine continued to be negligible, but he did not require ventilator use when sitting. Despite $EtCO_2$ of 45 to 50 mm Hg and SaO_2 of 88% to 92% when breathing unassisted, the $PaCO_2$ decreased to 33 to 38 mm Hg and the $SaO2$ was >95% within 2 minutes when using nasal IPPV, sitting or supine, on assist/control mode with a delivered volume of 1150 ml (pressure, 30 cm H_2O).

As he slept using nasal IPPV, part of the insufflation volume leaked out of his mouth, vibrating his lips, and decreasing the insufflation pressure to a minimum of 26 cm H_2O. At this pressure, the SaO_2 dropped to a low of 88% and $EtCO_2$ rose to the maximum of 49 mm Hg. The pressure varied from 26 to 28 mm Hg most of the night but was adequate to maintain a mean SaO_2 of 95%. His major complaint was that as soon as he stopped nasal IPPV in the morning, he became dyspneic for the rest of the day, but he resisted using daytime mouthpiece IPPV.

He did well until he was hit by a truck and incurred fractures of the left tibia and fibula in January 1991. Even though he had been unable to walk for 8 years, his fractures were set under general anesthesia. However, because he could not be weaned from the ventilator (he was left supine, a position in which he had no VFBT), he remained intubated, developed adult respiratory distress syndrome, self-extubated, and died while he was being re-intubated.

This patient demonstrated that:

1. Unessential surgery and general anesthesia should be avoided for individuals with GAH.
2. Because of failure to assess pulmonary function and ventilatory capacity with the patient recumbent, and failure to use inspiratory muscle aids in a timely manner, he had GAH for over 10 years, severe cor pulmonale, and ultimately fatal complications. Noninvasive IPPV alone can reverse cor pulmonale.
3. Hypoventilation can increase the risk of respiratory complications and hospitalizations when oxygen therapy is used instead of inspiratory muscle aids.
4. A variety of IPPV interfaces, oral and nasal, should be tried, and the patient allowed to choose.

Case 4: Failure to Evaluate or Use PCF as Criterion for Extubation

It has recently been appreciated that, irrespective of the extent of autonomous breathing ability or VC, the primary criterion permitting safe tracheal extubation for patients with neuromuscular ventilatory failure is the ability to generate at least 3 l/sec of PCF.[3] Three tracheostomized, autonomously breathing patients with spinal cord injury maintained normal SaO_2 while breathing room air and had VCs of 1.3, 1.7, and 2.1 liters, respectively. In each case, the tracheostomy tube was removed and a tracheostomy button was placed. All three developed dyspnea, oxyhemoglobin desaturations, diminution in VC, and, in two cases, hyperpyrexia, in <24 hours. The tracheostomy tubes were replaced, and the patients received aggressive mechanical insufflation-exsufflation through them. SaO_2 and VCs returned to baseline levels over a period of hours. Further examination revealed that one patient had tracheal stenosis, and two had vocal cord adhesions preventing full abduction.

Although it has been argued that prior to tracheostomy tube removal, all patients should undergo laryngoscopic evaluation of the upper airway,[13] in our experience, demonstration of the ability to generate PCF >3 l/sec ensures safe elimination of indwelling endotracheal tubes, irrespective of the extent of respiratory muscle paralysis.[3]

Case 5: Inappropriate Administration of Oxygen, Bronchodilators, and Chest Physical Therapy and Body Ventilator-Associated Obstructive Sleep Apneas

A patient with complete C4/C5 tetraplegia from a fall at age 14 in 1957 developed GAH in 1969. He complained of hypersomnolence from 1969 to 1974 that was treated by continuous home oxygen therapy. As a result, his $PaCO_2$ climbed to 70 to 80 mm Hg and his hypersomnolence worsened. He was first hospitalized for respiratory failure triggered by a respiratory tract infection in 1974. He was intubated, tracheostomized, and received IPPV for 3 weeks. Over the next 9 years, he was hospitalized on eight occasions and intubated three times for respiratory failure. In 1983, he developed cor pulmonale and had three respiratory arrests resulting in loss of consciousness during attempts to wean him from IPPV via a nasotracheal tube following urologic surgery. Chest shell ventilator use permitted extubation. He continued to use it nightly for 4 years and then switched to a negative-pressure wrap-style ventilator nightly until 1989. From 1983 to 1989, he was hospitalized on nine occasions and intubated eight times. He underwent bronchoscopic mucus removal on 13 occasions and had two grand mal seizure episodes associated with theophylline therapy.

In 1989, with a VC of 450 ml sitting and 580 ml supine, the patient had arterial blood gas analysis and continuous noninvasive blood gas monitoring performed to evaluate the effectiveness of nocturnal negative-pressure wrap ventilator use. His awake unaided $PaCO_2$ ranged from 55 up to 95 mm Hg during periods of fatigue late in the day. PaO_2 ranged from 40 to 50 mm Hg. Severe oxyhemoglobin desaturation occurred during sleep as well as throughout daytime hours. He was switched to nocturnal mouthpiece IPPV but refused to use a Bennett lipseal (Puritan-Bennett, Boulder, CO) because of his inability to independently remove the retention straps that would allow use of a sip-and-puff–activated telephone during the night. His blood gases were not optimal on nocturnal mouthpiece IPPV without a lipseal. Because he retained antigravity strength in his right biceps, a pulley system was set up that allowed him to remove lipseal straps independently (Fig. 25–2).

Theophylline, oxygen, and routine chest physical therapy were discontinued. Mouthpiece IPPV with lipseal retention normalized the nocturnal SaO_2 and alveolar ventilation as monitored by $EtCO_2$ measurements. He also discovered by using oximetry and occasionally capnography as biofeedback that daytime use of mouthpiece IPPV could normalize his SaO_2 and alveolar ventilation and relieve daytime fatigue and dyspnea. His VC increased to 720 ml sitting and 760 ml supine 4 months following initiation of noninvasive IPPV in December 1989, and his ventilator use requirement decreased from 24 to 14 hours/day. He has had no respiratory complications or hospitalizations over the last 6 years while using mouthpiece IPPV and mechanical insufflation-exsufflation to clear airway secretions during RTIs. He has had no further seizure activity. His maximum PCF are 0.9 l/sec unassisted, 1.2 l/sec with an abdominal thrust following a maximum insufflation of 1100 ml, and 6.9 l/sec by mechanical insufflation-exsufflation.[2]

This patient demonstrated the need for effective alveolar ventilation (noninvasive IPPV)

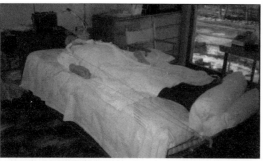

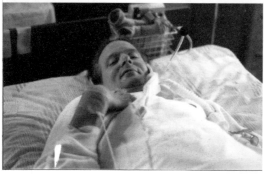

FIGURES 25–2. Spinal-cord-injured patient with late-onset chronic ventilatory failure using a pulley system to remove the lipseal retention system he uses for nocturnal mouthpiece IPPV.

around-the-clock and effective airway secretion management in order to prevent respiratory complications and hospitalizations. As in the other cases, oxygen therapy and theophylline were useless or harmful. As for 40 previously described patients, body ventilator use became increasingly inadequate, and this patient, too, needed to be switched to noninvasive IPPV and try various noninvasive IPPV interfaces.[7]

Case 6: Inappropriate Resort to Electrophrenic Pacing

The longest case of decannulation and dependence on noninvasive respiratory aids in a high-level spinal-cord-injured patient is that of a man, who at 17 years of age in March 1967, fell from a horse in a school gymnasium and sustained a fracture dislocation of C1 on C2 and complete C2 tetraplegia. He was immediately apneic and became permanently ventilator-dependent without VFBT. In March 1967, phrenic pacemakers were placed bilaterally but were ineffective. He remained in intensive care for 10 months because of pulmonary infections. He was transferred for rehabilitation in February 1968 with an indwelling tracheostomy tube and a cuff inflated with 12 ml of air. He developed severe trachiectasis with a cuff to trachea diameter ratio of 3:1. He continued to have frequent bronchial mucus plugging, which led to a respiratory arrest resulting in partial cortical blindness and in two near-arrests. He was very motivated for tracheostomy site closure.

He began using daytime mouthpiece IPPV with a portable pressure-cycled ventilator at a rate of 18/min and pressure of 20 cm H_2O in April 1968 with the tracheostomy tube plugged. He began nocturnal iron lung use in July 1968. Both methods provided him with normal alveolar ventilation and blood gases. Even with the tube plugged, however, tracheal site leakage prevented him from attaining more than 5 minutes of VFBT by combining glossopharyngeal breathing (GPB) and accessory muscle use. In April 1969, the tracheostomy site was allowed to close after another two episodes of pneumonia, and his pacemaker was removed. VFBT increased to >3 hours by GPB, and he developed a GPB maximum single breath capacity of 1700 ml.[6] The VC (without GPB) increased to 420 ml by accessory muscle use when sitting. He was converted from nocturnal iron lung to wrap ventilator use. He continues to use mouthpiece IPPV during the daytime and the Pulmowrap (Lifecare International, Inc, Westminster, CO) ventilator overnight. He has had two episodes of pneumonia resulting from respiratory tract infections over the last 27 years.

Although the pacemaker was placed in this individual 28 years ago, more recent results also fail to justify the resort to this expensive, invasive, and unphysiologic method except when noninvasive aids cannot be used.[4,8] All four traumatic tetraplegic ventilator-users with pacemakers and tracheostomy tubes whom we have decannulated and converted to noninvasive IPPV have permanently discontinued pacemaker use.

Case 7: Inappropriate Ventilator Use

A 24-year-old man sustained a spinal cord injury on 30 November 1979, was intubated and then tracheostomized, and used IPPV for 6 months with no VFBT. He was transferred for rehabilitation, where he developed VC of 340 ml and a maximum of 1 hour of VFBT by April 1980. VFBT gradually increased, and he was weaned to overnight IPPV in August 1980. He was discharged home and instructed to "never stop using nocturnal ventilatory support." He suffered two lung collapses and pneumonia in 1983 but had no further difficulties and underwent no further pulmonary function testing until presenting in January 1988 with a VC of 2920 ml sitting and 3170 ml supine. At that point he had been using nocturnal tracheostomy IPPV for 9 years. Nocturnal oximetry demonstrated a mean SaO_2 of 96% and a low of 91%. IPPV was discontinued and the tracheostomy site was allowed to close. His VC was 4200 ml sitting and 3600 ml supine in October 1992.

Case 8: Inappropriate Ventilator Weaning and Failure to Use Mechanical Insufflation-Exsufflation in a Timely Manner

A 67-year-old man with a 58-pack-year history of cigarette smoking had became a complete C4 ventilator-dependent tetraplegic in July 1992. He was weaned from ventilator use 2 months after injury and transferred for rehabilitation with an indwelling capped tracheostomy tube, receiving supplemental oxygen and with profuse airway secretions. Three days after admission, he developed pneumonia, was rehospitalized and ventilator-dependent for 3 weeks, and then once again weaned to oxygen supplementation and transferred for rehabilitation. At this time, his tracheostomy site was allowed to close, but secretions remained profuse and purulent and he

continued antibiotics and supplemental oxygen therapy. Subsequently, two episodes of hypercapnic coma necessitated two further hospitalizations and bronchoscopic removal of mucus plugs over the next 2-month period. He was then referred to a rehabilitation ventilator unit.

A review of earlier hospital and rehabilitation records revealed that his VCs had ranged from 750 to 1000 ml. At ventilator unit admission, his VC was 900 ml, oxygen therapy was discontinued, and baseline SaO_2 varied from 93% to 80% with $EtCO_2$ to >50 mm Hg. He was placed on mouthpiece IPPV with oximetry biofeedback and nocturnal nasal IPPV to normalize ventilation and provide deep breaths for assisted coughing. His maximum unassisted PCF were 1.2 l/sec. He had frequent sudden oxyhemoglobin desaturations below 80% that were corrected with the elimination of mucus plugs by mechanical insufflation-exsufflation (MI-E) coordinated with manually applied abdominal thrusts. With the initial application of MI-E, large volumes of mucus were eliminated, and his VC rose to 1200 ml. He required MI-E every 15 minutes during daytime hours for 2 days, at which point his airways became virtually free of sputum; his SaO_2 remained over 94% at all times; his VC increased to 1600 ml or by 77% in 2 days; and he discontinued nocturnal nasal IPPV. He was able to complete his rehabilitation program without further incident and return home without ventilatory support largely because of MI-E.

Case 9: Over-reliance on Tracheostomy, Failure to Deflate Cuff, and Failure to Evaluate Home Care

A patient with classic phenotypic Duchenne muscular dystrophy presented with pseudohypertrophic calves and characteristic biopsy and electromyogram findings. He had lost the ability to walk at age 10 and subsequently developed severe scoliosis and then symptomatic GAH at age 26, with a VC of 46% of predicted normal. He was placed on nocturnal mouthpiece IPPV, which he used without lipseal retention. By 1980, he required mouthpiece IPPV for increasing periods during daytime hours and used it 24 hours a day from 1981 to 1985, at which point his VC was 340 ml or 13% of predicted normal. Because he was never offered a lipseal retention system for nocturnal mouthpiece use,[7] he had frequent sleep arousals and was convinced by his physicians to undergo elective tracheostomy during his first hospitalization in 1985. Following tracheostomy, he developed pneumonia for which a Hickman catheter was placed for antibiotic therapy. His dysphagia worsened because the tube restricted the muscles of deglutition, malnutrition developed, and a gastrostomy tube was placed.

Once the patient's condition was stable, it was discovered that he could not be discharged home because his wife was a poliomyelitis survivor who could walk but had no upper extremity function and therefore could not perform tracheal suctioning. After a hospitalization of 6 months, the patient was forced to return to his parents' home. His tracheostomy tube cuff was never deflated, so he could no longer communicate.

In 1988, the family sent me a copy of his hospital records. He had continued to receive 24-hour oxygen therapy and tracheostomy IPPV with an inflated cuff. His Hickman catheter had been changed on two occasions. Overall, he had received 20 weeks of inhospital intravenous antibiotics and an additional 740 days of antibiotics at home. He no longer had sufficient stamina to sit in a wheelchair, and he had not been placed into one since hospital discharge 2.5 years earlier. He was extremely depressed because he could no longer live with his wife. I was told that the physicians had informed the family 2.5 years earlier that he was "being sent home to die, and the oxygen will make him more comfortable." He died in October 1988 when, as noted on his patient chart, he had developed sepsis from the Hickman catheter.

This patient's depression and ultimate demise were the result of unnecessary tracheostomy, unnecessary long-term cuff inflation, an unnecessary central line, and failure to consider postdischarge tracheostomy management. It has been shown that with an optimal tracheostomy tube diameter and some residual vocal cord function, virtually no GAH patient requires cuff inflation unless pulmonary compliance is very poor.[5] Virtually no patient with Duchenne muscular dystrophy requires a tracheostomy for ventilatory support.[1]

Case 10: Inadequate BiPAP Settings, Inappropriate Use of BiPAP instead of Volume Ventilators, Failure to Extend the Nocturnal Use of Noninvasive IPPV into Daytime Hours, Inappropriate Use of Oxygen, and Unnecessary Emphasis on Tracheostomy

A cognitively intact patient with Duchenne muscular dystrophy underwent Harrington rod placement for scoliosis in 1989 at age 14. He remained stable until February 1995, when a respiratory tract infection caused fatigue and cyanosis. His $PaCO_2$ was found to be 88 mm Hg. He was treated with BiPAP (inspiratory PAP 12 and expiratory PAP 6, or 12/6 cm H_2O) in a local emergency room with some improvement and then sent home using nocturnal BiPAP with supplemental oxygen. However, for 1 month, he complained of frequent nocturnal arousals with tachycardia, saying "breathe" to himself. He was therefore readmitted, but because the hospital had no policy regarding BiPAP, its use was not permitted. On the first morning after admission, he was found to be comatose with a $PaCO_2$ of 99 mm Hg. The physicians advised his parents to "let him go," but their advice was refused and he was placed back on BiPAP at 12/6 cm H_2O. He awoke with severe anoxic encephalopathy. I advised discontinuing oxygen therapy and increasing the BiPAP to 18/2 cm H_2O to normalize SaO_2 without supplemental oxygen therapy; however, 12/6-cm H_2O BiPAP and oxygen therapy were continued.

Because the patient remained precariously underventilated, his parents were pressured to accept his undergoing tracheostomy. At our urging against this, however, his parents insisted on his coming to our clinic. Because the hospital felt that it was hazardous to discharge or transfer the patient using BiPAP and the ambulance "did not have oxygen," his parents had to sign him out against medical advice and bring him themselves. We were advised to admit him for tracheostomy.

We converted him to the use of nasal IPPV using the assist control mode on a PLV-100 portable volume-cycled ventilator (Lifecare International Inc., Westminster, CO). He and his family were instructed in our noninvasive respiratory muscle aid protocol, which included discontinuing oxygen therapy and eliminating airway secretions by manually and mechanically assisted coughing methods. His SaO_2 returned to normal and remained normal in this manner. He has had no subsequent respiratory complications but remains too cognitively impaired to direct his own care.

This case demonstrates failure to use BiPAP at settings adequate for ventilatory assistance, inappropriate use of BiPAP rather than a volume-cycled ventilator for a patient requiring more than nocturnal aid, unnecessarily protracted hospitalization, failure to use expiratory muscle aids to eliminate airway secretions, hazardous use of oxygen therapy, and needless emphasis on tracheostomy.

Case 11: Hazardous Use of Oxygen and Overemphasis on Tracheostomy, with Increased Respiratory Muscle Endurance by Rest with IPPV

A floppy neonate was diagnosed with spinal muscular atrophy at 2 years of age in 1958. Despite never having had the ability to sit or walk and developing severe scoliosis, she achieved a PhD and worked full-time as a leisure counselor from 1979 to 1991, when severe carbon dioxide retention caused symptoms that prevented her continued employment. These symptoms included hypersomnolence with sleep episodes every 5 to 10 minutes, confusion, "black outs," depression, headaches, nightmares, frequent nocturnal arousals but difficult morning arousal, and polycythemia (hematocrit 55%). She had been evaluated by physicians in three Jerry Lewis Muscular Dystrophy Association clinics in Pennsylvania, prescribed continuous oxygen therapy that only exacerbated her hypercapnia and hypersomnolence, and was advised to undergo tracheostomy or die in a matter of weeks.

After reading an article about our approach, she came to our clinic. She was extremely depressed. Her VC (maximum effort) was 120 ml; weight, 37 lbs; and she had >120° of scoliosis. Her baseline SaO_2 on room air was 70% to 78%; on receiving 1 liter of oxygen, it was >94%, but $EtCO_2$ increased to >80 mm Hg. As she fell asleep, her baseline SaO_2 on room air was 37% to 44% and on oxygen it was 70%.

Oxygen therapy was discontinued, and she was instructed in the use of respiratory muscle aids and oximetry biofeedback. She was immediately able to maintain normal SaO_2 when using mouthpiece IPPV with room air when awake. She also maintained normal SaO_2 when using nasal IPPV during sleep. All symptoms of hypercapnia cleared and she returned to gainful employment in 1 month. Because her compensatory metabolic alkalosis cleared and her ventilatory drive normalized, she almost immediately became dependent on noninvasive IPPV with virtually no VFBT. However, after 1 to 2 months, she found that she could maintain normal SaO_2 for increasing periods of time up to 4 hours while breathing on her own. Despite increased ventilatory ability, no change was observed in her VC.

This case demonstrates the hazards of oxygen therapy and unnecessary insistence on tracheostomy. Also, it shows that VFBT (inspiratory muscle endurance) can initially be lost entirely while ventilatory drive resets, but it can subsequently increase with the inspiratory muscle rest provided by the continuous use of noninvasive IPPV over a period of weeks to months.

A second case illustrates these same principles. A 54-year-old high school teacher with a history of Pott's disease at age 3, severe kyphoscoliosis, and a 5-year history of shortness of breath, hypersomnolence, fatigue, and headaches was hospitalized for ventilatory failure, placed on continuous home oxygen therapy, informed that he would require a tracheostomy tube or he would not survive 2 months, and sent home. With oxygen therapy, $PaCO_2$ increased to 74 mm Hg and PaO_2 to 55 mm Hg. Dyspnea eased, but hypersomnolence and other symptoms of GAH worsened, and he complained that he frequently fell asleep while teaching classes. He had two additional hospitalizations for ventilatory failure over the next 4 months and continued to refuse to undergo tracheostomy, but he became very depressed and thought that he was dying. His respiratory therapist referred him to our program.

His mean nocturnal SaO_2 on room air was 71% ($EtCO_2$ was 53mm Hg); on 4 l/min of oxygen via nasal cannula, it was 89%; on nasal IPPV with room air, 91%; and on nasal IPPV with 2 l/min of oxygen, 95%. Supplemental oxygen use was discontinued to optimize nocturnal nasal IPPV.[9] Using oximetry for occasional biofeedback, he was able to maintain SaO_2 >94% during daytime hours by breathing deeper and using mouthpiece IPPV for periods of time. He has continued to use nocturnal nasal IPPV with a custom-molded nasal interface (*see* Fig. 24–11) and periods of daytime mouthpiece IPPV for 8 years. He continues to teach school without any symptoms of GAH.

Case 12: Over-reliance on Tracheostomy and Benefits of Glossopharyngeal Breathing

A 43-year-old journalist with limb-girdle muscular dystrophy had been using IPPV via a tracheostomy 24 hours a day with a VC of 200 ml and no VFBT for 5.5 years. During this time, she could not be safely left alone to work, and she had had numerous febrile episodes that were treated with intravenous antibiotics. In July 1992 her tracheostomy tube was removed, the site closed, and she was converted to using daytime mouthpiece and nighttime nasal IPPV (*see* Fig. 25–3). She also mastered GPB sufficiently for up to 8 hours of VFBT. This permitted her to work

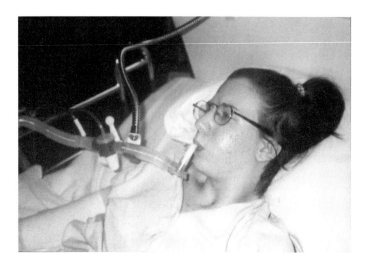

FIGURE 25–3. A 17-year-old complete C2 tetraplegic with a vital capacity under 200 ml and no ventilator-free breathing ability. She was switched from continuous tracheostomy IPPV to daytime mouthpiece IPPV and nocturnal nasal IPPV. She has achieved ventilator-free breathing only by glossopharyngeal breathing.

safely at home alone. With her maximum GPB single-breath capacity of 1200 ml, she was also better able to shout and cough.

A 17-year-old girl had a complete C1/C2 cervical spine injury in January 1993. She had a VC of just under 200 ml and no VFBT. Her tube was removed and the site closed in May 1993, and she was converted to daytime mouthpiece IPPV and nocturnal nasal IPPV (Fig. 25–3). She has achieved 20 to 30 minutes of VFBT by GPB.

Case 13: Unnecessary Endotracheal Intubation, with Extubation and Conversion to 24-hour Noninvasive IPPV

An 18-year-old man with Duchenne muscular dystrophy developed acute respiratory failure during an otherwise benign respiratory tract infection and was intubated in a local hospital. His VC decreased from 800 ml at baseline to 200 ml, and he had no VFBT. Despite this decrease, he previously had been instructed in use of the mouthpiece and nasal IPPV, and so he was extubated and switched directly to continuous noninvasive IPPV and use of MI-E. With aggressive MI-E, his VC immediately increased to 400 ml, but he continued to have no VFBT and airway secretions remained profuse for 5 days, at which point he weaned to nocturnal nasal IPPV and went home using MI-E as needed. He thus far has had four subsequent episodes of acute respiratory distress associated with respiratory tract infections which have been managed at home with continuous noninvasive IPPV and use of manually and mechanically assisted coughing methods. During one respiratory tract infection, nasal congestion rendered nasal IPPV ineffective, and he developed respiratory distress with a $PaCO_2$ of 55 mm Hg. When given the choice between switching to lipseal IPPV or using nasal decongestants, he chose the latter and had no further elevations of $EtCO_2$ or significant oxyhemoglobin desaturations. Despite temperature elevations to 104°F and leukocytosis during at least three of the five infections, he was never again hospitalized. Thus, a noninvasive aid protocol can be extremely effective in preventing or treating ventilatory failure.

Case 14: Over-reliance on Tracheal Suctioning

A 43-year-old man with C5 traumatic tetraplegia and a VC of 1900 ml maintained normal alveolar ventilation and SaO_2 when breathing unassisted; however, his tracheostomy tube had not yet been removed. While receiving physical therapy, he suddenly developed respiratory distress and his SaO_2 decreased to 75% to 79%. Aggressive chest percussion, postural drainage, and tracheal suctioning were administered, but these neither relieved his dyspnea nor improved his SaO_2. After continuing these efforts for about 10 minutes, he received MI-E through the tracheostomy tube (with the cuff inflated). A large mucus plug was immediately eliminated, his dyspnea cleared, and SaO_2 returned to normal. Thus, MI-E can be more effective than routine tracheal suctioning. Undoubtedly, the mucus plug originated from the left airways, airways that are often poorly cleared by suctioning via an endotracheal or tracheostomy tube.[10] This patient would otherwise have required emergency transfer to a local hospital for bronchoscopy.

Case 15: Noninvasive Nocturnal Blood Gas Monitoring, Need to Customize and Vary Interfaces, Oximetry Biofeedback, Improvement in Respiratory Muscle Endurance by Rest with IPPV

A ventilator-user, born in 1970, with severe, confirmed Duchenne muscular dystrophy stopped walking at 30 months of age. His VC plateaued at 1050 ml before 9 years of age. Spinal surgery was refused, and his spinal curve eventually became 114° to the left (Cobb technique) in 1994. From January 1985 to September 1987, he was hospitalized five times for dyspnea, difficulties managing airway secretions, and respiratory tract infections. His mother said that he had frequent "mucus attacks," described as episodes of profuse salivation, airway congestion, and uncontrolled drooling.

In October 1987, he presented with a temperature of 104°F, complaints of chronic headaches, difficulty swallowing, weight loss, VC of 280 ml, and profuse mucopurulent airway secretions. Manually assisted coughing was not effective because of severe scoliosis. He received antibiotics and required intravenous fluids because of dehydration. $PaCO_2$ on admission was 57 mm Hg. His SaO_2 varied from 89% to 94% when awake, with $EtCO_2$ from 50 to 54 mm Hg.

Trials of mouthpiece IPPV failed because of inadequacy of oropharyngeal muscles to grab the mouthpiece. He was taught and used nasal IPPV during the daytime with $EtCO_2$ and pulse oximetry biofeedback. In this manner, his $EtCO_2$ was maintained below 43 mm Hg and his SaO_2 over 94%. He napped using nasally delivered volumes of 560 ml (mask pressure, 23–25 cm H_2O) at a rate of 16/min. He received 500 ml while awake and with the mouth open or closed. During overnight sleep monitoring using nasal IPPV, his $EtCO_2$ varied from 40 to 47 mm Hg and his SaO_2 averaged 95%, with a low of 85%, and he had few oxyhemoglobin desaturations. He was discharged home using nasal IPPV nocturnally.

The following week his mother stated that he felt stronger, was eating better, and "mucus attacks" were less frequent and less severe. He no longer required daytime ventilatory aid to maintain SaO_2 >94%, except occasionally when tired. Repeat nocturnal sleep studies were routinely performed with delivered volumes of 1200 ml. The mean SaO_2 was 96%–97%, and the maximum recorded $EtCO_2$ was 40 cm H_2O. The low-pressure alarm, which was set at 14 cm H_2O, sounded often, but for only a few seconds, and about twice per night for longer periods. These alarms correlated with the SaO_2 dips that at no time were lower than 82%. He had excellent control of his secretions and his swallowing improved. His VC increased from 270 ml on 27 October 1987 to 330 ml on 3 February 1988. He gained weight and was able to sit in this wheelchair all day without fatigue.

This patient had four subsequent respiratory tract infections with oral temperatures exceeding 102°F, leukocyte counts exceeding 10,000/mm³, and profuse mucopurulent airway secretions during his first 15 months using nocturnal nasal IPPV. With each one, he was managed at home using continuous SaO_2 monitoring and 24-hour nasal IPPV with instructions to maintain normal SaO_2 by using nasal IPPV and cough assistance. On no occasion was supplemental oxygen administered. Sudden dips in SaO_2 that could not be corrected by taking large insufflation volumes were corrected by MI-E. With only 1 l/sec of unassisted PCF, he required MI-E about four times per hour during respiratory tract infections.

During an infection in August 1988, his SaO_2 ranged from 88% to 93%, PaO_2 ranged from 62 to 70 mm Hg, and $EtCO_2$ remained normal for 6 days as he used continuous nasal IPPV and frequent MI-E. Desaturations as low as 70% occurred with immediate rebound to a baseline of 91% to 93% following MI-E. The patient apparently had diffuse microscopic atelectasis that could not be identified on chest radiographs. As during the previous respiratory infections, MI-E was initially necessary about four times per hour and then less frequently needed for about 2 weeks, by which time the SaO_2 baseline returned to normal.

Except during respiratory tract infections, the patient used nasal IPPV only overnight and for short periods during the day until July 1989, when his total sitting time was down to less than 2 hours/day. He complained of extreme fatigue, frequent "mucus attacks," dysphagia, and weight loss. His VC was 250 ml. He then began to use nasal IPPV 24 hours a day. As a result, his symptoms once again cleared and he returned to being up in his wheelchair 16 hours/day and to maintaining an active lifestyle that included frequent interstate travel with his family.

Because of the need for 24-hour aid, he alternated the use of four different commercially available CPAP masks and two custom-fabricated nasal interfaces. Of the nasal interfaces, he initially tried using one fabricated from a SEFAM kit (available from Lifecare International Inc., Westminster, CO), but he found this interface to be heavy. For the last 3 years, he used only IVALs (Interface for Ventilator-Assisted Living)[12] (Fig. 25–4), which he alternated over 12-hour periods. This alternating use of devices sufficiently redistributed pressure around his nose to avert any discomfort or skin irritation, despite requiring increasingly higher pressures on the retention straps to avert insufflation leaks because mask pressures gradually increased to >40 cm H_2O.

Nocturnal SaO_2 monitoring, which was repeated every 12 months since August 1988, demonstrated a mean SaO_2 at ≥95% with a mean of 1.7 4% dips in SaO_2 per hour and infrequent dips below 90%. His unassisted PCF were <0.5 l/sec. With air stacking of the nasal insufflations, he generated PCF of 1.8 l/sec. Manually assisted coughing with an abdominal thrust timed to follow an air-stacking maneuver did not yield more than 1.8-l/sec PCF because of his severe scoliosis. His PCF generated by MI-E was found to be 9.23 l/sec.[2]

On 3 May 1995, the ventilator-delivered volumes were generating mask pressure averaging 52 cm H_2O, nocturnal mean SaO_2 had decreased to 92% (on room air), airway secretion production had increased, and he had become febrile with a leukocyte count of 16,000/mm³. A

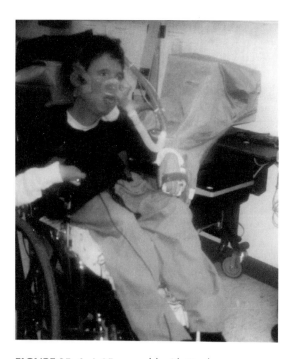

FIGURE 25–4. A 25-year-old with Duchenne muscular dystrophy and severe scoliosis who required 24-hour nasal IPPV for over 5 years. He used acrylic low-profile transparent nasal interfaces fabricated from plaster moulages.[12]

chest radiograph demonstrated a massive pneumothorax with complete collapse of the right lung. Considering the clinical picture of slowly increasing mask pressures without respiratory symptoms, this was felt to be an insidiously progressive process. Following chest tube placement, the patient's mild dyspnea was relieved and ventilator pressures normalized with the same delivered volumes; however, 7 hours later, he developed repeated episodes of ventricular tachyarrhythmias and died despite repeated attempts at resuscitation.

This patient demonstrates that:

1. Oximetry biofeedback and sleep monitoring are useful in patient management.
2. There is a need for switching between various nasal interfaces for IPPV.
3. Nasal IPPV can be used 24 hours/day long-term when the lips are too weak for effective mouthpiece IPPV and scoliosis is too severe for use of an intermittent abdominal pressure ventilator
4. Nasal IPPV can provide continuous ventilatory support, even when patients have no VFBT, pulmonary compliance is poor, and ventilator-delivered volumes generate mask pressures >40 cm H_2O.
5. VFBT can increase with the respiratory muscle rest provided by noninvasive IPPV.
6. Use of respiratory muscle aids can be critical for avoiding pulmonary complications and hospitalizations.
7. The volume-cycled ventilator gauge pressures should be monitored and chest radiographs performed regularly to treat any intercurrent pulmonary complications in a timely manner.
8. MI-E can be effective even when manually assisted PCF cannot exceed 3 l/sec.

Case 16: Failure to Discharge Conventionally Managed Patients to the Community

A 31-year-old Texan woman with a history of poliomyelitis at 4 years of age developed a respiratory tract infection and acute respiratory failure in April 1987. She suffered a cardiopulmonary arrest while on route to a local hospital. She was intubated and subsequently tracheostomized. Attempts at ventilator weaning failed, and she was reluctantly transferred to a chronic nursing care facility despite the fact that she required only nocturnal ventilatory support. Her VC in the sitting position was 1030 ml but only

630 ml supine. She was not permitted to return home to her husband who had a 9-to-5 job, because regulations prohibited tracheal suctioning by other than family members and licensed health care professionals, for which no funds would be allocated. She remained at the chronic care facility using nocturnal tracheostomy IPPV with an inflated cuff for 6 months. This caused severe tracheomalacia.

She was transferred to a rehabilitation facility for decannulation. On the first night, her cuff was deflated and the delivered ventilator volumes increased to compensate for insufflation leakage through the upper airway. This relieved the pressure on the trachea and permitted speech while using tracheostomy IPPV. Then, her tracheostomy tube was removed; a firm occlusive dressing was placed over the site; and the patient was placed on nocturnal nasal IPPV. She used this for 2 weeks until she complained of nasal bridge discomfort from the nasal interface. Once again, an attempt at weaning failed, when after 10 days off aid, severe fatigue and blood gas deterioration resulted in her being placed in an iron lung overnight for 2 weeks. She was converted to using a Pulmowrap Ventilator overnight and discharged home. Although this adequately assisted her inspiratory muscle function, it was inconvenient to don and she eventually switched to a strapless oral nasal interface for IPPV. She continues to use this strapless oral nasal interface for nocturnal IPPV and has not required rehospitalization.

In a second case, a 49-year-old woman with a congenital myopathy and a long history of fatigue, difficulties with concentration, dyspnea, and hypersomnolence developed pneumonia and was hospitalized and tracheostomized in February 1990. She was weaned from IPPV with the tracheostomy tube left open and placed on continuous supplemental oxygen therapy for 3 weeks, but she developed increasing hypercapnia ($PaCO_2$, 55–93 mm Hg). She could not tolerate plugging of the tube. Chronic fatigue lead to her being placed back on tracheostomy IPPV, and she continued to receive continuous oxygen therapy. Further attempts at ventilator weaning involved alternating the use of diminishing rate and periods of synchronized intermittent mandatory ventilation with CPAP. Her arterial blood gases typically demonstrated normal pH, PaO_2 of 130 to 170 mm Hg, $PaCO_2$ of 65 to 74 mm Hg, and elevated bicarbonate levels. This patient lived in a communal ashram, and her caregivers were not relatives. No one could or would be permitted to take responsibility for tracheal suctioning, and so she could not be discharged.

After 5 months of unsuccessful ventilator weaning, she was transferred for tracheostomy removal on 27 July 1990. Supplemental oxygen therapy, bronchodilators, and theophylline were permanently discontinued with no untoward effects. Using oximetry biofeedback, it was found that she could normalize SaO_2 and $PaCO_2$ by breathing deeper for short periods before tiring. The tracheostomy tube was removed, and she was ventilated by a chest shell ventilator for 18 hours while the tracheostomy site closed (*see* Chapter 22, Fig. 22–5). During overnight chest shell use, her mean SaO_2 was 89%, she had a maximum $EtCO_2$ of 55 mm Hg, and she had been uncomfortable and vomited twice. She felt better and maintained normal SaO_2 the next day by deep breathing supplemented by periods of mouthpiece IPPV and was placed on nasal IPPV for nocturnal ventilatory aid. Using nocturnal nasal IPPV, her mean SaO_2 was 97% with a low of 89%. The airway secretions that had been due to tracheostomy tube irritation were cleared by MI-E for the 2 days following tracheostomy site closure, at which point she no longer had sputum to clear. She was discharged home on the fourth day after admission using mouthpiece and nasal IPPV as described. Although at discharge, her VFBT was <2 hours, the maintenance of normal alveolar ventilation around the clock by IPPV kept her symptom-free. She returned to her very active career as a professional writer and counselor and thus far has used noninvasive IPPV 16 to 20 hours/day for 8 years without further respiratory difficulties.

Thus, access to a variety of noninvasive inspiratory muscle aids and IPPV interfaces can be important, and transition to their use can facilitate discharge to the community.

Case 17: Intubation Avoided by Noninvasive IPPV

A 15-year-old boy was hospitalized with C3 motor-complete tetraplegia and an odontoid fracture as the result of a diving accident in May 1988. His respiratory status deteriorated rapidly. Twenty-four hours after admission, he had a VC of 750 ml and $PaCO_2$ was 50 mm Hg. His physical examination and chest radiographs demonstrated no lung pathology. His increasing dyspnea was managed with the use of a chest shell ventilator (Fig. 25–5), which provided a tidal volume of 550 ml and normalized his blood

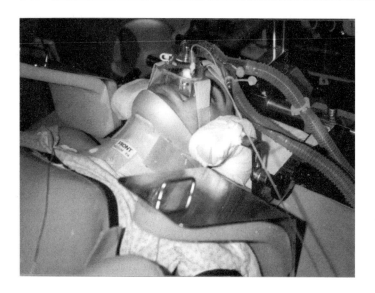

FIGURE 25–5. A 15-year-old spinal-cord-injured patient whose ventilatory failure was relieved by chest shell ventilator use. Because the chest shell had to be removed to accommodate a neck stabilizing brace, he was switched to noninvasive IPPV.

gases. Within 24 hours, he had no VFBT, his VC was <500 ml supine, and his unassisted tidal volumes were <200 ml.

His neck was temporarily stabilized with a Philadelphia collar, and he was transferred to a trauma center. Halo traction was to be placed on 2 June 1988, 4 days post-injury. At this time, his VC was 480 ml and he continued to have no VFBT. Because the halo could not be placed with the chest shell in place, he was switched to mouthpiece IPPV. He mastered the technique in <10 minutes. The chest shell ventilator was removed, and the halo traction unit was placed (Fig. 25–6). The ventilator settings of volume 890 and rate 16/minute maintained SaO_2 >94%, $PaCO_2$ <45 mm Hg, and complete relief of dyspnea. Because he had no VFBT and no neck or upper extremity movement, the mouthpiece had to be kept in his mouth. He switched from mouthpiece to nasal IPPV for sleep without changing ventilator settings.

He used noninvasive IPPV in this manner for 24 hours a day for 3 days. Nocturnal blood gas monitoring demonstrated no significant oxyhemoglobin desaturations. On 6 June 1988 at 1AM, he discontinued nasal IPPV because of nasal bridge irritation from CPAP mask pressure. Because no custom interface was available, he switched to lipseal IPPV (Fig. 25–7). It was strongly recommended that he use lipseal retention for mouthpiece IPPV, but at 3 AM he had the lipseal removed and continued mouthpiece IPPV without the lipseal. It was observed that during sleep, he maintained a firm oral grip on the mouthpiece, and insufflation leak-associated oxyhemoglobin desaturations remained infrequent.

The next day his VC was 660 ml supine (11%

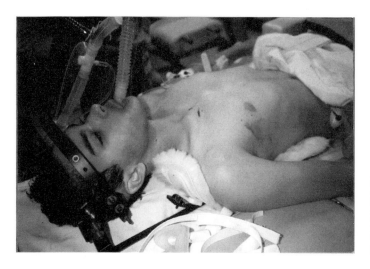

FIGURE 25–6. Once the chest shell was removed, a pressure ulcer became visible. He had no tactile sensation on his thorax. Here, he is using mouthpiece IPPV as the four-poster brace is being placed.

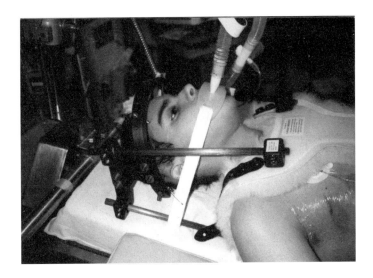

FIGURE 25–7. The same patient is seen using mouthpiece IPPV with lipseal retention for nocturnal ventilatory support. A single cloth retention strap was attached around each posterior poster by Velcro rather than having straps course above and below the ears.

of predicted), and he had approximately 1 minute of VFBT. He continued continuous mouthpiece IPPV from June 6th (VC 540 ml) through June 9th (VC 860). On 10 June 1988, his VC was 940 ml and he became free of ventilatory support during the daytime. On June 11th, with a VC of 1070 ml, he discontinued mouthpiece IPPV except for periodic deep insufflations to prevent atelectasis, maintain pulmonary compliance, and increase voice volume. He had no need for assisted coughing.

This patient would have been endotracheally intubated if noninvasive techniques had not been available to him. He also demonstrated the need for versatility in the use of noninvasive aids and that mouthpiece IPPV can at times be used even without a lipseal, as patients with intact chemotaxic drive develop reflex muscle activity during sleep to periodically decrease insufflation air leakage and maintain adequate blood gases.[9]

Case 18: Unnecessary Resort to Endotracheal Intubation and Tracheostomy

A 62-year-old man with chronic obstructive pulmonary disease (COPD), atherosclerotic heart and carotid artery disease, hypertension, peptic ulcers, and steroid-induced diabetes had a history of tachyarrhythmias and frequent hospitalizations and intubations for acute exacerbations of COPD, pneumonia, and respiratory failure. He signed a statement refusing further invasive interventions. During early April 1992, while he was on continuous oxygen therapy, his baseline $PaCO_2$ was 48 to 61 mm Hg. On 30 April 1992, he experienced severe dyspnea, tachypnea, disorientation, lethargy, and hypercapnia leading to severe obtundation. Since intubation

was not an option, nasal IPPV was tried. However, he was mouth breathing rapidly, and because of severe obtundation and depression of central chemotaxic centers by hypercapnia and oxygen therapy, he did not trigger the nasal IPPV and all delivered volumes leaked out of his mouth. Mouthpiece IPPV via a lipseal was then tried. With this essentially closed system of ventilatory support his carbon dioxide tensions decreased and he woke up. His SaO_2 increased to 94% to 95% after 30 minutes of lipseal IPPV at delivered volumes of 800 ml, assist control rate of 10 per minute, and FiO_2 of 30%. With improved chemotaxic responsiveness, he was then switched to nasal IPPV, with which he fell asleep and maintained a mean SaO_2 of 91% with the above settings. When awake, he used mouthpiece IPPV and maintained normal SaO_2 and $PaCO_2$ of 40 mm Hg with little supplemental oxygen. When he left his ventilator for any period of time, he became dyspneic whether or not using supplemental oxygen. He therefore had become dependent on 24-hour noninvasive IPPV. He weaned down to 6 hours of noninvasive IPPV per day, but this led to another episode of acute respiratory failure and hospitalization for reinstitution of 24-hour noninvasive IPPV, which he then continued for 2 years before dying suddenly. This patient used a rolling walker with a ventilator tray for daytime mouthpiece IPPV (Fig. 25–8).

We have subsequently had another instance of a severe lung disease patient with a history of 24 episodes of respiratory failure managed by endotracheal intubation who also had refused further invasive interventions. He, too, was resuscitated from hypercapnic coma by lipseal IPPV and subsequently maintained by 24-hour noninvasive IPPV for 14 months.

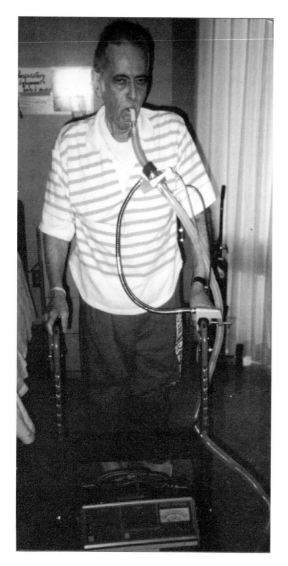

FIGURE 25–8. A 61-year-old man with COPD was maintained by using mouthpiece IPPV while rolling a walker with a ventilator tray during daytime hours and nasal IPPV overnight.

References

1. Bach JR: Management of neuromuscular ventilatory failure by 24-hour noninvasive intermittent positive pressure ventilation. Eur Respir Rev 3:284–291, 1993.
2. Bach JR: Mechanical insufflation-exsufflation: Comparison of peak expiratory flows with manually assisted and unassisted coughing techniques. Chest 104:1553–1562, 1993.
3. Bach JR: Amyotrophic lateral sclerosis: Predictors for prolongation of life by noninvasive respiratory aids. Arch Phys Med Rehabil 76:828–832, 1995.
4. Bach JR: Prevention of morbidity and mortality with the use of physical medicine aids. In Bach JR (ed): Pulmonary Rehabilitation: The Obstructive and Paralytic/ Restrictive Pulmonary Syndromes. Philadelphia, Hanley & Belfus, 1996.
5. Bach JR, Alba AS. Tracheostomy ventilation: A study of efficacy with deflated cuffs and cuffless tubes. Chest 97: 679–683, 1990.
6. Bach JR, Alba AS, Bodofsky E, et al: Glossopharyngeal breathing and non-invasive aids in the management of post-polio respiratory insufficiency. Birth Defects 23:99–113, 1987.
7. Bach JR, Alba AS, Saporito LR: Intermittent positive pressure ventilation via the mouth as an alternative to tracheostomy for 257 ventilator users. Chest 103:174–182, 1993.
8. Bach JR, O'Connor K: Electrophrenic ventilation: A different perspective. J Am Paraplegia Soc 14:9–17, 1991.
9. Bach JR, Robert D, Leger P, Langevin B: Sleep fragmentation in kyphoscoliotic individuals with alveolar hypoventilation treated by nasal IPPV. Chest 107:1552–1558, 1995.
10. Fishburn MJ, Marino RJ, Ditunno JF: Atelectasis and pneumonia in acute spinal cord injury. Arch Phys Med Rehabil 71:197–200, 1990.
11. Haber II, Bach JR: Normalization of blood carbon dioxide levels by transition from conventional ventilatory support to noninvasive inspiratory aids. Arch Phys Med Rehabil 75:1145–1150, 1994.
12. McDermott I, Bach JR, Parker C, Sortor S: Custom-fabricated interfaces for intermittent positive pressure ventilation. Int J Prosthodont 2:224–233, 1989.
13. Richard I, Giraud M, Perrouin-Verbe B, et al: Laryngotracheal stenosis after intubation or tracheostomy in neurological patients. Arch Phys Med Rehabil (in press).
14. Rochester DF, Braun NMT: Determinants of maximal inspiratory pressure in chronic obstructive pulmonary disease. Am Rev Respir Dis 132:42–47, 1985.

The Role of Ventilatory Muscle Training in Persons with Neuromuscular Disease

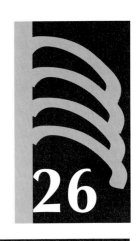

26

Ditza Gross, MD

Individuals with generalized neuromuscular diseases and others with paralytic or restrictive pulmonary syndromes have reduced ventilatory muscle strength and endurance (Table 26–1).[14] In addition, there is a real or relatively elevated respiratory load because of respiratory muscle weakness and decreased pulmonary compliance, and eventually these patients can develop chronic alveolar hypoventilation.[39] Thoracic cage deformities when present add to the presence of stiff lungs and chest walls in increasing the work of breathing. The inability to manage the increased workload leads to ventilatory muscle fatigue in a manner similar to that which has been described for the fatigue observed in cardiac and skeletal muscles.[17] Respiratory muscle dysfunction can eventually result in the development of pulmonary complications and potentially fatal acute or chronic ventilatory insufficiency.[26,32,35,36]

In earlier studies, it has been shown that the strength and endurance of the respiratory muscles can be improved by specific training.[12,28] This has been demonstrated in normal subjects,[9,21] in tetraplegic individuals,[18] and in patients with COPD[6,7,29] and muscular dystrophy.[13,14,40] The overall purpose of training the ventilatory muscles is to improve the muscles' ability to overcome the elevated respiratory loads caused by the disease. Because reduced ventilatory muscle performance can bring about respiratory complications and respiratory failure,[21] the goal is for respiratory muscle training to improve respiratory muscle function and possibly improve exercise performance. Such improvement may avert or delay the development of chronic respiratory muscle fatigue and pulmonary complications.

Effect of Training on Skeletal Muscles

Training modifies the structure and function of muscle in many ways. It increases maximum oxygen consumption, the capacity to extract more oxygen (arterial-venous oxygen difference) from the lungs, the number of capillaries per muscle mass, the amount of muscle myoglobin, and the size and number of mitochondria.[15,26,30] Hence, oxygen transport from the muscle capillary bed to the mitochondrial enzymes is enhanced.[21] All of these factors are important for the improved muscle endurance that becomes possible with muscle training.

Although strength and endurance are closely related, it is clear that muscles respond differently to strength and endurance training. Strength is determined by the density of the actomyosin filaments, the number of motor neuron units activated, and the impulse frequency, which, in turn, affects the pattern of innervation, the precontraction length of the muscle fibers, and the velocity of fiber shortening.[15,26,27,30] Strength training can be accomplished by performing three to seven weekly sessions of no more than 12 maximal contractions, each lasting 2 seconds or more.[14,26] Endurance training requires exercising at a sufficient load,

TABLE 26–1
Common Conditions Associated with Respiratory Muscle Weakness

Neurologic diseases
  Myelopathies
  Myasthenia gravis
  Poliomyelitis
  Guillain-Barré syndrome
  Motor neuron diseases
Muscle diseases
  Muscle dystrophies
  Congenital and metabolic myopathies
Connective tissue disease
  Polymyositis
  Systemic lupus erythematosus
Endocrine disorders
  Thyrotoxicosis
  Cushing's disease
Metabolic disorders
  Hypophosphatemia
  Hypocalcemia
  Hypomagnesemia
  Metabolic alkalosis

speed, and duration to overload the metabolic citric acid cycle and the electron transport systems.[13,21,22] Training can improve absolute endurance, defined as the amount of work that can be performed by muscle in a given time. It has, however, little effect on relative endurance, which is defined as the duration that a number of contractions at a fixed proportion of maximum can be repeated.[12,15,18]

All muscles consist of different fiber types. Two main types have been identified based on various staining techniques. They are called fast (FT) and slow (ST) twitch fibers. These have been further subdivided into FTa and FTb fibers. With regards to metabolic activity, the ST fibers are the more oxidative and the FT fibers the more glycolytic of the two. Thus, ST fibers are mainly recruited when working at low tension and FT fibers when working at higher tension.

The distribution of FT and ST fibers in the different muscles appears to be genetically determined, and it is unclear whether interconversion between the two types takes place with training. Nevertheless, in endurance-trained subjects, there is a greater proportion of FTa fibers, whereas strength training induces a greater proportion of FTb fibers.[2,22,40] The qualitative effect of strength training seems to be to increase the cross-sectional area of the FT fibers and improve the coordination of the various motor units. The general effect of endurance training appears to be to increase circulation

(increased capillary density) and improve oxidative metabolism.[15,26,30]

VENTILATORY MUSCLE TRAINING: EFFECT ON VENTILATORY CAPACITY

The field of respiratory muscle training is relatively new, with most of the important work having been done in the last 12 years. The muscle training principles used for the respiratory muscles are similar to those used in skeletal muscle training. Because the inspiratory muscles are the most important for quiet breathing, inspiratory muscle training has received the most attention.

METHODS OF INSPIRATORY MUSCLE TRAINING

Inspiratory muscle strength can be increased by regularly performing maximal inspiratory efforts.[12,24,31] Inspiratory muscle endurance can be improved by using resistive breathing training or isocapneic hyperpnea exercise.[18,24,29]

In training with the use of inspiratory resistive loading, the resistive loads are usually applied to the inspiratory muscles for 5- to 15-minute periods two to three times per day.[1,2,18] Several simple devices employing this approach are now commercially available.[7,10,11,18,38] The response to such training is measured either as an increase in the maximal tolerable resistance over a specified period of time or as an increase in the time a given load is tolerated. With such measurements, it is imperative that breathing strategy be monitored and controlled to ensure that the training stimulus is, in fact, being applied to the respiratory muscles.[7,11] Simple inspiratory resistive loading is usually provided by the patient breathing through a narrow orifice with an adjustable diameter. Thus, the greater the flow, the greater the resistance and the inspiratory effort required. An individual using this technique can decrease the workload of breathing by decreasing flows or prolonging the inspiratory effort. With inspiratory threshold training resistive breathing, the inspiratory pressure load is determined largely by the amount of pressure needed to open a spring assembly mounted on a one-way valve.[10] Thus, with this method, the patient must overcome a set pressure before the orifice opens to permit flow. The response is assessed by changes in the amount of time a subject can create flow against the relatively fixed load.

In voluntary isocapnic hyperpnea training,[6,24,29] individuals maintain high target levels of ventilation over periods of up to 15 minutes. The response is measured by changes in the maximum sustainable ventilatory capacity, which is the maximum level of ventilation that can be sustained in this manner for 15 minutes.

EFFECTS OF RESPIRATORY MUSCLE TRAINING ON PULMONARY FUNCTION

The effect of respiratory muscle training on pulmonary function varied greatly in various studies.[3,14,16,23–25,34,37] The main parameters that have been observed to improve with respiratory muscle training are forced vital capacity (FVC), peak expiratory flow rates (PEFR), and maximum voluntary ventilation (MVV). All three parameters correlate with either respiratory muscle strength (FVC and PEFR) or endurance (MVV).

In one study, normal subjects were asked to hyperventilate maximally for 15-minute periods.[18] It was found that they could significantly improve maximum sustainable ventilatory capacity. MBV also increased from 85% to 95% after 5 weeks of 30 minutes of hyperpnea per day. In another study, Keens and coworkers[23] showed 22% improvement in maximum sustainable ventilatory capacity in normal subjects after 25 minutes per day of hyperpnea for 5 days per week for 4 weeks.

The effect of respiratory muscle training in quadriplegic patients was first demonstrated by Gross and colleagues in 1980.[18] In that study, it was found that quadriplegics are predisposed to the development of inspiratory muscle fatigue owing to reduced respiratory muscle strength and endurance. In these individuals, inspiratory muscle training significantly increased both strength and endurance. It was suggested that this might protect them from the development of acute respiratory muscle decompensation and acute respiratory failure.

Respiratory muscle strength and endurance training has also been shown to be beneficial for patients with progressive neuromuscular diseases.[13,14,18,19,24,34] Training has consistently resulted in greater improvements in respiratory muscle endurance than in strength. This is possibly because respiratory muscle remains active continuously even when placed under added loads such as during exercise, when there is concomitant cardiac impairment, or during respiratory infections. Because respiratory muscles are most likely to fail when placed under added loads, training programs should be initiated early on to prepare patients to withstand such episodes or conditions.

A specific regimen of respiratory muscle strength and endurance training was found to improve the vital capacity and the MVV by a mean of 70% for progressive muscular dystrophy and spinal muscular atrophy patients.[13,14] Because respiratory insufficiency commonly occurs during the late stages of these conditions,[8,20] it is important to use any method that might improve baseline respiratory muscle function and reserve.

In one study,[19] the effect of ventilatory muscle training by resistive breathing on the pulmonary function of patients with various neuromuscular diseases was investigated. The main findings were significant increases in both strength and endurance parameters by 70% to

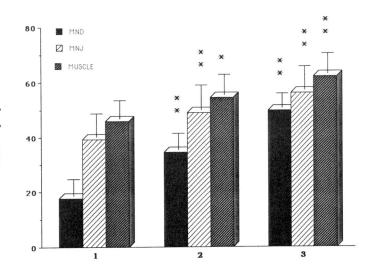

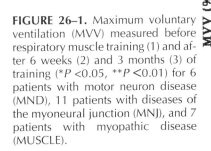

FIGURE 26–1. Maximum voluntary ventilation (MVV) measured before respiratory muscle training (1) and after 6 weeks (2) and 3 months (3) of training ($*P < 0.05$, $**P < 0.01$) for 6 patients with motor neuron disease (MND), 11 patients with diseases of the myoneural junction (MNJ), and 7 patients with myopathic disease (MUSCLE).

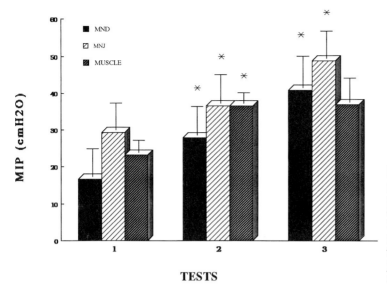

FIGURE 26–2. Maximum inspiratory pressure (MIP) measured before respiratory muscle training (1) and after 6 weeks (2) and 3 months (3) of training ($*P < 0.01$) for 6 patients with motor neuron disease (MND), 11 patients with diseases of the myoneural junction (MNJ), and 7 patients with myopathic disease (MUSCLE).

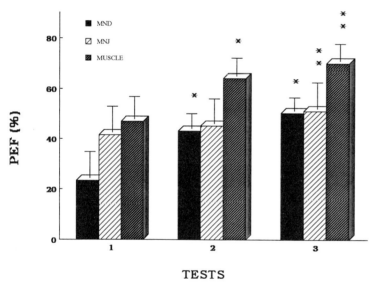

FIGURE 26–3. Peak expiratory flow rate (PEF) measured before respiratory muscle training (1) and after 6 weeks (2) and 3 months (3) of training ($*P < 0.05$, $**P < 0.01$) for 6 patients with motor neuron disease (MND), 11 patients with diseases of the myoneural juntion (MNJ), and 7 patients with myopathic disease (MUSCLE).

280%. This was reflected mainly by improvements in PEFR, MVV, and maximum inspiratory pressures (MIP). The most significant change was the improvement in MVV (an index of respiratory endurance and reserve) (Figs. 26–1, 26–2, and 26–3). In addition, the patients reported increased activities of daily living, and they experienced a subsequent reduction in the frequency of acute respiratory exacerbations.

This is not surprising because, for these patients, a small increase in the ventilatory load, such as occurs during upper airway infections, can cause acute respiratory failure.[34] It has also been demonstrated that patients with neuromuscular diseases can benefit from noninvasive

mechanical ventilatory assistance used nocturnally or for as much as 24 hours a day to improve or maintain normal arterial blood gases.[4,5] It is suggested that the mechanism by which this is effective is at least in part by resting respiratory muscles. This period of rest may also enable them to perform ventilatory muscle training more effectively during hours free of assisted ventilation. The combination of the use of rest and training has not been studied as yet, but from the author's experience it is highly effective in enhancing and maintaining ventilatory function and facilitating ventilator weaning. With improvements in daily activities and decreased fatigue, patients have been increasingly

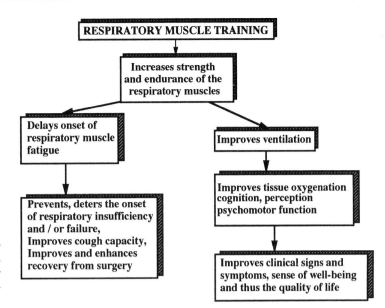

FIGURE 26–4. A schematic flow chart of the theoretic effects of ventilatory muscle training on pulmonary function and quality of life for patients with neuromuscular disease.

motivated to continue the respiratory muscle training and appear to derive further benefits long-term.

The author concludes that ventilatory muscle function can be significantly improved by inspiratory muscle training for individuals with neuromuscular disease. This can improve quality of life and most likely reduce the risk or incidence of respiratory failure and early mortality (Fig. 26–4). Such intervention should be a part of routine management for these patients.

References

1. Aldrich TK, Karpel JP: Inspiratory muscle resistive training in respiratory failure. Am Rev Respir Dis 131:461–462, 1985.
2. Andersen P, Henriksson J: Training induced changes in subgroups of human type II skeletal muscle fibers. Acta Physiol Scand 99:123–125, 1977.
3. Anderson JB, Dragsted L, Kann T, et al: Resistive breathing in severe chronic obstructive pulmonary disease, a pilot study. Scand J Respir Dis 60:151–156, 1979.
4. Bach JR: Pulmonary rehabilitation considerations for Duchenne muscular dystrophy: The prolongation of life by respiratory muscle aids. Crit Rev Phys Rehabil Med 3:239–269, 1992.
5. Bach JR, Alba AS: Pulmonary dysfunction and sleep disordered breathing as post-polio sequelae: Evaluation and management. Orthopedics 14:1329–1337, 1991.
6. Belman M, Mittman C: Ventilatory muscle training improves exercise capacity in COPD patients. Am Rev Respir Dis 120:273–280, 1980.
7. Belman MJ, Schadmehr R: A target feedback device for ventilatory muscle training. J Clin Monit 7:42–48, 1991.
8. Buchsbaum MW, Martin WA, Turino GM, Rowland LP: Chronic alveolar hypoventilation due to muscular dystrophy. Neurology 18:317–327, 1966.
9. Bye PT, Esau SA, Walley KR, et al: Ventilatory muscles during exercise in air and oxygen in normal men. J Appl Physiol 56:464–471, 1984.
10. Clanton TL, Dixon G, Drake J, et al: Inspiratory muscle conditioning using a threshold loading device. Chest 87:62–66, 1985.
11. Dekhuijzen PN, Folgerin HT, Van-Hawaarden CL: Target flow inspiratory muscle training during pulmonary rehabilitation in patients with COPD. Chest 99:128–133, 1991.
12. Delhez S, Bottin R, Thonon A, Vierset J: Modifications du diaphragme: Pression, volume maximum de l'appareil thoraco—pulmonaire aprè entrainment de muscle respiratorires par des exercises statique. Arch Int Physiol Biochim 74:335–336, 1966.
13. DiMarco AF, Kelling J, Sajovic M, et al: The effects of inspiratory resistive training on respiratory muscle function in patients with muscular dystrophy. Muscle Nerve 8:284–290, 1985.
14. Estrup C, Lyager S, Noeraa N, Olsen C: Effect of respiratory muscle training in patients with neuromuscular diseases and in normals. Respiration 50:36–43, 1986.
15. Faulkner JA: New perspectives in training for maximum performance. JAMA 205:741–746, 1968.
16. Gross D, Appelbaum A: Respiratory muscle training in health and disease in chronic pulmonary hyperinflation. In Grassino A, Rampulla C, Ambrosino N, Fracchia C (eds): Current Topics in Rehabilitation: Chronic Pulmonary Hyperinflation. New York, Springer-Verlag, 1991, pp 160–168.
17. Gross D, Grassino A, Ross D, Macklem PT: The EMG pattern of diaphragmatic fatigue. J Appl Physiol 46:1–7, 1979.
18. Gross D, Ladd HW, Riley EJ, et al: The effect of training on strength and endurance of the diaphragm in quadriplegia. Am J Med 68:27–35, 1980.
19. Gross D, Meiner Z: The effect of ventilatory muscle training on respiratory function and capacity in ambulatory and bed ridden patients with neuromuscular diseases. Monaldi Arch Chest Disease 48:322–326, 1993.
20. Guyton AC: Textbook of Medical Physiology, 5th ed. Philadelphia, WB Saunders, 1976, pp 130–147.
21. Holoszy JO: Adaptation of muscular tissue to training. Prog Cardiovasc 18:45–48, 1976.

22. Jansson E, Keijser L: Muscle adaptation to extreme endurance training. Acta Physiol Scand 100:315–324, 1977.

23. Keens TG, Krastins IRB, Wamamaker EM, et al: Ventilatory muscle endurance training in normal subjects and patients with cystic fibrosis. Am Rev Respir Dis 116:853–860, 1977.

24. Leith D, Bradley M: Ventilatory muscle strength and endurance training. J Appl Physiol 41:508–516, 1976.

25. Merrick J, Axen K: Inspiratory muscle function following abdominal weight exercises in healthy subjects. Phys Ther 61:651–656, 1981.

26. Muller EA: Influence of training and of inactivity on muscle strength. Arch Phys Med Rehabil 51:449–462, 1970.

27. Noble-Hamieson CM, Heckmatt JZ, Dubowitz V, Silverman M: Effects of posture and spinal bracing on respiratory function in neuromuscular disease. Arch Dis Child 61:178–181, 1986.

28. Panta C, Leith DE, Brown R: Maximal shortening of inspiratory muscles: Effect of training. J Appl Physiol 54:1618–1623, 1983.

29. Pardy RL, Rivington RN, Despas PJ, Macklem PT: Inspiratory muscle training compared with physiotherapy in patients with chronic airflow limitation. Am Rev Respir Dis 123:421–426, 1981.

30. Rach PJ, Burke RK: Kinesiology and Applied Anatomy: The Science of Human Movement, 6th ed. Philadelphia, Lea & Febiger, 1978, pp 349–360.

31. Reid WD, Warren CPW: Ventilatory muscle strength and endurance training in elderly subjects and patients with chronic airflow limitation: A pilot study. Physiol Can 36:305–311, 1984.

32. Rochester DF: Respiratory effects of respiratory muscle weakness and atrophy. Am Rev Respir Dis 134:1078–1093, 1986.

33. Rochester DF, Arora NS: Respiratory muscle failure. Med Clin North Am 67:573–597, 1983.

34. Rothman JG: Effects of respiratory exercises on the vital capacity and forced expiratory volume in children with cerebral palsy. Phys Ther 58:421–425, 1987.

35. Roussos CS, Fixley M, Gross D, Macklem PT: Diaphragmatic fatigue in man. J Appl Physiol Respir Environ Exerc Physiol 46:897–904, 1979.

36. Roussos CS, Macklem PT: Diaphragmatic fatigue in man. J Appl Physiol Respir Environ Exerc Physiol 43:189–197, 1977.

37. Sharp JT, Druz WS, Moisan T, et al: Postural relief of dyspnea in severe chronic obstructive pulmonary disease. Am Rev Respir Dis 122:201–211, 1980.

38. Sonne CJ, Davis JA: Increased exercise performance in patients with severe COPD following inspiratory resistive training. Chest 81:436–439, 1982.

39. Van Noord JA, Cauberghs M, Van de Woestijne KP, Demets M: Total respiratory resistance and reactance in ankylosing spondylitis and kyphoscoliosis. Eur Respir J 4:945–951, 1991.

40. Watt PW, Kelly FJ, Goldspink DF, Goldspink G: Exercise induced morphological changes in skeletal muscles of the rat. J Appl Physiol 53:1144–1151, 1982.

Dysphagia and Nutrition in Neuromuscular Disorders

27

Thiébaut Noël Willig, MD
Christian Gilardeau, MD
Marta S. Kazandjian, MA, SLP
John R. Bach, MD
Venance Varille, MD
Jean Navarro, MD
Karen J. Dikeman, MA, SLP

Dysphagia occurs in more than one-third of patients with spinal muscular atrophy (SMA),[100] in 41% of patients with myotonic dystrophy,[54,100] in at least 73% of patients with amyotrophic lateral sclerosis (ALS) before requiring ventilatory support,[62] and in virtually all patients with Duchenne muscular dystrophy (DMD) by 12 years of age.[49] Dysphagia is also the presenting sign of myasthenia gravis in neonates and in 6% to 15% of adult patients.[43] However, despite its very high prevalence, its potential for causing respiratory complications and nutritional deficits, and its role as the principal reason for tracheostomy in patients with neuromuscular disorders, the diagnosis of dysphagia is often delayed.

PHYSIOLOGY

Alimentation can be divided into prealimentary, taste and mastication, and deglutition phases. Prealimentation requires an appropriate appetite and depends on olfactory and metabolic parameters. Taste comprises differentia-

tion of saltiness, sweetness, bitterness, and sourness. Mastication involves the rotary action of the jaw in three planes.

Normal deglutition involves the coordinated function of the structures of the oral cavity, pharynx, larynx, and esophagus. Until 1 year of age, deglutition is characterized by suction, propulsion, deposition in the posterior pharynx, and initiation of the pharyngeal and esophageal reflexes that complete the swallowing process (*primary deglutition*). After 1 year of age, deglutition occurs 600 times per day and involves a bolus being formed in the mouth, chewed if necessary, and then propelled posteriorly to a point where the pharyngeal swallowing reflex is triggered (*secondary deglutition*). This reflex involves the circular, superior, medial, and inferior constrictor muscles, creating a peristaltic action to move the bolus through the pharynx to the esophagus. The muscle fibers of the pharyngeal constrictors are attached to the pterygoid plates of the sphenoid bone, the base of the tongue, jaw, soft palate, and larynx. The fibers attached to the thyroid cartilage of the larynx form the pyriform sinuses and end at the cricopharyngeus muscle, the pharyngoesophageal juncture. The cricopharyngeal fibers are contracted at rest to prevent gastric reflux and to keep air from entering the esophagus during respiration. During deglutition, the muscle relaxes to allow the bolus to flow into the esophagus, then returns to rest in a contracted state. The speed of the pharyngeal swallow is judged by observing laryngeal elevation.

Finally, esophageal peristalsis moves the bolus past the gastric sphincter into the stomach. The esophagus is 23 to 25 cm long and has striated muscle in the upper third, which is often most involved in myopathic conditions, striated and smooth muscle in the middle third, and smooth muscle in the lower third. The swallowing reflex and esophageal action are involuntary.

PATHOPHYSIOLOGY

All phases of swallowing can be affected by neuromuscular pathology. Children with DMD, SMA, and other pediatric neuromuscular diseases have difficulty achieving secondary deglutition due to muscle weakness and abnormal morphology of facial bony structures, which often includes shortening of the ramus of the mandible[4] and hypomobility and dysplasia of the temporomandibular joint. Spinal instrumentation and fusion to reverse spinal deformity, common in this patient population, may also hamper swallowing by altering the position and decreasing the flexibility of the neck.

For most individuals with neuromuscular dysfunction, initial difficulties are usually limited to mastication and decreased temporomandibular joint motion, and for pediatric patients, dental malocclusion and prognathism. Even in the presence of severe impairment of mastication, however, the risk of aspiration is very low when deglutition is intact. Weakness of lip and cheek muscles and tongue elevators become more pronounced subsequently. The often-present excessive cervical lordosis stretches the muscles that close the jaw and retract the mandible. The upper lip retracts, and neck flexion and rotation are reduced. Sitting balance difficulties, which can also hamper deglutition, are also affected by the presence of scoliosis and cervical and lumbar hyperlordosis.

Initially, patients complain of difficulties managing liquids. Although semisolid food facilitates bolus formation, it increases the risk of depositing residue. Pharyngeal swallowing reflexes are eventually delayed because of impaired elevation and retraction of the tongue.

Compensatory neck flexion and extension movements are used to trigger the reflex; however, reduction in flexion and rotation of the cervical spine eventually hamper this.

With advanced disease, aspiration of food and saliva, weight loss, and pulmonary complications occur (Fig. 27–1).[38] Appetite may also be decreased by diminished appreciation of taste, impaired emptying of the stomach, and salivary insufficiency. Anosmia may be linked to repeated nasal infections or may be part of the clinical picture of certain conditions. Because air does not pass through the upper airway, ventilator use via an indwelling tracheostomy tube prevents patients from smelling and therefore appreciating the taste of food. The chronic pathogenic bacterial colonization associated with indwelling tracheostomy tubes and associated impairment of physiologic airway secretion mechanisms may also alter taste. Fear of food aspiration can also decrease appetite.

CLINICAL ASSESSMENT

The team members who are vital in the assessment process are the treating physician, speech pathologist, radiologist, otolaryngologist, dietitian, and, in some cases, occupational therapist. The assessment process includes clinical, fiberoptic, and videofluoroscopic evaluations of swallowing.

Symptoms and Signs

Dysphagia symptoms should be anticipated as oromotor function deteriorates. A proactive approach depends on the patient learning to recognize the symptoms so that the use of compensatory techniques can permit oral feedings to be tolerated as long as possible. Because difficulties are often underestimated by the patient, the history should also be obtained from the family.

The patient and family are queried about difficulties in chewing and swallowing. Factors triggering or aggravating eating difficulties are determined, such as food textures, states, consistencies, and bolus sizes. Associated difficulties with salivation, breathing, endurance, or airway secretions are explored.

Evaluation

The *mouth* is examined for caries, gingivitis, ulcers, or other lesions. In addition, tongue size

Respiratory complications
per patient per year

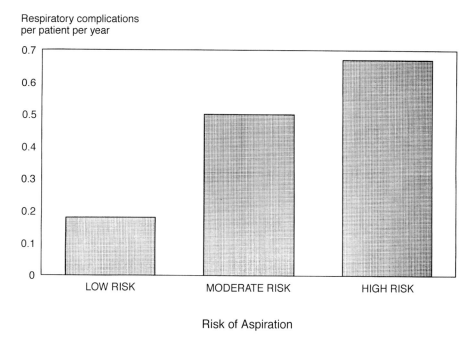

Risk of Aspiration

FIGURE 27–1. Risk of pulmonary complications from airway congestion as a function of aspiration risk.

can be assessed and classified as either normal, mildly enlarged (an imprint of the teeth can be seen on the lateral surface), or markedly enlarged (tongue protrudes through the incisors). The masseter, pterygoideus, soft palate, lips, tongue, and buccal muscles and the ability to create intraoral pressures are specifically evaluated.

The *orthopedic* examination includes assessment of contractures and the general morphology of the jaw and mandibular angle. Temporomandibular joint mobility, dental occlusion, lateral jaw movement and opening, and the power of labial occlusion are assessed. Neck stability and mobility, especially flexion and extension, are assessed. Posture, positioning, and sitting balance and stability are evaluated and optimized.

Patients with DMD and ALS commonly report impaired *smell* and *taste*. Therefore, olfaction and taste as well as pharyngeal, gag, and cough reflexes are evaluated.

The patient's ability to manage a variety of food textures and consistencies is evaluated during eating. The ability to masticate food and to move it through the oral cavity is documented. Repeated neck flexion and extension may be observed as the patient attempts to facilitate movement of the bolus posteriorly. Oral reten-

tion may be observed in the lateral sulci. Inadequate velopharyngeal seal can cause nasal regurgitation.

Although the clinical examination primarily assesses the oral phase of the swallow, repeated requests for sips of fluid with each mouthful suggest pharyngeal retention as the patient must alternate swallowing liquids and solids. It is also possible to judge the speed of the pharyngeal swallow by observing laryngeal elevation.

The presence of airway congestion can be highly suggestive of *aspiration*. Other symptoms suggestive of aspiration in the patient with bulbar muscle dysfunction include coughing, throat clearing, choking, nasal speech, wet vocal quality following the swallow, sudden episodes of dyspnea, and spitting. Aspiration is often first recognized when the patient experiences acute respiratory distress from associated airway encumberment.[38] This is because dysphagia and aspiration are usually not recognized early on and are compensated by the patient taking greater care during the early phases of swallowing and by optimizing food preparation. Furthermore, because the patient often has lost the ability to feed himself or herself by this time, the clumsy efforts of care providers also contribute in this regard.

Cervical auscultation is done to listen for the passage of the bolus through the pharynx in relation to airway opening.[96] Aspiration of liquids can occur without an accompanying cough (silent aspiration). Aspiration can also result from pooling of foods in the vallecula and pyriform sinuses when the initiation of pharyngeal swallow is delayed. This can occur for all food consistencies and may be accompanied by a laryngeal cough.

When a tracheostomy tube is present, a *methylene blue* or *vegetable dye test* is performed to assess for gross aspiration. Several drops of the colored substance are placed into a glass of water, and after the patient drinks the water, mechanical insufflation-exsufflation (MI-E) is performed through the tracheostomy tube with the cuff inflated. If any of the fluid was aspirated, the suctionate is correspondingly colored (positive methylene blue test), and further assessment of aspiration is undertaken with a videofluoroscopic barium swallow study. If an inflated tracheostomy tube cuff is being used for intermittent positive pressure ventilation (IPPV), the methylene blue test should first be performed with the cuff inflated, and then if the test is negative, the cuff is deflated, colored fluid again swallowed, then the cuff reinflated, and MI-E repeated to observe the suctionate. Care must be taken to increase the ventilator-delivered volumes to compensate for insufflation leakage out of the mouth and nose when deflating a tracheostomy tube cuff.[11] Shortness of breath should be avoided or swallowing cannot be accurately assessed.

When a cuff is initially deflated to continue tracheostomy IPPV with a deflated cuff, MI-E is used through the tube prior to cuff deflation. Once the cuff is deflated, after a few seconds, it is briefly reinflated for another short course of MI-E to eliminate the airway secretions that were resting on the cuff.[9] Airway suctioning is used if an In-Exsufflator (J.H. Emerson Company, Cambridge, MA) is not available.

A *fiberoptic evaluation* of swallowing provides objective information regarding airway protection capabilities. Airway patency, glottic competence, vocal cord mobility, the presence of any infectious or traumatic lesions, and any pooling of food or secretions are observed. Direct visualization of the pharynx and larynx is done during swallowing.[56] Methylene blue or vegetable dye in fluid or food is usually given to the patient while the scope is in position, and if aspiration is present, the dyed material is detected in the airway before or after the swallow takes place. Although useful, the fiberoptic study provides only limited information about the swallowing process.

The most comprehensive evaluation tool for swallowing assessment is *videofluoroscopy,* also known as a modified barium swallow or a swallowing study. Videofluoroscopy permits the identification of impaired propulsion of food, stasis with pooling of food in the pharynx, vallecula, or pyriform sinuses, and the presence of aspiration. It is especially useful for identifying aspiration of fluids with the head in high-risk positions, such as with the neck in hyperextension, due to fatigue or loss of concentration.

During videofluoroscopy, therapeutic maneuvers and postural changes are evaluated to optimize the patient's ability to swallow different food consistencies. The examination is typically carried out with a variety of barium-coated foods that include the most difficult for the patient to manage. A range of consistencies and bolus sizes are used. Patients who demonstrate inadequate airway protection for thin liquids or foods of other consistencies during videofluoroscopy are instructed to use liquid thickening agents. Oral preparation, bolus propulsion, pharyngeal passage of the bolus, location and quantity of pharyngeal retention, speed of initiation of the swallowing reflex, presence and timing of aspiration, and esophageal motility disorders can be documented. A more extensive esophagram may be recommended.

During videofluoroscopy, management techniques are tested for particular impairments. For example, if aspiration occurs before the initiation of the pharyngeal reflex because of weakness of the base of the tongue, the patient may be instructed to, and helped to, flex the neck. This has the effect of widening the vallecula (the space between the base of tongue and the epiglottis) so that more material can collect there until the pharyngeal swallow is triggered and the bolus is cleared. The technique also serves to elevate the larynx slightly, thus enhancing airway protection. Information is also obtained regarding pharyngeal peristalsis and possible cricopharyngeal malfunction. The last, however, is probably rare. Because videofluoroscopy captures swallowing function for only a short period, it may underestimate swallowing impairment. False-negative examinations can also be caused by poor patient concentration, anxiety, or fatigue.

Other useful tests include oximetry during the swallowing test and while eating, assessment of peak cough flows with a peak flow meter (Access Peak Flow Meter, Health Scan, Cedar Grove, N.J.),[12] manometry, pH monitoring for gastroesophageal reflux and dysfunction,[25] scintigraphy to quantify aspiration,[88] and ultrasound of the oral cavity to observe tongue function.

TREATMENT FOR DYSPHAGIA

Integral to the management program are patient education and dietary counseling. The patient is counseled to widen the variety of food flavors and odors to find greater pleasure in eating. Flexibility regarding etiquette is emphasized. Soft, easy-to-chew foods reduce fatigue. Caution is taken to avoid large mouthfuls. Food preparation must be done with the patient's limitations in mind. Numerous groups have made practical suggestions for the management of alimentation difficulties, and books of adapted recipes have been produced.[1] The care providers are given a list of foods to avoid.

Pureed foods are often not recommended because they fall apart and are hard to swallow. Soft foods such as custards tend to hold together and can be swallowed as a single bolus. Sticky foods, such as white bread, and substances that combine with saliva to create thick mucus, such as milk products and chocolate, should be avoided. Pills should be placed in gelatin cubes or custard to be swallowed as a single bolus.[28] Because a patient may fatigue during a large meal, and abdominal distention may be associated with delayed gastric emptying and dyspnea, more frequent and smaller meals may need to be recommended. Liquids often give the greatest difficulties because they require greater oropharyngeal skill to prevent aspiration than solids.

As dysphagia progresses, it is especially important to monitor the nutritional value and caloric adequacy of meals. Caregivers are also taught to observe for the symptoms and signs of aspiration. They are taught oximetry screening for aspiration as part of the respiratory muscle aid protocol.[10] When the gag reflex is diminished, an orogastric tube can be placed for each meal. Patients have passed these tubes for 6 months or more, up to five times a day, without apparent ill effect.[28]

Oral motor exercises and positioning devices to provide proper head and trunk support may be helpful. Cervical spine and temporomandibular joint contractures are minimized by range-of-motion exercises. If present, airway and nasal congestion, sinusitis, dyspnea, and fatigue should be treated. The patient is also counseled regarding future therapeutic options to facilitate future cooperation.

Factors aggravating aspiration are determined, and corrective therapy is initiated. Before eating, pooled saliva in the vallecula is cleared (Fig. 27–2). Cricopharyngeal myotomy has been used to decrease pyriform sinus and vallecula pooling.[28,55] This procedure is useful when there is a defect in relaxation of the superior sphincter of the esophagus with conservation of sufficient pharyngeal propulsion to carry the food to the back of the throat. Several groups have proposed orthodontic treatment or maxillofacial surgery for mandibular deformations and problems with dental articulation secondary to DMD or myotonic dystrophy,[68] but there is little experience with these procedures.

Seat belts should be loosened to decrease the risk of gastroesophageal reflux. Generally, the

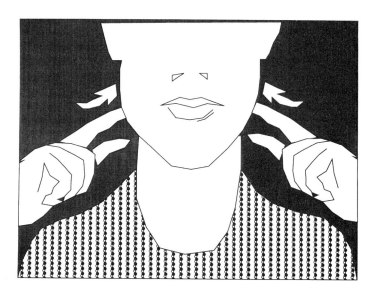

FIGURE 27–2. Clearing of the pharynx.

patient should be seated upright at 90° and the neck flexed approximately 30 to 40°. Repeated head flexion and extension to trigger the pharyngeal swallow reflex can be facilitated and fatigue reduced by having the patient lean his or her head against a headrest. Upper extremity assistive devices are introduced, including robotics,[14] to delay or eliminate the need for attendant care for feeding. This step can be important because the patient is often reluctant to resort to another's assistance for eating, which may contribute to malnutrition. Because manually assisted coughing can cause gastroesophageal reflux when the stomach is not empty, if aspiration or airway congestion occurs, mechanically assisted coughing can be critical to clear the airway.

Patients' ventilatory insufficiency is rarely recognized and treated before tachypnea and dyspnea hamper swallowing efforts. Weight loss correlates with swallowing impairment (Fig. 27–3). Weight almost invariably increases once adequate ventilatory assistance is provided. The use of noninvasive IPPV facilitates swallowing efforts, but the patient must be trained to coordinate the assisted breathing with swallowing. When tracheostomy IPPV is used, an inflated tracheostomy tube cuff anchors the strap muscles in the neck, hampering laryngeal elevation and neck rotation.[20,60] This results in reduced glottic closure and increased laryngeal penetration, increasing the chances of aspiration. Interference with relaxation of the cricopharyngeal sphincter, compression of the esophagus, and changes in intratracheal pressure can add to the problem.[20,60]

Many patients maintain adequate nutrition by intake of high-calorie thick liquid food supplements alone and have little or no aspiration despite severe bulbar muscle dysfunction. When full nutrition and hydration can no longer be taken by oral feedings, gastrostomy must be considered. Psychologic support should be provided. After a gastrostomy tube is placed, it is regularly evaluated for signs of obstruction, rigidity, or deterioration, and it is changed regularly.

Most commonly, the use of enteral nutrition does not preclude continuing some oral feedings, particularly with selected food consistencies in small quantities. Oximetry monitoring is used to ensure rapid detection of significant food aspiration and to monitor its elimination by manually or mechanically assisted coughing methods. MI-E should be used after every few swallows and for every aspiration-triggered oxyhemoglobin desaturation until the aspirated material has been eliminated and the oxyhemoglobin saturation returns to normal.

In general, noninvasive respiratory aid alternatives to tracheostomy are effective until severe

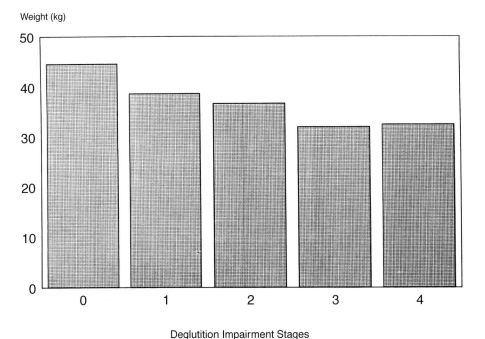

FIGURE 27–3. Weight as a function of deglutition impairment stage.

bulbar muscle dysfunction results in ongoing aspiration of food and saliva. When aspiration causes a decrease in oxyhemoglobin saturation baseline below 95% despite optimal use of assisted ventilation and coughing methods, bronchial mucus and food pooling result in episodes of pneumonia, and the prognosis is guarded. This is true whether or not the patient has an indwelling tracheostomy tube.

Attempts to decrease saliva production can include the use of small doses of amitriptyline (10 mg every 8 hours). Anticholinergic agents have not proved to be useful. Transtympanic sectioning of the corda tympani and tympanic plexus and parotid duct ligation,[28] procedures that can be done under local anesthesia, can reduce salivary production. When ongoing aspiration of saliva causes frequent choking and vocal cord dysfunction precludes verbal communication, whether or not ventilatory assistance is needed, tracheostomy and closure of the larynx can resolve the choking and aspiration.[8]

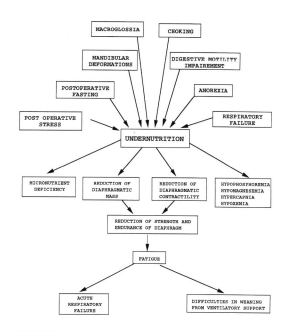

FIGURE 27–4. The consequences of undernutrition.

CONSEQUENCES OF DYSPHAGIA ON NUTRITION

Dysphagia-associated nutritional deficiencies are very common but rarely diagnosed early, and their management for patients with neuromuscular disorders is often considered to be of secondary importance. The consequences of malnutrition, however, can be severe on locomotion and respiratory function as well as on other bodily systems (Fig. 27–4). Even in individuals without neuromuscular disorders, severe malnutrition alone can lead to atrophy of respiratory muscles and hypercapnic coma.

Malnutrition can cause a reduction in the ventilatory response to hypoxia[15,30] and hypercapnia.[5] The pulmonary parenchyma can also exhibit lesions that are directly related to malnutrition[91] and to its effect on decreasing the synthesis of alveolar surfactant.[79] Humoral and cellular immunity are also altered,[15,63,67] and there is an increase in bacterial adhesion in the lower respiratory tract.[69] Undernutrition also reduces the diameter of the diaphragm's type 2 fibers and, to a lesser extent, its type 1 fibers,[17,58] resulting in loss of muscle mass.[2] Diaphragm force, contractility,[78] and endurance are decreased.[3,53]

Specific nutritional deficiencies can also have repercussions on respiratory function. Hypophosphatemia, which can be due to malnutrition or rapid glucose loading, can cause acute respiratory insufficiency or difficulty in weaning from assisted ventilation.[6] Fatty acid status, particularly the φ-3: φ-6 polyunsaturate ratio, can also influence respiratory function. Similarly, excessive carbohydrate intake can increase carbon dioxide production. For patients whose ventilatory status can not be improved, it has been recommended to increase the amount of energy derived from lipids to up to 55% of total caloric intake, but this maneuver can cause liver steatosis and pulmonary lipid deposition. Conversely, it has recently been shown that carbon dioxide production is increased more by high caloric intake than by a high percentage of carbohydrate in the diet,[92] especially if vitamin E tissue levels are low. Obesity, frequently encountered in some neuromuscular diseases, should also be avoided. It can compromise both ventilatory dynamics and the mechanisms of central regulation of spontaneous ventilation.[83]

ANTHROPOMETRIC TECHNIQUES AND MEASUREMENT OF BODY COMPOSITION

Anthropometry and reference methods for the measurement of body composition permit a precise description of normal growth and provide criteria for defining obesity and malnutrition. The situation is much more complex for neuromuscular diseases because they primarily affect the muscle mass, often during the growth period. In addition, height measurements can be imprecise, and it may be unreliable to correlate them with normal values, especially for patients with back deformities. Alternate measurements have been suggested: arm span, single arm length, and knee height.[90] Although the measurement of arm span permits prediction of height in childhood scolioses in general,[35] it does not seem to be applicable to individuals with DMD.[64]

Weighing the patient, especially the wheelchair-bound patient, is too often neglected, but it is the only means of detecting weight changes that can signal nutritional imbalance. A double weighing technique or use of weighing chairs that permit weighing of a patient while sitting may be necessary. Normal weight charts are not applicable to children with neuromuscular disease. The proposed mean values and standard deviations do not take into account disease-associated reduction of muscle mass. Specific weight charts for children with neuromuscular disease have only been described for DMD (Fig. 27–5).[41]

Skinfold thickness measurements are commonly used to estimate fat and fat-free body mass. Although the subcutaneous body fat may theoretically be represented by the adipose layer measured at the usual sites, there is often a peri- and intramuscular lipid infiltrate in dystrophic diseases that is not taken into account by these measures. Therefore, graphs[23,86] relating skinfold measurements as a function of age for physically intact children[35,80,93,99] and adults[19] must be used with caution.

Numerous techniques have been proposed to obtain precise measures of body composition. Table 27–1 summarizes the different techniques and studies that have been conducted on children with neuromuscular diseases. Magnetic resonance imaging and body impedance analysis are of particular interest. MRI is probably the most precise reference technique for neuromuscular diseases, but its applicability has been limited to research protocols. Body impedance analysis may also become a useful clinical tool. Early applications have indicated that new equations need to be developed for evaluation of lean body mass for individuals with neuromuscular disorders.

CONSIDERATIONS FOR SPECIFIC NEUROMUSCULAR DISORDERS

Duchenne Muscular Dystrophy

Although various reports have described the impaired deglutition for individuals with oculopharyngeal muscular dystrophy,[22] myotonic dystrophy, dermatomyositis, and ALS,[31,60,85] little attention has been given to DMD despite its high incidence and severity. However, in 1990, Jaffe et al. demonstrated evidence of severe dysphagia in an otherwise asymptomatic population of young DMD patients.[49] Because of the high prevalence of dysphagia and malnutrition in DMD, this disorder is a good model for understanding other neuromuscular disorders. A specific weight chart for children with DMD has been devised (Fig. 27–5).

In 1991 Gilardeau proposed a *classification for dysphagia* in DMD that takes into account the characteristics of the difficulty and the type of food involved (Tables 27–2 and 27–3).[38] For mastication, denticular apposition is incomplete early on, even though the muscles of mastication remain strong until advanced age. Thus, the average age of patients with both stage 0 and stage 1 masticatory dysfunction is 17 years of age, whereas stages 2 and 3 occur much later.

The average age at each level of functional impairment for deglutition is less than that for

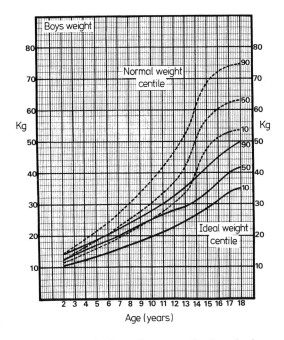

FIGURE 27–5. Ideal weight percentile chart for boys with Duchenne muscular dystrophy, based on data from Edwards et al.,[33] Edmonds et al.,[32] and Tanner et al.[93] It assumes a 4% per year decline in muscle bulk. (From Griffiths RD, Edwards RHT: A new chart for weight control in Duchenne muscular dystrophy. Arch Dis Child 63:1256–1258, 1988; with permission.)

TABLE 27–1
Techniques and Studies of Body Composition in Children with Neuromuscular Disease

Method	Parameters Analyzed	Patient Acceptance	Cost*	Precision†	Technical‡ difficulties	Duration of measurement (min)	Study (No. of Patients)
Skinfold thickness measurement	FM, LM, local measurements	Easy	1	1	1	10	Willig et al.,[99] 1993 (85)
Creatinuria	LM	Easy	1	3	4	24–72h	Edmonds et al.,[32] 1985 (20); Griggs et al.,[42] 1983 (31); Edwards et al.,[33] 1984 (21)
Body impedance analysis	TBW, ECW, ICW, LM, FM; or TBW ECM, BCM, LM, FM	Easy	2	4	1	5	—
Total body conductivity	TBW, LM, FM (ECS?)	Easy	3	4	2	10–15	—
Biphotonic absorptiometry	Calcium mass, LM, FM	Acceptable	3	4	3	15	—
Underwater weighing	LM, FM	Easy	3	4	3	60	—
Isotopic dilution (stable or radioactive)	TBW (D_2O,^{18}O, ^3H)	Easy	4	4	4	240–360	Edmonds et al.,[32] 1985 (20)
	ECW (BrNa, ^{82}Br, radioactive sulfate)		3	4	5	240	Edwards et al.,[33] 1984 (21)
Gamma camera	^{40}K, LM, FM	Easy	4	4	5	60	Edmonds et al.,[32] 1985 (20); Griggs et al.,[42] 1983 (31); Edwards et al.,[33] 1984 (21); Wagner et al.,[97] 1966 (82)
X-ray CT	Local measurements (LM, FM)	Difficult	4	?	5	Variable	Edwards et al.,[33] 1984 (21); Jones et al.,[51] 1983 (43)
MRI	FM,LM, local measurements	Easy	4	5	5	30	—
Echography	Subcutaneous fat mass (local measurements)	Easy	3	2	3	20–30	—
Neutron activation	FM, LM, calcium mass	Difficult	4	5	5	?	—

Abbreviations: LM, lean mass; FM, fat mass; TBW, total body water; ECW, extracellular water; ICW, intracellular water; BCM, body cell mass; ECM, extracellular mass.
*Cost is rated on a scale from 1 (low) to 4 (high).
†Precision and technical difficulty are rated on a scale from 1 (low) to 5 (high).

TABLE 27–2
Functional Classification of Masticatory Impairment

Stage 0	No difficulty—intact ability to bite, crunch, and tear
Stage 1	Little difficulty—moderate difficulty in biting; relatively intact crunching, munching, and tearing
Stage 2	Moderate difficulty—loss of functional biting and crunching; can tear bread
Stage 3	Severe difficulty—unable to bite, crunch, and tear; can malaxate and mix in the mouth

TABLE 27–3
Functional Classification of Deglutition Impairment

Stage 0	No Difficulty
Stage 1	Little difficulty—must exclude hard or large pieces of solids
Stage 2	Moderate difficulty—must exclude thin liquids and hard solids; aspiration rare
Stage 3	Considerable difficulty—alimentation limited to blended and pureed foods and moist bread; occasional aspiration
Stage 4	Great difficulty—alimentation limited to thick liquids; aspiration frequent

the corresponding stage for impaired mastication. Deglutition can be functional despite complete neck instability. The risk of pulmonary complications correlates with deglutition impairment (Fig. 27–6). With moderate or stage 2 impairment of deglutition, the risk of aspiration is related to associated masticatory dysfunction, types of foods used, care with which the patient eats, and any associated alimentary tract pathology.

Jaffe et al. found that by mean age 11 years, 8 months, all patients had significant dysphagia.[49] Difficulties included abnormalities of temporomandibular joint motion, dental malocclusion, prognathism, and cough and swallowing impairment. Moderate swallowing dysfunction appeared between ages 9 and 18 with muscle deficits predominating in the lip and cheek muscles and tongue elevators. The muscles of the soft palate and masticatory apparatus were relatively preserved until advanced age. Masticatory muscle dynamometry demonstrated a highly functional mean force of 5.4 kg at age 18, and this strength was relatively well retained subsequently. By age 15, however, head instability due to neck flexor weakness created difficulties. Prognathism was common, whereas retrognathism appeared to be rare.

By age 18, osseous asymmetry of the jaw is seen. The protrusion of the mandible, often seen in these patients, seems to be associated with macroglossia and weakness of the pterygoideus and superior constrictors of the pharynx. Osseous and articular malformations lead to malocclusion with only posterior dental apposition. Temporomandibular joint motion is limited and jaw opening is reduced to 3 cm (67% of normal). In contrast to commonly held notions, only 30% of DMD patients have macroglossia by age 18. Salivation is diminished and jaw closure is limited by articular limitations.

Advanced involvement occurs after age 18.[39] Dysphagia symptoms, weight loss, and aspiration become common at this point. DMD patients' ventilatory insufficiency is also rarely recognized and treated before tachypnea decreases oral phase time and respiratory fatigue further hampers swallowing efforts. Weight loss correlates with increasing impairment of deglutition. When the patient is at the point of requiring ventilatory support, weight is down to a mean of 70 lbs.[13] For individuals with DMD, the dysphagia symptoms are eased and weight increases once hypoventilation is diagnosed and treated by noninvasive IPPV. Very few DMD patients, even after 10 or more years of ventilator use, develop such severe dysphagia as to require a gastrostomy tube, and virtually no DMD patients require tracheostomy. Only 1 of our 52 DMD patients (mean age, 30 years) who have benefited from ventilatory assistance for a mean of 10 years (range, 2–24 years) required an indwelling gastrostomy tube, and 1 of 82 DMD ventilator-users required an indwelling tracheostomy tube. Many patients reach the point, however, of subsisting on thick hypercaloric fluids and requiring long periods to complete each liquid meal. If adequate caloric intake cannot be maintained in this manner, placement of a gastrostomy tube is warranted. For DMD patients, effective airway clearance can almost always be achieved by the use of manually and mechanically assisted coughing.[7,9,10]

Abnormalities in Body Composition in DMD

Important early changes in body composition have been correlated with abnormal utilization of substrates. An abnormally elevated fasting respiratory quotient (RQ) has been found by gas exchange measurements. There is preferential glucose utilization and poor lipid mobilization.[44,95] Glucose intolerance was first noted by Haymonds et al. during a 30-hour fast-

Respiratory complications per
patient per year

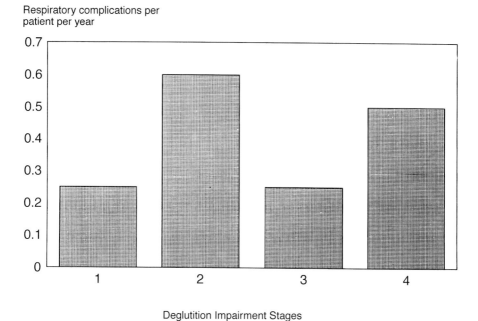

Deglutition Impairment Stages

FIGURE 27–6. Risk of pulmonary complications from airway congestion as a function of deglutition impairment stage.

ing blood glucose test, although insulin levels tended to be slightly higher in DMD patients than in controls.[46] An oral charge of glucose in animal muscular dystrophy models was followed by normal insulin secretion, but blood glucose normalization tended to be slightly slower.[66] In vitro, DePirro et al. found that receptor sensitivity to insulin was normal in DMD, but the number of receptors per cell was decreased.[29] In a study of glycolysis pathways, muscle cells from DMD patients, female carriers, and controls were incubated with glucose, and end products of metabolism were measured. It appeared that glucose was converted to fructose through the glucitol pathway. As a result, lactate formation was decreased and lipogenesis was accelerated in DMD boys and female carriers compared to controls,[34] but no major abnormality of blood glucose levels was found.

Our data indicate that the blood lipid profile of DMD patients appears normal. The substrate oxidation rate calculated from gas exchange measurements indicates poor fasting lipid mobilization at rest. During a 30-hour fast, ketone bodies increased as blood glucose decreased, testifying to the integrity of the mitochondrial enzymatic pathway. Increased ketone bodies are found during the end stages of any diseases with major muscle atrophy.[70] Abnormally high lipid synthesis from glucose has been found in vitro,[34] and decreased triglyceride mobilization, due to

the lack of physical exercise, may contribute to an increase in the fat mass of DMD patients.

Muscle biopsies have been used to measure the rate of muscle loss per year in DMD patients.[42,98] Although protein synthesis is normally increased during the first years of life, protein turnover using stable isotopes has been found to be decreased shortly afterward.[76] In fasting states, glyconeogenesis from alanine is low compared to that in healthy controls, perhaps because of low muscle mass.[46] No major protein catabolism has been observed in overweight DMD patients on a low-calorie diet.[33] Several abnormalities of body composition in DMD have now been thoroughly described. In addition to the muscular atrophy linked to the deficit in dystrophin, there is a lipid infiltrate in the muscles, representing up to 80% of the surface of sections of the triceps, and a replacement fibrosis, representing 26% to 70% of the muscular zones that have not been lipid-infiltrated.[51]

Energy Metabolism in DMD

Energy balance can be evaluated by measuring food intake, energy expenditure, and substrate oxidation rate. Food intake is usually recorded for 3 consecutive days. Although the best method would be to weigh the meal before and after eating and analyze the composition of a paired meal by bomb calorimetry, such studies are rare. Most of the time, dietitians estimate intake by using spoonful and glass measures of food with known caloric content. Average caloric intakes were generally found to be lower in patients than in controls, even in overweight patients. For example, caloric intakes in DMD patients were 1800 kcal/day in 9- to 13-year-olds compared to 2000±300 kcal/day for healthy controls.[44] The caloric intakes of older malnourished patients were 1000 to 1200 kcal/day.[72] The percentage of calories from protein was 14% or more of the total daily caloric intake, or about normal.[73]

Total daily energy expenditure is the sum of resting energy expenditure (REE), thermic effect of feeding (TEF), and energy expenditure for activity (EEA). Usually, REE represents 60% of total energy expenditure; TEF, 10%; and EEA, 30%. In patients with neuromuscular disease, reduced activity without decreased energy intake is probably the major cause of obesity, but uncertainty remains concerning the real value of REE and TEF and the possibility of their adapting to changes in caloric intake and physical activity. REE and TEF can be measured by open-circuit indirect calorimetry under a ventilated hood. Energy expenditure is calculated from gas exchange measurements and urinary nitrogen elimination using either the Ben-Porat or Weir formula.[50]

The REE of 7- to 9-year-old DMD patients with normal weight, who were still walking, was 1300±300 kcal/day and was similar to that for healthy controls. TEF after a mixed meal was similar in patients and in controls, with 60 cal/kcal ingested for patients and 52 cal/kcal ingested for controls.[95] Mean REE of 9- to 13-year-old children was 1233 kcal/day in overweight DMD patients and 1140 kcal/day in nonobese DMD patients, whereas REE in controls was 1313 kcal/day.[44] The REE of older, anorexic, malnourished DMD patients was 900±100 kcal/day.[72] The REE per kilogram of fat-free mass estimated in DMD patients from deuterium dilution space[95] or by body impedance analysis,[44] was greater than or equal to that in healthy controls.

Energy metabolism during physical exercise has been studied using ^{31}P-MRI.[16] DMD patients and female carriers were compared to healthy controls. They were asked to move a finger while ^{31}P metabolism and pH variation were measured before, during, and after movements. No major abnormality was observed, and mitochondrial function was apparently normal. The only anomalies observed were slower recovery and higher intracellular pH in patients than in controls. Data on REE are not yet available.

Dietary Recommendations

Obesity occurs in up to 44% of boys with DMD by age 13.[99] It is essential to warn the children and their families of this propensity and help them to achieve weight stabilization, notably by using the ideal weight curve adapted for DMD as a guideline (Fig. 27–5).[41] Excessive weight gain decreases mobility, complicates every day care, and can exacerbate ventilatory insufficiency. There is at present no simple method to predict the energy requirements of boys with DMD, except for the following equation which depicts spontaneous energy intake during periods of weight stability, especially for adolescent and young adult DMD patients[40]:

$$\text{Daily energy intake (kcal)}$$
$$= 2000 - \text{age (in yrs)} \times 50$$

Once obesity has set in, many physicians hesitate to recommend an overly restrictive diet for fear of aggravating muscle atrophy by relative fasting. However, surveillance of the body composition of two patients with very severe caloric restrictions did not demonstrate any deleterious effects on either body composition or muscular function.[33] Thus, it seems reasonable in practice to advise a moderate reduction in caloric intake that would lead to a monthly weight loss of 2 kg for obese patients with neuromuscular disorders.

For DMD patients, *malnutrition* begins at age 13 and affects 44% of young adults.[99] It is frequently unrecognized because of the regular progression of muscle atrophy and orthopedic, respiratory, and cardiac consequences of the disease. Initially, the main cause of malnutrition is the difficulty in utilizing cutlery, preparing the food, and bringing it to the mouth. This is caused by the combination of weakness and hand deformities that are frequently neglected.[97] Surgical correction of scoliosis may worsen the situation by increasing the distance between the head and hands, because of the postoperative fasting period and major blood losses (0.5 to 1.5 times blood volume), and because of hypercatabolism due to pain.

Chronic *ventilatory insufficiency* may also contribute to a defect in utilization of energy substrates. In this case, the restoration of normal blood gases, rather than an increase in caloric intake, can correct the problem.

The role of dystrophin deficiency-associated abnormalities in smooth muscle is unclear despite the occurrence of cases of chronic intestinal pseudo-obstruction.[57] Effects on the stomach may lead to two phenomena: a delay in gastric emptying that can affect the absorption of medication as well as food,[17] and repeated episodes of acute gastric dilatation requiring emergency gastric aspiration and intravenous rehydration.

Brown adipose fat is usually encountered in human neonates and in some species of rodents. It facilitates nonshivering thermogenesis. It is characterized by a high content of mitochondria and the presence of a decoupling enzyme that is responsible for massive heat production from energy substrates. An excess of brown adipose tissue was found in 12 young DMD adults who died from respiratory insufficiency.[48] Thus, a relative increase in energy expenditure can be another explanation for undernutrition in older DMD patients.

Spinal Muscular Atrophy

SMA is a disease with wide variability in severity and progression. Severe type 1 SMA neonates are ventilator-dependent and have virtually total bulbar muscle dysfunction in the neonatal period. Mild type 3 SMA patients begin to develop generalized weakness as young adults, and bulbar musculature remains functional throughout life.

More than one-third of SMA patients do not attain or lose the ability to bring food to the mouth.[100] Severe facial and bulbar muscle weakness and orthodontic deformities complicate the problem. Jaw opening sometimes becomes limited to 3 mm or less. Utilization of a neck collar to stabilize the cervical spine, a common practice for SMA, can also cause temporomandibular joint ankylosis.

Swallowing difficulties in type 1 patients involve both anterior and posterior swallowing phases and include weak sucking, weak or slow movements of the tongue, and stagnation of the food in the pharynx with no movement of the epiglottis.[71] The utilization of artificial alimentation techniques may be necessary in the neonatal period. Dividing the intake into small meals may improve tolerance for a child with respiratory insufficiency.[49] The possibility of the occurrence of acute gastric dilatation should also be explained to patients and their families, because this complication is not unusual in SMA, and it may be complicated by severe hypoglycemia and dehydration.

There have been few studies of body composition and energy requirements in SMA. One study confirmed the existence of growth retardation in this disorder.[94] There may also be precocious puberty due to extension of the disease to the diencephalon.[18,65] Caloric intake in 7- to 9-year-old SMA patients was found to be 1300 kcal/day or 35% lower than in healthy controls. Calories from protein were 14% of total caloric intake in both patients and controls.[95]

Mean REE in 7- to 9-year-olds with SMA measured by indirect calorimetry was 1230 ± 290 kcal/day, whereas healthy controls of the same body weight had an REE of 1330 kcal/day. TEF was 24 cal/kcal ingested in SMA patients, which was significantly lower than the control value of 52 cal/kcal ingested. Body composition was measured in both children and adolescents and showed a major increase in fat mass. REE per kilogram of fat-free mass was higher in patients than in controls.[95] Data on total daily energy expenditure are not available. The fasting respiratory quotient was lower in SMA patients than in controls.[95] These patients had poor fasting tolerance and rapidly developed ketone bodies. There is a secondary defect in the mitochondrial oxidation of fat,[45] and a low-fat diet with carnitine and coenzyme Q therapy seems to be beneficial for some patients.

Amyotrophic Lateral Sclerosis

About 73% of ALS patients experience swallowing problems prior to requiring ventilator use,[62] and a much higher percentage have difficulties subsequently. Despite differences in disease presentation, a general scheme of progression has been suggested, beginning with dysfunction of the lips and tongue, followed by dysfunction of the palate, chewing weakness, and paresis of the constrictors of the pharynx and buccinator muscles.[47] The patient may initially complain of choking on saliva while reclining or of postnasal congestion. This progresses to difficulties with liquid intake and eventually with solids, until enteral nutrition becomes necessary.

The only study on energy metabolism and caloric intake in a group of ALS patients using ventilatory assistance and enteral nutrition highlighted the problems of adjusting caloric intake, because three-quarters of the patients had excessive weight gain.[81] Perendoscopic gastrostomy seems to be the technique of choice for severely dysphagic ALS patients, at least for those who utilize ventilatory assistance.[36,78,84]

Other Neuromuscular Diseases

Swallowing difficulties also occur in other neuromuscular diseases. In *myotonic dystrophy,* alimentation problems occur in 41% of patients[100] and involve both anterior and posterior phases of swallowing.[27] Mastication problems may be caused by myotonia of the masticatory muscles, weakness, and mandibular deformation. Choking is very common and often underestimated by patients and their care providers.[100] Fluoroscopic studies can demonstrate severe difficulties during the posterior swallowing phase with irregular filling and delayed evacuation of pharyngeal recesses and deformation and ballooning of the pyriform sinuses and vallecula.[75] Silent choking can occur in these cases and may cause respiratory infections or death.[74] The pathophysiology of swallowing dysfunction seems to be mainly due to muscular weakness rather than to myotonia.[21]

Dysphagia is the first sign of *myasthenia gravis* in 6% to 15% of adult patients,[43] and the neonatal forms of disease are characterized by problems in sucking, deglutition, and weak or absent crying. Symptoms vary greatly from one patient to another and often from hour to hour. Dysphagia is frequently encountered with the first signs of acute respiratory distress. Therefore, care providers must be especially aware of these symptoms during myasthenic crises.

Dysphagia symptoms in *post-polio syndrome* include the sensation of food being retained in the hypopharynx, coughing, choking, nasal regurgitation of liquids, and nocturnal choking on secretions.[26] Radiologic studies have demonstrated tongue-pumping to initiate swallow, delayed initiation of the swallowing response, uncontrolled bolus flow into the pharynx, diminished laryngeal rise and epiglottic tilt, delayed pharyngeal constriction, diminished or absent peristaltic wave, unilateral transport of boluses through the pharynx, retention of boluses in vallecula and pyriform sinuses, "silent" laryngeal penetration, and laxity of pharyngeal walls.[24,26,59,89] Swallowing was studied specifically in 32 post-polio patients reporting recent decreases in limb strength. There were abnormalities in oropharyngeal function in 31 of the patients.[89] Thus, routine evaluation of swallowing is indicated for these patients.

Slonim et al. reported a significant improvement in muscle strength in a child with *acid maltase deficiency* after 4 months of using a high-protein diet.[87] Margolis and Hill reported an adult with severe ventilatory muscle weakness.[61] A high-protein diet (1.6 g/kg/day) together with a reduction in caloric intake appeared to induce significant improvement in respiratory function.[61] A high-protein diet may also be beneficial for other patients.

Spinal Cord Injury

Spinal cord lesions in which the region of injury extends into the brainstem can result in dysphagia; however, such individuals are rarely candidates for the use of noninvasive alternatives to tracheostomy and often have inadequate glottic control to prevent frequent aspiration of airway secretions. Individuals with C2 to C4 injury generally have adequate neck and bulbar muscle function and ability to generate assisted cough flows,[10] allowing them to use noninvasive alternatives to tracheostomy. For some, however, previous intubation and tracheostomy may have impaired glottic function, and food aspiration may preclude oral intake. For humanitarian reasons, however, it can be important to continue some oral feedings. We have succeeded in using oximetry feedback and MI-E after every few swallows to eliminate the aspirated food (Fig. 27–7).

The body composition assessment of spinal-cord-injured patients is difficult. Hydrodensito-

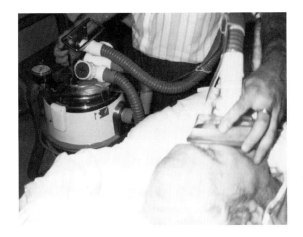

FIGURE 27–7. Seventy-two-year old man with C2 complete tetraplegia and no VFBT. He had hypomobility of the left vocal cord and severe dysphagia, which resulted in extensive aspiration of food. For humanitarian reasons, limited oral intake was permitted with the instructions to use MI-E after every few swallows to eliminate the aspirated food and reverse aspiration-induced oxyhemoglobin desaturations. When aspiration of food and airway secretions was excessive and mucus production increased, oral feeding was suspended for a few days until airway secretions (and, at times, mean oxyhemoglobin saturation levels) returned to normal.

metry was shown to lead to wrong estimations of fat-free mass.[37] Studies on short-term variation in body composition have highlighted a major increase in nitrogen excretion during the weeks after injury (235 g in 4 weeks), corresponding to a loss of 4 to 5.9 kg of muscle mass.[52] This is similar to levels observed in patients with Guillain-Barré syndrome and other acute generalized paralyses.

Body composition has also been studied for stable spinal-cord-injured patients. Most of them were found to be malnourished, with a reduction of body cell mass together with an increase in extracellular fluid,[82] caused by an infiltration of muscles by fat, water, and connective tissue. Anorexia, gastrointestinal dysfunction, and protein loss from decubitus ulcers were found to contribute to malnutrition.

In summary, dysphagia and malnutrition can cause, exacerbate, or result from ventilatory impairment. Management can be critical for the success of using noninvasive respiratory muscle aid alternatives to tracheostomy.

Acknowledgment

The authors thank Anne-Marie Brunel for typing the manuscript and Susan Cure for the English adaptation of the text.

References

1. Appel V, Calvin S, Smith G, Woehr D: Meals for Easy Swallowing. Tuscon, AZ, Muscular Dystrophy Association.
2. Arora NS, Rochester DF: Effect of body weight and muscularity on human diaphragm muscle mass, thickness and area. J Appl Physiol 52:64–70, 1982.
3. Arora NS, Rochester DF: Respiratory muscle strength and maximum voluntary ventilation in undernourished patients. Am Rev Respir Dis 125:5–8, 1982.
4. Ashby DW: Bone dystrophy in association with muscular dystrophy. BMJ 1:1486–1488, 1951.
5. Askanazi J, Rosenbaum SH, Hyman AI, et al: Effects of parenteral nutrition on ventilatory drive [abstract]. Anesthesiology 53:S185, 1980.
6. Aubier M, Murciano D, Lecocguic Y, et al: Effect of hypophosphatemia on diaphragmatic contractility in patients with acute respiratory failure. N Engl J Med 313:420–424, 1985.
7. Bach JR: Pulmonary rehabilitation considerations for Duchenne muscular dystrophy: The prolongation of life by respiratory muscle aids. Crit Rev Phys Rehabil Med 3:239–269, 1992.
8. Bach JR: Amyotrophic lateral sclerosis: Communication status and survival with ventilatory support. Am J Phys Med Rehabil 72:343–349, 1993.
9. Bach JR: Update and perspectives on noninvasive respiratory muscle aids: Part 2. The expiratory muscle aids. Chest 105:1538–1544, 1994.
10. Bach JR: Prevention of morbidity and mortality with the use of physical medicine aids. In Bach JR (ed): Pulmonary Rehabilitation: The Obstructive and Paralytic/Restrictive Pulmonary Syndromes. Philadelphia, Hanley & Belfus, 1996.
11. Bach JR, Alba AS: Tracheostomy ventilation: A study of efficacy with deflated cuffs and cuffless tubes. Chest 97:679–683, 1990.
12. Bach JR, Saporito LS: Indications and criteria for decannulation and transition from invasive to noninvasive long-term ventilatory support. Respir Care 39:515–531, 1994.
13. Bach JR, Tippett DC, McCrary MM: Bulbar dysfunction and associated cardiopulmonary considerations in polio and neuromuscular disease. J Neurol Rehabil 6:121–128, 1992.
14. Bach JR, Zeelenberg A, Winter C: Wheelchair mounted robot manipulators: Long term use by patients with Duchenne muscular dystrophy. Am J Phys Med Rehabil 69:59–69, 1990.
15. Baier H, Somani P: Ventilatory drive in normal man during semistarvation. Chest 85:222–225, 1984.
16. Barbiroly B, Funicello R, Iotti S, et al: ^{31}P-NMR spectroscopy of skeletal muscle in Becker dystrophy and DMD/BMP carriers: Altered rate of phosphate transport. J Neurol Sci 109:188–195, 1992.
17. Barohn RJ, Levine EJ, Olson JO, Mendell JR: Gastric hypomotility in Duchenne's muscular dystrophy. N Engl J Med 319:15–18, 1988.
18. Barois A, Estournet B, Duval-Beaupere G, et al: Amyotrophie spinal infantile. Rev Neurol (Paris) 145:299–304, 1989.
19. Bishop CW, Bowen PE, Richey SJ: Norms for nutritional assessment of American adults by upper arm anthropometry. Am J Clin Nutr 34:2530–2539, 1981.
20. Bonanno P: Swallowing dysfunction after tracheostomy. Ann Surg 174:29–33, 1971.
21. Bosma JF, Brodie DR: Cineradiographic demonstration of pharyngeal area myotonia in myotonic dystrophic patients. Radiology 92:104–109, 1969.
22. Bray GM: Ocular myopathy with dysphagia. Neurology 15:678–684, 1965.
23. Brook CGD: Determination of body composition of children from skinfold measurements. Arch Dis Child 46:182–184, 1971.
24. Buchholz D: Dysphagia in post-polio patients. Birth Defects 23:55–62, 1987.
25. Buchin PJ: Swallowing disorders: Diagnosis and medical treatment. Otolaryngol Clin North Am 21:663–676, 1988.
26. Coelho CA, Ferrante R: Dysphagia in postpolio sequelae: Report of three cases. Arch Phys Med Rehabil 69:634–636, 1988.
27. Cox MS, Petty J: A videofluoroscopy chair for the evaluation of dysphagia in patients with severe neuromotor disease. Arch Phys Med Rehabil 72:157–159, 1991.
28. DeLisa JA, Mikulic MA, Miller RM, Melnick RR: Amyotrophic lateral sclerosis: comprehensive management. Am Fam Pract 19:137–142, 1989.
29. DePirro R, Lauro R, Testa I, et al: Decreased insulin receptors but normal glucose metabolism in Duchenne muscular dystrophy. Science 216:311–313, 1982.
30. Doekel RC JR, Zwillich CW, Scoggin CH, et al: Clinical semi-starvation: Depression of hypoxic ventilatory response. N Engl J Med 295:358–361, 1976.
31. Donner M: Swallowing mechanism and neuromuscular disorders. Semin Roentgenol 9:273–282, 1974.
32. Edmonds CJ, Smith T, Griffiths RD, et al: Total body potassium and water, and exchangeable sodium in muscular dystrophy. Clin Sci 68:379–385, 1985.
33. Edwards RHT, Round JM, Jackson MJ, et al: Weight re-

duction in boys with muscular dystrophy. Dev Med Child Neurol 26:384–390, 1984.

34. Ellis DA: Intermediate metabolism of muscle in Duchenne muscular dystrophy. Br Med Bull 36:165–171, 1980.

35. Engstrom FM, Roche AF, Mukherjee D: Differences between arm-span and stature in white children. J Adolesc Health Care 2:19–22, 1981.

36. Gauderer MWL: Percutaneous endoscopic gastrotomy: A 10-year experience with 220 children. J Pediatr Surg 26:288–294, 1991.

37. George CM, Wells CL, Dugan NL: Validity of hydrodensitometry for determination of body composition in spinal injured subjects. Hum Biol 60:771–780, 1988.

38. Gilardeau C: Dystrophie à Évolution Rapide (stade non ambulatoire) et Troubles de la Déglutition-Mastication. Entretiens de Montpellier, Edition Masson, 1991.

39. Goldberg MH: Correction of facial skeletal deformities in two patients with facio-scapulo-humeral dystrophy. J Oral Maxillofac Surg 47:996–999, 1989.

40. Griffiths RD: Controlling weight in muscle disease to reduce the burden. Physiotherapy 75:190–192, 1989.

41. Griffiths RD, Edwards RHT: A new chart for weight control in Duchenne muscular dystrophy. Arch Dis Child 63:1256–1258, 1988.

42. Griggs RC, Forbes G, Moxley RT, Herr BE: The assessment of muscle mass in progressive neuromuscular disease. Neurology 33:158–165, 1983.

43. Grob D: Myasthenia gravis. Arch Intern Med 108:615–638, 1961.

44. Hankard R, Gottrand F, Turch K, et al: Resting energy expenditure in preadolescents with Duchenne muscular dystrophy [abstract]. J Clin Nutr 13(suppl 1):50, 1994.

45. Harpey JP, Charpentier C, Paturneau-Jouas M, et al: Secondary metabolic defects in spinal muscular atrophy type II. Lancet 336:629–630, 1990.

46. Haymonds MW, Strobel KE, Deviva DC: Muscle wasting and carbohydrate homeostasis in Duchenne muscular dystrophy. Neurology 28:1224–1231, 1978.

47. Hillel Ad, Miller R: Bulbar amyotrophic lateral sclerosis: Patterns of progression and clinical management. Head Neck 11:651–659, 1989.

48. Ito M, Sekine I, Fuji H, Ogawa M: Brown adipose tissue in Duchenne's progressive muscular dystrophy. Arch Pathol Lab Med 112:550–552, 1988.

49. Jaffe KM, Craig M, McDonald IE, Hass J: Symptoms of upper gastrointestinal dysfunction in Duchenne muscular dystrophy: Case-control study. Arch Phys Med Rehabil 71:742–744, 1990.

50. Jequier E: Assessment of energy expenditure and fuel utilization in man. Annu Rev Nutr 7:187–208, 1987.

51. Jones DA, Round JM, Edwards RHT, et al: Size and composition of the calf and quadriceps muscles in Duchenne muscular dystrophy: A tomographic and histochemical study. J Neurol Sci 60:307–322, 1983.

52. Kearns PJ, Thompson JD, Werner PC, et al: Nutritional and metabolic response to acute spinal-cord injury. JPEN 16:11–15, 1992.

53. Kelsen SG, Ference M, Kapoor S: Effects of prolonged undernutrition on structure and function of the diaphragm. J Appl Physiol 58:1354–1359, 1985.

54. Kiliaridis S: Muscle function and craniofacial morphology: A clinical study in patients with myotonic dystrophy. Eur J Orthod 11:131–138, 1989.

55. Lacau St Guilly J, Péréi S, Willig TN, et al: Swallowing disorders in muscular diseases: Functional assessment and indications of cricopharyngeal myotomy. Ear Nose Throat J 73:34–40, 1994.

56. Langmore SE, Schatz K, Olsen N: Fiberoptic endoscopic evaluation of swallowing safety: A new procedure. Dysphagia 2:216–219, 1988.

57. Leon SH, Schuffler MD, Kettler M, Rohrmann CA: Chronic intestinal pseudoobstruction as a complication of Duchenne's muscular dystrophy. Gastroenterology 90:455–459, 1986.

58. Lewis MI, Sieck GC, Fournier M, Belman MJ: Effects of nutritional deprivation on diaphragm contractility and muscle fiber size. J Appl Physiol 60:596–603, 1986.

59. Linden P, Siebens AA: Dysphagia: Predicting laryngeal penetration. Arch Phys Med Rehabil 64:281–284, 1983.

60. Logemann JA: Evaluation and treatment of swallowing disorders. San Diego, College-Hill Press, 1983, p 119.

61. Margolis ML, Hill RA: Acid maltase deficiency in an adult: Evidence for improvement in respiratory function with high-protein dietary therapy. Am Rev Respir Dis 134:328–331, 1986.

62. Mayberry JF, Atkinson M: Swallowing problems in patients with motor neuron disease. J Clin Gastroenterol 8:233–234, 1986.

63. McMurray DN, Loomis SA, Casazza LJ, et al: Development of impaired cell mediated immunity in mild and moderate malnutrition. Am J Clin Nutr 34:68–77, 1981.

64. Miller F, Koreska J: Height measurement of patients with neuromuscular disease and contractures. Dev Med Child Neurol 34:55–60, 1992.

65. Miranda-Nieves G, Campos-Castello J: Pathological findings in Werdnig-Hoffmann's disease with special remarks on diencephalic lesions. Eur Neurol 3:231–240, 1970.

66. Mokdarian A, Even PC, Decrouy A, et al: Réponse métabolique et bioénergétique au test d'hyperglycémie provoquée chez la sourir atteinte de dystrophie musculaire de Duchenne (MDX) [abstract]. In 5th Colloque National sur les Maladies Neuromusculaires. Strasbourg, France, Association Francaise contra les Myopathies, 1993.

67. Moriguchi S, Sone S, Kishino Y: Changes of alveolar macrophages in protein deficient rats. J Nutr 113:40–46, 1983.

68. Muller H, Punt-Van Manen JA: Maxillo-facial deformities in patients with dystrophia myotonica and the anaesthetic implications. J Maxillofac Surg 10:224–228, 1982.

69. Niederman MS, Merril WW, Ferranti RD, et al: Nutritional status and bacterial binding in the lower respiratory tract in patients with chronic tracheostomy. Ann Intern Med 100:795–800, 1984.

70. Nishio H, Wada H, Matsuo T, et al: Glucose, free fatty acid and ketone body metabolism in Duchenne muscular dystrophy. Brain Dev 12:390–402, 1990.

71. Nutman J, Nitizan M, Grunebaum M: Swallowing disturbances in Werdning-Hoffmann disease. Harefuah 101:301–303, 1990.

72. Okada K, Manabe S, Sakamoto S, et al: Predictions of energy intake and energy allowance of patients with Duchenne muscular dystrophy and their validity. J Nutr Sci Vitaminol (Tokyo) 38:155–161, 1992.

73. Okada K, Manabe S, Sakamoto S, et al: Protein and energy metabolism in patients with progressive muscular dystrophy. J Nutr Sci Vitaminol (Tokyo) 38:141–154, 1992.

74. Pruzanski W: Respiratory tract infections and silent aspiration in myotonic dystrophy. Dis Chest 42:608–610, 1962.

75. Pruzanski W, Profis A: Dysfunction of the alimentary tract in myotonic dystrophy. Isr J Med Sci 2:59–64, 1966.

76. Rennie MJ, Edwards RHT, Millward DJ, et al: Effects of Duchenne muscular dystrophy on muscle protein synthesis. Nature 296:165–167, 1982.

77. Rochester DF, Arora NS, Braun NMT: Maximum contractile force of human diaphragm muscle determined in vivo. Trans Am Clin Climatol Assoc 83:202–208, 1981.

78. Rozier A, Ruskone-Fourmestraux A, Rosenbaum A, et al: Place de la gastrostomie endoscopique percutanée dans la sclérose latérale amyotrophique. Rev Neurol (Paris) 147:174–176, 1991.

79. Sahebjami H, MacGee J: Effects of starvation and refeeding on lung biochemistry in rats. Am Rev Respir Dis 126:483–487, 1982.

80. Sempé M, Roy MP: Auxologie, méthodes et séquences. Paris, Théraplix Editions, 1979.

81. Shimizu T, Hayashi H, Tanabe H: Energy metabolism of ALS patients under mechnical ventilation and tube feeding. Clin Neurol 31:255–259, 1991.

82. Shizgal HM, Roza A, Leduc B, et al: Body composition in quadriplegic patients. JPEN 10:364–368, 1986.

83. Shneerson J: Disorders of Ventilation. Boston, Blackwell Scientific Publications, 1988, pp 179–213.

84. Short SO, Hillel AD: Palliative surgery in patients with bulbar amyotrophic lateral sclerosis. Head Neck 11:463–469, 1989.

85. Silbiger ML, Pilielney R, Donner MW: Neuromuscular disorders affecting the pharynx: Cineradiographic analysis. Invest Radiol 2:442–448, 1967.

86. Slaughter MH, Lohman TG, Boileau RA, et al: Skinfold equations for estimation of body fatness in children and youth. Hum Biol 60:709–723, 1988.

87. Slonim AE, Coleman RA, McElligot MA, et al: Improvement of muscle function in acid maltase deficiency by high-protein therapy. Neurology 33:34–38, 1983.

88. Sonies BC, Baum BJ: Scintigraphy and manometry. Otolaryngol Clin North Am 21:637–648, 1988.

89. Sonies BC, Dalakas MC: Dysphagia in patients with the post-polio syndrome. N Engl J Med 324:1162–1167, 1991.

90. Spender QW, Cronk CE, Charney EB, Stallings VA: Assessment of linear growth of children with cerebral palsy: Use of alternative measures to height or length. Dev Med Child Neurol 31:206–214, 1989.

91. Stein J, Fenigstein H: Anatomie pathologique de la maladie de la famine. 21–27, 1946.

92. Talpers SS, Romberger DJ, Bunce SB, Pingleton SK: Nutritionally associated increased carbon dioxide production: Excess total calories vs. high proportion of carbohydrate calories. Chest 102:551–555, 1992.

93. Tanner JH, Whitehouse RH, Takaishi M: Standards from birth to maturity for height, weight, height velocity, and weight velocity: British children, pt II. Arch Dis Child 41:613–635, 1966.

94. Vallestrazzi A, Ballardini D, Battistini N, Merlini L: Growth pattern and body composition in spinal muscular atrophy. In Merlini L, Granata C, Dubowitz V (eds): Current Concepts in Childhood Spinal Muscular Atrophy. New York, Springer-Verlag, 1989, pp 221–226.

95. Varille V, Barois A, Willig TN, et al: Dépense energétique post prandiale de enfants atteints de dystrophie musculaire de Duchenne de Boulogne ou d'amyotrophie spinale infantile de type II. Nutr Clin Métab 8(suppl 4):56, 1994.

96. Vice FL, Heinz JM, Giuriati G, et al: Cervical auscultation of suckle feeding in newborn infants. Dev Med Child Neurol 32:760–768, 1990.

97. Wagner MB, Vignos PJ, Carlozzi C: Duchenne muscular dystrophy: A study of wrist and hand function. Muscle Nerve 12:236–244, 1989.

98. Webster C, Blau HM: Accelerated age-related decline in replicative life span of Duchenne muscular dystrophy myoblasts: Implications for cell and gene therapy. Som Cell Mol Genet 6:557–565, 1990.

99. Willig TN, Carlier L, Legrand M, et al: Nutritional assessment in Duchenne muscular dystrophy. Dev Med Child Neurol 35:1074–1082, 1993.

100. Willig TN, Paulus J, Lacau St Guily J, et al: Swallowing problems in neuromuscular disorders. Arch Phys Med Rehabil 75:1175–1181, 1994.

Functional Interventions for Persons with Neuromuscular Disease

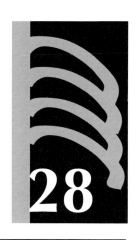

28

Joseph P. Valenza, MD, MCE
Susan L. Guzzardo, PT, MA
John R. Bach, MD

Regardless of the extent of physical disability, the goal of all persons with neuromuscular disease is to maximize quality of life.[41] An important part of the habilitation-rehabilitation process is the application of adaptive equipment to reverse the handicaps otherwise imposed by the disease. Specifically the goals of technology adaptation are to improve mobility, manipulation and control of the environment, activities of daily living (ADL), and, if needed, communication. Adaptive aids can permit individuals to perform lost or deteriorating functions. The restoration of independent functioning is critical for physically challenged individuals.[8] It results in improved self-esteem, more meaningful personal interactions, and enhanced satisfaction with life.

When considering assistive devices for individuals with neuromuscular disease, the following principles maximize outcomes:[33]

1. Interventions are designed to facilitate home management and ADL.
2. Interventions are based on a realistic evaluation and understanding of the patient's needs, capabilities (both physical and cognitive), and limitations, such as in strength, endurance, balance, and fitness of the care providers.
3. Cultural and social attitudes, timing, and patient and family acceptance are considered.

The premature introduction of a wheelchair can be rejected by an as yet unrealistic patient and family as an unwanted sign of "disability" or impending death.

4. Intervention is to maintain function rather than to improve strength.
5. Interventions are designed to make care providers' physical tasks easier. This can relieve the patient's feelings of being a burden and increase well-being.
6. Equipment must realistically fit into the patient's environment.[29] For example, it is important to know if a wheelchair can fit through the doorways of the individual's residence.
7. Both patients and care providers are properly trained in the use of adaptive equipment. Training may be necessary in the patient's home.
8. Patient and care provider creativity and ingenuity are encouraged. Patients and family are encouraged to develop practical substitution methods that can compensate for limitations. The major emphasis in the past was on controlling the patient's environment. Equipment was provided without encouraging patient and care provider initiative and creativity. Thus, sophisticated, expensive equipment can be found in closets, while simple, inexpensive adaptations and gadgets are being used.

9. Interventions and equipment are regularly reevaluated to determine their continued appropriateness in enhancing function or alleviating the physical demands on the care providers.[20]

Occasional home visits by physical or occupational therapists are usually needed for achieving these nine principles. The therapist's problem-solving ability and ingenuity can complement that of the patient and family in overcoming obstacles encountered during ADL. In addition, in-home instruction in the use of proper methods for assisting function and proper body mechanics can reduce safety risks to both patients and care providers.

MOBILITY

Ambulation

The ability to walk is important for independence. Individuals with neuromuscular weakness, including, at times, those who require continuous ventilatory support, may be able to walk only using walking aids as well as their ventilator. Depending on the degree of extremity weakness, a straight cane, a quad cane, a crutch, crutches, or a walker may be useful.

Walkers, Crutches, and Canes

Using assistive devices such as a cane, walker, or crutches requires adequate upper extremity strength, endurance, and coordination. The individual's gait is evaluated as different aids are tried. Devices offering the greatest stability are often bilateral in nature (i.e., walkers, pair of crutches). These enable both upper extremities to bear weight to compensate for weakness or lack of lower extremity mobility. For some individuals with poor upper extremity strength, a rolling platform walker or walker with a seat option may be necessary. For the individual with predominantly unilateral lower extremity involvement (most often postpoliomyelitis and motor neuron disease patients), a cane is often the best choice. Cane styles vary from the four- or three-point, wide-based or narrow-based quad canes to the one-point straight canes. As a general rule, when one cane is used for ambulation, it is used on the unaffected side. The reasons for cane placement contralateral to the involved side are twofold: to increase the base of support and, therefore, stability and to facilitate

a more biomechanically correct reciprocal gait sequence. In some cases, the added benefit of the placement of an assistive device on the uninvolved side permits a care provider to guard or support the patient on the weaker, more unstable side. This support provides the patient with maximum safety for ambulation.[34] For patients who require ventilatory support while walking, a rolling walker with a ventilator tray is necessary (Fig. 28–1). Skill and practice are required to ensure that these devices are used safely on all surfaces (i.e., stairs, ramps, curbs). A ventilator trolley may also be useful for home ambulation (Fig. 28–2).

Orthotics

Use of a cane or a walker may be sufficient for individuals with less severe lower extremity weakness, but lower extremity braces including ankle foot orthoses (AFOs) (Fig. 28–3), knee ankle foot orthoses (KAFOs), or rarely hip knee

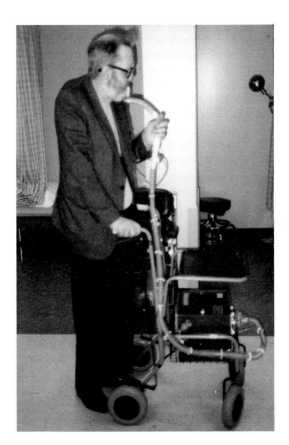

FIGURE 28–1. A 24-hour ventilator user was able to return to full-time employment using a rolling walker with a ventilator tray.

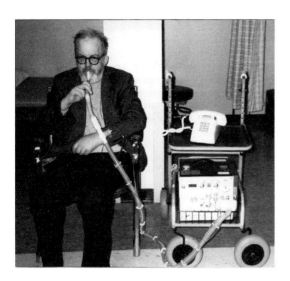

FIGURE 28–2. A ventilator trolley used for mechanical ventilation in the home.

ankle foot orthoses (HKAFOs) may be required for some patients with severe leg weakness. Careful monitoring of orthotics is necessary to prevent skin breakdown that can result from orthotic wear, especially for individuals with decreased sensation or circulation. Some individuals require both upper extremity aids and lower extremity orthoses to achieve independence in walking.

Orthotic prescription requires assessment of the individual's strength and function as well as of his or her potential for donning and doffing the orthoses. Orthoses can be used for any of the following reasons:

- *Stabilizing.* Allowing a secure base of support for a limb to enable a bipedal gait. An orthosis can compensate for muscular weakness or joint instability.
- *Motorizing.* Using the mechanical segment of an orthotic device to enhance a particular movement. An example would be to use a spring-loaded hinge near the ankle to assist foot dorsiflexion to prevent drop foot.
- *Corrective.* Minimizing orthopedic deformities. The developing bone and muscular structure of children may require support to attain correct biomechanical loading during gait. Bone growth is directly related to the forces imposed on the bone.[23] Correct orthotic prescriptions can prevent or at least minimize foot and lower extremity deformities and, at times, scoliosis.
- *Protective.* Relieving pressure or stress on a particular area. For example, an individual with skin breakdown on the foot may require an orthosis to prevent weight bearing on the involved skin while allowing ambulation and increased blood flow to the tissue to facilitate healing.[18]

Orthoses range in complexity from simple arch supports to bracing the entire extremity to the trunk. Consideration of the weight of the brace user, the brace's weight and appearance, and the circumstances of its donning and doffing is important for proper orthotic prescription. In the not so distant past, weighty braces constructed of heavy metals and leather were used. Now lightweight, durable plastics and metals (e.g., titanium) are used. An individual's

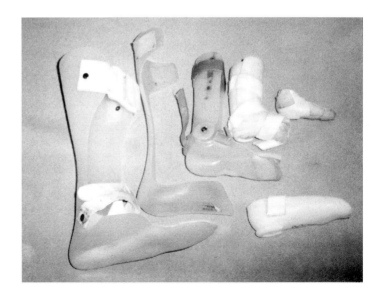

FIGURE 28–3. Orthotics, *from left to right:* solid ankle-foot orthosis (SAFO), posterior leaf spring orthosis, hinged ankle-foot orthosis, anti-crouch orthosis, superior malleolar orthosis (SMO), University of California at Berkeley heel cup (UCBL).

weight must be considered not only for the extent of bracing, but also for the materials to be used. When contemplating a long leg brace prescription, toileting must be considered. A care provider or user might not have the time or ability to remove the braces to allow prompt use of the toilet. Even the best orthotics are found in the closet if they are impractical for the user's daily functioning.

Heel cups and arch supports support the tarsal and metatarsal bones. They do not support the talocrural joint, although they can provide the alignment necessary to support foot functioning to minimize deformities. A supramalleolar orthotic (SMO) extends above the malleoli and can assist in the control of pronation and supination of the foot as well as support the pedal structures.

Solid AFOs are inflexible at the talocrural joint. This ensures a certain control of the foot in the brace that is particularly useful in the ankle with spasticity and positions the ankle for stability during weight bearing. By setting the brace in slight dorsiflexion, knee flexion is facilitated to decrease any tendency for genu recurvatum. Slight plantar flexion tends to increase knee extension.

Floor reaction braces require a user's ability to attain heel strike during gait. These braces transmit the force of heel strike anterior to the tibia to facilitate knee extension. They are particularly useful when the knee extension mechanism is weak.

AFOs can have a hinge mechanism at the ankle. Such braces allow for movement of the ankle into dorsiflexion or plantar flexion. A "stop" can be placed on the hinge to limit the motion at any angle. This can permit the tibia to continue to move forward during mid to late stance to provide better alignment and a better quality of ambulation, while supporting the foot and ankle. Further, a person with a footdrop who requires dorsiflexion support can walk with less fear of tripping on the toes.

The effect of the orthotic on body alignment must be carefully reassessed regularly. Uprights extended from the AFO to the thigh can provide support for the knee. Again, hinges or ratchets can be used. Drop locks can be used to lock the knee into extension for maximal stability during gait. Straps can be used to provide an extra force for varum or valgum correction at the knee.

A pelvic band can be attached to the upright laterally to provide for assistance for torsion forces at the hip (internal or external rotation). A pelvic band also has a hinge allowing flexion or extension of the hip. Braces that extend above the hip pose a challenge for toileting and hygiene, and the longer lever arm of the upright can cause excessive wear at the joint. Such braces are rarely if ever indicated for individuals with neuromuscular weakness and paralytic-restrictive pulmonary syndromes. The only exception of which the authors are aware is that of the patient with myelopathic paraparesis and chronic ventilatory insufficiency secondary to a combination of myelopathy, scoliosis, and obesity. For such a patient, particular attention to lower extremity alignment is necessary for standing and ambulation. AFOs are held in slight dorsiflexion, the knees are locked in extension, and medial and lateral uprights (Fig. 28–4) support alignment. Although the energy demand of this particular type of ambulation is high, it can increase an individual's functioning by allowing stair climbing with the use of upper extremity orthotics.

Primarily, although not exclusively, seen in the pediatric population, reciprocating gait orthotics (RGOs) can assist individuals with paraparesis or paraplegia to ambulate. These braces are constructed of AFOs, knee locks, uprights, pelvic/trunk bands, and cables. The cable system allows the advancement of one leg while the other is in stance. This is accomplished by weight shifting onto the stance leg and off the leg in swing.

The parapodium or standing tables are rigid devices that support the lower extremities and

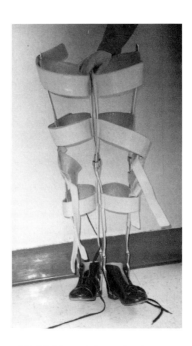

FIGURE 28–4. Long leg braces.

the entire body to maintain the user erect and to transmit weight through the skeletal frame. By enabling lower extremity weight bearing, orthopedic development and upright activities are facilitated. Continued erect posturing and ambulation benefit physiologic parameters,[22] enhance circulation to the lower legs and feet, discourage osteoporosis and disuse muscular atrophy, and retard the development of flexion contractures and possibly scoliosis.[43]

Besides the strollers (described later) that can be adapted to support the spines of small children with generalized weakness, orthoses can support children with generalized neuromuscular diseases, most commonly spinal muscular atrophy and congenital myopathies, who can sit. Total contact plastic thoracolumbar bracing is used to limit scoliotic progression and to allow normal early vertebral growth until age 6, at which point spinal instrumentation and fusion are often performed.[33,35]

CONSIDERATIONS FOR SPECIFIC DIAGNOSES

Duchenne Muscular Dystrophy

By the time patients with Duchenne muscular dystrophy experience respiratory complications, they are no longer able to walk. Before this point, however, AFOs can be useful to de-

crease pain and to give temporary ankle support as the patient returns to independent, brace-free ambulation following lower extremity musculotendinous surgery performed to prevent or correct contractures.[1] When patients are no longer able to walk, resting AFOs or KAFOs when used overnight can be useful to decrease the rate of contracture development. With the user sitting in a wheelchair, AFOs can support and protect the legs from injury as well as discourage contracture development. During the final stages of independent ambulation, AFOs can be used in conjunction with Lofstran crutches to support continued ambulation. Some physicians continue to use lower extremity musculotendinous surgery at the point at which the patient is about to become wheelchair confined. This approach necessitates the use of KAFOs for reambulation.[1] In general, AFOs are not indicated to assist ambulation in this population because they slow ambulation, hamper getting up from a chair because of loss of the ability to flex the knees, increase the weight on the extremity, and prevent use of the often strong plantar flexors.

Thoracolumbar bracing is never used to prevent scoliosis for individuals with Duchenne muscular dystrophy. Besides being ineffective, their use can delay effective surgical management to the point at which intervention may be precluded because of deterioration in cardiopulmonary function (Fig. 28–5).

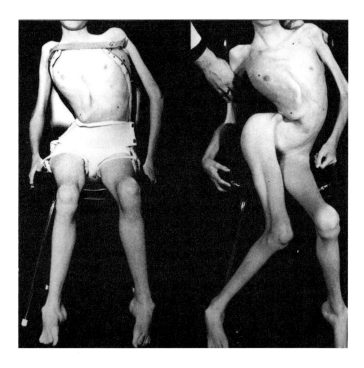

FIGURE 28–5. Patient with Duchenne muscular dystrophy who used thoracolumbar orthoses from age 10. This approach failed to prevent severe scoliosis, and surgical intervention was never undertaken because of the deterioration in pulmonary function while the brace was being used. At age 22, the orthosis provides some support to maintain seating balance.

Non-Duchenne Myopathies

Patients with non-Duchenne myopathies who most benefit from the use of lower extremity orthotics include those with adequate hip muscle strength to get up from a chair unassisted despite loss of knee mobility because of the brace. Patients with acid maltase deficiency, myotonic dystrophy, Becker muscular dystrophy, occasionally other muscular dystrophies, and certain generalized myopathies can often walk despite the need to use ventilatory assistance at least overnight and occasionally up to 24 hours a day. Because proximal muscle weakness is often severe, KAFOs rarely benefit myopathy patients; however, AFOs and crutches may be useful.

Multiple Sclerosis, Anterior Horn Cell Diseases, and Motor Neuron Diseases

The great majority of patients with motor neuron disease cannot benefit from the use of lower extremity orthoses because of the presence of severe weakness at the hips and because their conditions progress too rapidly for fabrication and ambulation training with AFOs to be practical. Some patients with relatively static or slowly progressive conditions have severe respiratory muscle involvement while still able to walk. These individuals may benefit from lower extremity bracing. Multiple sclerosis and post-poliomyelitis individuals can manifest any combination of respiratory and extremity muscle weakness. They not infrequently require ventilator use as well as AFOs or KAFOs for ambulation. Children with spinal muscle atrophy type 1 do not reach developmental milestones and require trunk orthotics and standing tables to optimize positioning and weight bearing. These individuals generally benefit only from the use of lower extremity orthotics to retard contracture development. Others with milder spinal muscular atrophies can on occasion benefit from lower extremity bracing when proximal (hip and shoulder) muscle strength is adequate.

Myelopathies

As noted previously, occasionally individuals with partial spinal cord lesions, particularly those occurring in the neonatal or early childhood period, can result in paraparesis and late-onset ventilatory insufficiency that requires ventilatory support. Such patients can benefit from lower and upper extremity orthoses for ambulation; however, motorized scooters are usually much more practical.

WHEELCHAIRS

For some individuals, ambulation is impossible or is limited by fatigue, poor safety awareness, weakness, balance difficulties, or high energy costs. Many types of strollers, wheelchairs, and scooters exist for such individuals. For maximal efficiency, a wheelchair needs to be of proper size and have accessories that increase the user's function and quality of life. The value of the wheelchair to the physically challenged individual cannot be overstated.

A wheelchair prescribed for someone who can walk with a cane, a walker, or an orthosis is used for traveling long distances in shopping centers or for transport over uneven terrain at outdoor events. The user should not spend any more time in the wheelchair than is necessary for transport. For such an individual, the ideal wheelchair is usually a light folding type for ease of transfer into an automobile (Fig. 28–6).

A more substantial wheelchair is needed when the individual is no longer able to ambulate independently. It can be either a manual or a powerwheelchair depending on the user's need. Which ever is chosen, it is imperative that the wheelchair be properly equipped and fitted to the user. Proper seating includes allowing enough room for wearing a coat and orthotics when applicable. Most wheelchairs have an overall width of 24 to 28 inches. Wider, more heavily constructed chairs can be made for obese individuals. A seat belt should be used for those with poor sitting balance or weak trunk musculature.

Rigid Frame Wheelchairs

Two types of lightweight wheelchairs are available, those with rigid and those with non-rigid frames (Fig. 28–6). A rigid frame refers to a solid, immovable wheelchair base. A solid axis connects one wheel to the other. These chairs are well suited for the active wheelchair user who uses the chair on a variety of often uneven surfaces and terrains. Because of the solid axis, these frames provide more stability, provide a smoother ride, and are more durable. Such wheelchairs can also support more weight and wheelchair accessories such as ventilators and robotics. A disadvantage of the rigid frame wheelchair is that it cannot be folded and put into a car. The wheels must first be removed and placed separately from the residual seat frame into a car. "Quick release" wheels, with a pin and a lock configuration, can be removed and replaced more easily. For the user who is inde-

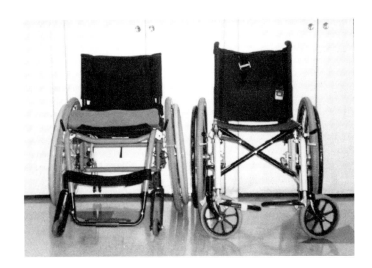

FIGURE 28–6. Rigid (*left*) and folding (*right*) frame wheelchairs.

pendent in all ADL, wheelchair durability is an important issue.

Nonrigid Frame Wheelchairs

The nonrigid frame wheelchairs have a cross bar connecting one side of the wheelchair to the other. The advantage of these wheelchairs is their ease of storage. They fold; thus their width is decreased in half. This is sufficient for placement on the backseats or in the trunks of cars. The cross frame, however, wears out with use, compromising the integrity and stability of the wheelchair. Nevertheless, wheelchair users may prefer a cross frame wheelchair because of its convenience. Because both are expensive, both the user and the caregiver should have the option to try both types of frames before purchase. Taking all factors into consideration, the rehabilitation team recommends the style most appropriate for the user's lifestyle and environmental restrictions.

One-Arm Drive

A one-arm drive wheelchair is available for individuals with only one functional upper extremity. A one-arm drive has two hand rims on the wheel. By manipulating one or both, the user can propel and turn the wheelchair.

Other Options

Most individuals with neuromuscular conditions require adjustable, removable leg rests with heel straps. Off-set foot plates and heel loops are used for individuals with severe ankle and foot deformities. The feet are maintained flat on the plates to discourage further deformity. Elevating foot rests often increase the turning radius of the wheelchair and are generally used only in conjunction with a reclining back for when lower extremity edema, postural hypotension, and skin pressure relief cannot be managed effectively in other ways. Individuals with poor endurance may also require a reclining seat (Fig. 28–7). The ability to recline with extended knees may also reduce the tendency to develop flexion contractures of the knee and hips, and the user can rest more comfortably, but, in general, these are insufficient indications for the prescription of such an option. A neck or head support can be necessary, especially for individuals with advanced motor neuron disease, infantile spinal muscular atrophy, and advanced Duchenne muscular dystrophy. Neck rests with a forehead strap provide both lateral and anterior-posterior support.

The user has the option of having full-length wheelchair arms or desk arms. Desk arms are usually preferred because they permit the user to approach and use tables. Full-length arms may be useful to support a lap tray. A lap board can facilitate the performance of school work, gainful employment, and recreational activities. Elevating arms are an option but are rarely required by users with neuromuscular weakness. The arms must be removable, however, to facilitate transfers.

Seating Systems

Special seating modifications are required for individuals with severe muscular weakness and

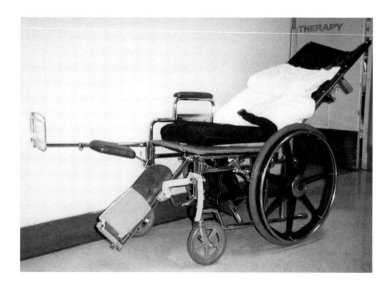

FIGURE 28–7. Wheelchair with reclining back, removable desk arms, elevating foot rests, and seat belt.

trunk, pelvis, or spinal instability or deformities. The individual must be positioned and aligned properly to discourage pelvic obliquity and other deformities. When bony prominences or pelvic obliquity are severe, a proper seating system can provide a stable surface while accommodating the deformities. The pelvis is supported by a firm seat cushion supporting both ischia to keep the pelvis level and balanced. For example, the Roho (Roho Inc., Belleville, IL), Jay (Jay Medical Ltd., Boulder, CO), and Avanti (Invacare, Inc., Elyria, OH) seating systems provide excellent pressure relief (Fig. 28–8). Clients should be evaluated on more than one system, and comfort and support must be optimized for any particular individual. An adductor wedge or, for those with a wide sitting base owing to excessive hip abduction, an abductor wedge or thigh strap can help maintain pelvis and lower extremity alignment. Padded inserts are made of materials that optimize comfort and maximize support to retard the development of contractures and deformities second-

ary to improper or asymmetric seating positions (Fig. 28–10). Lateral trunk supports may also be helpful. A fully contoured seat with integral arm, foot, and head rest is an option.[21]

Some seating systems permit users independently to vary their sitting positions, to adjust upright sitting posture, to increase head and upper extremity control, and to relieve skin pressure to avoid skin pressure ulcers. The Tilt-in-space seating mobility system (La Bac Systems, Inc., Denver, CO), which shifts the user and the wheelchair seat and back simultaneously, changes the seating orientation and shifts skin pressures. Users can operate the tilt themselves via a switch.

Motorized Wheelchairs

Motorized wheelchairs are heavy and costly but are essential for the independent mobility of many severely disabled individuals. The purchase of a motorized wheelchair must be closely

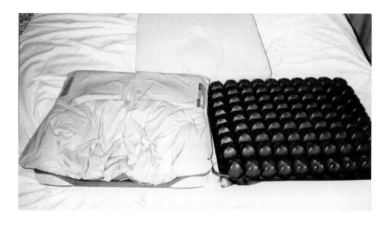

FIGURE 28–8. Adaptive seating, *from left to right:* Jay cushion, foam cushion with ischial cutout, Roho cushion

supervised by the rehabilitation team because of its expense and because of the many modifications to the chair needed to accommodate severe disability. There is no substitute for the practice sessions required to insure safety while using a motorized chair. The drive train chosen depends on the need of the particular patient. A front-wheel drive wheelchair is more maneuverable in the confined spaces of the home. A rear-wheel drive grips the ground better and is superior for outdoor use.

Many of the prescription considerations for standard wheelchairs also apply to power wheelchairs. The operation system is an additional consideration, however. Power wheelchairs can be operated by joy-stick controls. When hand function is absent, tongue, chin, and sip-and-puff controls can be used (Fig. 28–9). Daytime ventilatory support is conveniently provided by the delivery of intermittent positive-pressure ventilation (IPPV) via a mouthpiece fixed onto wheelchair controls adjacent to the mouth (Fig. 29–9). Other considerations when prescribing a motorized chair include its style for personal preference; adjustability of the control box for sensitivity of operation, programming chair speed, acceleration, and turning radius; noise; brake efficiency; tire treads and suspension system for smoothness of ride on flat, unlevel surfaces or on grass; curb jumping ability; range on a battery charge; durability; warranty; and price. Some motorized wheelchairs have the option of

standing the patient and being operated while standing. When it is estimated that daytime ventilatory assistance will be required within 3 years, any prescribed power wheelchair should have the capability of carrying a ventilator tray and holding additional batteries and possibly a charger.

Training

Family members or care providers are trained by physical or occupational therapists in the proper techniques of wheelchair mobility. This includes lifting and lowering the wheelchair onto and off of the curb and up and down ramps and propulsion on various surfaces including, possibly, on steps. Training in the propulsion systems of motorized wheelchairs is also important to prevent accidents and injuries for both the user and the care provider.

SCOOTERS

Other options for individuals with limited mobility are three-wheel and four-wheel scooters (Fig. 28–10). Many scooters have a maximum speed of 10 miles per hour, have a turning radius of about 20 inches, can ascend a grade of 30 degrees, and go about 20 miles on one battery charge. They have swivel seats and can have

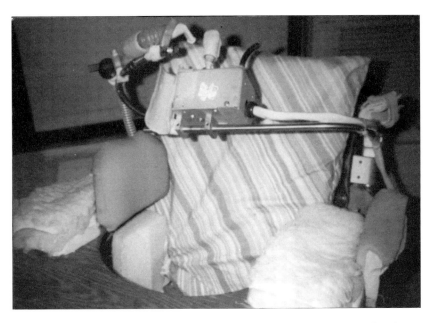

FIGURE 28–9. Chin control motorized wheelchair with mouthpiece set up adjacent to the chin controls for daytime ventilatory support.

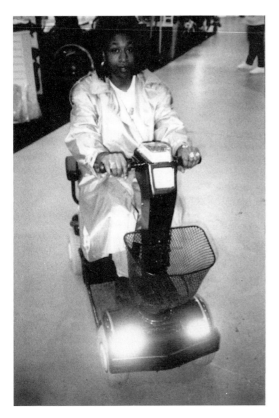

FIGURE 28–10. Motorized scooter. (Shoprider, Shoprider, Rosemont, PA.)

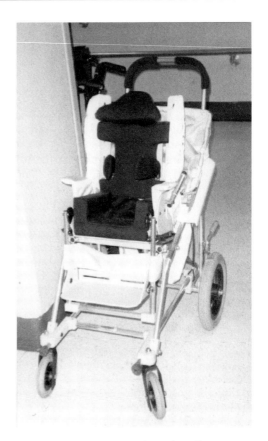

FIGURE 28–11. Adapted stroller.

elevating seats when this is necessary for transfers. They are longer, however, and require more maneuvering space than wheelchairs. When prescribed for community usage, it is important first to evaluate the presence of local curb contours because scooters cannot, in general, maneuver up curbs. Although scooters have seat belts, trunk and upper extremity musculature must be functional to transfer to and from and to operate a scooter. A wire basket is attached to the frame of the scooter for transporting objects. Although scooter use is not often thought to be appropriate for individuals with severe neuromuscular diseases, some Duchenne muscular dystrophy patients have adequate trunk and upper extremity strength to benefit from their use for 1 or 2 years before resort to a wheelchair is needed. Scooters are often more useful for individuals with milder or more slowly progressive conditions.

STROLLERS

Adapted strollers are available for children who are unable or are too young to propel a wheelchair and who require support to be positioned upright or when reclining (Fig. 28–11). Strollers provide an easy mode of transportation for a child. The parent can even use a wheelchair lift to get it onto and off city buses. Strollers are easily folded for storage. Their complexity can vary greatly. Similar to wheelchairs, the bases can have a "tilt-in-space" option that allows the parent to recline a child as necessary. Some strollers have a feature that permits the base to be reversed so that parents can conveniently monitor a child with seizures or who requires ventilatory support.

Seating systems are available that provide stability for the child while sitting. Head rests, lateral trunk supports, guides for hip placement, foot rests, and harness systems can be mounted to hold the child in place. Most seating cushions available for adults are also available in pediatric sizes (Jay, Roho, Avanti). While sitting with support, some children can use their upper extremities to operate communication systems, feed themselves, write, and do other recreational activities. Trays can also be mounted on strollers.

Growth considerations are important for all adaptive equipment for children. Seat depth, height, and width must be adjustable. The distance from seat to foot rest must also be extendable. Most pediatric wheelchairs and strollers can accommodate 4 to 6 inches of growth in each direction.

TRANSFERRING AND LIFTING

Transfers refer to getting an individual from one position or place to another. Depending on residual strength, the individual may assist with his or her transfers or may need to be lifted or transferred to and from bed; in and out of a wheelchair, car, or tub; and onto and off a toilet and require position changes day and night. The work involved may be taxing or impossible depending on the weight of the individual.

Guidelines for Transfers

The care providers responsible for moving a disabled child or adult need early, thorough, and ongoing instructions in the most efficient and safe way to accomplish it.[11] Some important guidelines should be stressed

1. Proper biomechanics are taught to prevent back strain. Lifting is done with the back straight and with a wide base of support to emphasize that the power comes from the legs to minimize stress to the back.
2. Conditions for transfers are optimized. This may require equalizing the height of the transfer surfaces.
3. The patient assists in the transfers as much as possible. The patient should also be comfortable in instructing others in performing their transfers.

4. Whether the individual can walk or not, long-leg orthoses are used when they aid in performing pivot transfers.
5. Individuals are evaluated for the use of transfer boards (Fig. 28–12). The wheelchair is apposed to the surface onto which the individual will be transferred and the board placed between the two surfaces. As the patient slides along the board, he or she maintains contact with the board throughout the transfer, minimizing the potential for falls.

Hoists, Ramps, and Door Openers

Mechanical hoists have a role in lifting and transferring heavy and severely disabled individuals. A variety of lifts are available, including the Hoyer lift and Translift (Guardian Sunrise Medical, Arleta, CA) and Barrier Free Lift (Barrier Free Lifts Inc., Manassus, VA). These facilitate transfers and can also greatly facilitate bowel evacuation by hoisting the patient over a commode as part of the bowel management program (Fig. 28–13).[5] Portable hoists are effective; however, in practice, they are often not used because they are cumbersome and bulky, and it can be difficult getting larger patients onto the hoist. They are also difficult to move between rooms. Ceiling lifts (Barrier Free Lifts, Inc.) have the advantages of permitting independent user transfers and multidirectional user transport and being battery powered. The Meyland-Carlift (Access Unlimited, Binghamton, NY), which can be fixed onto a car door, in a bathroom area or in any room in which it will be used, can lift the user into and out of a car, onto a toilet seat, and so forth. Ordinary car seats can be replaced by motorized car seats (Fig. 28–14). Stair glides can be used for people who can

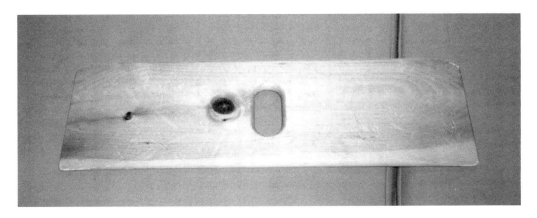

FIGURE 28–12. Sliding board.

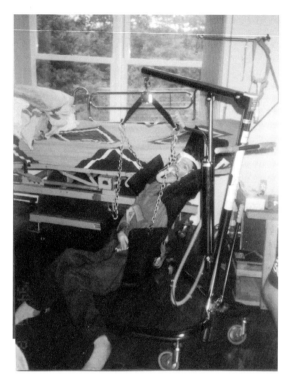

FIGURE 28–13. Duchenne muscular dystrophy ventilator user with no ventilator-free breathing ability being transferred from bed by Hoyer lift. With his feet on the ground, thighs applying pressure to the abdomen, and buttocks in optimal dependent position, his bowel movements are initiated and rapidly completed using the Hoyer lift in this manner as part of a bowel program.

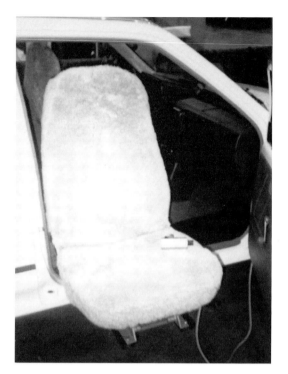

FIGURE 28–14. Motorized car seat to facilitate car transfers. (Merlin 360 degrees, Medgroup, Inc., Newbury Park, CA.)

be transferred onto and off of the glide (Fig. 28–15). For the individual unable to walk, these glides require another surface onto which to transfer. This might require the care provider to carry the wheelchair to the next flight of stairs. When the stairway has a wide platform, glides are available that also accommodate wheelchairs. Spiral stairs are a difficult obstacle for wheelchair users. Frequently, home remodeling is necessary for accessibility. Vertical platform lifts are other options when all else fails.

Portable folding and telescoping ramps can be custom-made to bypass stairs. Ramps may be needed to enter one's home as well as at school or in the place of work. Remote-controlled door systems can also facilitate wheelchair accessibility (Open Sesame, Inc., San Leandro, CA; Gentleman Door Co., Yorklyn, DE). The home visit of an occupational therapist can aid the physician in prescribing these useful devices and in-home modifications. Such an evaluation is necessary to assess room accessibility before ordering a wheelchair or a lift.

BEDS AND MATTRESSES

A major problem in caring for individuals with neuromuscular disease is the need for frequent overnight turning. Sleep disturbances have been documented in nonambulatory patients with neuromuscular disease even in the absence of chronic ventilatory insufficiency. These individuals awaken and require repositioning in bed from 2 to 10 times a night.[19,36] Spinal cord–injured individuals need repositioning every 2 to 4 hours to avert skin ulcers. The rehabilitation team can instruct and problem solve with the care providers to determine the safest, most effective ways to turn or position the individual.

Determining which mattresses provide the greatest comfort and reduce the nocturnal turning requirement is an empiric process. Various mattress surfaces are available that disperse pressure over large areas. Common mattress choices are egg crate, water, and air mattresses.

Egg crate–style soft foam with raised and recessed textures is commonly used because of its convenience and low cost. This mattress increases the effective surface area, thus decreasing the amount of pressure on the tissues. The foam can deform with pressure, however, allow-

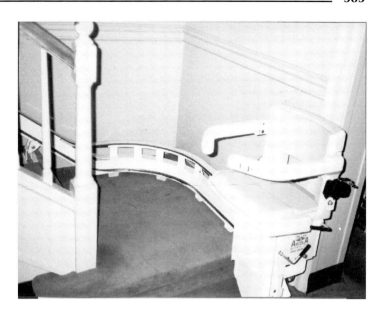

FIGURE 28–15. Stair glide.

ing pressure buildup to occur in spots. Therefore, careful skin monitoring must be continued.

Water mattresses can help regulate body temperature and disperse pressure. Expense and water leakage are common problems; for users with poor balance and trunk control, instability while lying on a water mattress can hamper activities such as dressing, grooming, and eating. Air mattresses can also be used to regulate body temperature and disperse pressure. These mattresses, and especially those that circulate the air, are even more expensive but lighter and simpler to maintain than water mattresses. They must also be assessed for air leakage, and, as with water systems, contact with sharp or angular surfaces must be avoided. This stipulation necessitates caution for the usage of some orthoses and ADL equipment while in bed.

Bed rails may be useful for some individuals to assist themselves in turning from side to side or for other bed mobility. Bed rails are either mounted to the bed frame or hooked under the mattress. For the independent individual, a secure bed rail must be raised or lowered with ease.

A hospital bed can raise or lower the head and feet. For ease of transfers, the bed height can also be raised or lowered. The mechanisms are usually at the foot of the bed or by push button control. Modifications for a sip/puff system are also available.

Regardless of mattress style, one or two overnight turns usually continue to be needed for comfort or skin ulcer prevention. The Motion Bed (Emerson Co., Cambridge, MA) is a bed that rotates the user slowly from side to side. This alleviates any need for turning. Not all patients can get used to or tolerate this continuous movement, and the movement can loosen nasal or lipseal interfaces. This might require occasional attention overnight.

In the authors' experience, alternating pressure pad air mattresses are most useful to decrease the nocturnal assisted-turning frequency of many neuromuscular patients. It is not effective, however, for every individual. The Motion bed can be remarkably effective, but it is not always tolerated. Candidates for the use of this bed should try it first for a few nights.

TOILETING

A raised toilet seat and bars attached to the wall or to the toilet seat can assist with toilet transfers.[25] The bars can be removable or fixed, depending on how long they will be needed and on whether or not permanently fixing objects into the walls or floor is permissible. Bars are available that can be suction cupped to surfaces. The height from the floor and the width of the bar must insure optimal usage and accessibility.

Commode chairs can also be used. They can be used at bedside or placed over a toilet or in some other convenient location. Some are available on wheels, so a care provider can easily move the user into and out of the bathroom. In general, commode chairs are narrower than wheelchairs and can more readily fit through doors. Self-propelled commode chairs allow independent access into the bathroom. Some models can be rolled into a shower. Commode chairs on wheels can also have seat belts, foot rests, and removable arm rests.

In many homes, the bathroom is not situated for easy access from the living or sleeping quarters. Urinals can be useful for male patients. Wheelchair-bound ADL-dependent patients' daily activities outside the home can be greatly facilitated by the use of a condom catheter urinary drainage system by males or a Foley or intermittent catheter system for females so that assistance with urination need not be sought during daytime activities.

For the pediatric patient, specially adapted potty chairs are available that provide support and positioning (Fig. 28–16). These vary from sophisticated systems to support the head, trunk, and pelvis to minimal systems consisting of a ring encircling the user's waist and a seatbelt. Some of these potty chairs can be placed onto the toilet, whereas others are used only on the floor. These systems have adjustable parts that allow for the growth of the child. The size and layout of the bathroom must be considered before ordering large pieces of bathroom equipment. The burden on the parents can be minimized by carefully selecting equipment with the most adaptability, durability, and practicality.

BATHING

Bathing can be a nightmare for the physically challenged individual and the care provider.

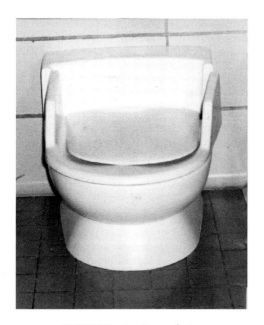

FIGURE 28–16. Potty chair.

Transfer to the tub can be dangerous and exhausting. Bath seats can make it feasible for patients with limited muscle strength to wash in a tub or shower (Fig. 28–17). Bath seats and tub benches can be fitted with seat belts for the individual with limited trunk balance. Seats with a hole in the center can allow for ease in bathing the perineum; however, it can make transferring off of the tub bench more difficult. Equipment should be evaluated with the patient using it for bathing whenever possible. Bathtub or wall-mounted rails can be useful. Portable lifts are the best solution for bathing heavy or severely disabled individuals. The use of the Hoyer lift for bathing, however, is often limited because of bathroom and doorway space limitations.

A water-powered bath chair (Bath Mate, Ontario, CA) lowers to within 2 inches of the tub bottom. After bathing, it rises and slowly returns the user to tub side. A hand-held shower head can enable the user to direct water during bathing. Water temperature must be carefully assessed for individuals with insensate areas.

When the bathroom can be remodeled, a roll-in shower can permit a rolling shower chair or commode chair to be wheeled into the shower. The only transfer necessary, in this case, is the one from the bed to the shower chair and back.

HYGIENE

Long-handled combs, brushes, and sponges; dressing sticks; toilet paper holders; shoe horns; flexible shower hoses and adapters; shower-tub transfer seats; high bath/shower chairs and raised toilet seats; bedside commode chairs; dressing aids; kitchen aids; and lifts can be used by individuals with muscle weakness.[7] Long-handled brushes are designed with numerous angles to eliminate the need to lift the arms above the head.

CLOTHING AND DRESSING AIDS

Many individuals are more easily dressed while in bed. The bed provides a stable surface for dressing activities. Some can gain independence for dressing activities using widely available self-help aids and a few clothing adaptations. The clothing must be sturdy in construction, loose enough to allow freedom of body movement, and easy to put on and to fasten.[24] Zippers are more manageable with a ring pull. Long pulls are used for zippers on the back

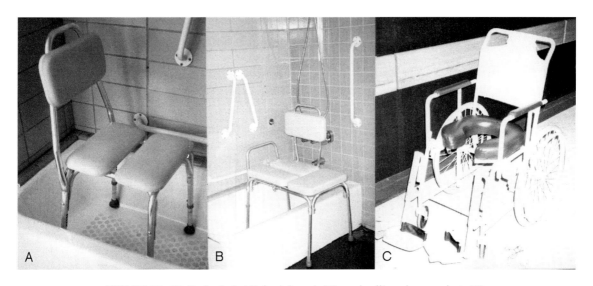

FIGURE 28–17. Bath chair (*A*), bath bench (*B*), and rolling shower chair (*C*).

of dresses. Shoes with elastic shoe laces or with Velcro closures are convenient. Flexible, long shoe horns can be helpful for some individuals. Socks one size too large are easier to put on than are otherwise appropriately sized socks.

Buttoned shirts should be one size too large. For patients with limited hand mobility, the stell hook of a button helper can facilitate zipping and buttoning. Velcro can also be used as a substitute for buttons and button holes on shirt cuffs. Bras can be hooked in front for easy donning or have Velcro closures. Occupational therapists can help resolve dressing problems.

Clothing adaptations are most acceptable when they are compatible with current styles and if they are adeptly concealed. Physically challenged individuals do not wish to appear differently from their peers. Specialized clothing catalogues with practical, yet fashionable solutions are available.

ADAPTIVE EATING

For individuals with some extremity function who have the potential to feed themselves with assistance, correct positioning and table height are important. A swivel spoon or fork can be used for individuals who cannot supinate or pronate. These maintain the spoon or fork surface horizontal regardless of upper extremity rotation. Lightweight utensils and utensils with large handles are often helpful. Plastic drinking cups and straws are useful. Built-up plate rims that clamp onto the plate can be used to help guide food onto the fork or spoon, and they help prevent spills. Plate guards snap onto the rim of a plate to keep food contained.

Individuals with advanced neuromuscular disease, who usually retain more distal than proximal upper extremity muscle function, can often use substitute movements such as bending the trunk forward to meet the hand. They may use objects as levers for the forearm so that the residual hand movements can be functional. Some individuals use their fingers to crawl up the opposite arm, dragging the weaker arm in this manner. Once vertical and balanced on the tip of the elbow, the forearm requires less effort to move.[27] A person who can use the arms against gravity for a limited period of time is instructed to rest the elbows on the table, eliminating gravity, and use the shorter lever arm to bring the hand to the mouth. Rather than bring the head forward to the food, the table surface can be raised so that the hand is closer to the mouth. Using a raised tray avoids having the table too high for other family members. If a utensil is difficult to hold, enlarged handles provide an increased gripping surface for the utensils (Fig. 28–18). A universal cuff holds a variety of eating and writing utensils in the palm of the hand (Fig. 28–19). When slipped onto a hand, no active grasp is required. An overhead sling, a motorized system of arm suspension,[27] or a ball bearing (balanced) forearm orthosis (BFO) or mobile arm support (Fig. 28–20)[42] may be useful for self-feeding and other activities when the shoulder, scapular, and elbow flexor muscle strength is less than antigravity. Elbow flexor strength greater than poor (Grade of 2) optimizes use of overhead slings and BFOs.[42]

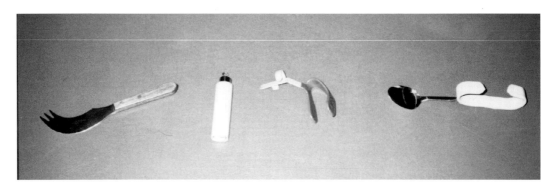

FIGURE 28–18. Adaptive utensils, *from left to right:* rocker knife, button loop, pen holder, adaptive spoon

When these mechanical devices can no longer be used for independent feeding, finger excursion alone can operate wheelchair-mountable, programmable robot arms (Figs. 28–21 and 28–22) as well as computers, environmental control systems, and motorized wheelchairs. Fortunately, finger movements are retained by Duchenne muscular dystrophy patients into their fifth decade even after 20 years or more of ventilatory support.[5] Most individuals with neuromuscular disease retain finger function despite having severe generalized weakness and requiring ventilator use. Thus, finger-operated robot arms can permit many individuals to continue to feed themselves, pick up objects from the floor, open doors, and perform many other upper extremity activities.[5,30,31] Such robot arms can be inexpensive or they can be expensive and extremely sophisticated.[30,39] They include: the Magpie, $1500 (Oxford Orthopaedic Engineering Ctr., Headington, Oxford, England); the Helping Hand, $10,000 (Kinetic Rehabilitation Instruments, Hanover, MA); and the Manus, $35,000–$40,000 (Exact Dynamics, Zevenaar, Holland). Voice-activated systems are also now available, e.g. DeVar, $60,000–$70,000 (Independence Works, Inc., Stanford, CA).

HOMEMAKING AND KITCHEN AIDS

Many assistive devices make cooking easier for the physically challenged. An under-the-counter jar opener permits jar opening with little effort. An all-purpose utility knob fits over most knobs, is easy to hold, and, because of its long handle, increases leverage for turning on or off stoves, televisions, and radios.[13,26] Doorknob extenders can make door opening easier. A one-handed cutting board secured to a work surface by suction cups has aluminum nails that

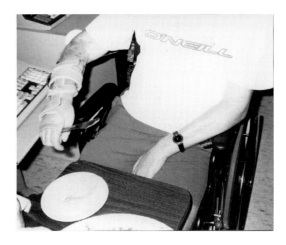

FIGURE 28–19. Universal cuff.

spear vegetables and other difficult-to-hold items. With this board, individuals with one weak arm can function as though they had two strong arms. A reacher is ideal for people restricted to wheelchair use. A light extension switch fits over any wall switch for easy on-off accessibility from a wheelchair.

When considering how much effort an individual should make to perform self-care activities, it should be kept in mind that severely physically challenged individuals whose time is better spent in gainful employment or other important activities should be encouraged to let their self-care be managed quickly and efficiently by personal care attendants.

COMMUNICATION AND COMPUTER ENVIRONMENTAL CONTROL

Speech recognition systems can provide the means for people with disabilities to write, often faster than many people can type. It can allow a

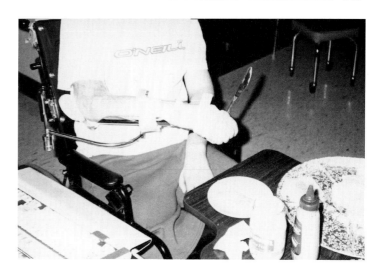

FIGURE 28–20. Balanced forearm orthosis.

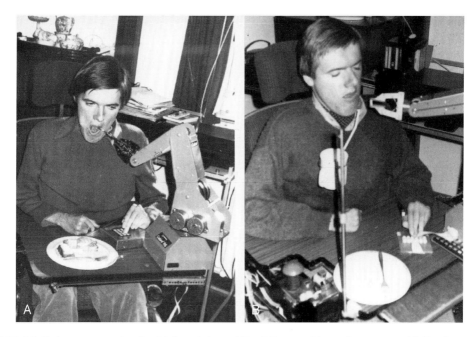

FIGURE 28–21. Robot arm used to feed (*A*) and shave (*B*) a 27-year-old ventilator user with Duchenne muscular dystrophy.

severely disabled ventilator user to be competitive in a wide variety of educational and employment situations. Individuals who are severely dysarthric or anarthric but who retain at least one reliable muscle movement, such as eye blink, can also be provided with methods for effective communication. A simple plastic or cardboard communication board can be used by the individual who has difficulty articulating or who speaks softly. This board has the letters of the alphabet as well as common words and phrases such as "yes" and "no" and the names of significant others. The person directs his or her eyes

or fingers to the letters on the board. Indicating the initial letter of a word in this manner enhances understanding, and the board can be used to spell out entire words as necessary.

Oversized keyboards can be used by some individuals with poor fine motor abilities. Miniature keyboards can be effective for people who have limited active hand movements without loss of fine motor control. Pointing devices can be used. These can have two functions: point, which can position a cursor on a computer screen, and select, which causes a certain function to be performed. The most commonly used

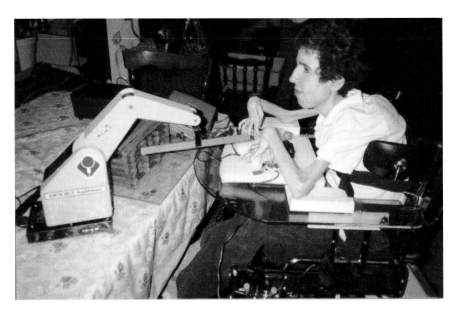

FIGURE 28–22. This ventilator user with Duchenne muscular dystrophy constructed the house pictured on the table in front of him using his robot arm alone.

pointing device is the mouse. A joystick or switch can be substituted for a mouse and can be modified and sized to be operated by any volitional muscle movement of the extremities (Fig. 28–23), chin, lips, or tongue.

For the person who is unable to hold a pen or a pencil without assistance, pencil holders include a pencil grip, sarong pencil holder, and click holder. These fit into a universal cuff. Many individuals have little wrist and finger mo-

tion but can write "from the shoulder" using gross motions. When there is no remaining upper extremity function, a mouthstick can be used. Typical mouthstick activities include writing, turning pages, painting, pressing buttons, keyboard control, and pushing or maneuvering small objects. The individual must be appropriately positioned to use these methods.

Many ventilator users with amyotrophic lateral sclerosis, severe spinal muscular atrophy, or

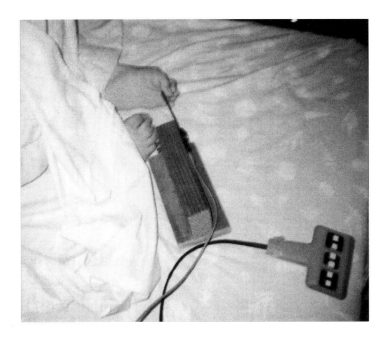

FIGURE 28–23. Toe switch used to operate computer software and environmental control system of an individual with Duchenne muscular dystrophy and no ventilator-free breathing ability who has used mouthpiece IPPV 24 hours a day for 15 years.

other severe conditions reach the point of having little more than residual eyelid and extraocular muscle function. Such individuals can blink to operate an eye switch activated by infrared limbus-pupil reflection. Other activation methods include the use of electro-ocular or finger-activated switches. In this way patients can use computer operated printers and voice synthesizers with the appropriate software (Words+, Inc., Sunnyvale, CA). With such a system users can create about 6 to 10 words per minute, store and quickly reproduce complex phrases, sentences, and paragraphs, and initiate communication as desired. The Eyegaze System (LC Technologies, Inc., Fairfax, VA) (Fig. 28–24) is operated by the user simply gazing at the desired letter or word on the computer screen for a fraction of a second. Although potentially effective, this system is expensive and requires careful positioning for accurate use. These activation methods permit individuals to use personal computers with keyboard emulator software to communicate with voice synthesizers and printers. The voice synthesizers can produce voices of different pitches, genders, and age groupings.

Phone systems can be programmed with automatic dialing functions initiated by striking a key or by sip-and-puff, finger switch, joy-stick, or voice-activation. A typical voice-activated speaker phone answers automatically once the patient says hello after the second ring and disconnects by itself. A sip-and-puff connects to the operator who can place a call (Temasek Telephone, Inc., San Francisco, CA), or voice-activated phones can be used with sip-and-puff dialing. Voice amplification is an option. A vast network of online services including food and clothes shopping can increase the independence of the user.

Voice, finger switch, eye movement, and blink activation can also be used for computer-operated environmental control so that the severely disabled individual can control all of the electrical appliances in the home (Fig. 28–25).[28] The computer can also be used for many other personal, educational, recreational, and vocational tasks. Increasingly, personal computers are being adapted and used in place of the specially designed adaptive equipment. Because technologic advances occur rapidly, however, devices often become obsolete in less than a year.[13] The major reasons for discarding assistive devices are ineffectiveness, malfunction, the use of substitute activities that render the device useless, aesthetic unacceptability, and availability of a more efficient device.[9]

DIAGNOSIS-RELATED FUNCTIONAL CONSIDERATIONS

Many patients with non-Duchenne myopathies such as myotonic dystrophy, certain mitochondrial myopathies, glycogen and lipid storage diseases, postpoliomyelitis, myasthenia gravis, obesity-hypoventilation syndrome, disorders of central chemotaxic sensitivity, and restrictive pulmonary diseases associated with lung and chest wall pathology are able to walk and retain considerable physical function despite requiring the use of nocturnal and occasionally around-the-clock ventilatory support. These patients often benefit from a wide range

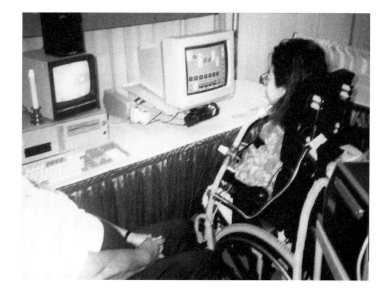

FIGURE 28–24. Eyegaze Systems use a low-power infrared-light–emitting diode mounted in the center of a video camera lens. This illuminates the eye and provides a bright image of the pupil and a bright spot reflecting off the cornea. Image processing software computes where on a control monitor screen the user is looking and enables the user to rapidly activate keys as small as 5/8 of a square inch (Eyegaze System, LC Technologies, Inc., 4415 Glenn Rose Street, Fairfax, VA). This technology permits much more rapid nonverbal communication and environmental control, albeit at a significantly greater cost.

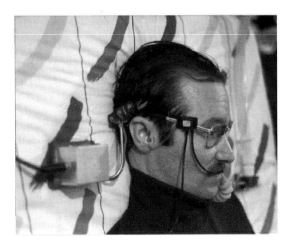

FIGURE 28–25. Ventilator user with no volitional movement below the neck, using an adapted telephone head set. Head rotation activates the system and contacts the operator. The speaker is in his ear and the small mouthpiece microphone is kept just over his lip and adjacent to his mouthpiece for ventilatory support.

of assistive devices and training in energy conservation.

Without the use of assistive devices, most children with Duchenne muscular dystrophy lose all ability to feed themselves by late adolescence. Subsequently, only hand movements permit continued function. These patients, however, can use finger movements (joy-stick controls) to operate computers, environmental control systems, robotics, and motorized wheelchairs. Fortunately, functional finger movements are usually retained by Duchenne muscular dystrophy patients into their fifth decade. Likewise, patients with spinal muscular atrophy, motor neuron disease, and most other neuromuscular diseases retain either functional finger excursion or other muscular activity with which to operate these critical systems.

High-level spinal cord–injured patients with complete lesions must rely on voice-activated or facial muscle–operated systems such as sip-and-puff, chin, and tongue controls.

Because about 95% of amyotrophic lateral sclerosis ventilator users retain eye-blink and extraocular movements, these are usually used to operate critical systems.[3] The 5% of amyotrophic lateral sclerosis ventilator users who lose these abilities generally lose all means of effective communication and functioning, are usually institutionalized, and may have a poor prog-

nosis because they are unable to communicate their airway suctioning needs.

SPLINTING

Static splints are used to rest joints or to prevent or retard the development of musculotendinous contractures, to support extremities to facilitate function, and to protect tissues.[15] Dynamic splints actively move body parts or vary tension during the user's active movements to enhance the function of weaker muscle groups. For example, hand splints include spring-loaded or rubber band–loaded finger extension assist splints that can bring the fingers back into extension to permit functional use of stronger finger flexors. Opposition splints position the hand with the thumb opposed to the palm to facilitate grasping conical or cylindric objects. Tenodesis splints assist individuals with active wrist extension but no finger control to have a functional grasp. As for lower extremity splinting, splints can be fabricated out of some combination of plastic (plastizote, polypropalene), fiberglass, plaster, and metal. A Dynasplint (Dynasplint Systems, Severna Park, MD) provides tension to stretch tight joints delicately and can be particularly effective for decreasing contractures. The tension imposed must be tolerable for the user to wear it for hours without skin irritation or breakdown.

Serial casting is the application of a cast over an extremity to decrease tone, stretch tight tissues, or facilitate proper bone growth (e.g., to counter equinovarus deformity). Precise positioning is required as the cast is applied. Casting materials are typically fiberglass or plaster. The cast is left on for a minimum of 1 to 2 days, and the patient's circulation and skin tolerance are frequently reassessed.[16,37]

WORK SIMPLIFICATION

The following principles may be followed to maximize energy conservation.

- Eliminate all unnecessary work.
- Place components of the task within easy reach, avoid straining and stretching, and organize tasks for minimum energy expenditure.
- Lay out work areas within easy reach.
- Use proper biomechanics when lifting and performing patient transfers. Slide, do not lift and carry. It is also usually easier to pull

an object toward oneself than to carry or push it. If it is necessary for the patient or care provider to lift an object, good spinal alignment is maintained, and the object is placed as close to the lifter as possible before lifting. Lifting with the legs straight or without an adequate lumbar lordotic curve places considerable stress on the back and causes repetitive stress injuries. The legs should provide the power for the lift. As the individual squats to the floor, the object is brought as close to the lifter as possible. With the back straight, the person then comes to stand while picking up the object. Twisting the back should also be avoided. It is better to lift and carry than to lift and twist. These guidelines are particularly important for patient transfers. Proper biomechanics should also be used when lifting children. Many people who use proper lifting techniques when picking up a 30-pound tool box improperly lean over to pick up a child. Besides helping to prevent care provider injury, the use of proper mechanics optimizes the safety of patient transfers.

- Minimize the amount of work done overhead because upper extremity muscles fatigue quickly, and exercise of the upper extremities places a great demand on the cardiopulmonary system.
- Have fixed work stations with all supplies for the given task on hand.
- Use the fewest tools possible.
- Avoid holding objects. Frequently put them down, preferably on a high stand.
- Let gravity work.
- Use small tools that can be grasped and used without bending and reaching.
- Place controls and switches within easy reach.
- Sit to work whenever possible. Strategically placed chairs allow for rest while using appliances.
- Modify work surface height for the best biomechanical advantage to the task.

SERVICE ANIMALS

People with motor disabilities are increasingly turning to service dogs as extra pairs of arms and legs.[38] The dogs undergo about 15 months of training to learn 60 commands. They go everywhere with the human partner. The Americans with Disabilities Act has established that service dogs be granted access virtually everywhere. One study showed that people with service dogs required an average of 72% fewer hours of human personal assistance time.[38] The service animals can retrieve items dropped on the floor and objects off high counters. They can operate wall switches, open and close doors, and go for help when needed. Trained dogs can also help companions dress, pulling garments up over the legs. Service dogs are used to power standard wheelchairs, thus often delaying the need for a motorized wheelchair until prolonged daytime as well as nocturnal ventilatory support is required. The Delta society (Renton, WA) publishes a Service Dog Directory listing the 70 or so training programs. All have waiting lists of 6 months to 5 years. For already trained dogs, fees are usually $10,000 or more. The cost of maintaining the dog is about $800 to $1000 a year, including food, grooming, veterinary care, and equipment. Insurance or rehabilitation services may ease the cost.

Service chimpanzees are less frequently available (Dr. M. Williard, Albert Einstein Medical School); and they are more difficult to domesticate and costly to maintain. However, they are more versatile than the dogs because of their fine hand motor skills. This permits them to operate finer environmental controls and manipulate small objects. For example, they can place a mouth stick in the patient's mouth, install a cassette, and feed the human companion. Chimpanzees have most often served high-level traumatic tetraplegic individuals.[14]

TRANSPORTATION

The ability to move about in the community is critical to remain active, independent, and productive. Mass transit, although economical, is often inconvenient, difficult, or impossible for the physically challenged individual to use consistently. To date, the most effective form of transportation is the adapted personal vehicle driven by the physically challenged individual or care provider. The problems associated with adapting a vehicle for use by a physically challenged driver are those of access, restraint, and control. Transportation needs can be assessed by certified driving instructors and occupational therapists to determine driving capabilities with adaptations or evaluating the wheelchair passenger transport set-up.

As a rule a sedan is less expensive to purchase, modify, and drive than a van. To use a sedan, it must be possible to transfer the patient into it and to load any needed equipment such as the wheelchair. The previously mentioned Meyland-Carlift (Access Unlimited, Bingham-

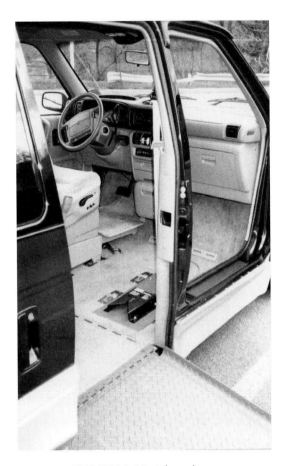

FIGURE 28–26. Adapted van.

ton, NY), which can be affixed to the car door, can facilitate such transfers. The least expensive adaptations for driving are levers, knobs, and extensions operated by either hand. If only one arm or leg is nonfunctional, an automatic transmission and power steering should be provided. A vehicle can be operated by upper extremity activity only. Air conditioning is critical for temperature control to avoid respiratory symptoms. Whether or not the physically challenged individual has sufficient residual muscle function to operate an appropriately modified vehicle or to be a passenger in one safely, can be certified by driving instructors and occupational therapists.

If the user cannot be transferred efficiently into an automobile, a van is the vehicle of choice (Fig. 28–26). A wheelchair-accessible van is particularly important for the transport of individuals with heavy motorized wheelchairs. Before 1984, the standard for accessibility was the full-sized van, equipped with a slow, noisy, and sometimes awkward lift. Once inside, the wheelchair passenger had limited headroom, visibility, and maneuvering room. Since that time, there have

been many advances. Today one has the option to purchase or rent a lowered floor accessible minivan. With the touch of a button, a sliding door opens, a folded ramp lowers, and the rear suspension lowers approximately 5 inches to decrease the ramp angle for easier access. Button touch then reverses the process (National Mobility Corporation, Elkhartz, IN). Urbanites may require a side lift to get into and out of the vehicle after parallel parking, whereas suburbanites often use a lift in the back. Although third-party payers rarely pay for the purchase of a van, governmental organizations such as the Division of Vocational Rehabilitation may provide funds for modifications.[3]

CONCLUSION

An extensive array of ADL, mobility, and communication assistive devices is available for individuals with neuromuscular disease. Firth, and colleagues,[19] however, noted that "practical" problems in daily care were the most frequently noted principal problems for 66 families of individuals with Duchenne muscular dystrophy.[19] "Service" problems caused by difficulties and delays in obtaining needed services were first, and personal assistance problems were second in frequency, and "emotional" problems ranked third. The specific problems in daily care cited most frequently were lifting (47%), housing (28%), bathing and toileting (19%), and lack of sleep owing to the need to turn the patient in bed at night (9%). Dressing and feeding were mentioned only rarely as problems. Although assistive devices can facilitate ADL and enhance independence, and this results in increased feelings of well-being,[31] the importance of family involvement cannot be overstated.

Organizations with periodicals that can provide valuable information about habilitation options for individuals with neuromuscular disease include the Jerry Lewis Muscular Dystrophy Association which is based in Tuscon, Arizona; Families of Children with Spinal Muscular Atrophy, Highland Park, Illinois; the National Easter Seal Society, Chicago, Illinois; the Polio Society, Washington, D.C.; the International Polio Network, whose publication *Gazette International Network Incorporated* is enormously useful for ventilator users with any diagnosis, St. Louis, Missouri; the ALS Association, Woodland Hills, California; the Myasthenia Gravis Foundation, Chicago, Illinois; the Charcot-Marie-Tooth Association, Upland, Pennsylvania; the National Ataxia Foundation, Wayzata, Minnesota; the National Support Group for Myositis, Cooperstown, New York; the Guillain-Barré Syndrome Foundation International, Wynnewood, Pennsylvania; the Malignant Hyperthermia Association of the United States, Westport, Connecticut; *New Mobility,* a magazine designed for individuals with spinal cord injury, North Hollywood, California; and the National Association for Ventilator Dependent Individuals, a newly formed social service organization dedicated to facilitating opportunities to enhance the quality of life of ventilator users, New York.

In 1879, Gowers said of Duchenne muscular dystrophy that it is "sad on account of our powerlessness to influence its course" and that "each year (it) takes (the patient) a step further on the road to a helpless infirmity, and in most cases to an early and inevitable death."[6] Over 100 years later, despite the often dramatic physical medicine interventions discussed in this book, this sense of therapeutic futility pervades and has been repeated word for word.[17] The failure to take a proactive approach to prevent orthopedic and especially respiratory complications pervades the medical establishment,[1,2] and patients have inconsistent access to the use of beds and mattresses; urinary drainage systems; computers; robots; physical medicine respiratory interventions; and other aids that can increase their comfort, function, and survival while easing care provider burden. Considering the fact that to this day more attention is being paid to thanatology[40] than to the use of noninvasive respiratory aids, individuals with neuromuscular disease continue to face an uphill battle to obtain vital information.

References

1. Bach JR: Standards of care in Muscular Dystrophy Association clinics. J Neuro Rehabil 6:67–73, 1992.
2. Bach JR: Ventilator use by muscular dystrophy association patients: An update. Arch Phys Med Rehabil 73:179–183, 1992.
3. Bach JR: Therapeutic interventions and habilitation considerations: A historical perspective from Tamplin to robotics for pseudohypertrophic muscular dystrophy. Semin Neurol 15:38–45 1995.
4. Bach JR, Barnett V: Ethical considerations in the management of individuals with severe neuromuscular disorders. Am J Phys Med Rehabil 73:134–140, 1994.
5. Bach JR, Zeelenberg A, Winter C: Wheelchair mounted robot manipulators: Long term use by patients with Duchenne muscular dystrophy. Am J Phys Med Rehabil 69:59–69, 1990.
6. Bonduelle M: Histoire de la neurologie: Aran-Duchenne? Duchenne-Aran? La querelle de l'atrophie musculaire progressive. Rev Neurol (Paris) 146:97–106, 1990.
7. Brammell CA: Assistive devices for patients with neuromuscular diseases: The role of the occupational therapy.

In Maloney FP, Burks JS, Ringel SP (eds): Interdisciplinary Rehabilitation of Multiple Sclerosis and Neuromuscular Disorders. Philadelphia, JB Lippincott, 1985, pp. 259–276.
8. Bregman AM: Living with progressive childhood illness: Parental management of neuromuscular disease. Social Work in Health Care 5:387–408, 1980.
9. Britell CW, Scott NG: Computer adaptive systems and technology for the disabled. In DeLisa JA (ed): Rehabilitation Medicine, 2nd ed. Philadelphia, JB Lippincott, 1993, pp 555–562.
10. Brooke MH: A Clinician's View of Neuromuscular Diseases, 2nd ed. Baltimore, Williams & Wilkins, 1986, pp 117–154.
11. Cherry DB: Transfer techniques for children with muscular dystrophy. Phys Ther 53:970–971, 1973.
12. Chyatte SB, Long C, Vignos PJ Jr: The balanced forearm orthosis in muscular dystrophy. Arch Phys Med Rehabil 46:633–636, 1965.
13. Congressional Office of Technology Assessment: Technology and Handicapped People. New York, Springer-Verlag, 1985.
14. Cotman CW, Nieto-Sampedro M, Gibbs RB: Enhancing the self-repairing potential of the CNS after injury. Central Nervous System Trauma 1:3–14, 1984.
15. Cusick B: Progressive Casting and Splinting for Lower Extremity Deformities in Children with Neuromuscular Dysfunction. Tuscon, Therapy Skill Builders, 1990, p 251.
16. Downie P: Cash's Textbook of Neurology for Physiotherapists, 4th ed. Philadelphia, JB Lippincott, 1986, pp 36–40.
17. Dubowitz V: Management of muscular dystrophy in 1977. Isr J Med Sci 13:235–244, 1977.
18. Edelstein J: Lower Limb Orthotics. New York, New York University Graduate School, 1986, pp 99–100.
19. Firth M, Gardner-Medwin D, Hosking G, Wilkinson E: Interviews with parents of boys suffering from Duchenne muscular dystrophy. Dev Med Child Neurol 25:466–471, 1983.
20. Gibson DA: Rehabilitation for children with neuromuscular disorders. Semin Orthop 2:173–181, 1987.
21. Gibson DA, Albisser AM, Koreska J: Role of the wheelchair in the management of the muscular dystrophy patient. Can Med Assoc J 113:964–967, 1975.
22. Granata C, Cornelio F, Bonfiglioli S, et al: Promotion of ambulation of patients with spinal muscular atrophy by early fitting of knee-ankle-foot orthoses. Dev Med Child Neurol 29:221–224, 1987.
23. Guyton A: Human Physiology and Mechanisms of Disease, 5th ed. Philadelphia, WB Saunders, 1992, pp 593–595.
24. Hall DS, Vignos PJ Jr: Clothing adaptations for the child with progressive muscular dystrophy. Am J Occup Ther 18:108–112, 1964.
25. Hartley FD: A nurse's view: Amyotrophic lateral sclerosis. J Neurosurg Nurs 13:89–95, 1991.
26. Huber SR: Therapeutic application of orthotics. In Umphred DA, (ed): Neurological Rehabilitation. St. Louis, CV Mosby, 1990, pp 773–789.
27. James WV, Orr JF: Upper limb weakness in children with Duchenne muscular dystrophy—a neglected problem. Prosthet Orthotics Int 8:11–13, 1984.
28. Kazandjian MS, Dikeman KJ, Bach JR: Assessment and management of communication impairment in neuromuscular disease. Semin Neurol 15:52–57, 1995.
29. Kortman B: Rehabilitation of patients with motor neuron disease: The occupational therapist's role. Aust Occup Ther J 34:114–118, 1987.
30. Kwee HH, Duimel JJ, et al: The Manus wheelchair-

mounted manipulator: System review and first results. In Proceedings of 2nd International Workshop on Robotic Applications in Medical and Health Care, Newcastle Upon Tyne, England, 1989, pp 1–11.

31. Lord JP, Lieberman JS, Portwood MM, et al: Functional ability and equipment use among patients with neuromuscular disease. Arch Phys Med Rehabil 68:348–352, 1987.

32. Mann W, Lane J: Assistive Technology for Persons with Disabilities: The Role of Occupational Therapy. Baltimore, American Occupational Therapy Association, 1991, p 11.

33. Merlini L, Granata C, Bonfiglioli S, et al: Scoliosis in spinal muscular atrophy: Natural history and management. Dev Med Child Neurol 31:501–508, 1989.

34. Palmer L, Toms J: Manual for Functional Training, 2nd ed. Philadelphia, FA Davis, 1986, p 264.

35. Phillips DP, Roye DP, Farcy JC, et al: Surgical treatment of scoliosis in a spinal muscular atrophy population. Spine 15:942–945, 1990.

36. Redding GJ, Okamoto GA, Guthrie RD, et al: Sleep patterns in nonambulatory boys with Duchenne muscular dystrophy. Arch Phys Med Rehabil 66:818–821, 1985.

37. Snedden J: Myasthenia gravis: A study of social, medical and emotional problems in 26 patients. Lancet 1:526–528, 1980.

38. Sowell C: Service dogs have their day. Quest 1:4–8, 1994.

39. Stanger CA, Anglin C, Harwin WS, Romilly DP: Devices for assisting manipulation: a summary of user task priorities. IEEE Trans Rehabil Eng 2:256–265, 1994.

40. Therapy For Childhood Neuromuscular Diseases (Course Brochure). Tuscon, Jerry Lewis Muscular Dystrophy Association, 1994.

41. Vignos PJ Jr, Archibald KC: Maintenance of ambulation in childhood muscular dystrophy. J Chron Dis 12:273–290, 1960.

42. Yasuda YL, Bowman K, Hsu JD: Mobile arm supports: Criteria for successful use in muscle disease patients. Arch Phys Med Rehabil 67:253–256, 1986.

43. Ziter FA, Allsop KG: The value of orthoses for patients with Duchenne muscular dystrophy. Phys Ther 59:1361–1365, 1979.

Psychosocial, Vocational, Quality of Life, and Ethical Issues

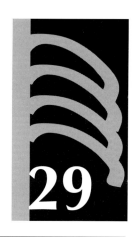

John R. Bach, MD
Vicki Barnett, PhD

"Throughout the ALS process, I have learned many things. I have learned that having ALS does not necessarily mean a death sentence, that I am not living with a life-threatening disease, but rather with a life-enhancing condition."—Justice Sam Filer, a ventilator-user, April 19, 1991.[5]

It is now clear that life can be greatly prolonged for many individuals with respiratory muscle weakness or paralysis by long-term ventilatory support and that such individuals can be maintained in the community. Little in the medical literature, however, concerns the productivity, social reintegration, and life satisfaction of ventilator-users with neuromusculoskeletal disorders. This chapter reviews the results of a questionnaire used to assess ventilator-users' employment and marital status, ventilator style preferences, respiratory complications, satisfaction with life, and related ethical issues. All respondents were maintained in the community with equipment supplied by a major manufacturer of portable mechanical ventilators (Lifecare International Inc., Westminster, CO). For comparison, health care professionals and autonomously breathing spinal-cord-injured (SCI) individuals were surveyed.

STUDY POPULATION

Six hundred ninety-five out of a mailing to about 1000 community-based ventilator-users responded to the survey. Four hundred ninety-four individuals were supported by noninvasive means, 92 by tracheostomy intermittent positive pressure ventilation (IPPV), and 35 either did not indicate by which means they were ventilated or did not answer the satisfaction index. Ninety-four of the 621 had used both tracheostomy and noninvasive aids and answered the questions from the perspective of the method they were currently using. Another 74 ventilator-users had also used both tracheostomy and noninvasive methods of ventilatory support but responded only to questions concerning ventilator style preferences. All 621 individuals who responded to all sections of the survey were wheelchair users, and 585 were unable to walk and were dependent on attendant care for virtually all activities of daily living (ADL). The 7 ventilator-users with intrinsic lung disease could walk very short distances using a rolling walker with a ventilator tray.

The diagnoses, mean ages, residual function, hours per day and years of ventilator use, and life satisfaction indices are listed in Table 29–1. There were 313 males with a mean age of 46.5 years and 306 females with a mean age of 52.2 years. Two individuals whose gender was not indicated had an average age of 41 years. The 621 ventilator-users had been dependent on ventilatory support for a mean of 21.1 years and, at the time of the survey, used aid a mean of 15.7 hours/day. The 46 autonomously breathing SCI individuals were randomly identified from the medical records of a rehabilitation facility.

TABLE 29-1
Duration of Ventilator Use and Life Satisfaction Index

Diagnosis	No. of Patients	Age(yrs)[a]	Residual Function	Years of Ventilator Use	Hours[b] per day	Life Satisfaction[c]
Individuals using noninvasive aids (n = 404)						
Poliomyelitis	336	54.5±8.9	1.2±0.9	27.8±12.6	15.4±9.7	5.2±1.6
DMD	47	27.3±7.2	0.6±0.5	7.6±5.0	18.0±6.8	5.1±1.5
Unknown[d]	29	54.3±16.2	1.6±1.3	14.2±12.7	13.9±6.7	4.8±1.3
Traumatic SCI	23	33.7±11.0	0.3±0.7	8.8±6.4	17.5±8.1	4.0±1.9
Non-Duchenne Myopathy	23	40.2±17.1	1.5±1.2	8.7±10.4	15.9±6.7	4.6±1.9
ALS	8	48.3±12.5	0.4±0.5	7.0±7.8	19.3±7.1	4.1±1.7
Intrinsic[e]	7	57.1±10.2	2.3±1.2	6.3±7.7	11.6±6.8	4.6±1.4
Myasthenia gravis	5	57.6±11.0	2.0±1.0	18.4±12.1	9.4±2.5	4.6±2.3
Kyphoscoliosis	4	60.3±13.7	2.8±0.5	9.5±3.0	8.5±1.3	4.7±1.9
Polymyositis	3	46.3±11.0	1.7±1.2	11.3±7.8	18.0±5.6	5.0±0.9
Obesity/hypoventilation syndrome	3	39.3±11.5	1.3±0.6	7.0±5.6	7.7±2.5	4.0±2.6
Myelopathy	3	54.7±13.7	0.0±0.0	10.9±10.1	18.2±10.1	5.5±1.5
Multiple Sclerosis	2	59.0±24.0	0.5±0.7	20.5±12.0	5.8±6.0	4.7±1.1
Arthrogryposis	1	26.0	2.5	11.0	8.0	5.5
Tracheostomy IPPV users (N = 92)						
Poliomyelitis	44	53.1±10.0	1.4±0.9	24.1±11.8	16.0±6.6	4.6±1.8
DMD[d]	13	30.8±4.8	0.6±0.5	5.0±3.0	20.8±5.5	4.8±1.3
Non-Duchenne Myopathy	12	34.2±13.6	1.3±1.0	9.4±6.5	19.9±6.7	4.9±1.6
ALS	5	51.8±21.7	0.6±0.9	11.4±20.5	20.2±6.1	2.5±1.5
Unknown[d]	5	50.8±20.5	2.4±0.5	8.2±1.5	11.8±7.1	5.5±2.6
Traumatic SCI	4	31.3±9.1	0.0±0.0	30.8±18.2	20.0±8.0	5.4±1.7
Polymyositis	2	41.0±9.9	1.0±1.4	4.0±1.4	23.0±0.0	3.0±2.8
Charcot-Marie-Tooth disease	2	53.5±0.7	1.5±0.7	6.5±4.9	24.0±0.0	4.5±3.5
Kyphoscoliosis	1	47.0	3.0	11.0	8.0	5.5
Myelopathy	1	40.0	1.0	27.0	8.0	5.5
Multiple Sclerosis	1	62.0	0.0	6.0	24.0	3.0
Spinal muscular atrophy	1	40.0	1.0	26.0	16.0	7.0
Polyneuropathy	1	17.0	0.0	7.0	24.0	5.5

[a]Age at the time of the survey.
[b]Hours per day of ventilator use.
[c]Patient satisfaction with life in general, where 1 is very dissatisfied and 7 is very satisfied.
[d]Not reported on the survey.
[e]Intrinsic lung disease, including pulmonary fibrosis and chronic obstructive pulmonary disease.

MARITAL STATUS

Two hundred seventy-seven (45%) ventilator-users, 157 males and 120 females, had not married. One hundred eighty-six (97 males and 89 females) were married prior to requiring ventilatory support and remained married and living with their spouses. This included 4 individuals who were widowed prior to requiring ventilatory support and later remarried while using support and 2 males who were divorced prior to requiring support and remarried while on aid. These 186 individuals had been using ventilatory support for a mean of 22.7 years and required 13.7 hours of support per day. Twenty other individuals were married prior to requiring ventilatory aid then were subsequently widowed. Thirty-six individuals (10 males and 26 females) were married prior to requiring ventilatory support and divorced and have remained so while using ventilatory aids. An additional 60 individuals (32 males and 28 females) who were single prior to requiring ventilator support married as ventilator-users and live with their spouses. Forty-two individuals did not respond to this question.

Therefore, 16.2% of the ventilator-users who were married before onset of ventilator dependence were divorced subsequently and have not remarried over a mean period of 22.7 years of ventilator use. This group became ventilator-users at the mean age of 28 years. The general nondisabled population has a divorce rate of 30% for people married at the mean age of 28 years.[41] Another 20% of ventilator users who were single before requiring ventilator use married for the first time after becoming ventilator-users.

The marital status of autonomously breathing SCI individuals has been reported.[49] Wilcox and Stauffer found that although equal numbers of paraplegic and tetraplegic individuals married, the divorce rate was higher among individuals with tetraplegia.[54] In a follow-up study of SCI individuals, DeVivo et al. found approximately a 6% rate of new marriages and a 6% to 15% divorce rate during the 2 years following injury.[21] Following injury, the long-term divorce rate was 25% for our autonomously breathing traumatic tetraplegics and 59% for the SCI ventilator-users, and the new marriage rate was 22% and 11%, respectively.

EMPLOYMENT STATUS

Two hundred thirty-four individuals (134 males, 99 females, and 1 whose gender was not indicated) were gainfully employed despite ventilator dependence (Table 29–2). Seventeen other ventilator-users reported being active daily as volunteers for various philanthropic causes, and 24 were students. In addition, 32 married female ventilator-users reported being housewives.

A 46% employment rate was found among individuals with tetraplegia in a study of employment after SCI in 286 individuals an average of 18.6 years postinjury.[34] A national study by Stover et al. found employment rates of 14% to 28% for SCI individuals.[49] The percentage of SCI ventilator-user respondents who were employed at the time of this survey (29%) was nearly as high as the percentage of employed autonomously breathing traumatic tetraplegics (32%). These figures are comparable to those reported by Stover et al.[49] It is of interest that the 14 employed and 8 student SCI ventilator-users who responded to this survey required ventilator use for a mean of 12.7 years, 17.5 hours/day. The occupations noted were teaching, computer analysis, accounting, telemarketing, ministering, office work, and administration. Twelve of these individuals used noninvasive ventilatory support, one's method of aid was not noted, and

TABLE 29–2
Occupations of Ventilator Users with Neuromusculoskeletal Conditions

Accounting/banking	28
Social work/counseling	27
Business owners	21
Teachers	18
Engineers/scientists	13
Business/corporation executives/administration	11
Journalism/freelance writers	10
Computer (programming, systems analysis)	10
Lawyers	9
College professors	8
Artists (including mouthstick)	8
Insurance sales	6
Investment brokers and analysts	4
Real estate brokers	4
Physicians	2
Architects	2
College administrators	2
Mail order sales	2
Dispatchers (police, trucking)	2
Speech language pathologist	1
Clergy	1
Receptionist	1
Librarian	1
Travel agent	1
Not Specified	42

one used tracheostomy IPPV. SCI individuals with regular occupational income score better on quality of life scales than those without employment.[38]

LIFE SATISFACTION

When asked to indicate how satisfied they were with their lives by circling a number from 1 to 7 (where 1 is very dissatisfied and 7 is very satisfied), the 615 individuals who responded had a mean of 5.1. The 586 individuals whose method of ventilatory support was known had a mean age of 49.4 ± 14 years (range, 16–84 years) and reported a mean satisfaction index of 4.98 ± 1.68. Two hundred forty-two nondisabled health care professionals with an average age of 33.0 ± 8 years (range, 21–59 years) reported 5.33 ± 1.2 for satisfaction with their own lives, with no one reporting 1. This was significantly different from the mean 4.98 score of the ventilator-users ($p < 0.005$). When asked how ADL-dependent, ventilator-dependent individuals would respond to this question, however, the health care professionals estimated the ventilator-users' responses to be 2.42 ± 1.37, significantly worse than the ventilator-users' actual responses ($p < 0.0001$).

Differences between individuals using noninvasive ventilatory aids and those on tracheostomy IPPV were found. Both groups were compared for level of upper extremity function in the following manner:

0, no upper extremity function;
1, sufficient finger movement to operate a motorized wheelchair;
2, adequate function to feed oneself;
3, normal or near-normal function.

The ages, levels of function, years of ventilator use, hours per day of use, and satisfaction index for the tracheostomy and the noninvasive groups are listed in Table 29–3. The noninvasive group was older than the tracheostomy group (50 vs 45.8 years, $p < 0.001$), had significantly less upper extremity function (1.13 vs 1.21, $p < 0.05$), used ventilatory support for fewer hours per day (15.5 vs 17.7, $p < 0.05$), but for more years (22 vs 17, $p < 0.005$). The tracheostomy IPPV group, however, had a mean satisfaction index of 4.68 as opposed to 5.04 for the noninvasive group ($p < 0.05$). These figures are compared for various diagnostic subgroups in Table 1.

None of the variables studied was significantly different at the 95% confidence level for

TABLE 29–3
Comparison of Tracheostomy IPPV and Noninvasive Ventilator-Users

Variable	Mean ±
Using Tracheostomy IPPV ($n = 92$)	
Age	45.8 ± 15.33
Function	1.21 ± 0.97
Ventilator use in yrs	17.05 ± 14.74
Ventilator use in hrs/day	17.65 ± 6.81
Satisfaction index	4.64 ± 1.85
Noninvasive ventilatory support ($n = 494$)	
Age	50.03 ± 13.69
Function	1.13 ± 0.97
Ventilator use in yrs	22.01 ± 14.29
Ventilator use in hrs/day	15.47 ± 8.95
Satisfaction index	5.03 ± 1.64

any of the diagnostic groups, except for the individuals with post-poliomyelitis. For this subgroup, age, years of ventilator use, hours per day of use, and level of function were not significantly different for the tracheostomy and noninvasive groups; however, the satisfaction index for the noninvasive group was significantly greater than that of the tracheostomy group (5.20 vs 4.55, $p < 0.02$).

QUALITY OF LIFE DOMAINS

The SCI,[16] post-polio,[12] and Duchenne muscular dystrophy (DMD)[13] ventilator-users and 273 health care professionals (controls) were asked to fill out Campbell's Scale of Life Domain Satisfaction Measures and his Semantic Differential Scale of General Affect in the manner described by Campbell et al.[18] In addition, the controls were asked how they thought ventilator users with little or no extremity function would respond. A summary of the responses is presented in Tables 29–4 and 29–5.

Ninety-three percent of Campbell's subjects, 91% of our health care professional controls, 87.5% of the ventilator-users with DMD, 85% of the ventilator-users with post-polio, and 69% of the SCI ventilator-users reported being satisfied with their lives (response of š4). The post-polio, DMD, and SCI ventilator-users were significantly less satisfied with their transportation, education, health, social lives, sexual lives, and life in general than were the controls. They were significantly more satisfied with their housing. There were no significant differences when comparing satisfaction with family life and em-

Table 29–4
Life Domain Satisfaction Measures*

Ventilator Users	Post-Polio	DMD	SCI	SCI Controls	Controls
Housing	386 5.7±1.7	78 5.6±1.4	42 5.6±2.1	47 5.0±1.5	263 5.2±1.5
Transportation	351 5.3±2.1	77 4.7±2.0	41 4.5±2.3	47 4.6±2.0	268 5.7±1.6
Education	388 5.2±1.9	82 5.2±1.5	42 4.6±2.1	46 4.8±1.8	266 5.5±0.1
Job	216 5.2±1.9	29 4.6±1.7	15 5.2±2.2	33 3.5±2.0	269 5.2±1.4
Health	384 3.9±1.9	82 3.8±2.0	42 4.1±2.1	47 3.9±1.7	269 5.7±1.2
Family life	364 5.6±1.8	77 5.6±1.7	41 5.7±1.7	47 4.9±1.8	268 5.6±1.4
Social life	360 4.8±1.8	75 4.4±1.9	41 4.5±2.0	47 4.4±1.9	268 5.4±1.4
Sexual life	324 4.1±2.2	51 3.6±2.3	36 3.1±2.2	46 3.2±2.0	227 5.5±1.5
Life in general	380 5.1±1.7	80 4.9±1.3	42 4.4±1.8	47 4.1±1.7	259 5.4±1.2
					268 2.5±1.7[†]

*Ventilator-users were asked to rate their satisfaction with the dimension under question from 1 to 7, where 1 indicates extreme dissatisfaction and 7 indicates extreme satisfaction. The SCI controls were autonomously breathing, spinal-cord-injured individuals. The controls were 273 health care professionals. Data are given as number of respondents to the dimension under question and mean ± SD scores (ranging from 1–7).
[†]Health professional controls' responses assessing the ventilator-users' satisfaction with life.

Table 29–5
Semantic Differential Scale of General Affect*

	Post-Polio (361–368)	DMD (250–256)	SCI (40–41)	SCI Controls[†] (44–46)	Controls[‡] (250–256)	Controls' Estimate of Ventilator-Users' Responses (233–239)
Boring—interesting	5.6±1.6	4.5±1.6	4.7±2.0	4.7±2.2	5.4±1.5	2.4±1.5
Miserable—enjoyable	5.6±1.5	4.9±1.5	4.9±1.9	4.5±1.6	5.7±1.2	2.4±1.4
Hard—easy	3.8±1.8	2.9±1.7	3.2±1.8	3.4±1.7	4.1±1.5	1.8±1.1
Useless—worthwhile	5.9±1.7	5.0±1.9	5.0±2.1	5.0±2.0	6.2±1.1	2.8±1.7
Lonely—friendly	5.9±1.7	5.3±1.7	5.1±2.3	4.9±1.9	5.8±1.4	3.0±1.9
Empty—full	5.5±1.6	5.0±1.5	4.8±1.8	4.6±1.8	5.8±1.2	2.7±1.4
Discouraging—hopeful	5.4±1.8	4.9±1.5	4.9±2.1	4.8±1.8	5.9±1.2	2.8±1.7
Tied down—free	4.0±2.0	3.5±2.1	3.2±2.1	3.8±2.0	5.0±1.6	1.8±1.2
Disappointing—rewarding	5.3±1.8	4.5±1.4	4.1±2.3	4.5±1.8	5.8±1.1	2.4±1.5

*Subjects were asked to indicate the extent that each heuristic dimension describes them by indicating a number from 1 to 7, where 1 and 7 reflect the extremes of the polar adjective pairs in a seven-point Likert-type scale. Data are expressed as mean ± SD. The range of the number of responses to each heuristic dimension is indicated in parentheses.
[†]SCI controls consisted of spinal-cord-injured autonomously breathing individuals.
[‡]The controls consisted of health care professionals.

ployment. Except for health (post-polio ventilator-users) and sexual activity (DMD and SCI ventilator-users), however, the ventilator users were generally satisfied in each domain, reporting a mean >4.0. The controls' estimation that the ventilator-users would report dissatisfaction with life in general was very significantly incorrect.

The controls felt that their lives were significantly easier, more worthwhile, fuller, more hopeful, freer, and more rewarding than the ventilator-users. The controls very significantly misjudged that the ventilator-users would give negative responses for each semantic differential (Table 5). In fact, the ventilator-users' mean responses were >4 for each differential except for "hard—easy" (post-polio, DMD, and SCI ventilator-users), and "tied down" (DMD and SCI ventilator-users). The post-polio ventilator-users even judged their lives to be more interesting and friendly than did the controls, although the differences did not reach statistical significance and there was also no significant difference in the "miserable–enjoyable" differential between the two groups.

VENTILATOR STYLE PREFERENCE: TRACHEOSTOMY IPPV VS NONINVASIVE PHYSICAL MEDICINE ALTERNATIVES

A survey of a subset of the population of 695 ventilator-users, that of the 168 with >1-month's experience in the use of both tracheostomy and noninvasive methods, was undertaken to compare their ventilator use preferences.[4] They had the following diagnoses: post-poliomyelitis, 135; non-Duchenne myopathies, 14; SCI, 13; severe kyphoscoliosis, 3; chronic obstructive pulmonary disease, 3; DMD, 2; Guillain-Barré syndrome, 2; and myasthenia gravis, multiple sclerosis, amyotrophic lateral sclerosis [ALS], and polymyositis, 1 each. They had a mean age of 54.7 ± 11.4 years and were using ventilatory support for 17.1 ± 6.5 hours/day and for 22.7 ± 13.1 consecutive years.

One hundred fifty-five of the 168 (92%) required both nocturnal and at least some daytime ventilatory aid. Over 155 had required 24-hour support for some period of time. They were divided into two groups: the 111 ventilator-users initially managed by noninvasive ventilatory support and subsequently switched to tracheostomy IPPV (noninvasive-first group), and the 59 ventilator-users switched from tracheostomy IPPV to noninvasive aids (tracheostomy-first group). There were no significant differences between the groups in age ($p = 0.22$), hours per day of ventilator use ($p = 0.11$), and years of ventilator use ($p = 0.10$). The noninvasive-first group used noninvasive aids for 13.7 ± 11.5 years before being switched to tracheostomy IPPV, which they used for another 10.5 ± 10.3 years. The tracheostomy-first group used tracheostomy IPPV for 1.6 ± 4.8 years before switching to noninvasive ventilatory aids for another 18.8 ± 14.8 years.

Besides tracheostomy IPPV, 84 respondents had used only body ventilator noninvasive aids for a mean of 14.3 ± 14.1 years overnight and 10.7 ± 14.1 years during waking hours; 24 respondents used only noninvasive IPPV for 9 ± 8.2 years for nocturnal support and 4.5 ± 7.5 years during waking hours, and 62 respondents used both body ventilators and noninvasive IPPV methods for a mean of 21.7 ± 10.0 years overnight and 21.7 ± 12.9 years during waking hours.

Figures 29–1 through 29–3 present the respondents' preferences for the quality of life issues surveyed. Table 29–6 demonstrates concordance of the principal caregivers' preferences with those of the ventilator-users. Other reasons cited for preferring tracheostomy or noninvasive aids are listed in Table 29–7. In addition, the ventilator users reported requiring tracheal suctioning a mean of 7.6 ± 8.3 times/day, with 27 patients (16%) reporting 10 or more times per day while they had indwelling tracheostomy tubes. Thirteen of the latter group cited numerous respiratory complications before switching to up to 24-hour use of noninvasive aids. Thirty-five percent of the tracheostomy IPPV users ex-

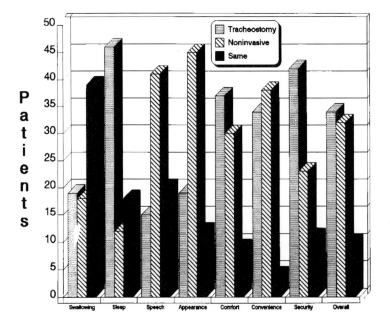

FIGURE 29–1. Preference of 76 ventilator-users switched from body ventilator use to tracheostomy IPPV (noninvasive-first or group 1). (From Bach JR: A comparison of long-term ventilatory support alternatives from the perspective of the patient and care giver. Chest 104:1702–1706, 1993; with permission.)

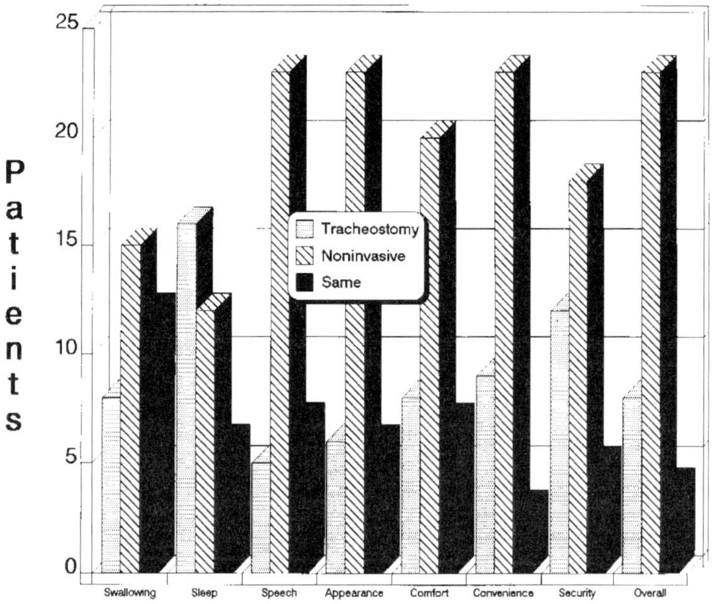

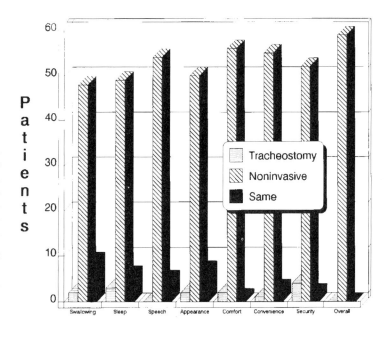

FIGURE 29–2. Preference of 35 patients switched from a regimen of body ventilators and/or noninvasive IPPV to tracheostomy (noninvasive-first or group 1). (From Bach JR: A comparison of long-term ventilatory support alternatives from the perspective of the patient and care giver. Chest 104:1702–1706, 1993, with permission.)

FIGURE 29–3. Preference of 59 patients switched from tracheostomy to noninvasive aids (tracheostomy-first or group 2), including 8 who switched to body ventilators, 18 to noninvasive IPPV methods, and 33 to a combination of body ventilators and noninvasive IPPV methods. (From Bach JR: A comparison of long-term ventilatory support alternatives from the perspective of the patient and care giver. Chest 104: 1702–1706, 1993; with permission.)

pressed the desire to return to noninvasive aids, whereas none of the respondents using noninvasive aids wished to switch back to tracheostomy IPPV. Two of the ventilator-users in the noninvasive-first group (2%) and 8 in the tracheostomy-first group (14%) had regular access to mechanical insufflation-exsufflation during respiratory tract infections. Twenty-eight of the ventilator-users in the noninvasive-first group (25%) and 22 in the tracheostomy-first group

(37%) mastered glossopharyngeal breathing (GPB) sufficiently to achieve or increase ventilator-free breathing time.

The ventilator-users were also surveyed for the number of times they were hospitalized for respiratory difficulties, and especially for pneumonia, before using ventilatory assistance, when using oxygen therapy, when using noninvasive aids for <16 hours/day versus >16 hours/day, and when having an indwelling tracheostomy

TABLE 29–6
Patient and Principal Caregiver Overall Preference for Tracheostomy or Noninvasive Ventilatory Aids

	Noninvasive	Tracheostomy	No preference
Noninvasive-first group			
Patients	55	42	14
Caregivers	50	38	23
Tracheostomy-first group			
Patients	59	0	0
Caregivers	48	1	8

TABLE 29–7
Other Reasons Cited for Preferring Tracheostomy Or Noninvasive Aids

	No.
For prefering tracheostomy:	
Facility in clearing airway secretions during respiratory tract infections	57 (31%)
Greater mobility in comparison with body ventilator use	8 (9%)
Better speech than with mouth IPPV	1 (1%)
For prefering noninvasive aids:	
Greater independence and control of breathing	24 (14%)
Facilitation of management in the community	17 (10%)
Suctioning no longer needed/absence of secretions	17 (10%)
Greater portability; less equipment, supply needs, and upkeep	14 (8%)
Greater mobility	11 (7%)
Fewer infections	11 (7%)
More natural	9 (5%)
Compatibility with GPB air stacking	3 (2%)

tube and receiving IPPV for any period of time daily. The ventilator-users were controlled for level of extremity function. Although this study is not yet completed, the initial results (statistically significant) indicate that the highest incidence of pneumonias and hospitalizations for respiratory complications was in the underventilated patients receiving oxygen therapy (28 patients), followed by those receiving IPPV via an indwelling tracheostomy (0.36 pneumonias/year and 0.45 hospitalizations/year over a mean 8.46-year period for 269 ventilator-users), and those using noninvasive aids <16 hours/day (0.08 pneumonias/year and 0.10 hospitalizations/year over a mean 14.09-year period for 202 ventilator-users). The population with the lowest incidence of complications and hospitalizations was the noninvasive aid users using aid >16 hours/day (0.04 pneumonias/year and 0.07 hospitalizations/year over a mean 17-year period for 296 ventilator-users). The fact that the lowest incidence of pulmonary complications was found in the noninvasive aid users with the greatest need for ventilatory support can be explained by their avoiding the complications associated with indwelling tracheostomy tubes; in addition, part-time ventilatory aid users are often underventilated and cannot increase insufflation volumes adequately to eliminate airway secretions as needed when not using their ventilators.

In miscellaneous survey questions, every ventilator-user without exception indicated that ventilatory assistance should be offered to every individual who could benefit from it; that finances should not be a consideration; and that each would have used ventilatory aid if it had to be done over again.

SOCIAL INTEGRATION

A total of 307 ventilator-users, or about one-half of the 621 total, maintained active and productive lives in their communities, as can be seen by reviewing the social and occupational activities of this group. The male/female ratio was equal. Because other activities, such as visits with friends or going to restaurants, sporting events, or other spectacles, were not surveyed, it is clear that over one-half of this population maintains a significant degree of mobility despite severe disability and ventilatory dependence. Technologic advances in environmental control systems, personal computers, and robot aids[11] as well as in ventilators and home health care delivery have also greatly facilitated a more active ventilator-user lifestyle. In addition, the federal government awards tax credits to businesses that hire disabled individuals and make physical modifications to accommodate them.

QUALITY OF LIFE AND LIFE SATISFACTION ASSESSMENT ISSUES

Campbell et al. recognized the difficulty in dealing with subjective perceptions of well-being in that reports of "excellent," "good," or "poor" overall quality of life may mean different things to different people. He concluded, nonetheless, that these subjective parameters yielded consistent results when compared between different populations and that they are essential for assessing individuals' personal values and their assessment of their own quality of life.[24] He found that the single-item measure of overall life satisfaction closely fit the measures of satisfaction with the specific domains of life, and as such, it was one of the most important measures. Kammann et al. also demonstrated that the items with the highest item validities were those which had a global frame of reference, such as feeling that life is going well in general.[32] The mean score of the overall life satisfaction item was 5.54 for Campbell's 2134 subjects as compared with 5.36 for our 273 health care professionals (controls). Although the approximately 5.0 mean scores of the ventilator-users was significantly <that of the physically able population, they were still very positive (>4.0) and significantly greater than those anticipated by the health care professionals in general (2.5).

Physicians' perceptions of the patients' quality of life are extremely variable.[42] This study demonstrated the extent to which health care professionals underestimate the severely disabled, ventilator-assisted individuals' satisfaction with life. This is important because physicians' assessment of patients' quality of life and about the relative desirability of certain types of existence determine the likelihood of individuals receiving therapeutic interventions.[3,20] Physicians consider patients' quality of life more often to support decisions to withhold therapy than to support decisions to use mechanical ventilation ($p < 0.01$).[42] This may be further seen in the fact that ventilator use is introduced to individuals with neuromuscular disease in only a very small minority of Jerry Lewis Muscular Dystrophy Association Clinics in the United States.[19] Some clinicians have gone so far as to say that "the use of chronic assisted ventilation should be avoided."[56] Others consider the long-term use of assisted ventilation for individuals with DMD to be "most controversial" and it "raises enormous ethical difficulties."[47]

It is surprising to many clinicians that individuals with such severe disability might be satisfied with their lives. However, habituation tends to produce a decline in the subjective pleasurableness or unpleasantness of any input.[32] Campbell et al. stated that "where an [unpleasant] situation is fixed for a person over a long term, there may be a tendency toward accommodation to it, reflected in gradual increases in satisfaction."[18] For ventilator-users with ever greater disability with time and decreasing expectations, habituation occurs along with, perhaps, maturity and acceptance to decrease the unpleasantness of the circumstances. Constricted horizons lead to satisfaction with the status quo.[18] In addition, the ventilator serves as a daily reminder of the tenuousness of human existence. Unless the patient is using nontracheostomy aids and is capable of GPB,[2] the ventilator is all that stands between the user and death. In a very concrete way, these individuals appear to appreciate that their quality of life is closely tied to their family lives and personal relationships, and their use of a ventilator takes on a positive aspect in permitting continued appreciation of these ties. Indeed, not one subject who expressed satisfaction with life in general was dissatisfied with his or her family life, and the strongest association for all ventilator-users groups was general life satisfaction with satisfaction with social life. Thus, severe disability may lead to a general scaling down of expectations and shifts in the importance of life domains. In addition, ventilator-users may come to experience life satisfaction as a consequence of cognitive dissonance.[50] They overcame the greatest of obstacles and challenges to simply be alive, so life *must* be meaningful and satisfying.

Whiteneck et al. studied the psychosocial outcomes of SCI individuals at least 20 years postinjury.[53] Three-quarters of the subjects rated their current quality of life as good or excellent on a 5-point scale. There were no significant differences by level of injury, but satisfaction correlated inversely with age. Whiteneck et al.'s group also demonstrated that SCI ventilator-users rated their quality of life higher than autonomously breathing traumatic tetraplegics, that fewer of the former than of the latter considered suicide at least once and six times or more, and that more of the former were happy to be alive, had greater self-esteem, and found sexual activity more satisfactory.[52] This chapter's survey was consistent with Whiteneck et al.'s findings in demonstrating that while the SCI ventilator-users were only dissatisfied with sexual function, autonomously breathing traumatic tetraplegics were dissatisfied (mean responses <4.0) with the domains of job satisfaction, health, and sexual functioning.[16] The SCI ventilator-users reported a significantly greater satisfaction with housing, job, and family life and a not statistically significant greater satisfaction with social life, health, and life overall by comparison with the autonomously breathing traumatic tetraplegics. They also felt that life was somewhat friendlier, more interesting, more enjoyable, fuller, and more hopeful than did the latter group. This level of psychosocial adjustment and well-being is remarkable considering that besides ventilator use, these SCI individuals also had less upper extremity function than the autonomously breathing tetraplegics. However, with less limited horizons because of greater residual upper extremity function, the latter are faced with more frustration in attempts to accomplish upper extremity tasks every day. In another study, the quality of life in older SCI veterans was reported to be better than that in similarly aged nondisabled males. This also implied that the level of disability is not as important a factor as aging in determining overall long-term life satisfaction.[23]

The more positive well-being measures of the post-polio and DMD patients than of the SCI ventilator-users may be explained by the fact that many of the former were initially managed by noninvasive methods of long-term ventilatory assistance, including use of intermittent abdominal pressure ventilators, chest shell ventilators, and mouth, nasal, and/or oral-nasal IPPV. The ventilator use requirement usually increased gradually, with the patient controlling the depth of each assisted breath and the duration of each period of ventilator use. They essentially "ventilated themselves" rather than "got ventilated," thus increasing their sense of control, mastery over their environments, self-esteem, and self-worth. Insidious late-onset chronic ventilatory failure has only been described for a few SCI individuals.[6] Thus, the post-polio and DMD populations had more time to adjust to both physical disability and ventilator use than did the SCI ventilator-users.

Campbell et al. noted that different life domains have different importance to different people. The downgrading of importance of any particular life domain can be explained by denial or adaptation to situations.[18] Likewise, it appears that family life and housing issues, domains less affected by physical disability, take on the greatest significance for ventilator-users. Campbell also found that satisfaction with family life was one of the most effective predictors of general life satisfaction in his study population. It correlated even more significantly with general life satisfaction for our ventilator-users.

PATIENT PREFERENCE: TRACHEOSTOMY IPPV VS NONINVASIVE PHYSICAL MEDICINE ALTERNATIVES

Individuals using noninvasive techniques of ventilatory support expressed greater satisfaction with their lives than tracheostomy IPPV users. There are many reasons for this. Ventilator-users with little ventilator-free breathing time using tracheostomy IPPV are fearful of sudden apnea resulting from tracheostomy disconnection or ventilator failure. These individuals also require ongoing tracheostomy care, including tracheal suctioning and regular uncomfortable tube changes. Sudden detachment of mucus plugs from the tube or cuff can cause acute respiratory distress. At least one individual also abandoned the use of phrenic nerve pacing in favor of positive pressure ventilatory support because of the absence of pacemaker alarms and fear of sudden apnea from not infrequent pacemaker failure. In addition, tracheostomy IPPV users with inflated cuff cannot use their sense of smell or taste their food, and they require supplemental humidification because air does not pass through the nasal passages and upper airway. They often complain of having unpleasant taste sensations that appear to be associated with chronic pathogenic bacterial colonization of the tracheostomy site and upper airways. It is also more difficult to obtain attendant care in the home for tracheostomized individuals.

Individuals using noninvasive aids, on the other hand, maintain more normal speech. These individuals do not require suctioning, and only require assisted elimination of airway secretions during respiratory tract infections. The alleviation of fear of tracheostomy disconnection or sudden ventilator failure may be accomplished by use of GPB. Physiologic use of the upper airway permits the noninvasive ventilator-user to maintain normal airway humidification, olfaction, and taste sensations. All of these factors facilitate self-confidence and more active community living and may have contributed to the noninvasive aid users having greater life satisfaction than the tracheostomy IPPV users.

Specifically, this survey demonstrated that ventilator-users who switched from tracheostomy to noninvasive IPPV considered the latter to be safer, more convenient, and more comfortable and to permit more normal speech production, swallowing, sleep, and appearance than the former. Both the ventilator-users and their principal caregivers unanimously preferred the noninvasive IPPV methods overall to tracheostomy IPPV. The results also demonstrated that except for sleep, those switched from a noninvasive aid regimen (including noninvasive IPPV) to tracheostomy, also preferred the former for every item evaluated.

This finding is contrary to the views of many clinicians, who feel that IPPV via an indwelling tracheostomy tube may facilitate voice production or swallowing or be safer than noninvasive methods by providing better control of ventilator-delivered volumes and a convenient portal for upper airway suctioning. On the contrary, the presence of an indwelling tracheostomy tube ties down the strap muscles in the neck and impedes swallowing.[17,35,37] When a cuffless tracheostomy tube or a deflated cuff is used to force exhaled air passed the vocal cords, speech is crescendo/decrescendo and dependent on the cycling ventilator. Rhythm and voice tone are also less natural than when using an intermittent abdominal pressure ventilator with GPB or noninvasive IPPV. The use of GPB for deep breaths to increase voice volume and improve cough efficacy and for safety in the event of ventilator failure is rarely possible when using tracheostomy IPPV.[9] Indeed, a lower percentage of effective glossopharyngeal breathers would be expected and was found in the group that was ultimately switched to tracheostomy IPPV. All of these factors have considerable bearing on quality of life.

The individuals who were switched from body ventilator use only to tracheostomy IPPV preferred use of the former for appearance, convenience, and speech, and the latter for comfort, security, swallowing, sleep, and overall. These ventilator-users were probably never exposed to noninvasive IPPV methods since nocturnal mouthpiece IPPV with a lipseal was used almost exclusively in one center[11] and nasal IPPV was not described until 1987, long after most of these ventilator-users had been switched.[10] Their general preference for tracheostomy IPPV was understandable since body ventilators are less effective and more restrictive than IPPV and, except for the chest shell ventilator and intermittent abdominal pressure ventilator, must be used while reclining.[8] Of the ventilator-users who "preferred" tracheostomy, none had mastered GPB and none had had access to mechanical insufflation-exsufflation. It is therefore not surprising that 31% of the ventilator-users who preferred tracheostomy IPPV indicated that this was so because of the use of tracheal suctioning to clear airway secretions during respiratory tract infections. Thus, when more than nocturnal ventilatory support was re-quired, resort to tracheostomy IPPV appeared to be indicated because noninvasive IPPV and effective noninvasive airway secretion clearance methods were unavailable.

Although only a small percentage of respondents had had access to mechanical insufflation-exsufflation for evacuation of airway secretions, none with access preferred tracheostomy over noninvasive ventilatory support methods. Timely and effective use of manually assisted coughing techniques[48] and mechanical insufflation-exsufflation[7] when necessary can be vital for avoiding pulmonary complications, hospitalizations, and need for resort to endotracheal intubation.

Thus, whether switched to or from noninvasive ventilatory support regimens that include noninvasive IPPV, these methods are considered by ventilator-users to be safer, to be more convenient, and to have less untoward effects on swallowing, speech, appearance, and comfort than tracheostomy IPPV.

ETHICS

Purtilo observed that most discussion of ventilator use has focused on the critically ill patient maintained by tracheostomy IPPV in intensive care units.[43] She pointed out that this has "fostered misconceptions and stereotypes" regarding other appropriate uses of ventilators. There is, likewise, great potential for "misunderstanding of the ethical issues involved in treating patients whose chronic maintenance depends on either positive or negative long-term ventilator support." Informed decisions about ethically and financially complex matters, such as long-term ventilator use, should be made by examining the life satisfaction of competent individuals who have already chosen these options. The great majority of severely disabled ventilator-users with neuromuscular disease are satisfied with their lives despite the inability to achieve some of the "usual" goals associated with quality of life in the physically able population. Their principal life satisfaction derives from social relationships, the reorganization of goals, and their immediate environment. Thus, clinicians have the responsibility of accurately portraying the lives of individuals using ventilators since these portrayals, and especially the clinician's bias, influence patients' acceptance and feelings about ventilator use.

The right of the disabled individual to live freely is often jeopardized by health care and societal issues. Zola described the "dehumanizing indignity in safety."[57] "Life entails risk, and to try to create an environment without risk ultimately devalues the person with the disability by suggesting that he/she is not capable of coping except in the most restrictive and supportive environment."[50] What is often appropriate and necessary in the protective environment of the acute care setting is not appropriate in the rehabilitation setting and has led many patients to express "intense frustration at the double messages given by rehabilitation professionals: you must learn to be independent as a disabled person, but we will make all your decisions for you."[50]

A common reason for constraining the actions of institutionalized individuals is to avoid risk to them and liability to the institution. However, this controlling focus does not always change once the individual returns home, since patients' daily care is often provided and therefore directed by licensed nurses contracted by professional nursing agencies. Thus, the severely disabled individual's activities continue to be circumscribed by the rules of institutional health care organizations that hamper the client's self-determination and individuality. The solution for this problem is in the formation of client-maintained personal assistance services (PAS) and the provision of adequate PAS for the severely disabled self-directed individuals who require them.

"Our people are still being warehoused without hope of ever having a home or family or lifestyle of their own. When you think about it, in contrast to the vast numbers of us demanding our rights to first-class citizenship, only a handful of disabled people have publicly sought death. Yet . . . laws are being passed at record speed to ease the way to our demise. Prominent 'experts' [argue] for our right to die . . . as defenders of our freedom, dignity, humane treatment, and even 'independence' . . . [yet, it] has taken almost 20 years of exhausting struggle to get a basic civil rights law for disabled people."[26]

Although the Americans with Disabilities Act (ADA) is seen as an important step to prevent discrimination against disabled individuals, it does little or nothing for the self-directed disabled individual who, like most patients with neuromuscular disorders, is either not informed or biased against ventilator use by his or her misinformed physicians (Fig. 29–4),[3] nor does it help those who are warehoused in institutions because of lack of a national PAS policy. The false beliefs that prohibitively expensive continuous nursing care is required and that disabled ventilator-users are unable to take responsibility for and manage their own care are the greatest obstacles to returning them to the community. This is ironic since the provision of PAS for the home care of ventilator-users can greatly reduce cost[14] as well as enhance quality of life.

One large group of ventilator-users with respiratory failure was institutionalized for 24 to 31 years before obtaining release to enter the community. The ventilator-users were authorized to develop a client-maintained organization, Concepts of Independence, Inc., which permits self-

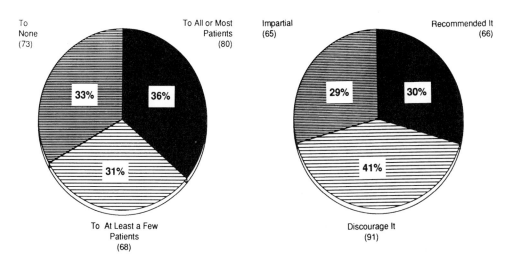

FIGURE 29–4. Muscular Dystrophy Association clinic directors attitudes toward ventilatory aid ($n = 222$ directors) and the number who discuss and offer ventilatory aids to Duchenne muscular dystrophy patients ($n = 221$ directors). (From Bach JR: Ventilator use by Muscular Dystrophy Association patients: An update. Arch Phys Med Rehabil 73:179–183, 1992, with permission.)

directed clients themselves to hire, train, direct, and dismiss their own personal care attendants.[45] Virtually all of the 50 ventilator-user clients of Concepts of Independence required 24-hour ventilator use and received attendant care 24 hours a day. With over 250 clients currently in this expanding program, there have been no significant accidents or litigation. Indeed, the home health care industry has had virtually no history of tort litigation.[44,45] The efforts of these courageous and tenacious ventilator-users succeeded in establishing a precedent for humanizing the care of severely disabled self-directed individuals in private domiciles and, in doing so, greatly increased the quality of their lives with 70% cost savings to the taxpayers of New York.[14]

The institutional control of chronic care, whether in an institution itself or in the community with PAS managed by nursing organizations, impersonalizes and dehumanizes care in the name of safety. It reduces the client's sense of personal control and self-efficacy and suggests inadequacy in coping except in the most restrictive and supportive environment. Physical medicine and rehabilitation specialists who train their patients in how to manage and take responsibility for their own care need to play a more active role in advocating for the procurement of the services needed to permit them to return to the community.

Typical counterproductive regulations include the prohibition of tracheal suctioning by unlicensed personal care attendants. In 46 states, young child relatives may perform tracheal suctioning but third-party payers and home nursing care agencies will not sanction this activity by trained PAS providers. Such regulations too often serve to protect private interests under the pretext of avoiding liability and ensuring the patient's safety. These restrictions continue despite the fact that the American College of Chest Physicians[27] and others[39] support the use of properly trained PAS providers as care providers for self-directed ventilator-users. So far, regulations have been modified to permit this only in Colorado, Massachusetts, and New York.[36]

We routinely close tracheostomy sites and convert ventilator-users to the use of noninvasive respiratory aids. Because this service is performed only by ourselves and in one other institution in this country,[51] most ventilator-users are never made aware of it, and many, without adequate family support, must remain institutionalized. Clearly, a responsibility of the rehabilitation specialist is to inform ventilator-users about noninvasive methods and to train them in the use of these methods, especially when their use can facilitate community living with PAS. "Without effective community options, we lose our humanity. More and more people are choosing to die rather than exist in institutions . . . warehoused for 'cost' and 'efficiency.' "[31] Further information concerning the need for and status of PAS is available.[1,36,55]

Although there is much consternation about growing medical costs, when it comes to mechanical ventilation, little is being done to limit costs and optimize care. For example, the initial costs of placement and training in the use of electrophrenic pacing (EPR) exceed $300,000 and EPR has only a 33% realistic success rate.[15] Further, patients using EPR must usually retain tracheostomy tubes. This creates an additional expense for disposable suction catheters, tracheostomy tube changes, related stomal care, and possibly home nursing services. This is in contrast to removing the tracheostomy tube, teaching GPB to free the patient from the ventilator, and using noninvasive ventilatory support alternatives such as mouthpieces ($3 each), nasal interfaces ($30–$500), and an Exsufflation Belt ($350; Lifecare International Inc., Westminster, CO). The $300,000 initial cost of EPR often comes out of a limited insurance policy. This money would often be much better used to provide ADL-enhancing equipment and personal care, but the profits from electrophrenic placement and use and the intensive marketing of this approach obscure the more reasonable but less immediately profitable resort to using noninvasive methods of ventilatory support. One still earns more money by putting in a tracheostomy tube or pacemaker than for removing them.

With the growing emphasis on cost-containment and reform of the health care delivery system in the United States, quality of life issues are being evoked to justify withholding life-sustaining medical interventions including mechanical ventilation.[3,42] Although it would appear that an intelligent, self-directed individual should be fully informed about therapeutic options and prognosis, in the frenzy of seeking a less-expensive health care delivery system, some physicians have suggested eliminating the patient from the decision-making process. Despite the fact that in 1983, the President's Commission for the Study of Bioethical Problems in Medicine and Behavioral and Biomedical Research reported that the principle of patient autonomy should guide treatment decisions, and the fact that some physicians have advocated for involving the patient in the decision-making process to use a ventilator,[29] as recently as 1989 it has been recommended that a physician's assessment of patient's quality of life be done "independent of the patient's feelings" to guide the clinician in whether or not to institute mechanical ventilation.[22]

Quality of life is difficult, if not impossible, to measure by objective criteria that can be applied to all individuals. Most efforts at measuring it, however, appear to have been based on factors relevant for physically able individuals.[33] However, Jonsen et al. noted that what is important is the subjective satisfaction experienced by an individual in physical, mental, and social situations, even though these may be deficient in some manner.[30] Thus, potential satisfaction with life and with the various aspects of one's existence should be considered if questioning the appropriateness of vital therapeutic options. It is particularly appropriate that the life satisfaction of individuals who have already chosen vital medical interventions and who are living the consequences of their decisions be considered when deciding about ethically and financially complex matters, such as long-term ventilator use for others.

Besides the fact that most physicians underestimate the life satisfaction of ventilator-users with neuromuscular disorders, the great majority of physicians caring for these individuals and having the responsibility of offering prolonged survival by noninvasive means are ignorant of these methods. It is not surprising, therefore, that many if not most physicians are biased against the long-term use of ventilatory assistance, which they wrongly associate with the need for an indwelling tracheostomy tube. This was recently documented in a survey of Muscular Dystrophy Association clinic directors.[3] Forty-one percent of 273 clinic directors discouraged ventilator use. Fifty-five percent of the directors cited "poor quality of life" to justify this view. Only 2 physicians who discouraged ventilator use were familiar with noninvasive IPPV. Not surprisingly, the directors who most underestimated the ventilator-users' life satisfaction were also the least likely to encourage ventilator use and be familiar with noninvasive respiratory aids. A manuscript demonstrating a 2-year prolongation of survival by the use of strictly noninvasive methods for individuals with ALS and no ventilator-free breathing ability was recently rejected from a reputed journal of neurology when one reviewer stated that, in his opinion, "these patients did not need to use ventilators." Was this statement a disbelief of the efficacy of the methods being discussed, the view that these patients were simply better off dead, or both?

Indeed, it appears that there are hardly any limits that some physicians will impose on their self-determined right to make life and death decisions for their patients. Ventilator use is a situation "in which the support system does not replace the diseased organ. The ventilator assists an organ system that is not primarily diseased. The model of renal dialysis [therefore] does not apply, since [in this case] the diseased organ is replaced by the function of the machine."[46] This rationale has been used despite the fact that the cost of ventilator use is about 30% that of renal dialysis and far less disruptive of a patient's day-to-day life. "Patients should be encouraged as much as possible to direct their own lives, but if they are incapable of reaching an unequivocal and seemingly rational decision, they should be able to trust their doctor to act in their best interest . . . the physician will consult the family and will look as objectively as possible at the quality of the patient's life."[28] Such physician attitudes make it imperative for patients to have sources other than their health care professionals to learn about their therapeutic options. Health care providers must avoid a paternalistic stance when working with a disabled individual. Self-directed individuals, once properly informed, should be treated as competent to make decisions regarding their welfare. Paternalism undermines the goals of rehabilitation.

When Does No Really Mean No?

It is now well established that a person's consent is necessary prior to initiating treatment. Informed consent requires that a competent, mature person make a decision, while cognizant of the consequences, without undue pressure from others. Consent requires that the patient be advised of all possible treatment choices and be knowledgeable of their benefits, consequences, and liabilities. Choices must include all alternative approaches that might provide equivalent clinical efficacy. Without complete knowledge of all feasible options, fully informed consent is not possible.

Thus, an individual must consent to use mechanical ventilatory assistance. There is frequent mention in the medical literature of the need for patients to make "crisis" decisions to initiate mechanical ventilation and to become dependent on it for the rest of their lives. However, the "crisis" decision has always referred to the institution of IPPV via endotracheal tubes, an invasive approach. Indeed, patients are encouraged to decide on whether or not these would be acceptable options well in advance by advanced directive, living will, and power of attorney mechanisms. Most patients prospectively refuse to consider undergoing tracheostomy for ventilatory support. However, "It is important to acknowledge, also, that the patient, his or her family, the physician, and other care providers may not be able to adhere to a planned decision to withhold [invasive] ventilatory support in the presence of impending respiratory failure, when the instinctive urge to preserve life supplants the rational conclusion that, in this particular instance, death is preferable to life under such profoundly altered conditions."[28] Indeed, the great majority of ALS patients and others with neuromuscular disease, when asked early on, indicate that they would rather die than use respiratory support. Most change their minds during episodes of acute respiratory failure, particularly when dyspnea can be relieved by the simple use of noninvasive respiratory muscle aids. As can be seen by the above quotation, the patient's attitude toward the use of ventilatory aids may more reflect his or her physician's attitude and the invasive nature of the treatment options being presented, rather than reflect an informed rational decision.[3]

The informed consent process almost invariably fails the patient with neuromuscular disease because these patients are virtually never made aware of noninvasive respiratory muscle support options. We have never had the experience of any individual with global alveolar hypoventilation refusing to use noninvasive respiratory muscle aids. This is because they are innocuous and always preferable to invasive options, and because they are usually introduced to individuals in nonemergency situations as means to expand the lungs and chest wall (range of motion) or as simple inspiratory and expiratory muscle aids to relieve symptoms of global alveolar hypoventilation and assist coughing. Patients gradually extend the simple therapeutic use of these methods on their own to their use for continuous ventilatory assistance. Noninvasive aids, thus, can postpone or entirely obviate the "crisis" of deciding whether or not to "go on a ventilator" (to undergo tracheostomy). Patients using noninvasive aids issue their consent at every stage of the treatment process as would any patient who is taking oral medications, and verbal consent rather than written consent is obtained. Indeed, in our clinic, patients and their families observe their use and are educated about them long before they are needed, and they are informed that their continual use may become necessary at some point in the future.

Without physical medicine interventions, the great majority of individuals with increasing ventilatory insufficiency experience episodes of acute respiratory failure triggered by mucus plugging and food or secretion aspiration. Unexpected respiratory failure allows little time for consideration of future disposition, and desperate, intubated patients are given a tracheostomy ultimatum which they accept with fear and anger. These patients and families feel overwhelmed, often inadequately counseled,[46] and rarely understand the wide-reaching financial, social, and, indeed, physical consequences of acquiescing to tracheostomy. Should we ignore their desire to live because "death is preferable to life under these conditions" or provide them with physical medicine alternatives? If severe bulbar muscle dysfunction makes tracheostomy necessary for continued survival, the experience individuals obtain in using ventilators for noninvasive aid allows them time to evaluate and to think through the ramifications of continuing ventilatory support via a tracheostomy when necessary.

PSYCHOTHERAPEUTIC INTERVENTIONS

Self-directed disabled individuals should be trained to take responsibility for their care during the rehabilitation process. The psychologist can assist in this by assessing and treating patients who require ongoing psychotherapeutic intervention and by providing family counseling. He or she can also foster a patient's resolution of disability/disease issues, empower the patient to make important treatment decisions, and can aid the physician in discussing particular topics, such as prognosis and the patient's expectancies, perceptions of, need for, and personal meaning of ventilator use. The patient who requires tracheostomy is encouraged to explore the anxieties inherent in the misconceptions concerning this option. Relaxation training, utilization of verbal and tangible cues, and positive self-talk can be helpful. Occasionally, intensive psychotherapeutic intervention may be warranted. Patients not infrequently become overly concerned about ventilator functioning and reflective of their own investment in life and their desire and will to live. In addition, SCI ventilator-users are often preoccupied with issues related to lack of physical functioning, mobility, bowel and bladder control, and sensation, and all ventilator-users are concerned about sexual functioning.

Ventilator use, itself, is rarely a source of ongoing stress. This may be due to the fact that breathing is taken for granted, whereas motor functioning is perceived as instrumental for achieving specified goals and is consciously initiated. The stressors resulting from ventilator use via an indwelling tracheostomy have been identified as feeling tied to the machine, and respiratory infections,[40] but the need for a surgical procedure to institute them and the inevitable fear of accidental tracheostomy tube disconnections and ventilator failure are also sources of ongoing stress.

For many patients, it can be beneficial to facilitate the transition from an instrumental to an interpersonal focus. The clinician fosters the patient's participation in relationships and acceptance of relationships as sources of productivity, self-esteem, and power. The development of healthy, supportive interpersonal relationships can be reframed as a goal, superseding that of physical independence, autonomy, and power over others. Caring for others and mutual empathy can be fostered. It may be necessary for the clinician to model healthy relatedness. Subordinate groups in society such as women, ethnic minorities, and the physically disabled may come to have difficulty identifying their needs and stating their preferences. Thus, reinforcing assertiveness and empowerment may be central to treatment so that the individual's desires are clearly heard and acknowledged.

We need to advocate for ventilator-users to obtain the PAS they require so that true independence can be achieved and self-actualization fostered. In the face of calls to limit entitlement spending, it should be noted that a society willing to provide free room, board, health care, legal and educational services, vocational training, and cable television for murders, rapists, drug dealers, and other felons at a cost of $60,000 per year for each has the ethical responsibility to provide PAS to those in need, some of whom are crime victims themselves.[14]

CONCLUSION

The use of noninvasive respiratory muscle aids can provide effective long-term support 24 hours a day; they can be used to avoid acute pulmonary morbidity, hospitalization, intubation, premature death, and undue expense; and they are greatly preferred over the tracheostomy alternative.[4] Further, the use of these methods eliminates the ethical considerations concerning suicide by withdrawal of ventilatory support since users of noninvasive methods are not passively attached to a respirator but actively control their alveolar ventilation. The individual's

personal sense of controlling his or her life is also enhanced by using these methods. We have the ethical responsibility of informing patients and giving them access to these physical medicine options.

Purtilo summed up an article on ethical issues concerning the management of ventilator-users by saying that misconceptions about the undesirability of "'going on a respirator' have far-reaching negative effects for persons now happily being supported on a respirator, and mitigate the positive effects it could have for some types of chronically impaired persons whose quality of life also could be enhanced by the use of a ventilator."[43] Freed stressed the importance of professionals not imposing their own concepts, values, and judgments onto the disabled person.[25] Clinicians should be cognizant of their inability to gauge disabled patients' life satisfaction and potential for social and vocational productivity and refrain from letting inaccurate and unwarranted judgment of subjective factors associated with quality of life in the general population affect patient management decisions.

References

1. Attendant Services Network: Personal Assistance for Independent Living. Oakland, CA, World Institute on Disability, 1988.
2. Bach JR: New approaches in the rehabilitation of the traumatic high level quadriplegic. Am J Phys Med Rehabil 70:13–20, 1991.
3. Bach JR: Ventilator use by Muscular Dystrophy Association patients: An update. Arch Phys Med Rehabil 73:179–183, 1992.
4. Bach JR: A comparison of long-term ventilatory support alternatives from the perspective of the patient and care giver. Chest 104:1702–1706, 1993.
5. Bach JR: Amyotrophic lateral sclerosis: Communication status and survival with ventilatory support. Am J Phys Med Rehabil 72:343–349, 1993.
6. Bach JR: Inappropriate weaning and late onset ventilatory failure of individuals with traumatic quadriplegia. Paraplegia 31:430–438, 1993.
7. Bach JR: Update and perspectives on noninvasive respiratory muscle aids: Part 2. The expiratory muscle aids. Chest 105:1538–1544, 1994.
8. Bach JR, Alba AS: Total ventilatory support by the intermittent abdominal pressure ventilator. Chest 99:630–636, 1991.
9. Bach JR, Alba AS, Bodofsky E, et al: Glossopharyngeal breathing and non-invasive aids in the management of post-polio respiratory insufficiency. Birth Defects 23:99–113, 1987.
10. Bach JR, Alba AS, Mosher R, Delaubier A: Intermittent positive pressure ventilation via nasal access in the management of respiratory insufficiency. Chest 92:168–170, 1987.
11. Bach JR, Alba AS, Saporito LR: Intermittent positive pressure ventilation via the mouth as an alternative to tracheostomy for 257 ventilator users. Chest 103:174–182, 1993.
12. Bach JR, Campagnolo D: Psychosocial adjustment of

post-poliomyelitis ventilator assisted individuals. Arch Phys Med Rehabil 73:934–939, 1992.

13. Bach JR, Campagnolo DI, Hoeman S: Life satisfaction of individuals with Duchenne muscular dystrophy using long-term mechanical ventilatory support. Am J Phys Med Rehabil 70:129–135, 1991.

14. Bach JR, Intintola P, Alba AS, Holland I: The ventilator-assisted individual: Cost analysis of institutionalization versus rehabilitation and in-home management. Chest 101:26–30, 1992.

15. Bach JR, O'Connor K: Electrophrenic ventilation: A different perspective. J Am Paraplegia Soc 14:9–17, 1991.

16. Bach JR, Tilton M: Life satisfaction and well-being measures in ventilator assisted individuals with traumatic tetraplegia. Arch Phys Med Rehabil 75:626–632, 1994.

17. Bonanno P: Swallowing dysfunction after tracheostomy. Ann Surg 174:29–33, 1971.

18. Campbell A, Converse PE, Rodgers WL: The Quality of American Life: Perceptions, Evaluations and Satisfactions. New York, Russell Sage Foundation, 1976, pp. 37–113.

19. Colbert AP, Schock NC: Respirator use in progressive neuromuscular diseases. Arch Phys Med Rehabil 66:760–762, 1985.

20. Crane D: Sanctity of Social Life: Physicians' Treatment of Critically Ill Individuals. New York, Russell Sage Foundation, 1975.

21. DeVivo MJ, Rutt RD, Black KJ, et al: Trends in spinal cord injury demographics and treatment outcomes between 1973 and 1986. Arch Phys Med Rehabil 73:424–430, 1992.

22. Dracup K, Raffin T: Withholding and withdrawing mechanical ventilation: Assessing quality of life. Am Rev Respir Dis 140:S44–S46, 1989.

23. Eisenberg MG, Saltz CC: Quality of life among aging spinal cord injured persons: Long term rehabilitation outcomes. Paraplegia 29:514–520, 1991.

24. Flanagan JC: Measurement of quality of life: Current state of the art. Arch Phys Med Rehabil 63:56–59, 1982.

25. Freed MM: Quality of life: The physician's dilemma. Arch Phys Med Rehabil 65:109–111, 1984.

26. Gill C: "Right to die" threatens our right to live safe and free. Mainstream 32–36, 1992.

27. Goldberg AI, Alba AS, Oppenheimer EA, Roberts E: Personal care attendants for people using mechanical ventilation at home [letter]. Chest 98:1543, 1990.

28. Goldblatt D: Decisions about life support in amyotrophic lateral sclerosis. Semin Neurol 4:104–110, 1984.

29. Hall CD, Howard JF, Donohue JF: The ventilator support of patients with neuromuscular disorders. In Charash LI, Lovelace RE, Leach CF, et al (eds): Loss, Grief, and Care. New York, Haworth Press, 1990, pp 185–191.

30. Jonsen R, Siegler M, Winslade WJ: Clinical Ethics: A Practical Approach to Ethical Decisions in Clinical Medicine. New York, Macmillan, 1982.

31. Kafka R: ADAPT Attendant Services Free our People. Denver, National ADAPT (American Disabled for Attendant Programs Today).

32. Kammann R, Christie D, Irwin R, Dixon G: Properties of an inventory to measure happiness (and psychological health). N Z Psychol 8:1–9, 1979.

33. Kolata G: Ethicists struggle to judge the 'value' of life. N Y Times 24 Nov 1992, C3.

34. Krause JS: Employment after spinal cord injury. Arch Phys Med Rehabil 73:163–169, 1992.

35. Leonard C, Criner GJ: Swallowing function in patients with tracheostomy receiving prolonged mechanical ventilation [abstract]. In International Conference on Pulmonary Rehabilitation and Home Ventilation, 1991, p 58.

36. Litvak S, Heumann JE: Attending to America: Personal Assistance for Independent Living—The National Survey of Attendant Services Programs in the United States. Berkeley, CA, World Institute on Disability, 1987.

37. Logemann JA: Evaluation and Treatment of Swallowing Disorders. San Diego, College-Hill Press, 1983, p 119.

38. Lundquist C, Siosteen A: Spinal cord injuries: Clinical, functional, and emotional status. Spine 16:78–83, 1991.

39. Make BJ, Gilmartin ME: Rehabilitation and home care for ventilator-assisted individuals. Clin Chest Med 7:679–691, 1986.

40. Miller JR, Colbert AP, Schock NC: Ventilator use in progressive neuromuscular disease: Impact on patients and their families. Dev Med Child Neurol 30:200–207, 1988.

41. National Center for Health Statistics: Vital Statistics of the United States, 1985: vol III. Marriage and Divorce. Washington, DC, Government Printing Office, 1989, p. 4–23,4–24 DHHS Publication No. (PHS) 89–1103.

42. Pearlman RA, Jonsen A: The use of quality-of-life considerations in medical decision making. J Am Geriatr Soc 33:344–352, 1985.

43. Purtilo R: Ethical issues in the treatment of chronic ventilator-dependent individuals. Arch Phys Med Rehabil 67:718–721, 1986.

44. Sabatino CP: Final Report: Lessons for Enhancing Consumer-Directed Approaches in Home Care. Washington, DC, Commission on Legal Problems of the Elderly, American Bar Association, 1990.

45. Schnur S, Holland I: Concepts—A unique approach to personal care attendants. Rehabil Gaz 28:10–11, 1987.

46. Sivak ED, Gipson WT, Hanson MR: Long-term management of respiratory failure in amyotrophic lateral sclerosis. Ann Neurol 12:18–23, 1982.

47. Smith PEM, Calverley PMA, Edwards RHT, et al: Practical problems in the respiratory care of individuals with muscular dystophy. N Engl J Med 316:1197–1204, 1987.

48. Sortor S, McKenzie M: Toward independence: Assisted cough [video]. Dallas, BioScience Communications of Dallas, 1986.

49. Dijkers MP, Abela MB, Gans BM, Gordon WA: The aftermath of spinal cord injury. In Stover SL, DeLisa JA, Whiteneck GG (eds): Spinal Cord Injury: Clinical Outcomes from the Model Systems. Gaithersburg, MD, Aspen, 1995, pp 185–212.

50. Trieschmann RB: Spinal Cord Injuries: Psychological, Social and Vocational Rehabilitation, 2nd ed. New York, Demos, 1988, pp 107–114.

51. Viroslav J, Sortor S, Rosenblatt R: Alternatives to tracheostomy ventilation in high level SCI [abstract]. J Am Paraplegia Soc 14:87, 1991.

52. Whiteneck GG, Carter RE, Charlifue SW, et al: A Collaborative Study of High Quadriplegia. Report to the National Institute of Handicapped Research. Craig, CO, Rocky Mountain Regional Spinal Cord Injury System, 1985, pp 29–33.

53. Whiteneck GG, Charlifue MA, Frankel HL, et al: Mortality, morbidity, and psychosocial outcomes of persons spinal cord injured more than 20 years ago. Paraplegia 30:617–630, 1992.

54. Wilcox NE, Stauffer ES: Follow-up of 423 consecutive patients admitted to the spinal cord centre, Rancho Los Amigos Hospital, 1 January to 31 December 1967. Paraplegia 10:115–122, 1972.

55. World Institute on Disability, Rutgers University Bureau of Economic Research: The Need for Personal Assistance. Oakland, CA, World Institute on Disability.

56. Ziter FA, Allsop KG: Comprehensive treatment of childhood muscular dystrophy. Rocky Mt Med J 72:329–333, 1975.

57. Zola IK: Social and cultural disincentives to independent living. Arch Phys Med Rehabil 63:394–397, 1982.

Index

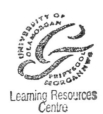